POCKET COMPANION TO TEXTBOOK OF CRITICAL CARE

POCKET COMPANION TO TEXTBOOK OF CRITICAL CARE

Senior Editor:

Ake Grenvik, MD, PhD, FCCM
Distinguished Service Professor of Critical Care Medicine
Director, Multidisciplinary Critical Care Training Program
University of Pittsburgh Medical Center
Pittsburgh, Pennsylvania

Editors:

Stephen M. Ayres, MD, FCCM
Professor of Medicine
Dean Emeritus, School of Medicine
Director, International Health Programs
Virginia Commonwealth University
Medical College of Virginia
Richmond, Virginia

Peter R. Holbrook, MD, FCCM
Professor of Anesthesia and Pediatrics
George Washington University School of Medicine
Chief Medical Officer
Children's National Medical Center
Washington, D.C.

William C. Shoemaker, MD, FCCM
Professor of Surgery, UCLA School of Medicine
Chairman, Department of Emergency Medicine
Vice Chairman, Department of Surgery
King-Drew Medical Center
Los Angeles, California

W.B. SAUNDERS COMPANY
A Division of Harcourt Brace & Company

Philadelphia • London • Toronto • Montreal • Sydney • Tokyo

W.B. SAUNDERS COMPANY
A Division of Harcourt Brace & Company

The Curtis Center
Independence Square West
Philadelphia, Pennsylvania 19106

Library of Congress Cataloging-in-Publication Data

Pocket companion to Textbook of critical care / [edited by] William Shoemaker . . . [et al.].

p. cm.

ISBN 0-7216-5833-4

1. Critical care medicine—Handbooks, manuals, etc.
I. Shoemaker, William C. II. Textbook of critical care.
[DNLM: 1. Critical Care—handbooks. WX 39 P7415 1996]

RC86.7.T453 1995 Suppl.

616′.28—dc20

DNLM/DLC 95-31495

POCKET COMPANION TO TEXTBOOK OF CRITICAL CARE ISBN 0-7216-5833-4

Printed in the United States of America.

Last digit is the print number: 9 8 7 6 5 4 3 2 1

Preface

The first edition of the *Textbook of Critical Care* was published in 1984 and contained 1063 pages. The second edition followed in 1989 with 1519 pages. The third edition was published in April 1995 with 1892 pages, almost double the size of the first edition. This heavy volume is too large to keep as a bedside reference. Therefore, the W. B. Saunders Company asked the editors to publish a companion book as well.

Less than a year after the appearance of the third edition of the *Textbook of Critical Care,* this pocket companion was published. The text emphasizes diagnostic work-up and patient management. It is designed as a pocketbook for house officers on intensive care unit (ICU) assignment. It is also meant for fellows in subspecialty training of critical care, particularly anesthesiologists, internists, and surgeons. Pediatricians may find the text useful, especially as it relates to older children. Medical students, ICU nurses, and student nurses should also find this pocketbook valuable in their daily ICU patient care activities.

The third edition of the original *Textbook of Critical Care* has 17 sections, almost all of which are summarized in separate chapters of this companion book. Wherever more detailed information is needed, please refer to the original textbook, where each section chapter has a detailed reference list. This companion book does not include any references in order to make it more compact.

As editors of both the third edition of the *Textbook of Critical Care* and this companion book, we dedicate this book to all physician and nurse trainees in the intensive care setting and wish all of you success in the management of your critically ill and injured ICU patients.

AKE GRENVIK, MD, PHD, FCCM
STEPHEN M. AYRES, MD, FCCM
PETER R. HOLBROOK, MD, FCCM
WILLIAM C. SHOEMAKER, MD, FCCM

Acknowledgments

The editors wish to thank all authors of the chapters in the *Textbook of Critical Care,* 3rd edition. Their work formed the foundation from which this pocket companion materialized. The names of the textbook chapter authors follow:

Edward Abraham, MD, FCCM

Norman S. Abramson, MD

Kareem Abu-Elmagd, MD

W. Keith Adkins, MD, PhD

Maurice S. Albin, MD, MSc(Anesth)

Charles G. Alex, MD

Harry L. Anderson, III, MD

Derek C. Angus, MB, ChB, MPH, MRCP(UK), FCCP

John M. Armitage, MD

Deborah K. Armstrong, PharmD, FCCM

Jeffrey S. Augenstein, MD, PhD

Raymond F. Austin, Jr., MD

Donald C. Axon, FAIA

Timothy J. Babineau, MD

Edward D. Ball, MD

Nils U. Bang, MD

Steven J. Barker, PhD, MD

William H. Barth, Jr., MD

Robert H. Bartlett, MD

Claudia Bartz, PhD, RN

Donald P. Becker, MD

Paul E. Bellamy, MD

Rinaldo Bellomo, MBBS, MD, FRACP

Michael K. Belz, MD

Marvin Bergsneider, MD

Gordon R. Bernard, MD

Bruce Beutler, MD

Morris I. Bierman, MD

Nicholas G. Bircher, MD

Carole Birdsall, EdD, RN, CCRN

Michael H. Bishop, DO

George L. Blackburn, MD, PhD

Thomas P. Bleck, MD, FCCM

Elana J. Bloom, MD

Glenn H. Bock, MD

Philip G. Boysen, MD, FACP, FCCM
Pierre G. Braquet, PhD, DSc
Gordon L. Bray, MD
David Bregman, MD, FACC, FACS
Kenneth L. Brigham, MD
Timothy J. Broderick, MD
Brian A. Broznick, CPTC
D. A. Bruce, MB, ChB
Christopher W. Bryan-Brown, MD, FCCM
Timothy G. Buchman, PhD, MD, FACS, FCCM
Ross Bullock, MD, PhD
David J. Burchfield, MD
Mitchell S. Cairo, MD, FAAP
James E. Calvin, MD, FRCPS, FACC
Wayne N. Campbell, MD
Robert L. Carithers, Jr., MD
Graziano C. Carlon, MD
Richard W. Carlson, MD, PhD
Adrian Casavilla, MD
Ned H. Cassem, MD
Donna A. Castello, DO
Leo A. Celi, MD
John M. Chandler, MD
Lakshmipathi Chelluri, MD
Bart Chernow, MD, FACP
John William Christman, MD
Michael J. Cinoman, MD
Cathleen Clancy, MD
Terry P. Clemmer, MD
Jacqueline J. Coalson, PhD
Patricia E. Cole, PhD, MD
Arthur H. Combs, MD, FCCM
Alasdair K. T. Conn, MD, FACS
James A. Cook, PhD
Arthur Cooper, MD
Lynn Coppage, MD
Paul Corso, MD, FACS, FACC
Joseph M. Darby, MD
Lakshmana Das Narla, MD
Joseph F. Dasta, MSc(Pharm), FCCM, FCCP
James Dauber, MD
Guy de Lisle Dear, MB, FRCA
R. Phillip Dellinger, MD, MSc

Margarida deMagalhaes-Silverman, MD
Robert H. Demling, MD
Michael A. DeVita, MD
Donald J. Deyo, DVM
David J. Diehl, MD
Bruce Dobkin, MD
Forrest Dodson, MD
Michael Donahoe, MD
Albert D. Donnenberg, PhD
John B. Downs, MD
John J. Downes, MD
Howard R. Doyle, MD
Jeffrey M. Drazen, MD
Rodney M. Durham, MD
Christopher Eager, MD
Thomas D. East, PhD
David H. Ebb, MD
Frederick J. Ehlert, PhD
Kenneth A. Ellenbogen, MD
I. Alan Fein, MD
Sandra L. Fein, MA, RN
Mitchell P. Fink, MD
Charles J. Fisher, Jr., MD, FCCM
Alpha A. Fowler, III, MD
Arthur M. Freedman, MD
Bradley P. Fuhrman, MD
John J. Fung, MD, PhD
T. James Gallagher, MD, FCCP, FCCM
Tomas Ganz, PhD, MD
Reed M. Gardner, PhD
Edward R. Garrity, Jr., MD
Raúl J. Gazmuri, MD, PhD
Todd W. B. Gehr, MD
Janet Geisel, MSN, RN
Jeffrey A. Gelfand, MD
Eileen R. Gillan, MD
Salvatore R. Goodwin, MD
A. Gerson Greenburg, MD, PhD
George A. Gregory, MD
Bartley P. Griffith, MD
Anthony H. Guarino, MD
Philippe Guinot, MD
Guillermo Gutiérrez, PhD, MD, FCCM

David W. Haas, MD
Steven M. Hall, MD
Perry V. Halushka, PhD, MD
Jiho Han, MD
Gary D. V. Hankins, MD
Robert L. Hardesty, MD
John M. Harlan, MD
Geoffrey O. Hartzler, MD, FACC
Maurene A. Harvey, RN, MPH, CCRN, FCCM
Andrea Hastillo, MD
Elizabeth A. Henneman, RN, MS, CCRN
Daniel A. Henry, MD
Lynn J. Hernan, MD
Carl Anthony Hess, MD
Michael L. Hess, MD
Rosemary Hickey, MD
Elizabeth Hingsbergen, MD
Chester B. Hollinger, Jr., MD
Karen W. Hollingsworth, RN, MS, CCRN
David Hosford, PhD
John W. Hoyt, MD, FCCM
Eric H. Hubli, MD
Christophe Van Huffel, PhD
Russell D. Hull, MBBS, MSc
Thomas K. Hunt, MD
Louis J. Ignarro, PhD
Robert M. Jackson, MD
Judith Jacobi, PharmD, FCCM
Michael R. Jacobs, MB, BCh, MRC Path
Khursheed N. Jeejeebhoy, MB, BS, PhD, FRCP(C)
Dennis M. Jensen, MD
Howard Jolles, MD
Robert M. Kacmarek, PhD, RRT
Allen B. Kaiser, MD
Peter W. Kakavas, MD
Yoogoo Kang, MD
Jill D. Kaplan, MD
Joan E. Kapusnik-Uner, PharmD
Robert Katz, MD
Elizabeth S. Kaufman, MD, FACC
Clifford J. Kavinsky, MD, PhD
Richard L. Keenan, MD
Stephen Keim, MD

Dennis L. Kelleher, PhD
John M. Kellum, MD, FACS
Andrew S. Kenler, MD
Gary J. Kerkvliet, MD
Michael B. Kesselbrenner, MD, FACC, FACP
Pavel L. Khimenko, MD, PhD
Anton I. Kidess, MBBS, MD
Thomas Killip, MD
Christina I. Klufas, MD
William A. Knaus, MD
Matyas Koltai, MD, PhD
Robert L. Kormos, MD
Harry B. Kram, MD, FCCM
David J. Kramer, MD
John W. Kreit, MD
Vladimir Kvetan, MD, FCCM, FCCP
Kenneth K. W. Lee, MD
Howard Levy, MD
Peter Linden, MD, DMD
Carl-Eric Lindholm, MD, PhD
Toby L. Litovitz, MD
Sandra Lookinland, PhD, RN
Thomas G. Luerssen, MD, FACS, FAAP
Philip D. Lumb, MBBS, FCCM
Ignazio Roberto Marino, MD
Lawrence F. Marshall, MD
G. Daniel Martich, MD, FCCP
Tom Masciangelo, MD
Henry Masur, MD
John E. Mazuski, MD, PhD
D. Robert McCaffree, MD
Jerry McCauley, MD
Joe M. McCord, PhD
David J. McConkey, PhD
Kristine M. McCulloch, MD
Mary McDonald, MD
Richard J. Melker, MD, PhD
Mark A. Mintun, MD
Cres B. Miranda, MD, FACC
Jerome H. Modell, MD
Richard E. Moon, MD, FACP, FCCP, FRCP(C)
Alan H. Morris, MD
William J. Morris, MD

Loren D. Nelson, MD
Dane J. Nichols, MD
Ronald Lee Nichols, MD, MS, FACS
J. V. Nixon, MD
Scott Norwood, MD, FACS, FCCM
Walter J. O'Donnell, MD
Steven L. Orebaugh, MD
Richard A. Orr, MD
Michele C. Papo, MD
Margaret M. Parker, MD
Joseph E. Parrillo, MD
M. H. Parsa, MD
William T. Peruzzi, MD
Sharon L. Pilmer, MD
Steven M. Pincus, MD, PhD
Graham F. Pineo, MD
Michael R. Pinsky, MD
Murray M. Pollack, MD
Fred Plum, MD
David T. Porembka, DO, FCCM, FCCP
David J. Powner, MD
Donald S. Prough, MD
Eric C. Rackow, MD
Louis Rakita, MD, CM, FACP, FRCP(C), FACC
David D. Ralph, MD
Jukka Räsänen, MD
Gary E. Raskob, BSc, MSc
Keith Reemstma, MD
H. David Reines, MD, FACS, FCCM
Jorge Reyes, MD
Camillo Ricordi, MD
William C. Roberts, MD
Dudley F. Rochester, MD
Robert M. Rogers, MD
Jonathan D. Root, MD
Allan H. Ropper, MD
Alan J. Rosenbloom, MD
Lewis J. Rubin, MD
Edward J. Ruley, MD
Edmund J. Rutherford, MD
Witold B. Rybka, MD
Peter Safar, MD
Michael Salem, MD

Merle A. Sande, MD
Mark H. Sanders, MD, FCCP
Andrew J. Satin, MD
Thomas J. Savides, MD
Joseph M. Scheller, MD
Stephen C. Schimpff, MD
Christine R. Schneyer, MD
Sidney H. Schnoll, MD, PhD
Luke O. Schoeniger, PhD, MD
Anton C. Schoolwerth, MD
Wolfgang H. Schraut, MD, PhD
Robert Selby, MD
Michael G. Seneff, MD
Curtis N. Sessler, MD
Barry A. Shapiro, MD
Leland Shapiro, MD
Marc J. Shapiro, MD
Ronald Shapiro, MD
William J. Sibbald, MD, FRCP(C)
Dean F. Sittig, PhD
M. Leon Skolnick, MD
Tod B. Sloan, MD, PhD
Robert C. Smallridge, MD, FACP
Howard S. Smith, MD
Robert A. Smith, MS, RRT, FCCM
Stephanie E. Spottswood, MD, MSPH
Sidney Starkman, MD
Thomas E. Starzl, MD, PhD
David L. Steed, MD
Michael L. Steer, MD
Keith L. Stein, MD, FCCP, FCCM
Steven M. Steinberg, MD
David M. Steinhorn, MD
Ronald A. Stiller, MD, PhD, FCCP
James K. Stoller, MD
Bryant W. Stolp, MD, PhD
Patrick J. Strollo, MD, FCCP
Susan A. Stuart, RN, BSN, CPTC
Dale Swift, MD
Karen N. Swisher, MS, JD
Richard A. Szucs, MD
Aubrey E. Taylor, PhD
Robert W. Taylor, MD

Patrick Tchou, MD
Charles Teo, MD
Jaime Tisnado, MD, FACR, FACC
Martin J. Tobin, MD
Satoru Todo, MD
Gail T. Tominaga, MD
Tor Inge Tønnessen, MD, PhD
Arthur L. Trask, MD, FACS
Steven J. Trottier, MD
Jonathan D. Truwit, MD
Andreas G. Tzakis, MD
Nicholas B. Vedder, MD
Dharmapuri Vidyasagar, MD
Sid M. Viner, MD
Thomas Vrobel, MD, FACP, FACC
Rade B. Vukmir, MD
Bertil K. J. Wagner, PharmD
John C. Wain, MD
John D. Ward, MD, FCCM
Kenneth Waxman, MD, FACS
Andrew S. Wechsler, MD
Lawrence R. Wechsler, MD
Richard E. Weibley, MD, MPH
Max Harry Weil, MD, PhD
Howard M. Weinberg, DO
Joel Weinthal, MD, FAAP
Randall C. Wetzel, MB, BS, FCCM, FAAP
Rodney A. White, MD
Peter Wilson, MD
Robert F. Wilson, MD, FACS, FCCM
Thomas C. Witt, MD
Ginger Schafer Wlody, RN, EdD, FCCM
Mark A. Wood, MD
David Woods, PharmD
Stuart J. Youngner, MD
David D. Zabel, MD
Barbara J. Zarowitz, PharmD, FCCP
Jack E. Zimmerman, MD
Janice L. Zimmerman, MD, FACP, FCCP, FCCM

Contributors

Edward Abraham, MD
Associate Professor of Medicine, Division of Pulmonary/Critical Care Medicine, University of Colorado Health Sciences Center; Section Head, Critical Care Medicine, and Director, Medical Intensive Care Unit, University of Colorado Health Sciences Center, Denver, Colorado
Cell Injury and Cell Death

Rinaldo Bellomo, MD, FRACP
Staff Specialist in Intensive Care Medicine, Austin and Repatriation Medical Center, Heidelberg, Melbourne, Victoria, Australia
Visceral Dysfunction and Renal Failure. Part B. Renal Failure

Charles F. Chandler, MD
Assistant Professor, Department of Surgery, University of California at Los Angeles, Los Angeles, California
Monitoring

Christiane C. Corriveau, MD
Assistant Professor of Anesthesia and Pediatrics, George Washington University School of Medicine; Director of Critical Care Fellowship Program, Children's National Medical Center, Washington, District of Columbia
Pediatrics

Joseph M. Darby, MD
Associate Professor of Anesthesiology/Critical Care Medicine, Internal Medicine, Surgery, and Neurological Surgery, University of Pittsburgh School of Medicine; Medical Director, Trauma/Neurosurgical Intensive Care Unit, Presbyterian University Hospital, Pittsburgh, Pennsylvania
Central Nervous System

Andrea Hastillo, MD
Associate Professor, Division of Cardiology, Department of Medicine, Medical College of Virginia; Director, Coronary Care Units, Medical College of Virginia Hospitals, Richmond, Virginia
Cardiovascular Issues

Michael L. Hess, MD
Professor of Medicine and Chairman, Division of Cardiopulmonary Laboratories and Research, Medical College of Virginia, Virginia Commonwealth University; Medical College of Virginia Hospitals, Richmond, Virginia
Cardiovascular Issues; Endocrinology and Metabolism and Pharmacologic Principles. Part B. Pharmacologic Principles

Herbert E. Jacob, MD, FACP, FCCP
Assistant Professor in Critical Care Anesthesia, Medicine and Medical Oncology, and Otolaryngology, University of Pittsburgh Medical School; Director, Critical Care Services, Magee Women's Hospital; Member, University of Pittsburgh Cancer Center, Pittsburgh, Pennsylvania
Hematology/Oncology

John A. Kellum, MD
Assistant Professor of Anesthesia and Critical Care Medicine, University of Pittsburgh School of Medicine; Staff Intensivist, Cardiothoracic and Liver Transplant Intensive Care Units, University of Pittsburgh Medical Center, Pittsburgh, Pennsylvania
Transplantation

Barbara A. Kerwin, MD
Transplant Intensivist, Oklahoma Transplantation Institute, Baptist Medical Center, Oklahoma City, Oklahoma
Respiratory Function

Joann I. Lamb, MSN, RN-C, FCCM
Vice-President, Patient Services, The Dobelle Institute, Columbia Presbyterian Medical Center, New York, New York
Patient Care, Organization, and Ethics

Kang H. Lee, MA, MBBChir, MRCP(UK)
Registrar and Clinical Teacher, Department of Internal Medicine, National University Hospital, Singapore
Respiratory Function

Thomas W. K. Lew, MBBS, MMed (Anes)
Clinical Teacher, National University of Singapore; Staff Anesthesiologist, Tan Tock Seng Hospital, Singapore
Central Nervous System

Peter Linden, MD, DMD
Assistant Professor of Anesthesiology and Medicine, University of Pittsburgh School of Medicine; Associate Co-Director, Liver Transplant Intensive Care Unit, Presbyterian University Hospital, Pittsburgh, Pennsylvania
Infectious Diseases

George V. Mazariegos, MD
Assistant Professor of Surgery, University of Pittsburgh Medical School; Co-Director, Liver Transplant Intensive Care Unit, University of Pittsburgh Medical Center, Pittsburgh, Pennsylvania
Transplantation

J. Harlan Meyer, MD, PhD
Assistant Professor, Division of Diabetes and Endocrinology, Scripps Clinic and Research Foundation, La Jolla, California
Endocrinology and Metabolism and Pharmacologic Principles. Part A. Endocrinology and Metabolism

Adelaida M. Miro, MD
Assistant Professor of Anesthesiology, Critical Care Medicine, and Medicine, University of Pittsburgh Medical Center, Pittsburgh, Pennsylvania
Respiratory Function

Juan B. Ochoa, MD
Chief Resident, Department of General Surgery, University of Pittsburgh School of Medicine and University of Pittsburgh Medical Center, Pittsburgh, Pennsylvania
Visceral Dysfunction and Renal Failure. Part A. Visceral Dysfunction

Sten Rubertsson, MD, PhD
Anesthesiology Fellow, Critical Care Medicine, University of Pittsburgh School of Medicine, Pittsburgh, Pennsylvania
Resuscitation

Michael D. Schwartz, MD
Instructor of Medicine, Division of Pulmonary/Critical Care Medicine, University of Colorado Health Sciences Center; Assistant Chief of Medicine, University Hospital, University of Colorado Health Sciences Center, Denver, Colorado
Cell Injury and Cell Death

Gail T. Tominaga, MD
Assistant Professor of Surgery, University of California at Irvine, Irvine, California; Assistant Professor of Surgery, University of California, Irvine Medical Center, Orange, California
Trauma

Kenneth Waxman, MD
Clinical Professor of Surgery, University of California, Irvine Medical Center, Orange, California; Director of Surgical Education, Cottage Hospital, Santa Barbara, California
Monitoring; Trauma

Contents

CHAPTER 1
Resuscitation

Sten Rubertsson, MD, PhD

CARDIOPULMONARY RESUSCITATION

Background

Each year, some 500,000 individuals suffer an episode of sudden cardiac death in the United States. Of these cardiac arrests, 100,000 are estimated to be reversible. Unfortunately, fewer than 3% of these victims leave the hospital alive and return to productive lives. In selected communities in the United States and abroad that have remarkably efficient emergency medical systems, however, as many as 30% of victims of sudden cardiac arrest survive. Prompted in part by these encouraging experiences, the American Heart Association introduced the concept of the Chain of Survival. It emphasizes that survival is contingent on the rapidity and sequence with which the resuscitation interventions are delivered. The Chain of Survival calls for specific, timely efforts:

- *Early* activation of the emergency medical system
- *Early* basic life support (BLS), including precordial compression and artificial ventilation
- *Early* defibrillation, ideally by the first responder
- *Early* advanced cardiac life support (ACLS), including intubation and medication

It is expected that such a tiered response would improve the dismal outcome of out-of-hospital cardiac arrest situations.

Because general outcome is still poor, however, cardiopulmonary resuscitation (CPR) researchers are trying to find alternative methods for treating cardiac arrest. The focus is on means to increase the perfusion pressure of both the heart and brain during CPR and immediately after restoration of spontaneous circulation. Promising new methods have emerged, including the following:

- Interposed abdominal compression
- Active compression–decompression
- Circumferential chest compression
- Intra-aortic balloon occlusion in combination with conventional closed-chest CPR
- Extracorporeal circulation using peripheral vascular access

Although no persuasive evidence yet exists that these new methods improve the long-term outcome of a cardiac arrest patient, it is hoped that hemodynamically more effective techniques may expand the time window for successful cardiac and cerebral resuscitation.

Management

Primary cardiac arrest

Ventricular fibrillation (VF)

Asystole

Secondary cardiac arrest

Asphyxia

Exsanguination

Signs of cardiac arrest

Unconsciousness

Apnea or gasping

Deathlike appearance

No pulse in the carotid and femoral arteries

For every victim the emergency medical services delivery team should estimate the following:

- Duration of cardiac arrest: Where and when was the victim found?
- Duration of CPR: When was basic life support (BLS) or advanced cardiac life support (ACLS) initiated?
- Duration of severe hypoxemia

Cardiopulmonary resuscitation consists of three phases:

- BLS—emergency oxygenation
- ACLS—restoration of spontaneous circulation
- Prolonged life support (PLS)—postresuscitative brain-oriented intensive care

Basic Life Support

Airway Control

- Backward head tilt, forward mandible displacement, open mouth
- Lung inflation attempts
- Manual clearing of mouth and throat—pharyngeal suctioning if available
- Oropharyngeal and nasopharyngeal tubes (airways)—use only in unconscious patient because they can promote vomiting and laryngospasm
- Endotracheal intubation—as soon as possible with a cuffed tube
- Cricothyrotomy—an alternative to endotracheal intubation performed by trained personnel
- Tracheotomy (below the cricoid cartilage)—should be an elective procedure
- Tracheobronchial suctioning—aspiration
- If massive aspiration—bronchoscopy and pharmacologic bronchodilation
- Gastric tube—inserted as soon as possible
- Immediate drainage of tension pneumothorax—confirmation by needle puncture in the midclavicular line of the second intercostal space of the affected side; should not be delayed until confirmation by radiography

Breathing Support

- Mouth-to-mouth ventilation—12 lung inflations per minute

  Mouth-to-nose ventilation if mouth-to-mouth ventilation is impossible

Mouth-to-adjunct ventilation; with or without oxygen (O_2)
Manual bag-mask (tube) ventilation; with or without O_2
Hand-triggered O_2 ventilation
Mechanical ventilation

- Once an endotracheal tube is in place, ventilation should be performed asynchronously at 12 to 15 ventilations per minute.
- If feasible, apply positive end-expiratory pressure (PEEP) titrated according to arterial and mixed venous oxygen values.

Circulation Support

- External chest compressions
  Depress lower sternum 1.5 to 2 inches (4–5 cm)
  Compression rate: 80 per minute
  Compression/relaxation ratio: 1:1
  One operator (patient not intubated): Alternate 2 lung inflations with 15 sternal compressions.
  Two operators (patient not intubated): Alternate 1 lung inflation with 5 sternal compressions.
- Manual control of external hemorrhage
  Tourniquet
  Pressure pants (military antishock trousers) for shock
  Trendelenburg position for shock; intravenous fluid

Open-Chest Cardiopulmonary Resuscitation

Open-chest CPR produces greater cerebral and coronary perfusion pressures than external (closed-chest) CPR but is limited to use by experienced physicians in hospitals.

Indications

1. Chest is already open (in the operating room).
2. Severe intrathoracic hemorrhage is suspected.
3. Cardiac tamponade is suspected.
4. Intra-abdominal exsanguination is suspected (for clamping of lower thoracic aorta).
5. Massive pulmonary embolism is suspected.
6. Hypothermic cardiac arrest has occurred (direct warming of the heart).
7. Chest or spine deformities are present and so external CPR fails to produce a carotid or femoral pulse.
8. Long duration of unwitnessed cardiac arrest is suspected, and optimal external CPR ALS is unable to restore spontaneous normotension within 5 to 10 minutes.

Technique

1. Intubate and ventilate the patient; add PEEP.
2. Cut through skin over the fourth or fifth left intercostal space.
3. Enter the chest bluntly and cut the intercostal muscles with Mayo scissors. Avoid the intercostal neurovascular bundle and the internal mammary artery.

4. Tear open the intercostal space with your fingers.
5. Insert a rib spreader, if available.
6. Stand on the patient's left side, facing cephalad. Without opening the pericardium, insert left hand through the thoracotomy incision, placing the thumb over the left (thick-walled) ventricle (posteriorly) and fingers 2 through 5 over the right (thin-walled) ventricle anteriorly. Take care not to pierce the atria or ventricles!
7. If feasible, compress the descending aorta with the other hand.
8. Heart compressions might be more effective by compressing the heart against the sternum or between one hand placed posteriorly and the other hand positioned anteriorly.
9. Compress about once per second and adjust compression force and rate to filling of heart.
10. Cool the patient's head if feasible.

Advanced Cardiac Life Support

Treat the patient, not the monitor!

- Electrocardiographic (ECG) monitoring should be established immediately. "Quick-look paddles" on defibrillators can be used initially to avoid delay.
  VF pulseless ventricular tachycardia (VT)?
  Asystole?
  Bizarre complexes (electromechanical dissociation [EMD])?

I. Ventricular Fibrillation and Ventricular Tachycardia

Possible Causes

Ischemia, infarction, hypoxia, hypothermia, acidosis, and electrolyte imbalance

Algorithm

Perform CPR until defibrillator attached

↓

Defibrillate three times if needed at 200, 200 to 300, and 360 J for persistent VF or VT → 1. Asystole—go to II
2. EMD—go to III
3. Restoration of spontaneous circulation

↓

Persistent VF or VT

↓

Continue CPR
Intubate

↓

Obtain IV access

↓

Epinephrine,* 1 mg IV push (10 mL of a 1:10,000 solution); repeat every 3 to 5 minutes

Consider sodium bicarbonate†

↓

Defibrillate at 360 J within 30 to 60 seconds

↓

Administer antifibrillatory agent‡
Lidocaine, 1.5 mg/kg IV push; repeat in 3 to 5 minutes to total dose of 3 mg/kg

↓

Defibrillate at 360 J 30 to 60 seconds after each dose of medication
Pattern: drug–shock, drug–shock

II. Asystole

Possible Causes

End result of VF, EMD, or heart block. Hypoxia, hyperkalemia or hypokalemia, severe metabolic acidosis, drug overdose, or hypothermia

Algorithm

Continue CPR
Intubate at once
Obtain IV access
Confirm asystole in more than one lead

↓

Consider immediate transcutaneous pacing

↓

Epinephrine,* 1 mg IV push (10 mL of a 1:10,000 solution); repeat every 3 to 5 minutes
Consider sodium bicarbonate†

↓

Atropine, 1 mg IV push; repeat every 3 to 5 minutes up to a total of 0.04 mg/kg

↓

If no response, consider termination of efforts

III. Electromechanical Dissociation

Possible Causes

- Hypovolemia: Start volume infusion (lactated Ringer's solution, dextran, albumin); administer norepinephrine and/or dopamine.
- Hypoxia: Start ventilation.
- Cardiac tamponade: Perform pericardiocentesis.
- Tension pneumothorax:
    1. Perform an immediate needle thoracostomy in the midclavicular line of the second intercostal space of the affected side.
    2. Insert chest tube (>36 French) in midaxillary line at intercostal space 4 or 5.
- Hypothermia
- Massive pulmonary embolism: Start thrombolysis, consider surgery.

- Drug overdose: Administer tricyclic antidepressants, digitalis, β-blockers, calcium channel blockers.
- Hyperkalemia
- Acidosis: Give sodium bicarbonate.†
- Massive acute myocardial infarction

Algorithm

Continue CPR
Intubate at once
Obtain IV access
Assess blood flow using Doppler ultrasound

↓

Epinephrine,* 1 mg IV push (10 mL of a 1:10,000 solution); repeat every 3 to 5 minutes
Consider sodium bicarbonate†

↓

If patient is experiencing absolute bradycardia (<60 beats/min) or relative bradycardia, give atropine, 1 mg IV push; repeat every 3 to 5 minutes to a total of 0.04 mg/kg.

---

*Epinephrine: The recommended dose is 1 mg IV push every 3 to 5 minutes. Higher doses of epinephrine, five to ten times greater than the standard dose, are more effective in animal models but have not proved effective yet in clinical studies.

†Sodium bicarbonate, 1 mmol/kg IV. Repeat not more than every 10 minutes and titrate as soon as possible according to arterial pH. Aim for arterial pH of 7.3 to 7.5 or to normalized calculated base deficit. Indications:

Known preexisting hyperkalemia

After prolonged arrest (at least 2 to 5 minutes) or CPR time to neutralize acidosis in order to prevent the arterial pH from decreasing below 7.2 during the early phase of restoration of spontaneous circulation

Tricyclic antidepressant overdose

‡Antifibrillatory agents—indicated in refractory or persistent VF:

Lidocaine: First choice. 1.5 mg/kg IV push, repeat in 3 to 5 minutes to total dose of 3 mg/kg. On restoration of spontaneous circulation, continuous infusion at 2 to 4 mg/min should be started.

Bretylium: When lidocaine and defibrillation fail to convert VF. 5 mg/kg IV push; repeat in 5 minutes at 10 mg/kg up to a maximum total dose of 30 to 35 mg/kg.

Procainamide: For refractory VF. 30 mg/min up to a maximum of 17 mg/kg.

Magnesium sulfate: For severe refractory VF. 1 to 2 g IV.

Administration of Medications During Cardiopulmonary Resuscitation

- Peripheral vein administration: Antecubital or external jugular vein should be first choice.
- Central venous line infusion: Internal jugular or subclavian vein is used because of more rapid arrival of drugs to their site of action.
- Endotracheal administration: If venous access is delayed, 2 to 2.5 times the recommended IV dose is diluted in 10 mL of normal saline or distilled water. Epinephrine, lidocaine, and atropine can be administered through the endotracheal tube.
- Intraosseous infusion: This is an excellent alternative. Re-

member to increase epinephrine doses 2 to 2.5 times the recommended IV doses.

When Not to Start and When to Stop Cardiopulmonary Resuscitation

- CPR should not be started when a patient is in the terminal stage of an incurable disease, when the order "do not resuscitate" (DNR) has been specified, or when another reason to withhold CPR is considered acceptable.
- When in doubt, BLS and ACLS should be initiated; there is no time for contemplation or consultation.
- Discontinuance of BLS and ACLS should be determined on the basis of cardiac death, not brain death.
- Cardiac death is evident when heartbeats cannot be re-established despite a maximum effort for at least 30 minutes.
- EMD is not a proof of irreversibility.
- As long as VF or VT is present, a chance to restore spontaneous circulation exists.

Prolonged Life Support

- Normotension (mean arterial pressure 90–100 mm Hg)—titration with fluids, vasopressor, or vasodilator as needed; arterial, central venous, and pulmonary artery catheter placement for hemodynamic monitoring
- Mechanical ventilation for about 12 hours; chest roentgenogram as soon as possible to evaluate endotracheal tube placement and potential pneumothorax
- Moderate hyperventilation ($Pa{CO_2}$ 25–35 mm Hg)
- Moderate hyperoxia ($Pa{O_2} > 100$ mm Hg)
- Arterial pH 7.3 to 7.5; arterial base deficit below 7 mmol/L (with sodium bicarbonate)
- Immobilization (partial neuromuscular paralysis) as needed
- Sedation (diazepam, barbiturates, narcotics) as needed
- Anticonvulsants (diazepam, phenytoin) as needed for seizure activity
- Normalization of hematocrit, electrolytes, osmolality, glucose
- Short-term steroids optional
- Normothermia—prevention of hyperthermia:
  - Permit spontaneous mild hypothermia of 34° to 36°C for about 12 hours.
  - Keep core temperature above 32°C.
  - Use standard intensive care for all vital organ systems.
  - Position head slightly elevated (30°). Turn trunk periodically from side to side.

When and How to Terminate Prolonged Life Support

- When contraindicated, PLS should be discontinued.
- Before brain death can be certified, more than 24 hours of extracerebral organ stabilization may be required.
- Irreversibility of vegetative state should be determined on

the basis of published predictive criteria, clinical judgment, and laboratory data.

- The decision to terminate treatment should be made by an experienced physician, who should also seek advice from consultants.

CRITICAL CARE MEDICINE AND THE OBSTETRIC PATIENT

Pregnant patients are unique because at least two patients, mother and fetus, must be considered.

Physiologic Changes of Pregnancy

Cardiovascular System

- Blood pressure: Both systolic and diastolic arterial pressures decrease until 28 weeks' gestation; thereafter, both increase to normal by term.
- Heart rate increases to 20% above normal.
- Cardiac output increases as early as 10 weeks of gestation, peaks at 30% to 50% (from about 4.5 to 6.5 L/min) over control values by late second trimester, and remains elevated through pregnancy (lateral decubitus position).
- Systemic vascular resistance decreases (peripheral vasodilation-reduced afterload).

Respiratory System

- Minute ventilation increases 40%, from 7.5 to 10.5 L/min, because respiratory rate is unchanged, primarily as a result of increased tidal volume.
- Tidal volume increases from about 500 to 700 mL.
- Vital capacity may be increased by 100 to 200 mL.
- Inspiratory capacity increases by about 300 mL by late pregnancy.
- Expiratory reserve volume decreases from 1300 to 1100 mL.
- Residual volume decreases from 1500 to 1200 mL.
- Functional residual capacity is reduced considerably (by 500 mL).
- Arterial blood gases: $Pa{CO_2}$ 27 to 32 mm Hg; pH 7.40 to 7.45; $Pa{O_2}$ 101 to 108 mm Hg early in pregnancy but 90 to 100 mm Hg near term.

Hematologic System

- Total blood volume increases 45% to 50%, mainly because of enhanced plasma volume. Serum albumin decreases, resulting in reduced plasma oncotic pressure. Capillary hydrostatic pressure increases. The consequence of these changes is an increase in interstitial fluid—edema.
- The clotting factors, particularly fibrinogen (50%), increase, and Factors VII, VIII, IX, and X have a marked increase at the beginning of the third trimester.

Urinary System

- Glomerular filtration rate increases approximately 50%.
- Renal plasma flow increases by 25% to 50%.
- Creatinine clearance increases about 50%.
- Urine volume is unchanged.
- Glucosuria occurs in more than 50% of pregnant women.

Gastrointestinal System

- Motility and smooth muscle tone are reduced, with the particular effect of delayed gastric emptying.

Trauma

Physical trauma complicates about 1 in 12 pregnancies. Trauma is the leading cause of death in women of reproductive age. It is not surprising, therefore, that trauma is the leading cause of nonobstetric maternal deaths.

Blunt Abdominal Trauma

Always consider the same organs are injured as in a nonpregnant woman.

ABRUPTIO PLACENTAE. Placental separation from the underlying decidua basalis complicates 1% to 5% of minor injuries and 40% to 50% of major life-threatening injuries.

FINDINGS

- Symptoms of shock (e.g., tachycardia and low blood pressure)
- Vaginal bleeding
- Intense abdominal and lower back pain
- Uterine tenderness (tetanically contracted)
- Fetal tachycardia, late decelerations, acidosis, bradycardia
- Fetal death

UTERINE RUPTURE. This is an infrequent (less than 1% of all injuries during pregnancy) but life-threatening complication.

FINDINGS

- Findings vary from only subtle signs to the extreme of rapid onset of maternal shock with possible fetal and maternal death.

DIRECT FETAL INJURY. The incidence is uncertain, since it is an uncommon event. Direct fetal injury most often involves the fetal skull and brain, and the most common mechanism involves simultaneous fracture of the maternal pelvis in late gestation when the fetal head is engaged.

GUNSHOT AND STAB WOUNDS. Visceral injuries to the mother complicate only 19% of gunshot wounds to the uterus, whereas the fetus is injured about 60% of the time. Any abdominal gunshot requires exploration. Stab wounds are limited by the length and width of the penetrating object. Observation is warranted in selected cases if both the mother and fetus are stable (low suspicion for intra-abdominal bleeding).

Management

Pregnancy should not restrict any of the usual diagnostic, pharmacologic, or resuscitative procedures or maneuvers. The first priority is the mother, since overlooking life-threatening maternal injuries lessens the likelihood of survival of both the mother and fetus.

UTERINE DISPLACEMENT. Deflection of the uterus off the inferior vena cava and abdominal aorta is important for improving perfusion of the uterofetal blood flow and maternal venous return in the supine position. This can be achieved by two approaches:

1. Placing patient in left lateral decubitus position.
2. Manually deflecting the uterus to the left and placing a wedge under the patient's right hip.

PERITONEAL LAVAGE. For evaluation of intraperitoneal bleeding. Open peritoneal lavage is preferred over blind needle insertion and has been shown to be safe, sensitive, and specific during pregnancy. Peritoneal lavage is unnecessary if intraperitoneal bleeding is clinically obvious.

ELECTRONIC FETAL MONITORING. In pregnant trauma victims beyond 20 weeks of gestation, electronic fetal monitoring may assist in the early diagnosis of abruptio placentae and should be initiated immediately after stabilization.

ULTRASONOGRAPHY. This is used to establish gestational age, to localize the placenta, to determine fetal condition, and to estimate amniotic fluid volume. It may help reveal intraperitoneal hemorrhage, but it is less sensitive for diagnosing abruptio placentae than is electronic fetal and uterine monitoring.

EXPLORATORY LAPAROTOMY. The fetus usually tolerates surgery and anesthesia well if maternal oxygenation and uterine perfusion can be maintained. The need to perform a laparotomy is not an indication to proceed with cesarean delivery. If the uterus has been penetrated and delivery is to be effected, a pediatric surgeon and a neonatologist should be present.

IMMUNOGLOBULIN D. Administration of 300 μg intramuscularly within 72 hours is recommended for D-negative trauma victims to prevent D-isoimmunization due to fetomaternal hemorrhage. The Kleihauer-Betke assay of excessive (>30 mL) fetomaternal hemorrhage should be performed to identify victims who will need additional immunoglobulin D.

Amniotic Fluid Embolism

Amniotic fluid embolism is a rare obstetric disorder that carries a maternal mortality rate as high as 80%. It has a dramatic presentation as cardiopulmonary collapse, pulmonary edema, or profuse hemorrhage, either individually or in combination.

Pathophysiology

For amniotic fluid embolism to occur, amniotic fluid must have a passage to the maternal circulation. This requires ruptured membranes, an opening in the maternal circulation such as occurs with a ruptured uterus, placenta accreta, cesarean section, retained placenta, abruptio placentae, or placenta previa.

Initial Response

Probably within the first 30 minutes:

- Pulmonary arterial pressure increases.
- Pulmonary capillary wedge pressure increases.
- Pulmonary vascular resistance increases.
- Resulting pulmonary shunting leads to arterial hypoxemia.

Secondary Phase

- Left ventricular failure—hypotension occurs.
- Pulmonary capillary injury—pulmonary edema occurs.
- Coagulopathy ranging from disseminated intravascular coagulation to minor disturbances in the coagulation system occurs in 40% of patients.

Clinical Presentation

- Sudden dyspnea, cyanosis, and acute respiratory failure occur.
- Variable hypotension occurs followed by cardiopulmonary collapse.
- Grand mal seizures occur in about 20% of cases.
- Bleeding diathesis is the presenting manifestation in 10% to 15% of cases. Venipuncture sites and surgical wounds bleed.

Laboratory Values

- Fibrinogen is decreased.
- Fibrin split products are increased.
- Partial thromboplastin and prothrombin times are increased.
- Thrombocytopenia is seen.
- Arterial P_{O_2} is decreased, arterial P_{CO_2} is increased, and arterial pH is decreased.

Management

Differential Diagnosis

- Septic shock
- Aspiration pneumonia
- Acute myocardial infarction
- Pulmonary thromboembolism
- Abruptio placentae with coagulopathy

Three Goals

- Oxygenation—Pa_{O_2} over 60 mm Hg (8.0 kPa), Sa_{O_2} over 90%

- Maintenance of cardiac output and blood pressure—systolic arterial pressure (SAP) over 90 mm Hg, urinary output over 25 mL/h
- Combating what is usually a self-limited coagulopathy

MONITORING

- Pulmonary arterial catheter and arterial line are recommended for guiding hemodynamic management.

TREATMENT

- If spontaneous breathing with oxygen is not sufficient or if the patient is unconscious, immediate intubation and mechanical ventilation with 100% oxygen and PEEP are required.
- Cardiac shock treatment with rapid volume infusion and early inotropic support with dopamine may be necessary.
- After initial resuscitation and correction of hypotension, fluid therapy should be restricted to minimize volume overload and pulmonary edema.
- Coagulopathy should be treated aggressively. *Avoid the temptation to re-explore the patient, even in the setting of intra-abdominal bleeding, until the coagulation defect has been corrected.*

Hypertension

Pregnancy-induced hypertension, which occurs in 5% to 10% of pregnancies, remains the second most common cause of maternal mortality in the United States. Pregnancy can induce hypertension in a previously normotensive woman or exacerbate blood pressures in a chronically hypertensive patient.

Pathophysiology

Regardless of the initial mechanism, preeclampsia is characterized by generalized vasospasm.

Classification

I. Pregnancy-induced hypertension
   A. Preeclampsia
      1. Mild
      2. Severe
   B. Eclampsia
II. Chronic hypertension—hypertensive disease that antedates pregnancy, is not associated with hydatidiform mole, or persists more than 6 weeks postpartum
III. Chronic hypertension with superimposed pregnancy-induced hypertension
   A. Superimposed preeclampsia
   B. Superimposed eclampsia

Signs and Symptoms

Mild Preeclampsia

- Blood pressure is 140/90 or higher or a rise occurs in diastolic blood pressure of at least 15 mm Hg or in systolic blood pressure of 30 mm Hg above prepregnancy baseline.
- Proteinuria is 300 mg or higher for 24 hours or 100 mg/dL in urine specimens 6 hours apart.
- Nondependent edema is usually visible in the face and hands and is associated with at least 5-lb (2.25-kg) weight gain per week.
- Laboratory values: hematocrit is increased; platelet count is decreased; serum glutamic-oxaloacetic transaminase is increased; prothrombin time and partial thromboplastin time are increased; and serum creatinine is increased.

Severe Preeclampsia

- Blood pressure is over 160/110 mm Hg.
- Proteinuria exceeds 5 g/24 h.
- Oliguria is below 400 to 500 mL/24 h.
- Cerebral or visual disturbances occur.
- Edema or cyanosis is present.
- Epigastric or right upper quadrant pain or impaired liver function may be seen.
- Hematologic: See laboratory values for mild preeclampsia.

Eclampsia

- Development of convulsions in a preeclamptic woman with no history of seizure disorder

IMPORTANT. Preeclampsia of any severity can rapidly evolve to eclampsia or severe preeclampsia.

Management

Prevent and treat seizures, treat hypertension, and provide meticulous fluid therapy and delivery.

Seizure Prophylaxis

- *Magnesium sulfate* ($MgSO_4$): Administer a loading dose of 4 g IV over 2 to 6 minutes, followed by a continuous IV infusion of 2 g/h. Maintain plasma magnesium levels of 4 to 7 mEq/L (4.8–8.4 mg/dL).
- Pay attention to magnesium toxicity: Hot flushes lead to loss of reflexes, which leads to respiratory depression and respiratory arrest, which can result in cardiac arrest.
- A Foley catheter is preferred. Measure urine output.
- Record and monitor intravenous and oral fluid administration.
- Monitor serum creatinine.
- Continue for a minimum of 24 hours postpartum if blood pressure elevation does not resolve.

Treatment of Eclamptic Seizure

- *$MgSO_4$:* Give 4 g IV over 2 to 6 minutes. If seizure activity continues, give another 2 g IV.
- *Secondary agent:* If seizure activity continues despite treatment with $MgSO_4$, give one of the following drugs:
  - Amobarbital, initial dose of 250 mg IV
  - Diazepam, initial dose of 1 to 10 mg IV
  - Thiopental, initial dose of 100 mg IV
  - Pentobarbital, initial dose of 100 mg IV
- Prevent injury and protect airway from aspiration.
- Once seizures are arrested, measure serum magnesium level and adjust $MgSO_4$ infusion accordingly.

Treatment of Hypertension

The goal is not normotension but prevention of extremes of blood pressure, because a profound decrease in blood pressure can result in uteroplacental insufficiency and subsequent fetal distress. Maintain diastolic blood pressure between 90 and 100 mm Hg.

- *Hydralazine:* Administer 5 mg IV bolus, followed by 5 to 10 mg every 20 to 30 minutes.
- *Labetalol:*
  1. Give 20 mg IV, followed by escalating doses every 10 minutes to a maximum cumulative dose of 300 mg.
  2. Give 0.5 mg/kg/h constant infusion with an increase in dose every 30 minutes by 0.5 mg/kg/h to a maximum of 3 mg/kg/h.
- *Diazoxide:* Administer 30-mg miniboluses IV.
- *Sodium nitroprusside:* Give 0.25 μg/kg/min, increasing by 0.25 μg/kg/min every 5 minutes to effect.
- *Nifedipine:* Administer 10 mg PO; repeat in 30 minutes if necessary.

Fluid Management

Patients with preeclampsia or eclampsia require strict monitoring of fluid intake and output. Invasive monitoring should be considered only when multiple compounding conditions are present along with preeclampsia, as in sepsis or underlying maternal cardiopulmonary disease.

- Foley catheter: Keep urine output above 30 mL/h.
- Keep fluid administration at or below 125 mL/h. If urine output is below 100 to 120 mL/4 h, give a *single* fluid challenge of 500 to 1000 mL normal saline.
- Administer IV furosemide if pulmonary edema or other signs of fluid overload are present.
- If invasive monitoring is indicated, use pulmonary artery catheter for monitoring of pulmonary capillary wedge pressure (not correlated with central venous pressure).
- Keep hematocrit above 25% to 30% with aggressive use of blood transfusion because of low tolerance for blood loss. The average blood loss is 500 mL with vaginal delivery compared with 1500 mL with cesarean delivery (corres-

ponding to one third of blood volume in preeclamptic woman).

Lumbar Epidural Analgesia

- This reduces pain, anxiety, and endogenous catecholamine levels, resulting in decreased peaks of hypertension.
- Hypotension with decreased uteroplacental blood flow as well as volume overload must be avoided.
- Epidural analgesia is contraindicated in patients with fulminant coagulopathy.

General Anesthesia

- This is the anesthetic technique of choice in cases of acute fetal distress.

THE SHOCK SYNDROMES

Of 2.1 million deaths annually in the United States, half are from acute illness and are associated with circulatory failure or shock and its sequelae (i.e., organ failures). Shock is routinely recognized and diagnosed by imprecise signs and symptoms, such as cold clammy skin, altered mental status, unstable vital signs (tachycardia, hypotension), and oliguria. Shock most often occurs as a complication of acute and life-threatening trauma, sepsis, neurogenic and cardiac conditions, or postoperative hypovolemia. It is the common pathway to death as well as the most common lethal and nonlethal complication of acute illness.

The conventional etiologic approach to shock lists signs and symptoms (which are essentially the same for each cause); laboratory data (which are not diagnostic); pathophysiology (which is one dimensional and therefore fails to identify cardiac, pulmonary, and tissue perfusion interactions); and therapy (which is based on a one-dimensional view of physiology and is suboptimal).

The conventional therapeutic approach to shock is to normalize the symptoms used to recognize shock, but this does not correct underlying circulatory deficiencies and does not provide information needed to improve outcome. Invasive monitoring is generally accepted as the gold standard for critically ill patients, but these measurements are often made too late, when shock is irreversible.

Pathophysiology

Hypoxia from poor tissue perfusion is the basic underlying physiologic defect of all shock syndromes. Tissue hypoxia can be initiated by either low blood flow or irregularly distributed flow at the microcirculatory level from uneven vasoconstriction. This occurs early in the course of shock and stimulates physiologic mechanisms (initial increase in cardiac index [CI] and oxygen delivery [DO_2]) and biochemical mediators (stimulating oxygen free radical production) that lead to inadequate tissue perfusion, local tissue hypoxia, organ dysfunction, and subsequently end-organ failure. Death from shock usually is a result of multiple organ failure.

Management

Monitoring

- ECG—heart rate, arrhythmias, and ischemia
- Arterial catheter—blood pressure and arterial blood gases. *Note:* Peripheral arterial blood pressure (e.g., radial or femoral artery) might be considerably lower than central arterial blood pressure because of vasoconstriction due to shock response or vasopressor treatment.
- Pulmonary arterial catheter—pulmonary artery pressures, mixed venous blood gases, and cardiac output
- Central venous catheter—right atrial pressure (equals central venous pressure) and fluid management
- Foley catheter—urine output above 30 mL/h
- Laboratory—routine blood chemistry testing including hemoglobin, hematocrit, and coagulation studies; cardiac enzymes; smears and cultures
- Imaging studies—radiography (including chest), computed tomography (CT), angiography for organ and vascular injury

Optimal Therapeutic Goals

- CI*—4.5 L/min/m^2, 50% higher than normal (2.8–3.6)
- Do_2*—600 to 1000 mL/min/m^2, higher than normal
- Oxygen consumption (Vo_2)*—170 mL/min/m^2, 30% higher than normal
- Blood volume*—500 mL in excess of the norm (i.e., 3.2 L/m^2 for men, 2.8 L/m^2 for women)

Note: Patients who are severely traumatized, stressed, cirrhotic, burned, or in septic shock may require even higher values. Cardiac patients have lower values.

Treatment

VOLUME THERAPY

- The first and most important goal is to restore blood volume. Colloids, which expand plasma volume without overexpanding interstitial water, are preferred.

INOTROPIC AGENTS

- After maximum effect of fluids has been obtained, inotropic agents can be used.
- Dobutamine: Start at 2 to 5 μg/kg/min and titrate dose to optimal response (CI increased, Do_2 increased, Vo_2 in-

---

*For more detailed description of cardiorespiratory variables, see Table 13–2 in the *Textbook of Critical Care.*

creased, systemic vascular resistance decreased, peripheral vascular resistance decreased).

Vasodilators

- Use vasodilators if a patient has normal or high mean arterial blood pressure (MAP) with a high systemic vascular resistance.
- Nitroglycerin, nitroprusside, labetalol, hydralazine, or prostaglandin E_1 alprostadil (PGE_1) can be titrated to achieve improved CI without production of hypotension (i.e., MAP > 80 mm Hg, SAP > 110 mm Hg).

Vasopressors

- Vasopressors are indicated for hypotension after volume therapy has been given.
- Dopamine, norepinephrine, epinephrine, or a combination can be titrated to the smallest dose needed to maintain satisfactory blood pressure while avoiding vasoconstriction and reduced microcirculatory blood flow.

Algorithm

Preliminary evaluation of high-risk critically ill patients is by routine intensive care unit workup, which includes arterial blood gas analysis, chest radiography, routine blood chemistry studies, ECG, and coagulation studies. These tests should either have been performed or be in progress, and the observed defects should be corrected.

STEP 1. Measure CI, DO_2, VO_2, and blood volume to determine whether the patient has reached the optimal therapeutic goals (see earlier). If not, proceed to step 2. If the goals are reached, the objective of the algorithm has been achieved; reevaluate patient and repeat measurements at intervals to maintain these goals.

STEP 2. Measure pulmonary artery wedge pressure; if above 20 mm Hg, proceed to step 3; if below 20, proceed to step 4.

STEP 3. If pulmonary artery wedge pressure is over 20, give furosemide at increasing dose levels (20, 40, 80, 160 mg IV) if there is clinical or radiographic evidence of salt and water overload or if there are clinical findings of pulmonary congestion. If not, consider administering vasodilators, nitroglycerin, or nitroprusside if MAP is above 80 mm Hg and SAP is above 120 mm Hg. Repeat to titrate the dose as needed to reduce wedge pressure to below 15 mm Hg but to maintain MAP above 80 mm Hg. If unsuccessful, place patient on a cardiac protocol.

STEP 4. If the hematocrit is below 33%, give 1 unit of whole blood or 2 units of packed red blood cells. If the hematocrit is over 33%, administer a fluid load (volume challenge) consisting of one of the following (depending on clinical indications of plasma volume deficit or hydration state): 500 mL of 5% plasma protein fraction; 500 mL of 5% albumin; 100 mL of 25% albumin (25 g); 500 mL of 6% hydroxyethyl starch; 500 mL of 6% dextran-60; or 1000 mL of lactated Ringer's solution or normal saline.

STEP 5. If the blood or fluid load improved any of the optimal therapeutic goals (see earlier), proceed to step 6; if none was improved, proceed to step 7.

STEP 6. If goals are not reached, repeat steps 2 through 6 until these goals are met or until the pulmonary capillary wedge pressure exceeds 20 mm Hg.

STEP 7. If MAP is between 70 and 100 mm Hg, give dobutamine by constant IV infusion in doses to increase CI, Do_2, and Vo_2.

STEP 8. Titrate dobutamine, beginning with 2 to 5 μg/kg/min and gradually increasing the dosing rate of up to 20 μg/kg/min or greater provided that CI, Do_2, and Vo_2 improve or until the goals are met.

STEP 9. If the goals are reached, re-evaluate and recycle. If the goals are not reached or if it becomes evident that higher doses of the drug are not more effective or that they produce hypotension and tachycardia, continue dobutamine administration at its most effective dosing range.

STEP 10. If MAP exceeds 100 mm Hg, give a vasodilator (e.g., nitroglycerin, nitroprusside, labetalol, hydralazine, or PGE_1) in gradually increasing doses provided improvement in CI, Do_2, or Vo_2 occurs.

STEP 11. Titrate vasodilators to decrease MAP and to increase CI, Do_2, and Vo_2. If no improvement in CI, Do_2, and Vo_2 occurs with vasodilator use or if hypotension ensues (MAP $<$ 70 mm Hg, SAP $<$ 110 mm Hg), discontinue vasodilator use. If improvement occurs in CI, Do_2, or Vo_2, titrate the vasodilator to maximum effect consistent with satisfactory arterial pressure.

STEP 12. If the goals are reached, re-evaluate and recycle at intervals.

STEP 13. If the goals are not reached and if MAP is below 80 mm Hg and SAP is below 110 mm Hg, give dopamine or another vasopressor.

STEP 14. Titrate the vasopressor in the lowest possible doses to maintain arterial pressures (MAP $>$ 80 mm Hg, SAP $>$ 110 mm Hg) and to optimize CI, Do_2, and Vo_2. If the goals and the pressures cannot be maintained, the patient is considered to be a protocol failure.

STEP 15. If the goals are reached, re-evaluate and recycle. Consider additional therapy to further increase CI, Do_2, and Vo_2, assuming greater than expected tissue hypoxia from poor tissue perfusion.

CLINICAL ALGORITHMS FOR RESUSCITATION IN ACUTE EMERGENCY CONDITIONS

The resuscitation and immediate management of high-risk, life-threatening emergencies require expeditious diagnostic work-up, physiologic monitoring, and fluid therapy of shock as well as definitive therapy of the specific injury or disease state. These activities must be rapidly planned and expeditiously coordinated as the patient moves from the emergency department to the operating room or to the intensive care unit.

Clinical algorithms in this section are for the following:

1. Initial fluid resuscitation of emergency hypotensive patients in the emergency department
2. Subsequent fluid management of the critically ill patient being monitored with a central venous pressure catheter
3. Management of blunt and penetrating wounds of the chest and abdomen

Abbreviations

ACLS = advanced cardiac life support
CPR = cardiopulmonary resuscitation
CT = computed tomography
CVP = central venous pressure
D_5RL = dextrose 5% in lactated Ringer's solution
MAP = mean arterial blood pressure (diastolic + [systolic − diastolic] ÷ 3)
RL = lactated Ringer's solution
SAP = systolic arterial blood pressure

Initial (First Hour) Fluid Resuscitation of a Hypotensive Emergency Patient

STEP 1. If the MAP is zero or nearly zero, determine whether cardiac arrest has occurred and begin CPR immedi-

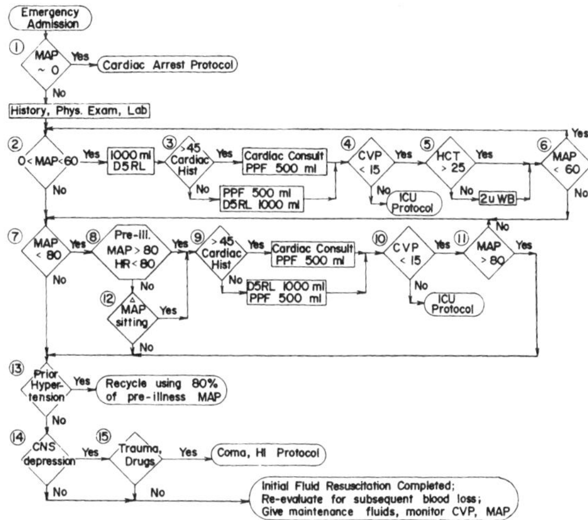

Figure 1–1. Clinical algorithm for the initial (first-hour) resuscitation of emergency admissions. This algorithm was designed for resuscitation of the acute emergency patient to restore circulatory integrity as rapidly as possible without producing fluid overload.

ately. If the MAP is below 20 mm Hg, alert personnel to a possible cardiac arrest.

STEP 2. If the MAP is below 60 mm Hg, immediately start administration of RL or D_5RL (dextrose 5% in RL), 1000 mL, and run as rapidly as possible, especially if the MAP is below 50 mm Hg.

STEP 3. If the patient is less than 45 years old and does not have a history of cardiac disease, place a CVP line and start another infusion of D_5RL, 1000 mL, plus 500 mL of plasma protein fraction or artificial colloid through a third intravenous line. If the patient is more than 45 years of age, go to step 9.

STEP 4. Monitor the CVP at frequent intervals during the rapid infusion of these three solutions so as not to exceed 15 cm H_2O. If the CVP exceeds 15 cm H_2O, go directly to the intensive care protocol.

STEP 5. If the hematocrit is below 25%, give 2 units of O-negative or type-specific blood. When crossmatched blood becomes available, transfusions of whole blood or packed red cells should be given to maintain the hematocrit over 33%.

STEP 6. Rapid restoration of the MAP to 60 mm Hg is the titration endpoint for fluids in this section. If the MAP is below 60 mm Hg, recycle from step 2 through step 6. If a MAP over 60 mm Hg has been achieved, proceed to step 7.

STEP 7. If the MAP is below 80 mm Hg, go to step 8; if not, proceed to step 13.

STEP 8. If the MAP is below 80 mm Hg, determine the patient's normal pre-illness control MAP by asking the patient or the patient's family or by consulting a previous hospital record. If the MAP is below 80 mm Hg and the heart rate is over 80 beats/min, measure orthostatic blood pressure (see step 12).

STEP 9. As in step 3, a cardiac patient requires less salt and water but more colloid. If the patient is more than 45 years old or if he or she has a history of cardiac disease, administer 500 mL of colloid; if the patient is less than 45 years old and he or she has no history of cardiac disease, give 1000 mL of D_5RL plus 500 mL of colloid.

STEP 10. Fluids may be given safely if the CVP is below 15 cm H_2O; if this is exceeded, go to the intensive care unit protocol and continue to give fluids as needed to restore circulatory integrity, provided wedge pressures of 18 mm Hg are not exceeded.

STEP 11. If the MAP is over 80 mm Hg without exceeding a CVP of 15 cm H_2O, the objective of this cycle has been achieved. If the MAP is below 80 mm Hg, recycle steps 7 through 11.

STEP 12. Orthostatic blood pressure is measured. If a 10-mm Hg change in MAP occurs on sitting or standing, this is presumptive evidence of a blood volume deficit of at least 1000 mL.

STEP 13. After the MAP has been restored to the normal value (>80 mm Hg), it is still necessary to be sure that the pre-illness blood pressure was normal. If a prior hypertension was observed, the patient should be cycled through steps 7 through 13 again, using 80% of the pre-illness value as the criterion for the adequacy of resuscitation.

STEP 14. Examine the patient for evidence of central nervous system depression, drug poisoning, or drug abuse.

STEP 15. Examine the patient for evidence of head injury or other trauma. If head trauma is present, the patient should be treated in accordance with a coma–head injury protocol.

Fluid Management of Patients with Central Venous Pressure Catheters or Suspected Hypovolemia

Complete Routine Work-Up

- Chest radiography
- Complete blood count and differential, routine electrolytes and blood chemistries (M300)
- Twelve-lead ECG and urinalysis
- Hematocrit and coagulation studies if significant blood loss or bleeding tendency
- Other indicated radiographic and laboratory studies
- If evidence of sepsis exists—blood, urine, or sputum culture; site drainage; and cerebrospinal fluid testing, if appropriate

STEP 1. Assess arterial blood gases. If abnormal, proceed with respiratory protocol.

STEP 2. If MAP is below 80 mm Hg, heart rate is over 100 beats/min, or urine output is below 30 mL/h, measure CVP

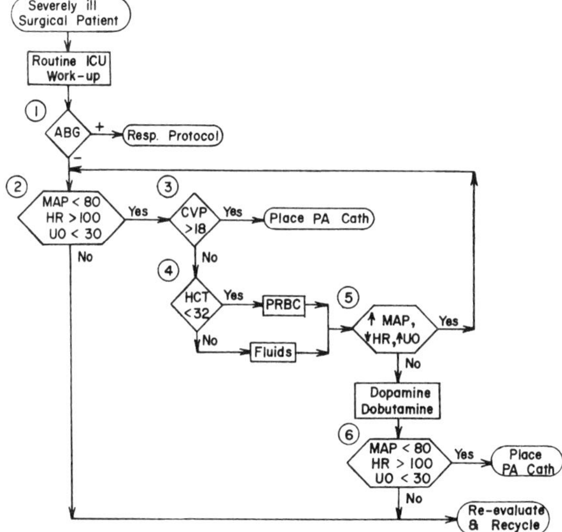

Figure 1–2. Algorithm for subsequent continuing fluid management in patients with CVP catheters.

and proceed to step 3, since inadequate hydration is a likely possibility. If MAP is over 80 mm Hg, heart rate is below 100 beats/min, and urine output is over 30 mL/h, re-evaluate at frequent intervals.

STEP 3. If CVP is over 18 mm Hg, place a pulmonary artery catheter; if CVP is below 18 mm Hg, measure hematocrit.

STEP 4. If hematocrit is below 32%, give 2 units of packed red blood cells or 1 unit of whole blood. If hematocrit is over 32%, give 1 L of RL or 500 mL of plasma protein fraction.

STEP 5. If the fluid load given improves MAP, heart rate, or urine output, it is evidence of hypovolemia or dehydration; proceed to step 2 to test adequacy of fluid load. If the criteria of step 2 (MAP > 80 mm Hg, heart rate < 100 beats/min, urine output > 30 mL/h) are met, re-evaluate at intervals; if not, recycle steps 3 to 5. This fluid cycle may be repeated as long as (1) there is continued improvement and (2) CVP does not exceed 18 mm Hg. It is also necessary, however, to search for continued fluid losses. If the fluid load as described does not improve MAP, heart rate, or urine output, dehydration and hypovolemia are unlikely. Start administration of an inotropic agent such as dobutamine or vasopressors in low doses and titrate gradually to achieve the optimal result.

STEP 6. If MAP is over 80 mm Hg, heart rate is below 100 beats/min, and urine output is above 30 mL/h, re-evaluate at frequent intervals. If these goals are not reached, place a pulmonary artery catheter.

Management of Blunt and Penetrating Wounds of the Chest and Abdomen

General Principles and Concepts

1. If the patient is hypotensive or in shock, immediate resuscitation and surgical exploration are mandatory.
2. If the MAP does not immediately respond to adequate volumes of fluids (5–10 L), urgent surgical exploration is mandatory to control the bleeding source. Fluid resuscitation is continued vigorously during the surgical attempts to control bleeding.
3. Gunshot wounds, except tangential or grazing wounds, should be explored.
4. Stab wounds without abdominal findings, except for localized tenderness at the wound site, can be considered for conservative (nonoperative) management to avoid negative explorations and to shorten the hospital stay.
5. Cardiac tamponade must be considered in stab and gunshot wounds of the chest as well as the upper abdomen, flank, and back; about 2% of penetrating chest wounds have tamponade. Elevated CVP is usually the first monitored sign of tamponade.
6. Patients with blunt abdominal trauma and peritoneal signs should be surgically explored urgently with or without diagnostic peritoneal lavage to repair lacerated solid or perforated gastrointestinal injuries.

7. CT scans can be done in hemodynamically stable patients with questionable abdominal signs and in patients with head injuries, coma, or ethanol intoxication.
8. Thoracoabdominal injuries require special considerations and should be explored with less rigorous indications, including hypotension, abdominal tenderness, guarding and rebound tenderness, or CT findings.
9. Repeated physical examinations provide important information in questionable cases.
10. Penetrating abdominal wounds are often overdiagnosed and unnecessarily explored, whereas blunt trauma is more frequently underdiagnosed and explored too late.

Common Problems

- Cardiac or respiratory arrest
- Respiratory distress
- Circulatory shock
- Laceration of the heart with or without cardiac tamponade
- Cardiac contusion
- Pneumothorax, tension pneumothorax, hemothorax
- Lacerations of the trachea, bronchus with air leak
- Sucking chest wound
- Fractures of the ribs with or without flail chest
- Pulmonary contusion
- Injury to great vessels
- Laceration or rupture of esophagus, stomach, small bowel, colon, or bladder
- Laceration of diaphragm
- Laceration or rupture of liver, spleen, kidney, or pancreas
- Vascular injuries
- Fractures of pelvis, spine, and long bones
- Retroperitoneal, mesenteric, or omental hematomas

General Work-Up

- Rapid physical assessment—parallel to resuscitation
- Blood type and crossmatch
- Hematocrit, complete blood count, routine electrolytes, coagulation studies
- Portable chest radiography
- Glucose, blood urea nitrogen, creatinine, and urinalysis
- Abdominal radiography, arterial blood gas measurement
- Additional blood chemistry testing (such as calcium and amylase) and other tests if indicated

STEP 1. If the patient has any physical signs (penetrating wounds, contusions, swelling, extremity weakness, or sensory loss) of blunt or penetrating neck injury or has any neck pain, maintain external cervical immobilization, obtain lateral spine radiographs to screen for major cervical injury, and continue resuscitation.

STEP 2. If respiratory arrest occurs, intubate patient and begin mechanical ventilation.

STEP 3. If respiratory distress or depressed level of consciousness is present as defined by one or more of the following criteria, proceed to steps 4 through 8: tachypnea (respiratory rate $\geq$ 30 breaths/min), bradypnea (respiratory rate $\leq$ 8 breaths/min), sternal retraction, use of accessory

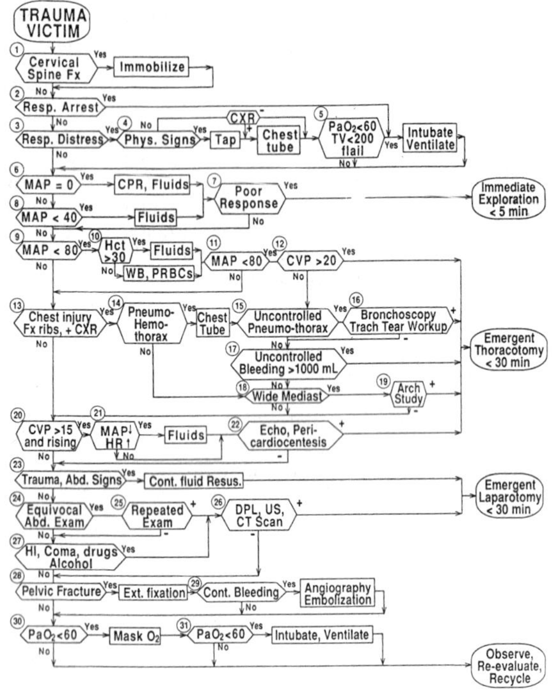

Figure 1–3. Algorithm for the clinical management of blunt and penetrating thoracic and abdominal injuries.

breathing muscles, flaring of nasal alae during respiration, cyanosis of the lips or skin, or Glasgow Coma Score of 9 or less.

STEP 4. If physical signs of pneumothorax are present, such as hyperresonance, distant or decreased breath sounds, or open chest wounds, perform an immediate needle thoracostomy in the midclavicular line of the second intercostal space of the affected side. Then, place a no. 36 or no. 40 chest tube in the affected hemithorax at intercostal space 4 or 5 in the midaxillary line and proceed to step 5. If no physical signs of tension pneumothorax are observed, obtain a portable chest radiograph. If this is negative, proceed to step 5. If the radiograph shows a hemothorax or pneumothorax, perform tube thoracostomy and go to step 5. If 1000 mL of blood is obtained immediately from the tube, however, clamp the tube and obtain a chest radiograph. If, after drainage of 1000 mL of blood, the radiograph shows an estimated 500 mL or more of blood still in the hemithorax (massive hemothorax), transport the patient to the operating room for further chest drainage and possible thoracotomy. (Letting chest drainage continue in the emergency department may precipitate a hypovolemic cardiac arrest). Colloids (5% albumin or hydroxyethyl starch) should be infused rapidly while the patient is prepared for the operating room.

STEP 5. Intubate the patient and start mechanical ventilation if one or more of the following conditions exist: PaO_2 is below 60 mm Hg on 40% O_2 delivered by facemask; $PaCO_2$ is over 45 mm Hg; spontaneous tidal volume is below 200 mL; expiratory rate is more than 30 breaths/min or below 8 breaths/min; flail segment exists; or Glasgow Coma Score is less than 9. Adjust ventilator settings to maintain arterial oxygen saturation at 93% or over or PaO_2 at 60 mm Hg or over and $PaCO_2$ at 45 mm Hg or less. Proceed to step 6.

STEP 6. If the patient has a detectable pulse and blood pressure, proceed to step 8. If the patient has no detectable blood pressure (MAP of zero), rapidly administer 3 to 5 L of fluids and 2 to 4 units of O-negative blood or packed cells while simultaneously initiating the ACLS protocol. With large-bore IV lines, 1 L of fluid can be given in 2 to 5 minutes. Inserting IV tubing through cutdowns into the greater saphenous, antecubital, or basilic vein establishes effective resuscitation lines. Proceed to step 7.

STEP 7. If, with fluid resuscitation and ACLS, a detectable pulse returns and the MAP rises to at least 40 mm Hg, proceed to step 9. If a response is obtained but the MAP remains below 40 mm Hg, transport the patient to the operating room for immediate exploration. *If no detectable pulse or blood pressure is obtained with resuscitation, proceed as follows:*

For penetrating truncal wounds: If the patient had signs of life at some time in the field or the emergency department, perform a left anterior thoracotomy. This is done to relieve pericardial tamponade, to perform direct cardiac massage, to cross-clamp the descending thoracic aorta and increase blood flow to the coronary arteries and brain, and to stop other intrathoracic bleeding. The incision may be easily extended to a transsternal thoracotomy (if necessary) to control hemorrhage from the right hemithorax. If the penetrating injury is on the right thorax, a right anterior thoracotomy can be done first to control bleeding from the wound.

For blunt injuries: Continue maximal volume infusion; perform bilateral needle thoracostomy immediately followed by bilateral tube thoracostomy (midaxillary line, intercostal space 4) to relieve tension pneumothorax; and perform pericardiocentesis to diagnose cardiac tamponade. If cardiac tamponade is present, perform left anterior thoracotomy, if either tube thoracostomy drains 1000 mL of blood and flow continues, clamp the tube, continue transfusions, and transport the patient to the operating room for thoracotomy. Allowing the tube output to continue may increase intrathoracic hemorrhage and lead to rapid cardiac arrest from hypovolemia.

STEP 8. If the MAP is over 40 mm Hg, proceed to step 9. If the MAP is below 40 mm Hg or the SAP is below 60 mm Hg, insert two large-bore IV (≥16-gauge) catheters (either percutaneously or by cutdown), and rapidly infuse 3 to 5 L of fluid. If inferior vena caval injury is suspected, use at least one upper extremity vein for volume infusion. If the MAP remains at or below 40 mm Hg for more than 5 minutes, transport the patient to the operating room for exploration. If the MAP rises to above 40 mm Hg, continue expectant volume loading and proceed to step 9.

STEP 9. If the MAP is over 80 mm Hg, proceed to step 13. If the MAP is below 80 mm Hg or SAP is under 100 mm Hg, administer IV fluids and proceed to step 10.

STEP 10. Measure hemoglobin, hematocrit, or both. If the hematocrit exceeds 30%, continue infusing IV fluids. If it is below 30%, administer two units of packed red blood cells or two units of whole blood. Proceed to step 11.

STEP 11. If, after resuscitation, the MAP rises to over 80 mm Hg, proceed to step 13. If the MAP remains below 80 mm Hg, insert a CVP catheter and go to step 12.

STEP 12. If the patient's CVP is below 20 mm Hg, proceed to step 13. If the CVP is 20 mm Hg or higher, continue resuscitation and repeat both MAP and CVP measurements at 5-minute intervals. If, for three consecutive measurements, the CVP remains above 20 mm Hg with the MAP remaining below 80 mm Hg, presume cardiac tamponade is present and transport the patient to the operating room for exploratory thoracotomy. If the CVP is 20 mm Hg or higher and the MAP has risen to above 80 mm Hg, reduce the rate of fluid infusion by 50% and recheck both the CVP and MAP at 5-minute intervals. If the CVP subsequently rises to over 24 mm Hg, presume cardiac tamponade is present and transport the patient to the operating room for exploratory thoracotomy. Otherwise, proceed to step 13.

STEP 13. Obtain a portable chest radiograph. If a hemothorax or pneumothorax is present, proceed to step 14. If a "sucking" chest wound is present, cover the injury with petroleum-impregnated gauze and place a chest tube on the affected side. If the radiograph is normal and no other clinical signs of thoracic injury are present, proceed to step 23.

STEP 14. If a hemothorax or pneumothorax is present, place a chest tube (>36 French) in midaxillary line at intercostal space 4 or 5. Replace lost blood using an autotransfusion device if the tube output is greater than 200 mL. Proceed to step 15. If the patient has no hemothorax or pneumothorax, proceed to step 18.

STEP 15. If a pneumothorax persists despite the proper performance of tube thoracostomy or if an air leak persists, place a second chest tube and go to step 16.

STEP 16. If the pneumothorax or air leak persists after a second tube thoracostomy has been performed on the affected side, proceed with bronchoscopy to evaluate for major tracheobronchial injury. If injury is diagnosed, proceed with thoracotomy and repair. If the second tube thoracostomy controls the air leak, or if the bronchoscopy reveals no tracheobronchial injury, proceed to step 17.

STEP 17. If, after the initial hemothorax is drained, the chest tube accumulates more than 100 mL of blood per hour for 3 hours or more, proceed with exploratory thoracotomy. If bleeding is controlled, proceed to step 18.

STEP 18. If the mediastinum appears to be of normal width on the chest radiograph and no other signs of a thoracic great vessel injury exist (e.g., pleural cap, indistinct aortic arch, obliteration of aortopulmonary window, displacement of nasogastric tube or mainstem bronchus), proceed to step 20. If the mediastinum appears widened on the chest radiograph or if one or more of the other signs of great vessel injury are present, proceed to step 19.

STEP 19. Obtain an aortic and great vessel angiogram. If it demonstrates great vessel injury, proceed with emergent thoracotomy and repair. For blunt injuries and penetrating thoracoabdominal wounds, a peritoneal tap and lavage should be performed in the operating room before thoracotomy to rule out intra-abdominal hemorrhage. For patients needing thoracotomy who are also suspected of having intracranial lesions that require operative intervention, a rapid CT head scan can be obtained before thoracotomy, or diagnostic bur holes can be made simultaneously with thoracotomy. If the great vessel angiogram has a negative result, go to step 20.

STEP 20. If the patient has clinical signs of cardiac tamponade, such as distended neck veins or distant heart sounds, or a penetrating injury in proximity to the precordial region, insert a CVP catheter in a subclavian or internal jugular vein. Perform three simultaneous CVP and MAP measurements over a 15-minute period. If the CVP is persistently below 15 mm Hg, go to step 23. If the CVP is above 20 mm Hg for three consecutive readings or is above 15 mm Hg and rises for three successive measurements, proceed to step 21.

STEP 21. If, after the three readings in step 20 have been performed, the MAP is below 80 mm Hg or the heart rate is over 110 beats/min, administer 500 mL of 5% albumin or hetastarch (Hespan) over 10 minutes. After the infusion is initiated, proceed to step 22. If the MAP remains above 80 mm Hg and the heart rate is below 110 beats/min, proceed to step 22 without giving an additional fluid bolus.

STEP 22. Obtain an echocardiogram or perform pericardiocentesis or subxyphoid window creation. If blood is found in the pericardial sac, assume cardiac tamponade is present and proceed with exploratory thoracotomy or median sternotomy. Also, if the patient's MAP falls more than 15 mm Hg in 5 minutes at any time, assume cardiac tamponade is present and proceed with exploratory thoracotomy or median sternotomy. If no blood is found in the pericardial sac, based on the results of echocardiography, pericardiocentesis, or subxyphoid window creation, proceed to step 23.

STEP 23. If the patient has an abdominal or thoracoabdominal gunshot wound (except one with a tangential grazing trajectory that could not possibly penetrate the abdominal cavity) or if he or she has a stab wound with hypotension (MAP < 80 mm Hg), diffuse tenderness, rebound tenderness, decreased bowel sounds, or other abdominal findings, exploratory laparotomy should be performed within 30 minutes. Patients with blunt injury and diffuse peritoneal irritation should undergo exploration. If the patient does not have diffuse peritoneal signs, proceed to step 24.

STEP 24. If the patient has a blunt injury or stab wound and has equivocal abdominal examination findings, proceed to step 25.

STEP 25. Perform at least three sequential abdominal examinations during a 15-minute period. If the patient's abdomen becomes tender, proceed to step 27. If equivocal results persist, proceed to step 26.

STEP 26. Proceed as follows:

For blunt injury: Perform peritoneal tap and lavage or triple-contrast abdominal and pelvic CT; if either test has positive results, perform exploratory laparotomy within 30 minutes. If results are negative, proceed to step 27.

For a stab wound over the rectus sheath: Perform local wound exploration. If the wound extends through the anterior rectus sheath, perform either peritoneal tap and lavage or triple-contrast abdominal and pelvic CT. If either test yields positive results, perform exploratory laparotomy within 30 minutes. If the anterior rectus sheath has not been penetrated or if diagnostic test results are negative, proceed to step 27.

For a stab wound between the lateral rectus sheath and the midaxillary line: Either peritoneal tap and lavage or triple-contrast abdominal and pelvic CT should be performed. If either test yields a positive result, perform exploratory laparotomy within 30 minutes. If the patient has a stab wound posterior to the midaxillary line, perform triple-contrast abdominal and pelvic CT. If either test has a positive result, perform exploratory laparotomy within 30 minutes. If diagnostic test results are negative, proceed to step 27.

STEP 27. If the patient has evidence of a head injury, drug ingestion, or ethanol intoxication, a normal abdominal examination may be inaccurate. Therefore, the patient should undergo either peritoneal tap and lavage or triple-contrast abdominal and pelvic CT. If either has a positive result, proceed with exploratory laparotomy within 30 minutes; if results are negative, proceed to step 28.

STEP 28. If no pelvic fracture is present, proceed to step 30. If the patient has a pelvic fracture, evaluate its stability. If the fracture is stable, proceed to step 29. If the fracture is unstable, immediately either place military antishock trousers or obtain an emergency consult with an orthopedic surgeon for external fixation.

STEP 29. Perform serial hemoglobin and hematocrit measurements every 30 minutes. If the patient's values drop and he or she needs more than 6 units of packed red cells within 6 hours of admission to maintain hemoglobin over 10 g/dL or hematocrit over 30%, perform pelvic vessel angiography for possible embolization. Proceed to step 30. If hemoglobin and hematocrit remain stable, proceed to step 30.

STEP 30. Obtain measurements of arterial blood gases. If the patient's Pao_2 is below 60 mm Hg on room air, administer 40% O_2 by facemask and proceed to step 31. If, on room air, the patient's PaO_2 is greater than 60 mm Hg, observe him or her for subsequent signs of respiratory distress, hypotension, and new symptoms of thoracic or abdominal injury.

STEP 31. After 40% O_2 has been administered for 10 minutes, obtain a repeat set of arterial blood gas measurements. If the PaO_2 is still below 60 mm Hg, intubate, ventilate, and re-evaluate for thoracic or abdominal injury. If the PaO_2 is above 60 mm Hg, observe the patient and re-evaluate periodically.

CHAPTER 2

Cell Injury and Cell Death

Michael D. Schwartz, M.D. • Edward Abraham, M.D.

REGULATION OF GENE EXPRESSION

Genes and Gene Expression

Genes are loci of developmental information associated with heritable characteristics. One gene is responsible for one enzyme. Ribonucleic acid (RNA) is the intermediate between genetic DNA and protein. RNA is transcribed from a DNA template by a DNA-dependent RNA polymerase. RNA may then be modified into a messenger form (mRNA) capable of being translated into a polypeptide, a process called post-transcriptional modification. Ribosomes translate the mRNA into a polypeptide. Proteins are then formed by various combinations of polypeptide chains into more complex structures.

In the nucleus, DNA consists of two strands of polymerized deoxyribonucleic acid that are directed in antiparallel orientation. mRNA is likewise directional, but consists of a single strand homologous to one of the DNA strands and complementary to the other, the latter DNA having served as the template from which the RNA was synthesized. This DNA strand homologous to the RNA is known as the coding strand or coding sequence. The most critical region regulating transcription, known as the promoter region, lies immediately adjacent to the transcription start site, the site at which expression of genes begins.

Gene Expression in the Intensive Care Unit

The broad scope of critical care medicine includes diseases that are related to gene expression. Congenital errors of gene expression include abnormal or aberrant hemoglobin synthesis, as seen in sickle cell anemia, in β-thalassemia, or in a congenital deficiency of factor VIII production, causing hemophilia. Recessive disorders (both genes absent or abnormal) may be corrected by replacement of a defective gene with a normal gene, by replacement of a cell carrying the normal gene and its product (e.g., exchange transfusion for sickle cell anemia), or by administration of the correct gene product itself (e.g., factor VIII infusion for hemophilia). Restoration of a gene product to 1% to 10% of normal levels may suffice to correct the biochemical defect. Acquired errors of gene expression may occur after viral infection, when new viral genes are acquired, and can induce a dysregulation of cell behavior, replication, or survival that results in malignant transformation. Finally, and most commonly for the intensivist, is abnormal expression of a normal gene, such as the up-regulation of proinflammatory cytokine genes that is felt to occur before or during multiple organ dysfunction syndrome.

Gene Expression in Cell Injury

No single "shock" or "injury" gene has been identified; hundreds of them exist. Gene expression can be used to define in operational terms:

Injury = A change in the external environment of a cell that is sufficient to trigger changes in gene expression.
Signal = An environmental change leading to change in gene expression. Some signals can penetrate the cytoplasmic membrane (e.g., steroid hormones), whereas other signals cannot, and therefore they must be transduced through a receptor molecule extracellularly displayed at the membrane.

MECHANISMS REGULATING GENE EXPRESSION

Initiation and Regulation of Transcription

Mechanisms that regulate the initiation of transcription control the expression of many genes. RNA polymerase II is the most important enzyme for gene transcription. In the nucleus, DNA is normally complexed with histone proteins and compacted into globular structures called nucleosomes. Each nucleosome includes about 180 base pairs of DNA and must be displaced in order for RNA polymerase II to effect gene transcription. Eukaryotic cells maintain a few persistently nucleosome-free regions through tight, sequence-specific binding of nonhistone proteins to DNA. This arrangement characterizes heat shock gene expression. More commonly, however, nonspecific activating proteins displace histones from DNA zones that include the promoter for a certain gene. These induced displacement zones are then occupied by sequence-specific DNA-binding proteins called nuclear factors.

The promoter has at least two functional regions where the nucleosomes have to be displaced. The core region serves as a scaffolding on which RNA polymerase II and other initiation factors can form the transcription complex. The core promoter region contains a crucial thymine- and adenine-rich region of DNA known as the TATA box. The second region includes DNA target sequences for the specific nuclear factors that regulate the rate at which RNA polymerase II initiates additional rounds of transcription at the core promoter region. These target sequences, or regulatory elements, are typically 6 to 20 base pairs in length and often have dyadic symmetry. RNA polymerase II adds about 50 nucleotides per second to nascent templates and is limited by the requirement to free DNA from nucleosomes. The activation of nuclear factors to initiate binding to regulatory elements must be very fast and tightly controlled and often is dependent on protein phosphorylation.

Three important nuclear factors are NF-κB, AP-1, and CREB. NF-κB is a heterodimeric protein that regulates gene expression in response to phorbol esters, antigens, cytokines, UV radiation, reactive oxygen species, and viral infection.

The heterodimer consists of two subunits, p50 and p65, which are themselves normally bound in the cytoplasm by a third, inhibitory protein, IκB. When phosphorylated, IκB dissociates from the heterodimer, and p50/p65 translocates to the nucleus, binds to its response element, and activates gene transcription. The nuclear factor AP-1 is a collection of homodimeric and heterodimeric complexes of the products of two genes called *fos* and *jun*. AP-1 binding is critical to the expression of many genes, including those of the acute phase response. CREB is a nuclear factor that activates genes in response to increasing cAMP levels by binding to the cAMP response element (CRE).

Whereas all genes have promoters, the transcription of some genes is further regulated by enhancers and locus control regions. Enhancers differ from promoters by virtue of their nonadjacency to the transcription start site and the sometimes great distance over which they can influence a particular gene. Locus control regions are similar to enhancers, but they typically regulate the expression of multiple gene loci during normal growth and development.

Transcript Processing: Appearance of Messenger RNA

Soon after transcription begins, three modifications to the RNA transcript occur to confer function as mRNA. A methylated cap structure is added to the 5′ end, a polyadenylate (polyA) tail is added to the 3′ end, and splicing occurs in organelles called splicosomes. Only after these three modifications can the transcript be identified as mRNA and transported to the cytoplasm. These modifications also affect the stability of the newly synthesized mRNA molecule; mRNA degradation is another regulatory step in the process of gene expression.

Translation

Translation of mRNA into protein is a complex process that consists of three stages: initiation, elongation, and termination. Initiation is the rate-limiting step. Elongation is a cyclic process in which transfer RNA molecules add additional amino acid residues to the c-terminal end of the nascent polypeptide chain. Termination is the release of the completed polypeptide from the ribosome, the organelle in which translation occurs.

MACROPHAGE FUNCTION

Macrophages play a central role in host defense against pathogenic microbes; in the development of immunity; in the pathogenesis of septic shock, acute and chronic infection; and in the processes of wound healing, tissue remodeling, and fibrosis.

Morphology and Development

Macrophages are mononuclear phagocytes, cells with a single, nonsegmented nucleus and the ability to ingest particles into cytoplasmic membrane-lined vacuoles. Most macrophages originate from bone marrow precursors that develop into blood monocytes, which, after a few days in the circulation, enter tissues and mature into macrophages. Monocytes and macrophage numbers are controlled by hematopoietic hormones, especially interleukin-3 (IL-3), granulocyte-macrophage colony–stimulating factor (GM-CSF), and macrophage CSF (M-CSF). The largest numbers of macrophages are found in the liver, small bowel, and colon when the weight of the organs is taken into account.

Macrophage Cytotoxicity

Unlike other phagocytes (e.g., neutrophils, eosinophils, monocytes), macrophages are resident in noninflamed tissues and thus are likely to interact with microbes during the earliest stages (first few hours) of infection. Macrophage response to microbial invasion consists of chemotaxis (movement toward the microbe), phagocytosis (recognition and ingestion), killing, and finally recruitment of additional effector cells, which produce amplification of the inflammatory response.

Chemotaxis

Movement of macrophages to the site of invasion is induced by a gradient of concentration of chemotactic substances that results in a higher occupancy of receptors on the leading edge of the macrophage as compared with the trailing edge. The chemotactic substances may include prokaryote-derived formylated peptides, complement fragment C5a, leukotriene B_4 (LTB_4), and others.

Phagocytosis and Antigen-Presenting Function

Receptor-mediated interactions on the surface of the macrophage trigger a cytoskeletal rearrangement that results in the invagination of the organism into the cell. Macrophage receptors involved in recognition include Fc receptors that recognize specific antibody covering the microbe, complement receptors C3b or C3bi, lectins, and receptors for endotoxin. After phagocytosis and proteolytic digestion by macrophages, microbial peptide fragments are associated with major histocompatibility complex class II molecules (MHC II) and are displayed on the macrophage membrane. This complex then binds to T cell receptors and activates T cells.

Killing

The macrophage creates a highly biotoxic environment within the interior of its phagocytic vacuoles through generation of reactive oxygen species, microbicidal and cytotoxic proteins, hydrolytic enzymes, nutrient deprivation, and low pH. The phagosomal membrane contains NADPH-oxidase, which reduces molecular oxygen to superoxide, which in turn is dismutated to microbicidal hydrogen peroxide.

Recruitment of Additional Effector Cells and Macrophage Activation

Macrophages release products that are chemotactic for neutrophils (LTB_4, IL-8) and lymphocytes (IL-8) to the site of infection or inflammation. Activation refers to a temporary and generalized enhancement of macrophage inflammatory response and includes morphologic and biochemical changes such as increased membrane ruffling and content of hydrolytic enzymes, reactive oxygen species, and MHC II molecules. Interferon-γ and TNF-α can activate macrophages, and transforming growth factor-β (TGF-β) can deactivate macrophages.

Scavenging and Secretory Function

Macrophages remove or degrade dust in the lungs, necrotic cells in wounds, intravascular particulates, and devolving structures during embryogenesis. Macrophages in atherosclerotic plaques ingest lipids and cholesterol, forming foam cells. Foreign body giant cells seen in areas of chronic antigenic or inflammatory stimulation are composed of macrophages. Macrophages are also potent secretory cells that perform a critical signaling function in the local and systemic inflammatory response (Table 2–1).

OXYGEN-DERIVED FREE RADICALS

A free radical is any molecule containing a single, unpaired electron; it may be viewed as a molecular fragment formed by homolytic cleavage of a bond. Oxygen has a great affinity for four more electrons, and the process of taking away electrons is called oxidation because oxygen does this so readily. The substance receiving electrons is said to be reduced. The family of reactive oxygen species (ROS) resulting from incomplete reduction of oxygen includes superoxide radical, hydrogen peroxide (H_2O_2), and hydroxyl radical, and occasionally the term is used to include singlet oxygen and even hypochlorous acid (HOCl) produced from H_2O_2 by neutrophil myeloperoxidase.

Iron Exacerbates Free Radical Injury

Iron is the most common redox-active transition element in biologic systems, and it may exacerbate any oxidative stress. Iron catalyzes a combination of reactions known as the Ha-

Table 2–1. SUBSTANCES SECRETED BY MACROPHAGES

Activity	Substances (Examples)
Chemotactic for neutrophils	LTB_4, IL-8
Growth factors (wound healing)	TGF-β, platelet-derived growth factor
Angiogenic factors	Basic fibroblast growth factor, TGF-α
Growth factors (hematopoietic)	GM-CSF, G-CSF
Acute-phase response, fever, signs of sepsis	TNF-α, IL-1, IL-6
Microbicidal substances	Lysozyme, hydrogen peroxide
Cytotoxic substances	TNF-α, hydrogen peroxide, nitric oxide
Macrophage regulatory factors	TNF-α, TGF-β
Lymphocyte regulatory factors	IL-1, IL-6
Lytic enzymes	Plasminogen activator, collagenase, elastase
Enzyme inhibitors	α_2-Macroglobulin, α_1-antitrypsin

ber-Weiss reaction or as superoxide-driven Fenton chemistry:

$$O_2^{\bullet -} + Fe^{3+} \rightarrow O_2 + Fe^{2+}$$

$$\frac{Fe^{2+} + H_2O_2 \rightarrow Fe^{3+} + HO^{\bullet} + OH^-}{O_2^{\bullet -} + H_2O_2 \rightarrow O_2 + HO^{\bullet} + OH^-}$$

Iron is stored in the ferric state (Fe^{3+}) by ferritin and transferrin, but superoxide radical is capable of reducing ferritin-bound iron to the ferrous state (Fe^{2+}), whereupon it is released and is free to catalyze the Haber-Weiss chemistry. Ferrous iron and ROS, especially hydroxyl radical, can attack structural macromolecules, cause DNA strand breaks, and initiate lipid peroxidation.

Superoxide and Bactericidal Action by Phagocytes

A multicomponent, reduced form of nicotinamide-adenine dinucleotide phosphate oxidase (NADPH-oxidase) is located in the plasma membrane of the neutrophil and macrophage. This enzyme may be the only enzyme in the body that produces superoxide by design rather than by accident. This enzyme enables neutrophils to produce superoxide in response to bacterial challenge and two additional potent antimicrobial metabolites of superoxide, H_2O_2 and HOCl. The neutrophil is thus equipped to fight against a broad spectrum of pathogens. Release of these substances generates much of the tissue injury that occurs with infection and the subsequent inflammatory response, whether local (the signs of redness, swelling, pain, and loss of function) or systemic (as seen in the adult respiratory distress syndrome [ARDS]).

Ischemia-Reperfusion Injury and Free Radical Production

In buffer-perfused isolated organ preparations in which no neutrophils are present, ischemia produces massive catabolism of the adenine nucleotide pool owing to the low-energy status of the tissue. Adenosine is broken down to inosine and then to hypoxanthine, which accumulates in abundance. Although about 10% of any tissue's xanthine dehydrogenase (XD) exists as an oxygen-utilizing, superoxide-generating xanthine oxidase (XO), ischemia-induced proteolytic conversion appears to result in even more of the oxygen radical–producing form of the enzyme. Hence, a period of ischemia is followed by production of XO (preexisting or newly converted) and an abundance of its purine substrate, hypoxanthine. At reperfusion, the remaining substrate, molecular oxygen, reenters the tissue and a burst of superoxide production ensues. Reperfused organs are dramatically protected by inhibition of XO or by superoxide dismutase (SOD), which dismutates superoxide into hydrogen peroxide and oxygen. There are also XO-independent mechanisms of superoxide production, most likely resulting from ischemic injury to mitochondria. There are also significant interspecies and intertissue differences in the content of XD/XO.

It is important to note that in vivo ischemia-reperfusion injury invariably involves subsequent neutrophil-mediated inflammation, because a small, localized amount of superoxide formation may initiate neutrophil chemotaxis and activation, amplifying the inflammatory response.

PROSTAGLANDINS, THROMBOXANES, LEUKOTRIENES, AND OTHER PRODUCTS OF ARACHIDONIC ACID

Arachidonic acid (AA), dihomo-γ-linolenic acid, and eicosapentaenoic acid are precursors of prostaglandins (PG), thromboxane (TX), and leukotrienes (LT). The name *eicosanoids* is used generically to name the products of these fatty acids (Table 2–2).

Sites of Synthesis and Pharmacologic Activity of the Eicosanoids

The pathway for the metabolism of AA is shown in Figure 2–1. PGA, PGB, and PGC are nonenzymatic dehydration products of PGE_2 and are considered artifacts of the extraction procedures.

Arachidonic Acid Release

Release of AA from membrane phospholipids is the rate-limiting step in the formation of eicosanoids in nonpathologic states. Activation of phospholipase A_2 (PLA_2) results in release of AA from the Sn2 position of phosphatidylcholine and phosphatidylethanolamine. Diacylglycerol can also release AA in a phospholipase C–dependent pathway.

Prostaglandin Synthase (Fatty Acid Cyclooxygenase)

PGH synthase catalyzes the committed step in the conversion of AA to the PG endoperoxides PGG_2 and PGH_2. PGH_2 is the direct precursor of primary PGs and TXA_2. PGH synthase is an integral membrane protein concentrated in the endoplasmic reticulum, nuclear envelope, and plasma membrane. Although it is found in most of the organs of all mammalian species, it is not found in all cell types. PGH synthase converts AA to PGG_2 and then peroxidizes PGG_2 to PGH_2. PGH_2 forms a substrate for the enzymes responsible for the synthesis of prostaglandins D_2, E_2, $F_{2\alpha}$, I_2, and TXA_2. Arachidonic acid is the most common substrate for PGH synthase in vivo. Aspirin and the nonsteroidal anti-inflammatory drugs (NSAIDs) inhibit PGH synthase.

Induction of Prostaglandin Synthase

PGH synthase may reside in two distinct pools: a constitutive pool (PGH synthase–1) and an inducible pool (PGH synthase–2). Endotoxin induces PGH synthase–2, and this enzyme is inhibitable by corticosteroids.

Table 2–2. EICOSANOIDS

	Site of Synthesis	Function	Putative Role in Septic Shock	Relevant Metabolites
PGD_2	Mast cells Platelets	Bronchoconstriction Vasoconstrication of PA Vasodilation (lower doses) Platelet antiaggregatory	?	
PGE_2	Kidney Platelets Vasculature	Vasodilatory Natriuretic Diuretic Uterine contraction Gastric acid secretagogue	Increased	
$PGF_{2\alpha}$	Various	Bronchoconstriction Venoconstriction Uterine contraction	Increased	

PGI_2 (Prostacyclin)	Endothelium Macrophages Lung Kidney	Vasodilation Platelet antiaggregatory		6-Keto-$PGF_{1\alpha}$
TXA_2	Platelets Macrophages Monocytes Lung	Potent vasoconstriction Potent bronchoconstriction Platelet aggregation	Markedly increased	TXB_2
LTB_4	Leukocyte Macrophage Synovial cells	Chemotaxin for leukocytes	Increased	
LTC_4	Lung Leukocytes Macrophages	Vasoconstriction Bronchoconstriction Increased permeability Increased mucus secretion	Increased in sepsis Increased in ARDS	LTD_4 LTE_4

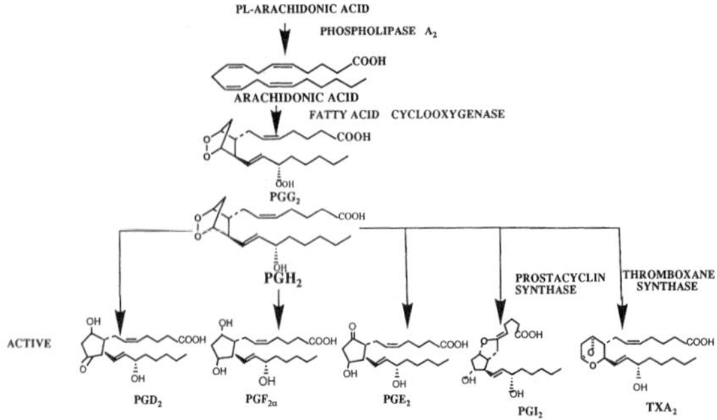

Figure 2–1. Metabolism of arachidonic acid. (From Wagner TR, Halushka PV, Cook JA: Cyclooxygenase products in septic and endotoxic shock. *In*: Handbook of Mediators in Septic Shock. Neugebauer EA, Holaday JW [Eds]. Boca Raton, CRC Press, 1993, pp 395–418. Used with permission.)

Increased Synthesis of Eicosanoids in Endotoxemia and Sepsis

Increased synthesis of eicosanoids in response to endotoxemia and sepsis occurs in several animal species and in humans. Increases in plasma levels of TXB_2 and 6-keto-$PGF_{1\alpha}$ can be demonstrated in a number of animal species with experimental endotoxemia and sepsis, and the relative amounts of TXB_2 and 6-keto-$PGF_{1\alpha}$ are influenced by both the frequency and route of endotoxin administration. 5-Lipoxygenase products are also increased in endotoxemia in animals and patients with sepsis and ARDS (5-HPETE, 5-HETE, and LTA_4). Bronchoalveolar lavage fluid of patients with ARDS demonstrates increases in sulfidopeptide leukotrienes and LTB_4.

Effect of Eicosanoid Synthesis Inhibitors and Receptor Antagonists

Numerous NSAIDs have been evaluated as potential therapies in endotoxemia and sepsis in animal models. When used as pretreatment they have generally been found to improve survival or survival time and to reduce cardiopulmonary dysfunction and indices of tissue injury. Ibuprofen, in addition to inhibiting fatty acid cyclooxygenase, also alters neutrophil function, inhibiting chemotaxis and adherence. Similarly, pretreatment with TXA_2 synthase inhibitors or TXA_2 receptor antagonists has improved survival time in endotoxemic animals. Most studies, however, have not shown such improvement(s) if the drug was given after endotoxin administration.

Therapeutic Approaches in Patients

The NSAIDs may have beneficial effects in the treatment of patients with trauma or sepsis. In one randomized, prospective study of surgical patients, patients receiving indomethacin exhibited improved markers of cell-mediated immunity (delayed-type hypersensitivity responses, mitogen-induced lymphocyte transformation) and a lower rate of opportunistic infections. Another study in severe sepsis showed that ibuprofen therapy decreased levels of metabolites of TXB_2 and 6-keto-$PGF_{1\alpha}$, along with febrile response, heart rate, and peak airway pressure; shortened the time to reversal of shock; and did not impair renal function.

CELLULAR SIGNALING AND CELL DEATH

Apoptosis is a process of regulated cell deletion that mediates many important physiologic and pathologic phenomena. It is the single most important cell death pathway of clinical relevance.

Occurrence of Apoptosis

A number of critical physiologic processes are mediated by apoptosis. Normal physiologic cell turnover, cell loss due to aging, and hormone-induced tissue atrophy all occur through apoptosis. Apoptosis also occurs in the setting of pathologic cell death induced by toxic chemicals, irradiation, and hypo- and hyperthermia, in which physical damage triggers a secondary apoptotic response. Apoptosis also probably mediates T cell depletion in AIDS, neural degeneration in Huntington's, Parkinson's, and Alzheimer's diseases, islet cell depletion in diabetes, and tissue injury due to inflammation.

Morphologic, Biochemical, and Molecular Mechanisms in Apoptosis

During apoptosis, a series of morphologic changes occurs within apoptotic cells that can be readily distinguished from those observed in cells undergoing necrotic cell death. Apoptosis is characterized by cell shrinkage: plasma and nuclear membrane blebbing and a consequent loss of volume. Relocalization and compaction of organelles and condensation of chromatin follow. Numerous membrane-enclosed fragments (apoptotic bodies) form. Apoptotic cells and bodies are then recognized and phagocytized by adjacent cells and tissue macrophages before a loss of membrane integrity. Thus, cell deletion occurs without consequent inflammation. Necrosis, in contrast, is characterized by obvious cell swelling, plasma membrane disruption, organelle dilation, and inflammation.

Apoptosis is a suicidal cellular response that involves gene expression, and it commonly can be blocked by inhibitors of protein (cycloheximide, puromycin) or mRNA (actinomycin D) synthesis. Several oncogenes have important roles in regulating apoptosis. Apoptotic machinery is constitutively present in most cell types.

The most characteristic biochemical feature of apoptosis is activation of an endogenous nuclear endonuclease, causing cleavage of host chromatin at internucleosomal "linker" regions, producing fragments that appear as a "ladder" after agarose gel electrophoresis. Necrotic cells do not demonstrate the formation of this DNA ladder; when DNA fragmentation occurs in necrosis, it constitutes a postmortem event because of random DNA cleavage and forms a "smear" cleavage pattern. The endonuclease responsible for apoptosis is constitutively present, is dependent on Ca^{2+} and Mg^{2+}, and likely causes chromatin condensation in apoptotic cells.

Cell Signaling in Programmed Cell Death

Endonuclease is strongly Ca^{2+} dependent. Series E prostaglandins and pharmacologic agents that elevate cAMP induce endogenous endonuclease activation in lymphocytes. Glucocorticoids and cAMP can also act synergistically to promote apoptosis. Other important cell signaling mechanisms include inositol triphosphate (which mobilizes Ca^{2+}) and diacylglycerol (DAG), which activates protein kinase C (PKC). It is important to note that TNF stimulates apoptosis in cells that bear the 55-kD TNF receptor.

CYTOKINES

Cytokines are intercellular messenger polypeptides that modulate many biologic responses and are involved, directly or indirectly, in the pathogenesis of many diseases. They are small, with molecular mass between 8 and 30 kD, and are biologically active at low concentrations (picomolar or less). Unlike classic endocrine hormones, they are produced by many cell types rather than by discrete organs, are usually produced de novo in response to stimuli, are often induced in response to exogenous (not endogenous) stimuli, and frequently have autocrine and paracrine effects. To date, more than 30 cytokines have been described (Table 2–3).

Cytokines and Sepsis (Systemic Inflammatory Response Syndrome)

Sepsis is currently listed as the 13th leading cause of death in the United States, and its incidence is increasing. It is the leading cause of death in noncoronary intensive care units. Mortality from the syndrome has not changed significantly during the past 30 years. Several definitions are important:

Bacteremia = The presence of bacteria in the blood, confirmed by culture

Septicemia = Bacteremia with significant clinical manifestations

Sepsis = Evidence of infection with a systemic response

Sepsis syndrome = Clinical evidence of infection, with a systemic response sufficient to produce adverse organ function such as respiratory insufficiency, renal dysfunction, acidosis, altered mental status, or other organ dysfunction

Table 2–3. SELECTED CONDITIONS ASSOCIATED WITH INCREASED CYTOKINE PRODUCTION

Condition	Example(s)
Infectious disease	Infection due to gram-positive or gram-negative bacteria, fungi, protozoa, viruses, and mycobacteria
Trauma	Burn injury, systemic inflammatory response syndrome, ARDS
Autoimmunity	Rheumatoid arthritis, systemic lupus erythematosus, vasculitides
Neoplasia	Many solid and hematologic malignancies
Circulating drugs/medications	Amphotericin B
Cryptogenic inflammatory disease	Sarcoidosis, Kawasaki syndrome, inflammatory bowel disease
Cardiac disease	Acute myocardial infarction, congestive heart failure syndrome
Production of endogenous substances	Cytokines, activated complement components, immune complexes

Septic shock = Sepsis syndrome associated with hypotension (systolic blood pressure < 90 mm Hg or a decrease of > 40 mm Hg from baseline if hypertensive)
Refractory septic shock = Septic shock lasting longer than 1 hour with no response to volume resuscitation or pharmacologic therapy
Systemic inflammatory response syndrome (SIRS) = A more general term for the clinical consequences of a widespread state of inflammatory endothelial activation, which is not limited to the presence or suspicion of infection; SIRS can occur as a result of trauma or pancreatitis, for example.

An emerging model of sepsis is illustrated in Figure 2–2. Several points bear mention:

1. Tumor necrosis factor (TNF) and IL-1 orchestrate the pathophysiology of the septic stage by their effects on thermoregulation, vascular resistance and permeability, cardiac inotropy, energy metabolism, and bone marrow function. TNF and IL-1 act both individually and synergistically in the septic state. TNF induces IL-1 in vivo.
2. Many of the effects of cytokines are mediated at target tissues by other mediators such as nitric oxide, eicosanoids, and the complement, coagulation, and kinin cascades.
3. TNF and IL-1 stimulate the production of other cytokines, producing an amplification of the inflammatory response, often termed a "cascade."
4. Although many of the cytokines produced have proinflammatory effects (TNF, IL-1, and IL-8, which recruits and activates neutrophils), some cytokines liberated in the process down-regulate the inflammatory response (IL-4, IL-6, IL-10, and TGF-β).

Tumor Necrosis Factor and Interleukin-1 in Sepsis

Intravenous infusion of endotoxin, IL-1, or TNF can replicate the physiologic effects of septic shock. In animal and human models of bacteremia and endotoxemia, TNF levels rise rapidly and peak at 60 to 90 minutes, followed by an increase in IL-1 levels that peak at 180 minutes (Table 2–4).

Selected Anticytokine Strategies

There are several potential advantages to anticytokine therapy in infectious or inflammatory diseases:

1. Broad applicability to many such diseases, because therapy is directed at the final common pathway of inflammation.
2. High specificity of some possible anticytokine agents, such as soluble cytokine receptors, which have a much higher affinity for their respective ligand than do monoclonal antibodies.
3. Small risk of immunogenicity, because many are naturally occurring substances.

Interventions specifically designed to modulate cytokine activity in sepsis have yet to produce clinical benefit in

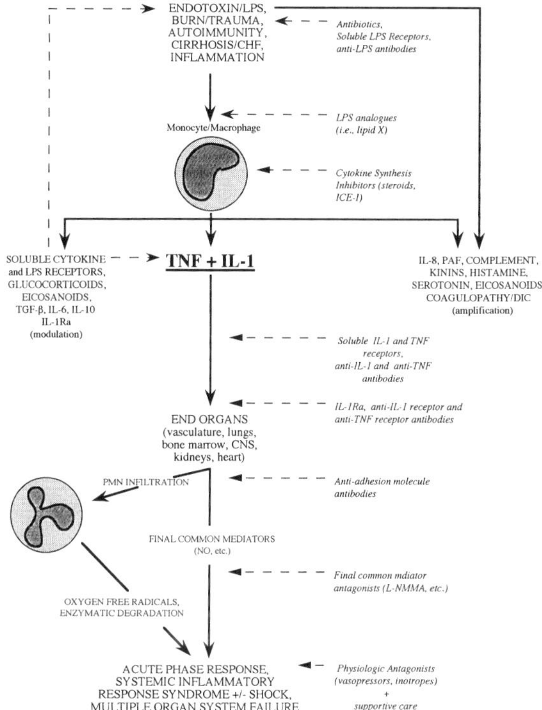

Figure 2–2. Any of a number of initiating factors can interact with mononuclear leukocytes and other cells to stimulate secretion of the key proinflammatory cytokines TNF and IL-1. In sufficiently high circulating concentrations, these two cytokines synergistically orchestrate all the phenomena of the systemic inflammatory response syndrome by proceeding to various end-organs and inducing specific final common mediators of organ dysfunction. Additionally, adhesion molecules are induced with subsequent recruitment and activation of polymorphonuclear leukocytes (aided by the chemotactic cytokine IL-8), which contribute to tissue damage. Amplification and diminution of the inflammatory responses proceed concomitantly with TNF and IL-1 production as shown. Also shown are possible targets for therapeutic intervention. *Abbreviations*: CHF = congestive heart failure; CNS = central nervous system; ICE-I = interleukin-1–converting enzyme inhibitor; IL-1Ra = interleukin-1 receptor antagonist; L-NMMA = L-N-monomethylarginine; NO = nitric oxide; PAF = platelet-activating factor; PMN = polymorphonuclear leukocyte; TGF-β = transforming growth factor beta; *solid arrow* = proinflammatory response induction; *dashed arrow with notched head* = naturally occurring down-regulatory responses; *dashed arrow with flat head* = possible areas of therapeutic intervention *(italics)*.

Table 2–4. PROINFLAMMATORY CYTOKINES, ANTI-INFLAMMATORY CYTOKINES, AND SOLUBLE TUMOR NECROSIS FACTOR RECEPTORS

Cytokine (Mass in kd)		Major Sources	Principal Activities
Proinflammatory	IL-1 (17.5)	Monocyte/macrophage, lymphocyte, neutrophil, endothelium, fibroblast, keratinocyte	Activation of T cells, B cells, natural killer cells, neutrophils, osteoblasts, and endothelium. Induces fever, sleep, anorexia, adrenocorticotropic hormone release, and hepatic acute-phase protein synthesis. Leads to myocardial depression, hypercoagulability, hypotension/shock, and death. Stimulates production of TNF, IL-8, and IL-6. Suppression of cytochrome P_{450}, thyroglobulin, and lipoprotein synthesis
	TNF (17.5)	Monocyte/macrophage, lymphocyte, neutrophil, endothelium, fibroblast, keratinocyte	Activation of T cells, B cells, natural killer cells, neutrophils, osteoblasts, and endothelium. Tumoricidal activity. Induces fever, sleep, anorexia, catabolism, adrenocorticotropic hromone release, hepatic acute-phase protein synthesis. Leads to myocardial depression, hypercoagulability, hypotension/shock, and death. Stimulates production of IL-1, IL-8, and IL-6. Suppression of cytochrome P_{450}, thyroglobulin, and lipoprotein lipase
	IL-8 (8)	Monocyte/macrophage, lymphocyte, endothelium, fibroblast keratinocyte	Recruitment and activation of neutrophils, chemotactic for lymphocytes, angiogenesis

Anti-inflammatory	IL-10, TGF-β (35, 12.5)	T cell, fibroblast	Suppression of B cell and T cell proliferation. Inhibition of LPS-induced monocyte IL-1 and TNF production. Induction of IL-1 Ra
	IL-6 (21–28)	Monocyte/macrophage, T cell, endothelium, fibroblast, keratinocyte	Induction of fever and the hepatic acute-phase response. Stimulates cortisol production. Decreases IL-1 and TNF production. Participates in activation and proliferation of B and T cells, facilitates immunoglobulin production by B cells
	IL-1ra (17.5)	Monocyte/macrophage, fibroblast	Specifically inhibits IL-1 effects, including SIRS due to endotoxin or *Escherichia coli* in animal models
Soluble TNF receptors—derived from TNF receptors p55 and p75 (30 and 40, respectively)		Unknown, but monocyte/macrophage and neutrophil are likely	Specifically inhibits TNF effects, including SIRS due to endotoxin or *Escherichia coli* in animal models

humans, and anticytokine agents are currently being investigated. Therapeutic trials in septic shock using monoclonal antibody to TNF, as well as treatment with soluble TNF receptors, are in progress. A recent trial of IL-1 receptor antagonist showed no significant survival benefit when given to patients with sepsis with or without shock.

ENDOTOXIN-INDUCED FACTORS THAT PROVOKE SHOCK AND THEIR RECEPTORS

Endotoxic shock could not occur in the absence of cells or factors of hematopoietic origin. Macrophages are the principal cellular mediator of endotoxic shock. Macrophages possess at least three sets of receptors for endotoxin. One set, CD14, recognizes endotoxin, also known as lipopolysaccharide (LPS), bound to a serum factor, LPS-binding protein (LBP). CD14 receptor activates the secretion of macrophage mediators. Another class of LPS receptors, CD18, includes multifunctional receptors subdivided as CD11a/CD18, CD11b/CD18, and CD11c/CD18. In relation to LPS, CD18 receptors may be important for nonopsonic (complement and antibody-free) phagocytosis of gram-negative bacteria and/or removal and degradation of LPS from the body. The third receptor type may be the scavenger receptor that internalizes acetylated low-density lipoprotein.

Tumor Necrosis Factor Ligand Family

Abundant evidence points to the involvement of TNF in mediation of shock. TNF-α (also known as cachectin), TNF-β (also known as lymphotoxin), and lymphotoxin-β are encoded by tightly linked genes that lie within the major histocompatibility complex. Although TNF-α and TNF-β are largely secreted, the former can also exist in a membrane-associated form. Lymphotoxin-β is entirely membrane-associated, and it may act to maintain TNF-β in close proximity with the cell membrane. The TNFs are trimeric proteins. Although the majority of effects elicited by TNF-α and TNF-β are identical, the two proteins are produced in response to entirely different stimuli and by different types of cells: TNF-α is produced largely by macrophages, whereas TNF-β is produced exclusively by lymphocytes. The pathogenetic role for TNF-α in shock is certain, but the role played by TNF-β is inferential and less well documented, because TNF-β is not known to be produced in vivo in response to LPS.

Regulation of Tumor Necrosis Factor Biosynthesis: Host-Sensing Mechanism

The activation of TNF biosynthesis is a paradigm for the study of pathways activated by endotoxin. Endotoxins are of variable structure, but they feature a disaccharide backbone containing two phosphate groups and a number of interlinking acyl chains. A polysaccharide moiety of variable size confers antigenicity to the LPS molecule but does not mediate toxicity. Toxicity is a function of the lipid moiety, which engages specific receptors on cells. In addition to activation of the TNF gene by LPS, lipoteichoic acid (from gram-positive organisms) and lipoarabinomannose (from mycobacteria) may also act as inducers of TNF synthesis.

The best-characterized receptor for LPS is CD14, residing on the membrane of macrophages and other cell types. It may also exist in a secreted form. By directly engaging LPS, or LPS and LBP, CD14 effectively concentrates the agonist in plasma or in tissues. High concentrations of LPS can also bypass CD14-coupled signaling.

LPS potently induces cytokine production via activation of the transcription factors NF-κB and AP-1, which initiate and enhance cytokine gene transcription.

INTRACELLULAR pH AND ELECTROLYTE REGULATION

Mechanisms Involved in the Regulation of Cytosolic pH

Although the most commonly ordered laboratory tests are electrolytes and pH, these measurements largely reflect the extracellular milieu, and what happens intracellularly is not known to clinicians. As a result of metabolism, ~20,000 mmol of carbon dioxide (CO_2), ~1500 to 4500 mmol of lactic acid, and ~100 to 200 mmol of other nonvolatile acids are formed each day. Additionally, intracellular pH is not uniform. Cytosolic pH (pH_i) is in most cells slightly lower (0.02 to 0.03 pH units) than extracellular pH (pH_o). Organellar pH is markedly different from cytosolic pH: lysosomes are very acidic (pH of 4.5 to 5.5), endosomes and Golgi apparatus more alkaline (pH of 5.5 to 6.5), and the nucleus slightly more acidic than the cytosol. Although these pH differences appear small, they are not. Recall that pH is a logarithmic scale. At pH 7.1 compared with pH 7.4, the amount of free protons is doubled (40 nmol/L at pH 7.40, 80 nmol/L at pH 7.10). Imagine what would happen if the patient's Na^+ or K^+ were suddenly doubled!

To maintain precise regulation of pH despite a very heavy acid load and the pH sensitivity of a number of cellular processes, the body employs four major buffering mechanisms:

1. Physiochemical buffers in extracellular fluid (ECF) and intracellular fluid (ICF)
2. Transport of acid and base across cell membranes
3. Removal of volatile acid by respiration
4. Removal of nonvolatile acid and absorption of base by the kidney

Physiochemical Buffering

EXTRACELLULAR BUFFERING

The main buffers in the blood and interstitial fluid are proteins, phosphate, and bicarbonate. Although the bicarbonate buffer system has a pK value of 6.1, it is quantitatively the most important extracellular buffer because of its high concentration (~25 mmol) and the fact that the "weak acid" CO_2 is effectively removed by respiration. ECF phosphate concentration is ~1 to 2 mmol, and it is less important as a physiologic buffer. ECF protein concentration is ~2 to 4 mmol, but each protein has many buffering residues, making them important buffers.

INTRACELLULAR BUFFERING

The main buffering of CO_2/H_2CO_3 takes place intracellularly. The main intracellular buffers are also proteins, organic phosphate, and bicarbonate. Bicarbonate ion constitutes ~50% of buffering capacity in the ICF. In RBCs, hemoglobin is a particularly effective buffer because of its high concentration and its many histidine residues, the only amino acid with significant buffering power near neutral pH. Deoxyhemoglobin has a higher affinity for protons than oxyhemoglobin has—a property known as the Haldane effect. Because of the high permeability of CO_2 across cell membranes, intracellular CO_2 concentration is under most circumstances equal to extracellular CO_2 concentration. Specific cell membrane transporters for HCO_3^- also exist. Since CO_2 is removed by respiration, intracellular H_2CO_3 is effectively regulated. The components of the bicarbonate buffer system (CO_2 and HCO_3^-) thus can be independently regulated by the body, making the bicarbonate buffer system particularly effective for both intra- and extracellular buffering. Given these relationships, every HCO_3^- ion can buffer two to four times better than any other physiologic buffering system.

Transmembrane Transport of Acid and Base

To transport molecules across its hydrophobic interior, the lipid bilayer of the plasma membrane employs a number of specialized membrane transport proteins: carrier proteins and channel proteins. Carrier proteins bind to the specific solute and undergo a conformational change to transfer the solute across the membrane. Channel proteins form water-filled "pores" that extend across the lipid bilayer and can be closed or open. If open, electrolytes traverse according to channel specificity and transmembrane gradient of the solute.

All channel proteins and many carrier proteins allow only passive transport (facilitated diffusion): the direction of transport is determined by the electrochemical gradient. Transport of a solute against its electrochemical gradient occurs only with carrier proteins and is either

- primary active transport (coupled to hydrolysis of ATP), or
- secondary active transport (coupled to simultaneous or sequential transfer of another solute with a more favorable electrochemical gradient).

Symport refers to transport of both solutes in the same direction; *antiport* refers to solutes exchanged in the opposite

Table 2–5. ELECTRONEUTRAL AND ELECTROGENIC PROCESSES

Electroneutral Processes	Electrogenic Processes
1. Na^+/H^+ antiport	1. Na^+-HCO_3^- symport
2. Na^+-coupled Cl^-/HCO_3^- antiport	2. Proton translocating ATPase
3. Na^+-independent Cl^-/HCO_3^- antiport	
4. H^+/K^+ ATPase	
5. H^+/lactate$^-$ symport	

Abbreviations: ATPase = adenosine triphosphatase; Na^+ = sodium ion; H^+ = hydrogen ion; Cl^- = chlorine ion; HCO_3^- = bicarbonate ion; K^+ = potassium ion.

direction. Voltage-gated channels are carrier proteins regulated by the electrical status of the cell. Ligand-gated channels are carrier proteins regulated by humoral mediators (Table 2–5).

Mechanisms of Transmembrane Acid and Base Transport

Electrolyte transport is an integrated part of pH regulation. See Figure 2–3. Certain carrier proteins contribute to maintenance of steady state pH_i. These are

- Na^+-coupled Cl^-/HCO_3^- antiport ($NaCO_3^-/Cl^-$)
- Hydrogen ion/lactate symport (in cardiac and skeletal muscle cells, placenta)
- Na^+-independent Cl^-/HCO_3^- antiport (HCO_3^-/Cl^-)

There are major differences in the relative numbers and proportions of these carrier proteins in different cell types.

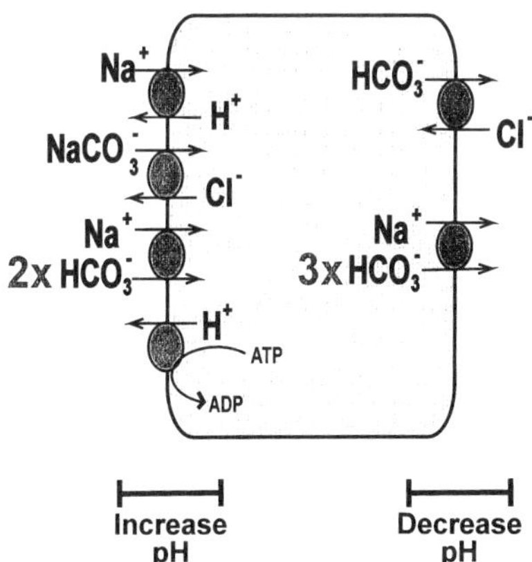

Figure 2–3. The most common mechanisms for transmembrane transport of acid and base.

Cooperation Among pH_i-Regulating Mechanisms: Bicarbonate Therapy in Systemic Acidosis

Based on experimental data, it is known that

1. In most cells, pH_i is higher in the presence of bicarbonate. Intracellular buffering power is approximately doubled in the presence of HCO_3^-. Furthermore, the activity of the Na^+-coupled Cl^-/HCO_3^- antiport or Na^+/HCO_3^- symport tends to increase, raising pH_i.
2. Recovery from both an acid and an alkali load is faster in the presence of bicarbonate than in its absence.
3. Bicarbonate is readily transported across the plasma membrane by specific carrier mechanisms.
4. In the setting of metabolic acidosis, administration of bicarbonate increases extracellular HCO_3^-, pH_o, and PCO_2. Because CO_2 is freely membrane-permeable, an immediate intracellular acidification takes place if extracellular PCO_2 is increased. This acidification is very short-lived, because the bicarbonate treatment has increased the pH_o, making the condition very favorable for a high activity of the Na^+/H^+ antiport and the Na^+-coupled Cl^-/HCO_3^- antiport. Within minutes, pH_i is higher than before treatment with bicarbonate. Despite a short-lived acidification, bicarbonate treatment does increase pH_i in cases of metabolic acidosis.

Role of pH_i-Regulating Mechanisms for Excretion of Acid by Respiration

Because of the high intracellular content of carbonic anhydrase, CO_2 is processed much more rapidly to H^+ and HCO_3^- inside erythrocytes than in plasma. Simultaneously with CO_2 entering the cells, O_2 leaves and hemoglobin, now deoxygenated, can buffer more acid (Haldane effect). The Haldane effect enables the body to double the amount of CO_2 transported. Moreover, erythrocytes possess abundant Na^+-independent Cl^-/HCO_3^- antiport protein ($\sim 1 \times 10^6$ molecules/cell), causing rapid export of HCO_3^- from the red cell into the plasma (Fig. 2–4).

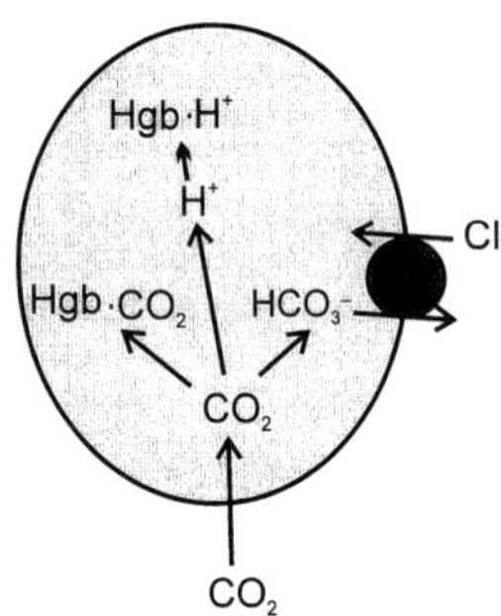

Figure 2–4. Mechanisms of CO_2 transport by red blood cells.

Role of pH_i-Regulating Mechanisms in Renal Handling of Acid-Base Balance

Due primarily to metabolism of food, there is a daily production of 40 to 200 mmol of nonvolatile acids. The renal excretion of H^+ and preservation for HCO_3^- involves two processes:

- The reabsorption of virtually all filtered bicarbonate (99.9%).
- The reclamation of bicarbonate consumed in the buffering of fixed acids in the blood.

Regulation of Cell Volume and Electrolyte Concentration

Cell volume is strictly regulated. The plasma membrane of most cells is highly permeable to water, and osmotically active solute, both intra- and extracellular, therefore determines cell volume. Swollen cells reduce volume by loss of KCl and water, known as a regulatory volume decrease. Shrunken cells increase volume by net uptake of NaCl. Na^+ is then exchanged with K^+ by Na^+/K^+-ATPase, eliciting a net gain of KCl and a concomitant gain of water and volume, known as a regulatory volume increase. Cells increase their volume before cell division. In the setting of hyponatremic hypotonicity, the compensatory volume decrease also decreases pH_i, because both the Na^+/H^+ and Na^+-coupled Cl^-/HCO_3^- antiporters have less favorable gradients under these conditions.

Regulation of Intracellular Ion Concentration

Regulation of ion concentration is closely related to regulation of cell volume. In most human cells, K^+ is the predominant intracellular cation, and its concentration, which varies little among different cells, appears to be mainly controlled by the activity of Na^+/K^+-ATPase. Anion concentration varies considerably, however, in different cells. Internal Cl^- concentration may be far above its electrochemical equilibrium, due to activity of the Na^+-K^+-$2Cl^-$ symport.

Role of pH_i-Regulating Mechanism in Pathophysiologic Conditions

Metabolic Acidosis

Metabolic acidosis is caused by several disorders. Lactic acid production under normal conditions is approximately 15 to 30 mmol/kg/day. The maximum capacity of the liver to convert lactate to glucose via gluconeogenesis or to CO_2 via the citric acid cycle is 3.5 mol/day. If this capacity is exceeded, a lactic acidosis will ensue, as in the case of severe liver failure.

Under conditions of aerobic metabolism, glycolysis goes via pyruvate to the citric acid cycle and then to oxidative phosphorylation. Under anaerobic conditions, however, the reduced form of nicotinamide adenine dinucleotide (NADH) formed during glycolysis builds up because it is not used in the citric acid cycle. This buildup depletes the cell of NAD^+, halting glycolysis. To regain NAD^+, and therefore resume production of ATP, lactic acid is formed:

$$\text{Pyruvate} + \text{NADH} + H^+ \leftrightarrow \text{lactate} + NAD^+$$

This anaerobic pathway generates 2 mol of H^+ per mol of glucose. Lactate dehydrogenase (LDH) is regulated by pH_i such that acidosis tends to decrease its activity, whereas alkalosis increases it. Respiratory alkalosis can thus increase lactate production. There is evidence that an H^+/lactate symport exists and markedly increases the transport of protons and lactate in heart and muscle cells.

In cases of systemic metabolic acidosis, HCO_3^- in the blood and interstitial fluid buffers acids by forming CO_2, which is removed by respiration, causing HCO_3^- to decrease. Bicarbonate ion tends to exit from the cell, primarily by the Na^+-independent Cl^-/HCO_3^- antiport, elevating pH_o and lowering pH_i. This action is functionally equivalent to a net transport of H^+ into the cell. Thus, even though cell membranes are poorly permeable to H^+ per se, an effective intracellular buffering of extracellular acidosis may be accomplished by the Na^+-independent Cl^-/HCO_3^- antiport. This indirect internalization of H^+ by exporting HCO_3^- via the antiport is likely an important defense mechanism in systemic acidosis. Compensation for metabolic acidosis is therefore hyperventilation, renal resorption of bicarbonate, and transport of acid equivalents, resulting in intracellular buffering.

Respiratory Acidosis

In cases of respiratory acidosis, PCO_2 is increased, rapidly crosses cell membranes, yielding H^+ and HCO_3^-. pH_i decreases, activating Na^+/H^+ antiport and, in certain cells, Na^+-coupled Cl^-/HCO_3^- antiport, causing a compensatory increase in pH_i. The net effect, however, is that the decrease in pH_o is more pronounced than the fall in pH_i. Renal compensation then occurs over a longer time period.

Metabolic Alkalosis

Metabolic alkalosis is clinically separated into chloride-responsive and chloride-unresponsive types. The former type is due to excess loss of chloride (vomiting, nasogastric suction, diuretic therapy), whereas the latter may be due to excess alkali loads or excess mineralocorticoid effects. Cells can compensate for intracellular alkalosis by exporting HCO_3^- in exchange for Cl^- via the Na^+-independent Cl^-/HCO_3^- antiport. This antiport is activated at alkaline pH and is driven by anion gradients. The intracellular compartment will thus buffer an extracellular alkalosis. Because of a higher buffering capacity intracellularly than in the extracellular space, pH_i will remain lower than pH_o.

Respiratory Alkalosis

Because of the high membrane permeability for CO_2, pH_i is rapidly elevated in respiratory alkalosis, to which the cells respond by activating the Na^+-independent Cl^-/HCO_3^- antiport. pH_i deviation is less than the change in pH_o, due to the high buffering power of the intracellular compartment. In chronic respiratory alkalosis, enhanced renal secretion of bicarbonate also occurs.

Cardiovascular Function

Effect of pH on Cardiac Function

Acidification of isolated cardiac muscle by a pH of ~0.2 has a severe negative inotropic effect, reducing contractility by ~40% to 50%. In vivo reflex sympathetic activation compensates for this negative inotropy, but norepinephrine's stimulatory effect is decreased at pH 7.2, and at pH 7.00 the stimulatory effect of epinephrine is completely lost. At low pH, the effects of catecholamines are more of tachycardia and peripheral vasoconstriction than of increased inotropy.

Vascular Function

Many vasoconstrictor agents (norepinephrine, epinephrine, serotonin, endothelin, and vasopressin) stimulate the Na^+/H^+ antiport and increase pH_i in the absence of HCO_3^-. The most common effect of in vivo acidosis is dilation of systemic vessels, whereas alkalosis is associated with vasoconstriction. The pulmonary vascular response to acidosis, however, is generally vasoconstriction.

Ischemia

During ischemia, not only is the supply of oxygen jeopardized, but also the removal of products of metabolism such as lactic acid, CO_2, and protons is severely limited. Hydrolysis of ATP yields protons, acidifying the cell. Phosphocreatine prevents the development of acidosis, since it can transfer phosphate to ADP, regenerating ATP and utilizing protons. In resting muscle cells, where phosphocreatine is abundant, ATP will be present for 1 to 2 hours of complete ischemia. Myocardial cells, despite phosphocreatine stores, deplete ATP within 10 to 20 minutes of ischemia, while neurons, containing even less phosphocreatine, can be irreversibly damaged by 5 minutes of severe ischemia.

T AND B CELL FUNCTION IN CRITICAL ILLNESS

Important alterations in T and B cell function are associated with critical illness, producing a relatively immunocompromised state.

T Cell Activation and Proliferation

T cells can be divided into two subsets, $CD4^+$ and $CD8^+$, on the basis of the presence of these T cell receptor (TCR) adjacent-surface molecules. Subpopulations of $CD4^+$ T cells have "helper" functions in augmenting T and B cell proliferation and activation. "Suppressor" $CD8^+$ T cells have been identified that can down-regulate T and B cell activation, and they also have cytotoxic functions, killing tumor cells as well as cells infected with viruses, bacteria, and fungi. In general, protein antigens require intracellular processing before being presented to T cells. Polysaccharide antigen, common on bacteria, can be recognized by immunoglobulin on B cells and directly presented to T cells. Tissue dendritic cells, B cells, and macrophages can all function as antigen-presenting cells (Fig. 2–5).

Substantial evidence indicates that many steps in T cell activation may be affected by critical illness, resulting in decreased T cell help in augmenting immune response, and in a predominance of suppressive T cell effects. The antigen-presenting ability of macrophages, especially important in viral, fungal, and intracellular bacterial antigen presentation, as well as macrophage expression of MHC class II molecules, decreases following hemorrhage and injury. The ability of both $CD4^+$ and $CD8^+$ T cells to be activated in an antigen-specific or nonspecific manner is diminished after hemorrhage, burns, and trauma.

Cytokines

A large number of cytokines are produced by T cells and macrophages (Table 2–6).

Recent evidence indicates that $CD4^+$ T cells can be divided

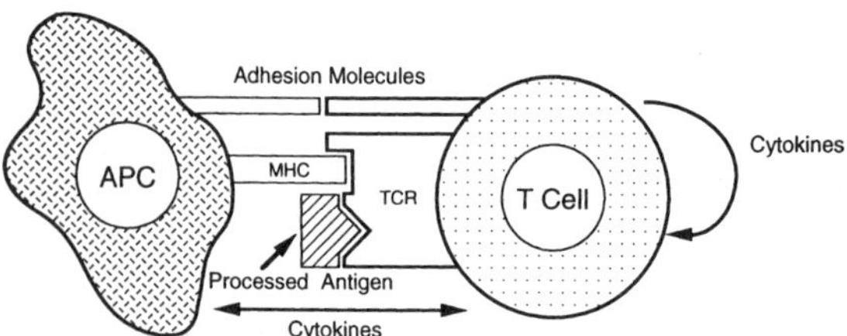

Figure 2–5. T cell activation involves presentation of antigen in a major histocompatibility complex (MHC)–specific manner to engage an antigen-specific T cell receptor (TCR) on the T cell surface. Interaction between the antigen-presenting cell (APC) and the T cell is promoted by adhesion molecules on the surfaces of both cells. Cytokines produced by the T cell and antigen-presenting cell (e.g., interleukin-1, interleukin-2, and others) can modulate the activation state of both cells. In particular, T cell–produced cytokines, such as interleukin-2, can promote further activation of T cells by up-regulating receptor numbers on the surfaces of T cells as well as receptor affinity.

into two subpopulations based on their cytokine profiles. Th1 cells are involved in inflammatory functions and produce TNF-α, IL-2, and IFN-γ, whereas Th2 cells provide B cell help and produce IL-4, IL-5, and IL-10. IL-10 has an important feedback role in that it down-regulates the production of Th1 cytokines and the production of cytokines by macrophages and monocytes (IL-1α, IL-6, IL-8, and TNF-α), and decreases macrophage expression of MHC class II molecules.

After trauma and blood loss, injured patients and animals demonstrate a decrease in Th1-associated cytokines and an increase in Th2-associated cytokines. In particular, IL-2 and IFN-γ production decrease after hemorrhage, whereas IL-4 and IL-10 production are increased. Decreased IL-2 results in depressed resistance to infection. Mucosal surfaces, such as lung and intestine, appear to be particularly vulnerable to bacterial colonization and infections in critically ill patients.

B Cells

B cells, through the production of antibodies, have a central role in resistance to extracellular organisms. Secretory antibodies, primarily IgA, are present at mucosal surfaces such as intestine and lung. Circulating antibodies are usually IgG and IgM, which coat bacteria, facilitating complement-mediated killing (unlike IgA), and enhance phagocytosis by neutrophils and macrophages, which use their Fc receptors to recognize antibody on the bacterial surface.

As B cells leave the bone marrow, they are already committed to producing antibody specific for a single antigen. Most B cells die before encountering their specific antigen, but the B cells that do are activated, proliferate, and secrete antibody. Some of these activated B cells remain as "memory" cells. An adequate antibody response to infection depends on the numbers of antigen-specific resting B cells (B cell clonal precursors) that are present at the time of infection and that can then be activated and recruited into the antibody-secreting plasma cell pool. Activation of B cell clonal precursors is affected by $CD4^+$ and $CD8^+$ T cells, as well as by cytokines such as IL-2, IL-4, IL-5 (enhancement) and TGF-β, and IFN-γ (inhibition). Critical illness profoundly decreases the numbers of bacterial antigen-specific resting B cells, particularly at mucosal sites such as the lung and intestine. These alterations in B cell repertoires result in inadequate levels of secretory antibody at mucosal sites, which may contribute to the increased incidence of bacterial colonization at these surfaces.

NEUTROPHIL–ENDOTHELIAL CELL INTERACTIONS

The adherence of neutrophils to endothelium is a critical early event in host defense against microorganisms and in the repair of injured tissues. Neutrophils are armed with a diverse array of effector mechanisms to carry out their normal function in host defense and repair. Neutrophils are

Table 2–6. MAJOR CYTOKINES AND THEIR PRIMARY ACTIVITIES

Cytokine	Actions
Interleukin-1	Induces fever, acute phase proteins; activates endothelial cells; stimulates T cell proliferation
Interleukin-2	Activates macrophages, stimulates natural killer cell activity, stimulates B cell proliferation and differentiation, activates T cells, stimulates T cell proliferation and differentiation
Interleukin-3	Stimulates eosinophil activity, B cell differentiation, in vivo hematopoiesis
Interleukin-4	Activates macrophages, T and B cells; stimulates B cell proliferation and differentiation; induces IgE receptors on B cells; stimulates T cell proliferation
Interleukin-5	Stimulates eosinophil activity, activates B cells, stimulates IgA isotype selection
Interleukin-6	Induces acute phase proteins; activates T cells; stimulates T cell proliferation and differentiation, B cell differentiation, and antibody production
Interleukin-7	Stimulates T and B cell proliferation
Interleukin-8	Chemotactic for neutrophils, induces neutrophil activation, inhibits neutrophil adhesion to endothelium
Interleukin-10	Suppresses cytokine production by Th1 cells and macrophages/monocytes, diminishes delayed hypersensitivity, suppresses monocyte/macrophage antigen-presenting cell function, down-regulates expression of MHC class II molecules on monocytes/macrophages, suppresses production of reactive nitrogen oxides by macrophages/monocytes, up-regulates MHC class II expression on B cells, augments proliferation and differentiation of B cells

Tumor necrosis factor-α	Activates macrophages; stimulates granulocyte activity, T cell proliferation; induces expression of intracellular adhesion molecules (e.g., ICAM-1); activates endothelial cells; induces fever and acute phase proteins
Transforming growth factor-β	Inhibits proliferation of hematopoietic precursors, inhibits activation and proliferation of T and B cells, stimulates growth of fibroblasts and osteoblasts, produces isotypes switching to IgA
Interferon-α	Induces a cellular antiviral state; stimulates natural killer cell activity, B cell proliferation and differentiation; inhibits T cell proliferation; induces fever
Interferon-β	Induces a cellular antiviral state, stimulates natural killer cell activity, enhances MHC class I expression, induces fever, stimulates B cell proliferation
Interferon-γ	Induces acute-phase protein production, stimulates isotype selection (IgG2a), inhibits B cell activation, activates macrophages
Granulocyte-macrophage colony–stimulating factor	Activates macrophages; stimulates granulocyte activity, eosinophil activity, T cell proliferation, in vivo hematopoiesis
Granulocyte colony-stimulating factor	Stimulates granulopoiesis and granulocyte activity

Abbreviations: IgE = immunoglobulin E; IgA = immunoglobulin A; MHC = major histocompatibility complex.

capable of generating reactive oxygen species (ROS), proteases, peptides, lipid mediators, and vasoactive substances. Neutrophils differ from macrophages, as seen in Table 2–7.

Neutrophil adherence to endothelium plays a pivotal role in neutrophil-mediated defense and repair as well as in neutrophil-mediated vascular injury. Important stimuli for neutrophil–endothelial cell adhesion and neutrophil aggregation include TNF-α, C5a, IL-8, platelet-activating factor (PAF), endotoxin, and bacterial chemotactic peptide (Fig. 2–6).

Mechanisms of Adhesion

Both neutrophils and endothelial cells (EC) are involved in adhesion, and there are two major categories of adhesion molecules. Selectin receptors are lectin-containing proteins that recognize specific carbohydrate counterstructures. Selectin receptors mediate the initial transient adherence of neutrophils that occurs at sites of inflammation, manifested as neutrophil "rolling" under conditions of blood flow. Once slowed by selectin-carbohydrate interactions, further inflammatory stimuli subsequently activate the neutrophil to produce firm integrin-immunoglobulin adhesion, the second category of adhesion molecules. This second interaction mediates firm adhesion, diapedesis, and migration at sites of inflammation (Fig. 2–7).

Integrin/Immunoglobulin-Mediated Adhesion

β_2 INTEGRINS: INTEGRIN SUPERFAMILY ADHESION RECEPTORS

The CD11/CD18 complex consists of three heterodimeric glycoprotein subunits. Each subunit consists of a light or β-chain polypeptide common to all three subunits, designated CD18, and a distinct heavy or α-chain polypeptide, designated CD11a, CD11b, or CD11c. The three CD11 α-chains and CD18 β-chains are members of the integrin superfamily of adhesion receptors:

- *CD11a/CD18 (LFA-1).* Found on all leukocytes.
- *CD11b/CD18 (Mac-1, Mo-1, or CR3).* Found on phagocytes and natural killer cells, but not on most lymphocytes. CD11b/CD18 appears to be the integrin most responsible for the firm adhesion of neutrophils, although CD11a/CD18 is also involved. CD11b/CD18 exists constitutively on the cell surface of neutrophils and in its secondary and tertiary granules. After stimulation, these granules translocate to the cell surface and increase CD11b/CD18 concentration by three- to tenfold. The heterodimer also undergoes a critical conformational change, resulting in high-affinity binding to its ligand.
- *CD11c/CD18 (p150.95).* Found on phagocytes and natural killer cells, but not on most lymphocytes.

IMMUNOGLOBULIN SUPERFAMILY LIGANDS

The endothelial counterstructures for the CD11/CD18 complex include intercellular adhesion molecules ICAM-1

Table 2–7. COMPARISON OF MACROPHAGES AND GRANULOCYTES

Property	Macrophages	Granulocytes
Differ by organs and tissues	Yes	No
Mature cells can divide	Yes	No
Life span in tissues	Days to weeks	About 1 day
Phagocytosis	Yes	Yes
Generate reactive oxygen intermediates	Yes	Yes
Contain microbicidal proteins	Few known	Yes
Preformed cytoplasmic granules	Unusual	Abundant
Constitutive secretion	Yes	No
Secretion by degranulation	Limited	Prominent
Protein synthesis	Very active	Minimal
Deoxyribonucleic acid synthesis	Moderate	Inactive
Present antigen to T lymphocytes	Yes	Unknown

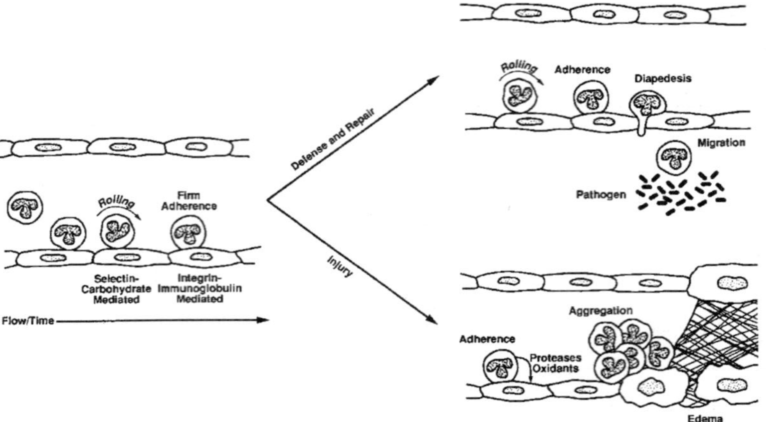

Figure 2–6. Diagram of the sequential events that occur at a site of inflammation as neutrophils leave the laminar flow stream of a postcapillary venule in the systemic circulation. Initial selectin/carbohydrate-mediated rolling along the surface of the endothelium is followed by integrin/immunoglobulin-mediated firm adherence. These two events are required either for neutrophil emigration in the setting of defense and repair or for neutrophil-mediated endothelial injury in pathologic conditions.

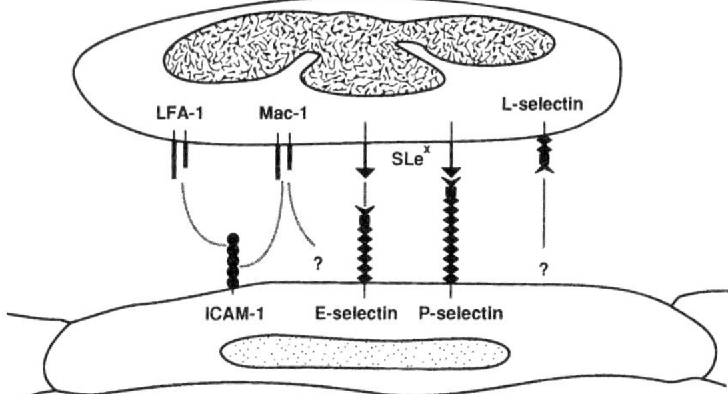

Figure 2–7. Diagram of the known neutrophil-endothelial adhesion receptors. The β_2 integrin receptors on neutrophils, LFA-1 (CD11a/CD18) and Mac-1 (CD11b/CD18; both represented as α/β dimers) bind to intercellular adhesion molecule-1 (ICAM-1 [CD54], represented with its five immunoglobulin domains) and another (other) as yet unidentified ligand (ligands) on the endothelial cell. Endothelial E-selectin (CD62E) and P-selectin (CD62P; represented with their N-terminal lectin domain, epidermal growth factor domain, multiple complement regulatory repeat sequences, transmembrane domain, and cytoplasmic domain) bind to carbohydrate ligands, particularly Sialyl Lewis X antigen (SLe^x; CD15s), expressed on glycoproteins or glycolipids of neutrophils. L-selectin (CD62L) on neutrophils binds to as yet unidentified carbohydrate ligand(s) on endothelium in the systemic vasculature.

and ICAM-2, members of the immunoglobulin superfamily. ICAM-1 is recognized by CD11b/CD18. ICAM-1 is expressed at low levels on resting EC in vivo and in vitro, and it is up-regulated over a period of hours in response to stimuli such as endotoxin, IL-1β, and TNF. Monoclonal antibodies to ICAM-1 inhibit neutrophil adherence to EC after stimulation, although to a lesser extent than monoclonal antibodies to CD11b or CD18.

Selectin/Carbohydrate-Mediated Adhesion

Recent evidence suggests that selectin-mediated adhesion is relatively resistant to shear forces and plays an important role in the initial rolling of neutrophils along the endothelium. The three selectin receptors are:

- *L-selectin (LAM-1, Leu-8, or LECAM-1).* Expressed only on leukocytes. Binds to carbohydrate ligand on EC. Constitutively expressed on neutrophils and can be shed in response to stimulation. The ligand for L-selectin on the endothelium is unknown.
- *E-selectin (ELAM-1).* Localized to EC; binds to carbohydrate ligand on neutrophils, usually Sialyl Lewis X (SLe^x). Requires de novo protein synthesis and does not reach peak surface expression for 4 to 6 hours after stimulation by endotoxin, IL-1β, or TNF-α.

- *P-selectin (GMP-140, PADGEM, CD62).* Found on platelets and EC. Binds to carbohydrate ligand on neutrophils, usually SLe^x. Stored within Weibel-Palade bodies in EC, P-selectin–mediated adhesion is a likely first step in initially slowing neutrophils, causing them to roll, before firm integrin-mediated adherence can take place.

In Vivo Models of Neutrophil-Mediated Injury

Multiple animal studies have examined the role of neutrophil-mediated injury in the setting of ischemia/reperfusion and inflammation/immune-mediated injury. No human clinical trials using specific agents to inhibit neutrophil-endothelial adhesion have been completed to date, however (Table 2–8).

RECEPTOR PHYSIOLOGY

The concept of a "receptor" explains the remarkably selective and potent effects that some natural and synthetic chemicals have on biologic tissues. Drugs do not create new responses in tissues; rather, they start, stop, or modulate natural physiologic functions.

Relationship Between Receptor Occupancy and Response

The reversible binding of a drug to its receptor usually obeys the following law of mass action:

$$D + R \leftrightarrow DR \qquad \textbf{[Equation 1]}$$

where D is the drug concentration, R is the receptor concentration, and DR is the drug-receptor complex. At equilibrium:

Table 2–8. ANTIADHESION THERAPY IN EXPERIMENTAL MODELS OF VASCULAR AND TISSUE INJURY*

Ischemia/Reperfusion	Inflammatory/Immune
Intestinal ischemia	Inflammatory skin lesions
Tissue reperfusion injury	Edema in meningitis
Shock/resuscitation	Endotoxic shock
Myocardial ischemia	Allergic asthma
Skeletal muscle ischemia	Autoimmune diabetes
Central nervous system ischemia	Pulmonary oxygen toxicity
	NSAID-induced gastric injury
	Burns
	Graft rejection
	Inflammatory lung injury

*Experimental models in which monoclonal antibodies that block neutrophil-endothelial adhesion molecules have been shown to be effective at attenuating injury. These studies fall into two major groups: processes of an inflammatory or immune origin, and those involving ischemia-reperfusion.

Abbreviation: NSAID = nonsteroidal anti-inflammatory drug.

$$[DR] = [D]R_T/[D] + K_d \qquad \textbf{[Equation 2]}$$

where R_T is the total concentration of receptor and K_d is the equilibrium dissociation constant of DR. K_d has units of concentration and is equivalent to the concentration of drug required for half-maximal receptor occupancy. K_d is thus a measure of affinity of a drug for a receptor: the lower the K_d, the higher the affinity.

The size of the response elicited by a drug depends on its intrinsic efficacy and the percentage of receptors that it occupies. In the absence of drugs, most native receptors are silent. An agonist is a drug that binds to the receptor, turns it on, and triggers a response. The property that enables the agonist to turn on the receptor is called intrinsic efficacy. An antagonist is a drug that lacks intrinsic efficacy but is capable of binding to the receptor. Drugs having a small or intermediate level of intrinsic efficacy are called partial agonists. Several dose-response curves are shown in Figure 2–8. When an agonist is capable of eliciting a maximum response at submaximal levels of receptor occupancy, the situation is referred to as spare receptors; only a fraction of the total functional receptor population needs to be occupied to elicit a maximum response.

Because antagonists lack intrinsic efficacy, all that is necessary to describe their interaction with a receptor at equilibrium is the K_d. The K_d of the antagonist can be estimated from the shift in the dose-response curve, using the following equation:

$$DR - 1 = [A]K_A \qquad \textbf{[Equation 3]}$$

in which DR (dose ratio) is the concentration of agonist causing a half-maximal response in the presence of antagonist divided by that measured in its absence, and [A] is the concentration of the antagonist.

Receptor Families

Physiologic receptors can be divided into four families on the basis of structural and functional properties:

1. G protein–linked receptors
2. Ligand-regulated transcription factors
3. Ligand-regulated enzymes
4. Ligand-gated ion channels

G Protein–Linked Receptors

The largest family of cell surface receptors is functionally linked to a specific class of intracellular molecules called G proteins. The cell surface receptors are members of the seven-pass transmembrane protein family, so called because the protein snakes back and forth across the membrane seven times, creating extra- and intracytoplasmic loops. The third intracytoplasmic loop is the most variable and selects for the particular G protein that will generate a second messenger. The G protein–linked family includes receptors for a number of endogenous neurotransmitters, including

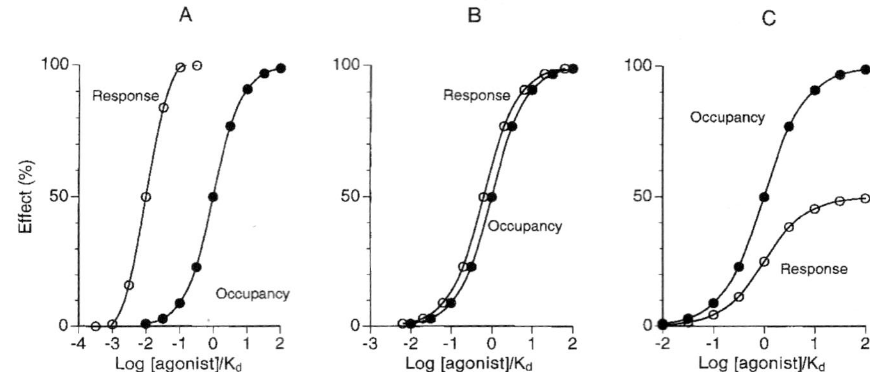

Figure 2–8. Relationship between receptor occupancy (●) and response (○) for a highly effacacious agonist (*A*), a less efficacious agonist (*B*), and a partial agonist (*C*). Both occupancy and response are expressed as percentages of their maximum values and are plotted on the ordinate scale. The concentration of the agonist is expressed on the abscissa as a log of the ratio of the agonist concentration divided by its K_d.

muscarinic acetylcholine, catecholamines, histamine, serotonin, as well as eicosanoids and some peptides. Members of this family of receptors also mediate the special sensory functions of vision, taste, and olfaction.

G Protein Structure and Mechanism

G proteins are heterotrimers consisting of α, β, and γ subunits. The β and γ subunits form a tightly bound complex common to all G proteins, and thus it is the specific α subunit that defines precisely the activity of a G protein. More than 20 different types of α subunits have been cloned. Alpha subunits also characteristically bind guanyl nucleotides and hydrolyze guanosine triphosphate (GTP) into guanosine diphosphate (GDP). When the α subunit has GDP in its binding site, it is quiescent. Binding of a ligand to a seven-pass transmembrane receptor stimulates the G protein to partially liberate the α subunit from the β/γ complex, which in turn allows replacement of the resident GDP by GTP. The α subunit becomes fully dissociated, freeing it to activate other effector molecules, in particular adenyl cyclase. Recall the importance of adenylate cyclase in making cAMP, a critically important second messenger.

Once cATP rises within the cell, it can mediate a variety of effects through allosteric binding to protein kinase A (PKA). Protein kinase A activation is well known to regulate metabolic pathways acutely by phosphorylating target enzymes. Protein kinase A also regulates gene expression by phosphorylating DNA-binding proteins that act as transcription factors. The turn-off mechanism for cAMP is phosphodiesterase, which rapidly hydrolyzes cAMP to AMP.

Some α subunits ($G\alpha_s$) stimulate their effector, and others ($G\alpha_i$) inhibit theirs. Cholera toxin, for example, attacks $G\alpha_s$ after GTP binding and prevents hydrolysis to GDP. This particular G protein stimulates adenylate cyclase. The massive diarrhea associated with cholera infection is directly attributable to the consequent sustained high levels of cAMP in intestinal epithelium. In contrast, pertussis toxin attacks G_i and G_o, which prevents receptor-mediated activation of Gi and Go. G proteins also regulate the activity of phospholipase Cβ, which is closely associated with the important second messengers diacylglycerol (DAG) and inositol triphosphate (IP_3), which activate protein kinase C and cause release of intracellular calcium, respectively. Some of the major transduction mechanisms of G protein–linked receptors are listed in Table 2–9.

Ligand-Regulated Transcription Factors

This receptor superfamily comprises a large group of soluble receptors that bind to DNA and regulate the activity of specific genes in a ligand-dependent manner. This family includes receptors for thyroid and steroid hormones, vitamin D, and retinoids. Most of these receptors are located in the nucleus. It is not surprising that the ligands for these receptors can readily penetrate the plasma membrane, and access to the receptor is controlled by hormone-binding proteins.

Table 2–9. SIGNALING MECHANISMS OF G PROTEIN–LINKED RECEPTORS

Representative Receptors	G Protein Family	Effector
β_1-and β_2 adrenergic D_1 dopamine H_2 histamine	G_s	Stimulate adenylate cyclase, open calcium channels
M_2 and M_4 muscarinic D_2 dopamine α_2 adrenergic	G_i and G_o	Open potassium channels, close calcium channels, inhibit adenylate cyclase, stimulate PIP_2-PLC, stimulate PLA_2
M_1, M_3, and M_5 muscarinic α_1 adrenergic Angiotensin II	G_q	Stimulate PIP_2-C
Rhodopsin	G_T	Stimulate cGMP phosphodiestease

Abbreviations: PIP_2-PLC = phosphatidylinositol-4,5-bisphosphate-specific phospholipase C; PLA_2 = phospholipase A_2; cGMP = cyclic guanosine monophosphate.

Many of these receptors have a DNA-binding region composed of two loops held in place by a zinc atom, known as the "zinc finger" domains. The site on DNA where binding occurs is called the hormone response element (HRE).

Ligand-Regulated Enzymes

This huge superfamily of receptors exhibits a unifying structural feature: the presence of an extracellular ligand-binding domain that regulates the activity of an intracellular catalytic domain. The two domains are connected by a single transmembrane-spanning region. This superfamily includes receptors for a variety of growth factors, cytokines, and peptides. One major group of receptors within this superfamily has a tyrosine kinase intracellular domain. Activation of these receptor tyrosine kinases (RTK) causes a variety of cellular events, including DNA synthesis, cellular replication, increased protein synthesis, stimulation of ion and glucose transport, and other cytoskeletal and morphologic changes. Receptors for atrial natriuretic peptide, nerve growth factor, and TNF are members of the ligand-regulated enzyme superfamily.

Ligand-Gated Ion Channels

This large superfamily contains receptors for the nicotinic acetylcholine receptor $GABA_A$, glycine, and various excitatory amino acids, such as glutamate and aspartate. Members of this superfamily are ion channels that open up and conduct an ionic current when a ligand binds to them. In the case of excitatory amino acid receptors, the ionic current is caused by both sodium and calcium, whereas inhibitory amino acid receptors (GABA and glycine) carry a chloride current. The overall structure of ligand-gated ion channels shows homology with many of the voltage-regulated ion channels.

Ligand-gated ion channels are widespread throughout the central and peripheral nervous systems and are responsible for rapid synaptic transmission. Nicotinic acetylcholine receptors, present at the neuromuscular junction, elicit skeletal muscle contraction from α-motoneurons and are the target of neuromuscular blocking agents. $GABA_A$ receptors are important targets for drugs used to treat anxiety, seizures, and insomnia.

PHYSIOLOGIC AND PATHOPHYSIOLOGIC SIGNIFICANCE OF NITRIC OXIDE

Pharmacology

Nitric oxide is a potent vascular smooth muscle relaxant, affecting veins as well as arteries. Its mechanism of action is fairly well established. Nitric oxide binds to the heme prosthetic group of the cytosolic form of guanylate cyclase and activates the enzyme, catalyzing the conversion of GTP to cGMP. Cyclic GMP acts as an intracellular messenger to cause a rapid decrease in the levels of free calcium and to inactivate myosin light chain kinase. Thus the contractile activity of vascular smooth muscle is paralyzed, and the muscle relaxes. Clinically useful nitrovasodilators include nitroglycerin, nitroprusside, and isoamyl nitrite; all work by stimulating NO and cGMP formation. Nitric oxide also relaxes nonvascular smooth muscle, including that in airways, gastrointestinal tissue, and the uterus.

Nitric oxide has a diverse number of other vital roles in biologic systems. Nitric oxide is a potent inhibitor of platelet aggregation induced by adenosine diphosphate, thrombin, and arachidonic acid. This action of NO is also cGMP dependent. Nitric oxide is a nonadrenergic-noncholinergic (NANC) neurotransmitter in numerous tissues. Nitric oxide is endothelium-derived relaxing factor (EDRF). In the central nervous system, NO plays a neurotransmitter role. Additionally, it has important effects on vascular smooth muscle proliferation.

Chemistry

Nitric oxide is one of the ten smallest molecules found in nature. It contains an odd number of electrons, and because of this unpaired electron it acts as a free radical. Nitric oxide is a water- and lipid-soluble gas. Biologically active concentrations of NO range from 1 to 100 nmol. Although it is very lipophilic, it has a short half-life of less than 3 to 5 seconds because of its spontaneous reactivity with molecular oxygen to yield nitrite (NO_2^-) and nitrate (NO_3^-), both of which are relatively inactive. Oxyhemoglobin (HbO_2) can catalyze the rapid inactivation of NO primarily to NO_3^-, and forms methemoglobin (met Hb) in the process:

$$HbO_2 + \cdot NO \rightarrow metHb + NO_3^-$$

Hemoglobin inactivates NO by sequestration, and thus restricts the biologic action of NO on nearby cells. In view of its short half-life, NO must elicit its biologic effects at sites that are very close to its site of biosynthesis, i.e., a paracrine or autocrine effect (Fig. 2–9).

At very high concentrations, NO not only binds to and reacts with iron in proteins but knocks the iron out of the protein, disrupting enzyme and cellular function. This reactivity with iron constitutes one of the pathophysiologic mechanisms by which NO elicits cytotoxicity. Some iron-containing proteins altered by NO include the mitochondrial enzyme aconitase and NADPH oxidoreductase enzymes. Another pathophysiologic mechanism involves the reaction of NO with superoxide to yield peroxynitrite anion ($ONOO^-$) and related radicals that promote lipid peroxidation and cell damage.

Biosynthesis of Endogenous Nitric Oxide

A number of different mammalian cells use NO synthase to synthesize NO from L-arginine (Fig. 2–10). Heme plays a key role in the electron transfer steps, as well as in the reversible inhibition of NO synthase, producing negative

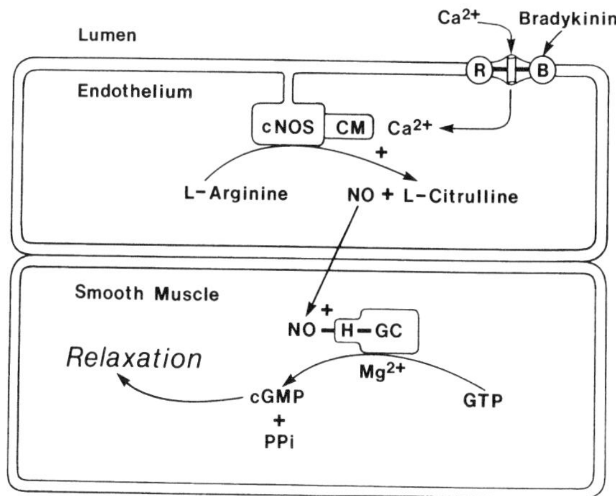

Figure 2–9. The interaction between endothelium-derived NO and vascular smooth muscle. In this example of endothelium-dependent vascular smooth muscle relaxation, bradykinin in the blood interacts with selective receptors (B) on the luminal surface of endothelial cells to trigger calcium ion (Ca^{2+}) influx. Other chemical agents in the blood may also interact with their own selective receptors (R) to trigger Ca^{2+} influx. Intracellular Ca^{2+} forms a complex with calmodulin (CM) that is bound to the constitutive isoform of NO synthase (cNOS), thereby causing enzyme activation (+). cNOS catalyzes the conversion of L-arginine to NO plus L-citrulline. The NO generated diffuses readily across membrane barriers into adjacent smooth muscle cells and forms a complex with heme (H) that is bound to the cytosolic guanylate cyclase (GC), thereby causing enzyme activation (+). GC catalyzes the conversion of GTP to cyclic GMP (cGMP) plus inorganic pyrophosphate (PPi) in the presence of magnesium ion (Mg^{2+}). cGMP acts as an intracellular second messenger to effect smooth muscle relaxation.

feedback regulation of NO on its own biosynthesis. Both constitutive (cNOS) and inducible (iNOS) isoforms exist in mammalian cells. Calcium and calmodulin regulate cNOS, such that increases in intracellular free calcium from 0.1 to 1 μmol activate cNOS and turn on NO production. In contrast, iNOS is not regulated by calcium or calmodulin. The inducible isoform of NOS is important in mediating the cytotoxicity of macrophages, neutrophils, and hepatic Kupffer cells. Endotoxin, IL-1, TNF, and IFN-γ all can activate the synthesis of iNOS. Four to six hours later, detectable quantities of NO and L-citrulline are formed, reaching a maximum after about 24 hours. In the setting of septic shock, iNOS induction and NO production appear to mediate the profound vasodilation characteristic of this syndrome.

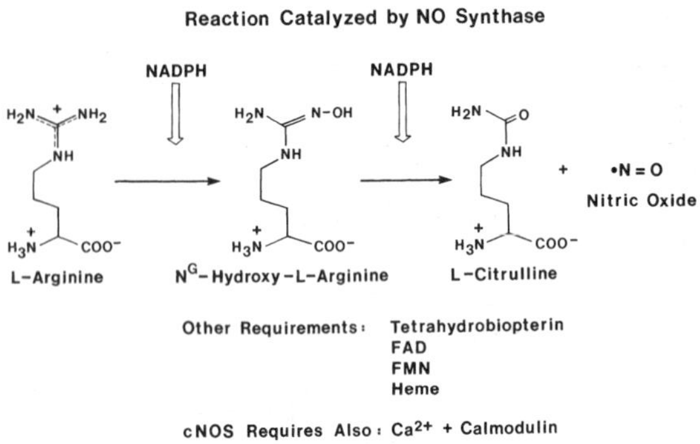

Reaction Catalyzed by NO Synthase

NADPH → NADPH

L-Arginine → N^G-Hydroxy-L-Arginine → L-Citrulline + •N = O Nitric Oxide

Other Requirements: Tetrahydrobiopterin
FAD
FMN
Heme

cNOS Requires Also: Ca^{2+} + Calmodulin

Figure 2–10. Characteristics of the biosynthesis of NO from L-arginine catalyzed by NO synthase. L-Arginine is a basic amino acid in which one of the two equivalent amino nitrogen atoms is oxidized and cleaved to yield NO (·N = O) plus L-citrulline. One of the reaction intermediates is known to be N^G-hydroxy-L-arginine. Nicotinamide-adenine dinucleotide phosphate (reduced form) (NADPH) is a required cofactor for the reaction as illustrated. Additional cofactors required for catalysis include tetrahydrobiopterin, flavin adenine dinucleotide (FAD), flavin mononucleotide (FMN), and heme, all of which function in electron transfer to accommodate the complicated five-electron oxidation of L-arginine to yield NO plus L-citrulline. Molecular oxygen is incorporated into both the NO and L-citrulline reaction products. Both the constitutive and inducible isoforms of NO synthase possess similar cofactor requirements. In addition, cNOS requires Ca^{2+} and calmodulin for enzyme activation.

Metabolism of Endogenous Nitric Oxide

Whereas the half-life of NO is 3 to 5 seconds in aqueous solutions, its biologic half-life is less than 1 second in tissues that contain biologic oxidants and oxyhemoproteins. This extreme chemical lability means that there is no need for complex enzymatic degradative or reuptake mechanisms for inactivation of NO. Its reactivity, coupled with its lipophilicity, means that NO readily elicits its effects in target cells adjacent to the cells of origin.

Physiologic and Pathophysiologic Roles of Nitric Oxide

The two most widely appreciated biologic roles for NO are vascular smooth muscle relaxation and inhibition of platelet-induced thrombosis. In vitro, acetylcholine interacts with muscarinic receptors on the extracellular surface of endothelial cells (EC) to trigger an increase in the concentration of intracellular free calcium, activating cNOS and producing NO. In flowing blood, tangential shear forces on vascular EC trigger NO synthesis, a process known as flow-dependent dilation. There may be a mechanoreceptor-coupled calcium channel responsible for the activation of cNOS in this setting. Electrical field stimulation also causes vascular smooth muscle relaxation in vitro. In vivo, autacoids such as bradykinin, histamine, and serotonin trigger NO production as well (Fig. 2–11).

Nitric oxide is also believed to retard or inhibit the proliferation of vascular smooth muscle cells. Activation of cytosolic guanylate cyclase by NO results in inhibition of thymidine incorporation into DNA in vascular smooth muscle cells in culture. Thus intact EC may retard or regulate proliferation of underlying smooth muscle cells; at sites of endothelial damage, such as an atherosclerotic plaque, smooth muscle hyperplasia may occur.

Nitric oxide–mediated neurotransmission may be a completely novel signal transduction mechanism in the nervous system. In the brain, glutamate-induced neuronal toxicity appears to occur as a result of stimulation of the local

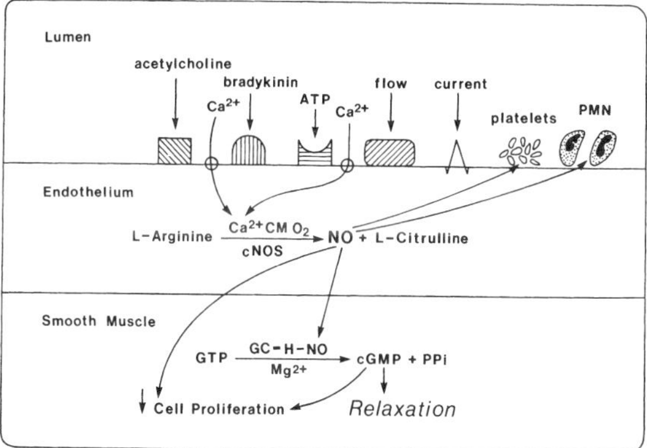

Figure 2–11. Multiple factors that stimulate formation of endothelium-derived NO and multiple vascular functions of endothelium-derived NO. Various chemical agents in the blood (acetylcholine, bradykinin, adenosine triphosphate [ATP]) as well as mechanical (flow) and electrical (current) forces can interact with selective membrane surface receptors to trigger the influx of Ca^{2+} into endothelial cells. Intracellular Ca^{2+} forms a complex with CM that is bound to cNOS. Oxygen is one of several requirements for catalysis. The NO generated diffuses in all directions. In the underlying smooth muscle, NO causes relaxation by cGMP-dependent mechanisms. NO forms a complex with heme (H) that is bound to GC, thereby causing enzyme activation and formation of cGMP plus PPi. NO also causes inhibition of smooth muscle cell proliferation, but the role of cGMP in this action of NO is unclear. At the luminal surface, NO interacts with platelets and polymorphonuclear leukocytes (PMN) to prevent both adhesion to the endothelial surface and cellular aggregation. These functions of NO are likely mediated by cGMP formed in the platelet and PMN.

production of NO. In a laboratory model of stroke, in which *N*-methyl-D-aspartate (NMDA) causes calcium-dependent, glutamate receptor–mediated neurotoxicity, the toxic action of NMDA was found to be mediated by NO and prevented by NO-synthase inhibitors.

PLATELET-ACTIVATING FACTOR IN SEPTIC SHOCK

Platelet-activating factor (PAF), characterized structurally as 1-O-alkyl-2(R)-acetyl-glycero-3-phosphocholine, is a potent phospholipid autacoid implicated in inflammation, ischemic disorders, and shock. It is produced by a variety of cells, including endothelial cells, neutrophils, platelets, monocytes, basophils, eosinophils, mast cells, and lymphocytes. Released from membrane phospholipids by activation of phospholipase A_2 (PLA_2), PAF mimics the shock state by producing hypotension, thrombocytopenia, myocardial depression, and multiple organ failure. Both animal and human data suggest huge increases in circulating nonpancreatic PLA_2 levels in the setting of septic shock. Endotoxin is a potent stimulus for PAF release and may produce many of its toxic effects through release of PAF. The primary target of PAF, but not its inactive metabolite lyso-PAF, is the endothelial cell (EC). PAF triggers the release of inositol triphosphate (IP_3), which modulates many calcium-dependent signals within cells.

Possible Mechanism of Platelet-Activating Factor–Induced Effects in Septic Shock

When activated by inflammatory stimuli, macrophages produce TNF-α and IL-1, which induce PAF synthesis in EC, neutrophils, and macrophages. Platelet-activating factor itself stimulates cytokine production, causing a positive feedback loop. In general, the cytokine/PAF interaction produces a bell-shaped concentration-effect curve. For example, after stimulatory agonist concentrations that usually produce a concentration-dependent increase in mediator release, a higher agonist concentration suppresses mediator release. PAF can thus exert down-regulatory effects on cytokine production.

Two inhibitors of PAF are BN 52021 and BN 50739, which demonstrated some protective efficacy in several animal models of septic shock, particularly in its later phases, and appear to decrease levels of circulating thromboxane A_2.

COLONY-STIMULATING FACTORS

Colony-stimulating factors (CSFs) are a family of glycoprotein hormones that potently regulate production and differentiation of hematopoietic cells. The CSFs comprise a complex family of cytokines, often referred to as hematopoietic growth factors. The nomenclature for the CSFs is arrived at by the generic CSF preceded by a prefix that indicates the main cell type stimulated by the specific CSF, e.g., G-CSF, which exerts its actions on the granulocyte lineage (Table 2–10).

Biology of Hematopoiesis

Hematopoiesis is a complex process that begins with an uncommitted pluripotent hematopoietic stem cell, which has the ability to self-renew, proliferate, and differentiate into all of the hematopoietic lineages. The ultimate result of this process is a mature, lineage-restricted circulating effector cell (Fig. 2–12). Each individual hematopoietic growth factor is coded for by a unique gene, many of which are located on chromosome 5 (which has also been implicated in myeloid leukemia and myelodysplastic syndromes).

General Properties of the Colony-Stimulating Factors

All the CSFs are glycoproteins in the 14 to 19 kD range. They are all monomeric proteins (except for M-CSF and IL-5, which are homodimers), and all are heavily glycosylated. They have high biologic activity, with concentrations in the picomolar range.

Granulocyte-Macrophage Colony–Stimulating Factor

Granulocyte-macrophage CSF (GM-CSF) enhances the effector function of mature neutrophils, eosinophils, and macrophage/monocytes, including augmentation of oxidative metabolism, chemotaxis, phagocytosis, leukotriene release, degranulation, and antibody-dependent cellular cytotoxicity. It also enhances macrophage antigen processing and cytokine production. Following GM-CSF administration in humans, there is a transient leukopenia (neutrophils, eosinophils, and monocytes) and pulmonary neutrophil sequestration, followed by a leukocytosis secondary to neutrophil demargination, increased marrow production, and increased circulating half-life.

GM-CSF has been used to treat refractory aplastic anemia, following bone marrow transplant, and in myelodysplastic syndrome. Therapy is generally well tolerated. Side effects include bone pain, myalgia, fever, rash, flushing, and elevated transaminases; a generalized capillary leak syndrome has been seen as well.

Granulocyte Colony-Stimulating Factor

Granulocyte CSF enhances mature neutrophil function. It is produced primarily by mature macrophages but is also produced by endothelial cells, fibroblasts, and mesothelial cells. Granulocyte CSF can be stimulated by TNF, endotoxin, IL-1, GM-CSF, IL-3, IL-4, and IFN-γ. Granulocyte CSF can produce a rapid release of bone marrow neutrophils into the circulation and reduce granulocyte maturation time. Additionally, it enhances the effector function of neutrophils (oxi-

Table 2–10. COLONY-STIMULATING FACTORS

Cytokine	Chomosome Location	Protein (kd)	Cellular Source	Progenitor Cell Target	Mature Effector Cell Target
G-CSF	17q11.22	18–22	Monocytes, fibroblasts, endothelial cells	CFU-GEMM, CFU-GM, CFU-G	Neutrophils
GM-CSF	5q21.32	14–35	T lymphocytes, monocytes, fibroblasts, endothelial cells, osteoblasts, smooth muscle cells, mast cells	CFU-GEMM, CFU-GM, CFU-G, BFU-E, BFU-Eo	Neutrophils, eosinophils, monocytes
M-CSF (CSF-1)	1	47–90	Fibroblasts, monocytes, endothelial cells, placenta	CFU-GM, CFU-M	Monocytes, neutrophils, eosinophils, basophils
(MGF, SCF, SLF, KL)	12q14.3	26	Fibroblasts, endothelial cells	PPSC, CFU-GEMM	No known effects
IL-1-α IL-β	2q13 2q14	17 17	Monocytes, lymphocytes, neutrophils	PPSC, lymphoid stem cell	Monocytes, lymphocytes, neutrophils, osteoclasts, endothelial cells, hepatocytes

IL-3 (multi-CSF)	5q23.31	28	T lymphocytes, monocytes	PPSC, CFU-GEMM, CFU-GM, CFU-M, CFU-G, CFU-Baso, CFU-Meg, CFU-Eo, BFU-E, CFU-E	Eosinophils, neutrophils, basophils, monocytes
IL-6 (INF-β-2) BSF-2)	7p15	19–26	T lymphocytes, B cells, monocytes, fibroblasts, endothelial cells	PPSC, CFU-GEMM, CFU-GM, BFU-E	B cells T cells
I-11		20	Fibroblasts, endothelial cells	CFU-GEMM, BFU-E, CFU-G, CFU-Meg, CFU-E	Platelets
EPO	7	14–39	Renal tubular cells, hepatocytes	CFU-GEMM, BFU-E, CFU-E	

Abbreviations: CSF = colony-stimulating factor; SCF = stem cell factor; G = granulocyte; M = macrophage; MGF = mast cell growth factor; SLF = steel factor; KL = *Kit* ligand; IL = interleukin; EPO = erythropoietin; CFU = colony-forming unit; GEMM = granulocyte, erythrocyte, macrophage, megakaryocyte; PPSC = pluripotent hematopoietic stem cell; Baso = basophil; Meg = megakaryocyte; E = erythrocyte; Eo = eosinophil; BSF = B cell–stimulating factor.

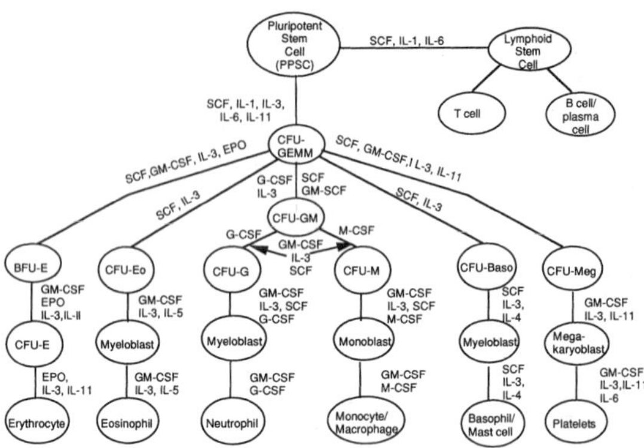

Figure 2–12. Colony-stimulating factors in hematopoiesis. *Abbreviations:* SCF = stem cell factor; IL = interleukin; CSF = colony-stimulating factor; CFU = colony-forming unit; GEMM = granulocyte, erythrocyte, macrophage, and megakaryocyte; GM = granulocyte-macrophage; G = granulocyte; M = macrophage; Eo = eosinophil; Baso = basophil; Meg = megakaryocyte; BFU-E = burst-forming unit–erythroid; EPO = erythropoietin.

dative metabolism, chemotaxis, and phagocytosis). It is well tolerated; the most common side effect is bone pain. Granulocyte CSF treatment shortens the duration and depth of neutropenia in patients receiving chemotherapy, resulting in a decreased incidence of fever and infection, a reduced use of antibiotics, and a reduced hospital stay. A number of animal studies have demonstrated improved survival in infection and sepsis when animals are treated with G-CSF and antibiotics versus antibiotics alone.

Erythropoietin

Erythropoietin (EPO) is a sialoglycoprotein hormone that regulates red blood cell production (erythropoiesis). Ninety percent of EPO is produced by the kidney and ten percent by the liver, in response to anemia or hypoxemia. Human recombinant EPO was first used in patients with chronic renal failure and has since been used in the setting of AIDS, cancer, and preoperative collection of autologous blood for elective surgery. Hypertension has been one of the few side effects noted.

Macrophage Colony-Stimulating Factor

Macrophage CSF was the first myeloid CSF to be defined and was originally called CSF-1. T lymphocytes do not produce M-CSF, unlike other myeloid CSFs. In addition to its hematopoietic effects, it also enhances the effector function of mature macrophages and monocytes. Macrophage CSF enhances intracellular killing of *Mycobacterium avium-intra-*

cellulare and *Candida albicans* and stimulates production and release of cytokines, eicosanoids, and superoxide dismutase. Dose-related thrombocytopenia has been observed, and a study of M-CSF in the setting of invasive fungal disease is under way.

Multicolony-Stimulating Factor/Interleukin-3

IL-3 has a broad range of target cells and synergy with other growth factors. IL-3 is currently being studied in myelodysplastic syndrome. It is unique in that it also induces megakaryopoiesis. Hematopoietic synergy also exists among other cytokines such as IL-1, IL-6, and stem cell factor (SCF).

CHAPTER 3

Monitoring

Charles F. Chandler, M.D. • Kenneth Waxman, M.D.

INTRAVASCULAR ACCESS AND LONG-TERM CATHETER MAINTENANCE

Vascular access is often essential for monitoring and treating critically ill patients. This section describes principles of catheter maintenance as well as the prevention, recognition, and management of complications.

Intravenous Access

Insertion of Peripheral Vein Conduits

Peripheral veins can be distended by appropriate application of a tourniquet prior to attempting cannulation. In a nonurgent setting, the site should be shaved and prepared with an iodine antiseptic solution and sterilely draped. After catheter insertion, the skin site should be covered with a clean dressing and checked daily. Peripheral intravenous access sites often become thrombosed within 4 days. To decrease the incidence of infection, the Centers for Disease Control and Prevention recommends changing peripheral access sites every 3 days. The possibility of septic thrombophlebitis must be kept in mind during fever work-up of hospitalized patients; thus all intravenous sites must be regularly examined.

Insertion of Central Venous Catheters

There are several possible approaches to cannulation of the superior vena cava; these are via the infraclavicular approach to the subclavian vein, the supraclavicular approach to the subclavian vein, and cannulation of the internal jugular vein. The superior vena cava can also be cannulated via an external jugular approach; this is particularly useful in patients with bleeding diathesis. The subclavian and internal jugular approaches are preferred for long-term central venous catheterization. The placement of a femoral venous line can provide rapid access and large-bore cannulation to provide rapid resuscitation. Although useful in the emergency situation, these lines are more prone to infection and thus should be removed after other access has been established.

Table 3–1 lists the relative merits of various central venous approaches. In general, the high internal jugular approach yields a somewhat lower success rate with regard to cannulation but has a decreased risk of hemothorax or pneumothorax as opposed to other superior vena cava approaches; however, the possibility of pneumothorax must still be kept in mind. Anterior, central, and posterior approaches to the internal jugular vein are reviewed in the *Textbook*. The internal jugular vein is usually deep to the belly of the sternoclei-

Table 3–1. RELATIVE MERITS OF ROUTES OF CENTRAL VENOUS ACCESS

Route	Advantages	Potential Problems
External Jugular	Preferred route if coagulopathy is present No risk of pneumothorax No risk of arterial puncture	High failure rate of access to central circulation (up to 50%) Difficult if patient is obese or edematous Patient discomfort
Internal Jugular	Second choice if coagulopathy is present Pneumothorax rare if high IJ approach	Poor landmarks if patient is obese or edematous Carotid puncture possible Brain infarction secondary to carotid injury or venous thrombosis Needle injury to trachea, esophagus, phrenic or vagus nerve Difficult access/catheter care if tracheostomy is present Patient discomfort
Infraclavicular	Anatomic landmarks constant High success rate Most patient comfort Ease of long-term catheter maintenance	Pneumothorax 2%–5%, highest in cachectic patients Poor control of bleeding if arterial puncture or coagulopathy Brachial plexus injury by needle stick or hematoma
Supraclavicular	Anatomic landmarks constant High success rate	Pneumothorax Poor control of bleeding if arterial puncture or coagulopathy Brachial plexus injury by needle or hematoma Patient discomfort Risk of chylothorax (left side)
Femoral	High success rate Can be placed despite ongoing CPR, intubation, or tracheostomy Second choice if coagulopathy is present	Risk of infection Occult retroperitoneal hemorrhage if above inguinal ligament

domastoid muscle, lateral to the carotid artery. In all internal jugular approaches, inadvertent cannulation of the carotid artery is possible. Although dissection or thrombosis is rare, it can be catastrophic. The operator must always palpate and be aware of the position of the carotid pulsation prior to attempting venous cannulation. Internal jugular approaches are in general preferred to subclavian approaches in patients with coagulation or platelet defects; with severe coagulopathy, the external jugular approach to central cannulation is the safest, but the rate of successful cannulation of the superior vena cava via this approach is only approximately 50%. The subclavian vein can also be approached by either the supraclavicular or infraclavicular approach, as detailed in the *Textbook.*

Subclavian cannulation is better tolerated in terms of patient comfort and catheter maintenance than are jugular approaches. Radiographs should be obtained routinely after internal jugular or subclavian approaches to assess tip placement and rule out pneumothorax. In all internal jugular and subclavian approaches, proper patient positioning, including the Trendelenburg position to increase venous distention and therefore increase the rate of success as well as decrease air embolization, must be stressed. Additionally, proper sterile technique, including gown, mask and gloves in nonemergency situations, is important for minimizing line sepsis. Whenever difficulty is encountered in any given approach in cannulating the vein, a second approach should be used or more experienced help should be obtained. It is convenient to prepare the infraclavicular, supraclavicular, and internal jugular access sites in the original sterile field.

The femoral approach is usually reserved for establishment of rapid access in emergency situations or when the superior vena cava sites are exhausted. The site of needle tip cannulation of the femoral vein must be below the inguinal ligament; otherwise, occult life-threatening retroperitoneal hemorrhage can occur.

Venous Cannulation by Cutdowns

When percutaneous establishment of venous cannulation is not safe due to severe coagulation defects, when percutaneous attempts fail, or for establishment of reliable rapid access, cutdown techniques can be employed to expose veins for direct cannulation with catheters, or directly with IV tubing. Again, if emergency lines are placed in this manner without meticulous sterile technique, these must be removed when other access is established. When used in emergency situations, it is stressed that a senior operator be available for assistance and that the primary surgeon has adequate experience in this technique prior to being primarily responsible for it in the emergency situation. With regard to emergency fluid resuscitation, the largest diameter and shortest catheter must be used, as flow is inversely related to catheter length and is also inverse to the third power of the radius of the cannula. IV tubing can be used in a saphenous vein cutdown. If the vein diameter will not allow this, 14-gauge cannulas can be used. The same principles apply in percutaneously achieved venous cannulation in emergency situations; introducer sheaths work well for rapid resuscitation via the femoral approach.

Complications of Intravenous Access

There are several risks in placement and maintenance of central venous access. Proper patient positioning and meticulous sterile technique are essential to minimize these risks. Table 30–5 in the *Textbook* delineates risk factors; Table 30–7 outlines risks of complications with regard to various placement approaches. Table 3–2 here summarizes these findings.

Inadvertent Arterial Puncture

Inadvertent arterial puncture can occur in any approach to central venous cannulation. The risk of this complication in most series is approximately 2%. Awareness of this possibility, prompt recognition should it occur, and application of

Table 3–2. RISK FACTORS IN CENTRAL VENOUS CATHETERIZATION

Inadvertent Arterial Puncture
- Hypertension
- Coagulopathy
- Long and large-bore needles
- Inexperienced operator
- Poor patient positioning
- Hypovolemia

Inadvertent Puncture of Lung Apex
- Emaciation
- Obesity
- Pulmonary disease (apical blebs, COPD, TB)
- Mechanical ventilation with high PEEP/tidal volume

Air Embolus
- Inappropriate patient position
- Hypovolemia/low venous pressure
- Accidental disconnection/opening system to air, especially if patient is upright
- Labored inspiratory effort
- On removal of catheter if patient is upright/hypovolemic

Catheter-Related Infection
- Contaminated insertion or maintenance
- Prolonged catheter use
- Immunocompromised patient
- Malignancy

Thrombosis
- Catheter malposition
- Hypercoagulable state
- Long-term catheterization
- Irritative catheter or infusion

Accidental Removal
- Restless/uncooperative patient
- Inexperienced patient care or transportation
- Inadequately secured, or suture too tight/necrosis at skin

Catheter Erosion of Vessel
- Tip at right angle to vessel wall
- Stiff catheters

pressure should it occur are essential. With subclavian approaches, significant or even life-threatening hemorrhage can occur. It is preferable to correct coagulopathy and severe thrombocytopenia prior to placement of these catheters. If not possible, alternative approaches should be used.

The carotid artery can be inadvertently punctured during attempted internal jugular vein cannulation. The seriousness of this complication is diminished if this is done with a 19-gauge finder needle only and not a larger-bore cannula. It is sometimes difficult to distinguish arterial versus venous blood; if there is any question, differentiation should be made by arterial blood gas determination or pressure tracing prior to dilating the vessel and placement of the large-bore cannula.

Lymphatic Duct Puncture

Lymphatic duct puncture at the thoracic outlet during cannulation of either internal jugular or subclavian veins can occur. This most commonly occurs when the supraclavicular approach is used to the left subclavian vein. It can be recognized by the aspiration of clear or milky fluid. It may not be recognized until later with leakage of clear or milky fluid around the catheter. If this should occur, removal of the catheter and application of a pressure dressing are indicated.

Pneumothorax

The overall risk of pneumothorax when placing superior vena cava lines via the internal jugular or subclavian approach is approximately 2%. This risk is somewhat diminished by the internal jugular versus subclavian approach, especially with high internal jugular venous approaches. The risk of this complication is increased in obese patients and is very much increased in cachectic patients. This is due to the loss of the fat pad between the dome of the pleura and the subclavian vessels in the cachectic patient. Pneumothorax may be recognized by aspiration of air in the syringe when attempting to find the vein. Clinically significant pneumothorax or tension pneumothorax is rare unless the patient is on positive-pressure ventilation. It is, however, possible to have significant hemodynamic compromise in this situation demanding definitive therapy prior to radiographic confirmation of the diagnosis.

Clinical as well as radiographic follow-up of all patients is essential after internal jugular or subclavian lines have been placed. A small pneumothorax (< 10%) may be followed expectantly, particularly if the patient is not on positive-pressure ventilation. Oxygen supplementation by nasal cannula or mask may aid in the washout of nitrogen and subsequent resolution of pneumothorax. Insertion of a thoracic vent with a one-way valve or placement of a chest tube may be required if a pneumothorax persists or increases. Treatment is particularly important if the patient is or will be placed on positive-pressure ventilation, as this may initiate tension pneumothorax.

Air Embolus

Air embolus is another potential and dangerous complication of central venous catheter placement. Most air emboli occur during the puncture of the vein and initial catheterization. They can also occur by inadvertently disconnecting existing central venous catheters open to air, or during catheter removal. Proper position of the patient (Trendelenburg) is important when placing catheters in the IJ or subclavian position, and it is preferable during their removal as well.

Malposition of Catheters

Catheter tips can inadvertently pass up the neck from the subclavian approach or out the arm from the internal jugular approach. The patient may complain of pain near the ear on the affected side should the wire pass up the neck. This can be minimized by proper positioning of the patient, including turning the head away from the side of venous puncture prior to beginning, and attention to the position of the bevel of the catheter as well as the curvature of the J wire in a direction toward the heart. Wires should be withdrawn back into the needle, and attempts should be made to reposition prior to placing the catheter should the patient complain of pain in and around the ear. Malpositioned catheters have an increased incidence of thrombosis as well as catheter erosion through the vessel wall. Correct position should be verified radiologically prior to use. If there is persistent malpositioning of the catheter despite the preceding maneuvers, the guidewire and catheter may need to be repositioned under fluoroscopic guidance, while maintaining meticulous sterile technique.

Extravascular Catheter Tip Malpositions

Extravascular catheter tip malposition in soft tissues, pleural space, or peritoneal cavity can occur from perforation of vessels during insertion. Perforations can also occur later by erosion when the tip is against the wall of the vessel, especially by catheters inserted from the left side and with stiff catheters, sometimes with disastrous results. Tips identified to be resting at right angles to the central veins should be withdrawn into better positions or replaced. Subclavian or internal jugular dialysis catheters or other central venous catheters are rarely placed inadvertently into the pleural space. This should be recognized by failure to obtain aspiration blood flow through the finder needle and catheter. This possibility reemphasizes the need for radiologic confirmation of placement prior to use of these catheters.

Catheter-Induced Coagulation and Thrombosis

Intravascular catheters induce clot formation to a variable extent, depending on factors related both to the individual catheter and to the patient's state of coagulability. Larger and more rigid catheters induce a greater degree of clot formation. Long-term use also increases the risk of thrombosis, and with long-term use and multiple catheters all accessible veins may become thrombosed. In patients with hypercoagulability states, anticoagulation therapy may prolong the duration of venous patency.

Neurologic Complications

Peripheral nerves and ganglia in proximity to veins can be injured directly, or indirectly by the pressure of hematoma resulting from inadvertent arterial puncture. Central nervous system complications can also result from venous thrombosis originating from internal jugular thrombosis or from injury to the carotid artery during attempts at placement of internal jugular catheters.

Catheter and Guide Wire Embolism

Two principles need to be observed to avoid these complications. First, never force a catheter or guide wire through a needle when undue resistance has been encountered during advancement. Second, never pull out a catheter or guide wire that has been forced in and does not come out easily. If this should occur, the needle is first pulled back. If the catheter or guide wire still resists removal, operative removal by exposure of the resistant site must be attempted. Additionally, when placing catheters by the Seldinger technique, it is essential to control the guide wire either proximally or at the skin site at all times. If embolization of the guide wire or a catheter fragment occurs, it may be retrieved using invasive radiologic techniques.

Infection

The risk of catheter-related infection can be reduced, but not eliminated, by rigorous sterile technique in placement and proper catheter care. Protocols should be used that stress routine changes of central venous catheters every 5 to 7 days and routine changes of PA catheters every 3 to 5 days. It remains controversial, however, whether frequent changes of lines decrease the overall long-term infectious complication rate. Overall duration of central venous catheterization does correlate with risk of line-associated infectious complication. Some centers utilize routine catheter changes over a guide wire; this reduces the number of catheter placement complications (as opposed to placing all catheters at new sites), but it is not as effective in reducing the rate of catheter-associated infections, and it may be no more effective than leaving catheters in place with regard to infection. Line-related sepsis or positive blood cultures are absolute indications for changing all central venous and arterial lines. Table 3–3 outlines other factors related to increased risk of catheter-associated infections.

Pulmonary Artery Catheters

The pulmonary artery balloon-tipped (Swan-Ganz) catheter provides many hemodynamic measurements useful in the

Table 3–3. FACTORS RELATED TO CATHETER-ASSOCIATED INFECTIONS

Prolonged catheter use
Poor sterile technique in insertion or maintenance
Insertion under emergency conditions or during operative interventions
Intravenous tubing or fluids exposed to unsterile technique
Sutures too tight at insertion site with local tissue necrosis
Insertion close to infected or contaminated sources
Short distance between skin and vein puncture sites
Immune deficiency
Advanced cancer

management of critically ill patients. With regard to placement, several technical factors merit discussion.

Strict sterile technique must be adhered to when placing pulmonary arterial catheters, including widely draped and prepped fields, as well as use of sterile gloves, a cap, and mask by the operator. Either the internal jugular or subclavian approach is used. Again, proper positioning of the patient, including Trendelenburg position, with the head turned away from the side of line placement and a shoulder roll placed prior to beginning the procedure, is important. The femoral approach may also be useful if neither jugular nor subclavian access is feasible.

Once a 16-gauge catheter is successfully introduced into the vein, a guide wire should be advanced only 20 to 25 cm to avoid disturbance of cardiac rhythm. A cardiac monitor should be continuously observed during this maneuver; any change in ventricular rhythm must be followed by immediate withdrawal of the wire until the rhythm is restored. Once the wire is in place the catheter is withdrawn, and a small skin incision is made prior to advancing an introducer (dilator) over the guide wire. If the introducer is easily advanced over the guide wire it is then withdrawn, care being taken always to control the guide wire. The sheath is then placed over the introducer and these are advanced together over the wire, again taking care to neither lose control of the wire nor advance it too far during these maneuvers. The introducer and sheath are then fully advanced, and the introducer and wire subsequently removed.

Prior to inserting the PA catheter an assistant should flush the catheter and test the balloon, and proper function of the monitor should be insured by reviewing tracings as the catheter is manipulated prior to insertion. The catheter should be advanced with the balloon deflated to 15 to 20 cm in adults prior to inflating the balloon. The catheter is then advanced and pressure tracings observed during this maneuver. Right atrial, right ventricular, and finally PA tracings should be observed, and finally the catheter should advance to a wedge position. The balloon is deflated after reaching the wedge position, and the tracing must revert to a PA tracing to ensure proper placement; this avoids the possibility of pulmonary infarction due to excessively distal tip position "overwedging." Additionally, the tip placement must be verified by chest radiograph after placement of the catheter. Again, care should be taken to avoid placement too distal.

Complications of Pulmonary Artery Catheters

Technical complications specific to PA catheters include failure to pass the catheter, especially in patients in shock and low-flow states. Ventricular tachyarrhythmias can occur, usually when the tip of the catheter is in the right ventricle; this demands that the catheter be withdrawn into the superior vena cava and repositioned. Rare complications of PA catheters include knotting of the catheter or rupture of pulmonary arteries. Catheters should never be withdrawn with the balloon inflated. If there is any resistance to withdrawing catheters, they should not be forced, as they can, rarely, become ensnared and knotted in cardiac valves or chordae. Finally, PA catheters should not be kept in place more than 5 days, to minimize infection rates; if continuing PA catheter monitoring is necessary, a new catheter should be placed through a new site.

The incidence of catheter tip erosion through a PA vessel wall may be reduced by using soft and pliable catheters. A sheath is best used as the conduit for Swan-Ganz catheterization; it can also be used for a conduit for rapid or emergency resuscitation; it should not be left in place following cessation of Swan-Ganz monitoring or acute resuscitation.

Insertion of central venous and PA catheters is contraindicated in patients with severe coagulation defects. Coagulation defects and severe thrombocytopenia should be corrected if possible prior to catheter placement. In the emergency situation, catheterization via an external jugular or femoral approach can be attempted.

If atrial or ventricular arrhythmias occur during catheter placement, the wire or Swan-Ganz catheter should be withdrawn back into the superior vena cava position, taking care to deflate the balloon of the Swan-Ganz catheter. Such withdrawal will lead to cessation of most ventricular arrhythmias; rarely lidocaine or defibrillation is necessary.

Finally, hypovolemia or low-flow states may greatly increase the difficulty of floating the Swan-Ganz catheter to a proper position. Additionally, acutely hypovolemic and acidemic patients are at increased risk of arrhythmias during Swan-Ganz placement. Patients should thus always have acute resuscitation initiated prior to placement of Swan-Ganz catheters.

Arterial Cannulation

Accessible arteries for cannulation include the radial, dorsalis pedis, femoral, brachial, and axillary arteries in the adult, and the umbilical artery in the newborn. The radial artery is used most frequently because cannulation and maintenance are easy to achieve. Before cannulation of the radial artery, the adequacy of ulnar palmar circulation must be assessed by the Allen test. If the patient does not have adequate collateral flow, the radial artery on that side should never be cannulated, as distal ischemia can be catastrophic in this setting. In the absence of collateral circulation to either hand, the dorsalis pedis is the second choice. Femoral arterial catheterization is possible but less desirable due to infectious complications and, rarely, ischemic complications. The axillary artery can be cannulated safely by those experienced in this technique; distal ischemic sequelae are rare (due to collateral flow around the shoulder) but can be catastrophic. Because of the higher risk of distal ischemia, brachial artery catheterization should not be used unless other sites are exhausted or unobtainable.

PHYSIOLOGIC MONITORING (INVASIVE AND NONINVASIVE)

Physiologic monitoring allows recognition of and response to treatment of physiologic derangements. The extent of monitoring necessary is dictated by the risk of a given patient and a given physiologic insult, as well as clues obtained by less invasive monitoring. Discovery of physiologic derangements can lead to institution of early corrective therapy, as well as ongoing corrective therapy in severely ill patients. Serial measurements can provide the temporal pattern of acute circulatory problems, as well as the responses to therapeutic interventions. Finally, monitored circulatory and physiologic values of survivors may be useful in guiding therapy of future patients.

The uncomplicated elective surgical patient is often monitored postoperatively by vital signs, urine output, serial hemoglobin or hematocrit levels if significant blood loss is a possibility, arterial blood gas determination, and electrocardiogram and central venous pressure monitoring in older patients or those with known cardiac disease or suspected intraoperative cardiac events. More extensive invasive hemodynamic and oxygen transport monitoring may be used pre- and postoperatively in evaluation of high-risk surgical patients; in patients with suspected acute circulatory compromise based on less invasive monitoring; in patients with myocardial infarction, sepsis, or blood loss; in patients with major chest, abdominal, or head trauma; and most importantly to direct therapy in patients with acute or persistent shock syndromes and other life-threatening conditions. Criteria for defining high-risk surgical patients are delineated in Table 31–1 of the *Textbook*.

Invasive hemodynamic and oxygen transport monitoring can identify correctable physiologic deficiencies in their early stages. A high index of suspicion in appropriate patients and recognition of derangements of values given by less invasive monitoring are useful guides to initiate invasive hemodynamic and oxygen transport monitoring. This information can then identify correctable physiologic deficiencies in the early stages and provide the basis for initiation of therapy. This next section summarizes various circulatory parameters from routine, noninvasive surveillance and screening techniques to invasive hemodynamic and oxygen transport monitoring methods.

Vital Signs

Arterial pressure, heart rate, temperature, and respiratory rate are the so-called vital signs and are the simplest, most easily, and most commonly monitored noninvasive circulatory variables. These measurements, along with hemoglobin and urine output, may serve as adequate screening tools for routine postoperative patients. If these measurements identify unexpected derangements, or if modest changes in vital signs do not respond in the expected fashion to therapy, more invasive monitoring should be instituted.

Arterial pressure measurements do not directly reflect changes in blood flow or volume status. Rather, changes in arterial blood pressure reflect the failure of circulatory compensations if derangements of blood flow or volume status have occurred. Changes in arterial pressure may be particularly late in an otherwise healthy young patient. If arterial blood pressure falls, however, it may serve as a clue to blood or fluid loss, cardiac failure, or the onset of sepsis. If postoperative or post-traumatic hypotension is not easily explained and does not respond immediately to simple therapeutic measures, it demands further evaluation and more invasive monitoring and therapy.

Normal arterial blood pressure is age dependent and is approximately 120/80 mm Hg for young healthy adults; this value gradually increases with age. It may be lower in teenage females, who may normally have a blood pressure as low as 90/60 mm Hg. Such a pressure, however, must not be assumed to be normal in a trauma or postoperative patient, or if sepsis is a possibility, until other explanations are ruled out. Additionally, it is important to remember that in surgical intensive care unit patients and in other postoperative surgical patients, changes in blood pressure may reflect a wide range of physiologic derangements; identification and treatment of these physiologic derangements are needed, as opposed to merely titrating blood pressure to desired values.

Mean arterial pressure is defined as the sum of the diastolic pressure plus one third of the pulse pressure. Mean arterial pressure is also measured directly in various invasive and noninvasive recording systems. Although differences in systolic and diastolic pressures may exist between cuff pressures and arterial line pressures, if each system is properly calibrated the mean arterial blood pressure should be identical.

Indications for continuous arterial pressure measurements via an indwelling arterial catheter include shock, hemorrhage, critical illness, and intraoperative and postoperative monitoring when values may change quickly and demand rapid titration of therapy. Likewise, arterial catheters can be useful if frequent arterial blood gas determinations are required.

In shock and trauma patients, arterial pressure decreases only after compensatory mechanisms are exhausted; this may occur long after the precipitating event. Severely reduced cardiac output for prolonged periods may exist prior to significant reduction in arterial pressure, particularly in young patients. Additionally, arterial pressure may be restored by saline or another crystalloid solution well before cardiac output and oxygen transport are corrected. A high index of suspicion must be maintained in these patients and more definitive physiologic values obtained if significant derangements are a possibility.

Heart Rate

Heart rate is likewise a nonspecific hemodynamic variable. However, increases in heart rate may occur prior to changes in blood pressure in response to a multitude of stressors. In surgical patients, increases in heart rate may reflect changes in blood flow or blood volume deficits; but the rate may also increase with infection, anxiety, pain, fever, delirium tremens, and other nonspecific stressors. Again, significant increases in heart rate may or may not reflect significant physiologic derangements; this always demands reevaluation by the physician.

Bradycardia of less than 50 beats per minute may be a response to inferior myocardial infarction, may be secondary to vasovagal response (acute gastric or bladder distention), or may be normal. Changes in rate are more important diagnostic clues than is any given absolute value.

Temperature

Body temperature may be assessed orally, rectally, or with a central core determination. Pulmonary arterial temperature, reflecting core temperature, is provided on a continuous basis by pulmonary artery thermodilution catheters.

An elevated temperature is often a clue to an infectious source but may also be a response to tissue necrosis, malignancy, hyperthyroidism, malignant hyperthermia, intracranial bleeds, or systemic inflammatory response (sepsis syndrome). Elevated temperature should alert the clinician to search for an infectious focus, although fever does not always represent an infectious source. Low-grade fever often results from atelectasis in surgical patients, but it can also result from surgical trauma, retroperitoneal or other hematomas, foreign bodies, fistulas, or urinary extravasation.

Hypothermia may occur in some patients with septic shock, hypothyroidism, malnutrition, severe anemia, and cold exposure. Like arterial pressure and heart rate determination, temperature measurement is a useful but nonspecific screening test.

Hemoglobin and Hematocrit

Serial hemoglobin or hematocrit determination is a useful screening test for hemorrhage in postoperative patients; it is also sometimes useful but not sensitive as an indicator of acute hemorrhage in the trauma patient. Additionally, serial determinations are important in patients with consumption coagulopathies, as well as in optimizing hemoglobin concentration to improve oxygen delivery in critically ill or septic patients.

A decreased percentage of red blood cells is an indirect effect of blood loss produced by compensatory transcapillary refilling of plasma volume by interstitial water. This compensation takes a considerable and variable amount of time to occur. If a patient rapidly exsanguinates within a few minutes, the first and last drops of blood may have nearly the same hematocrit. Additionally, serial hemoglobin or hematocrit determinations cannot distinguish among the conflicting effects of fluids administered intravenously, compensatory movement of interstitial water into the plasma space, red cell transfusion, or red cells dropping out of circulation via formation of cell aggregates or microthrombi. Thus while rapid drops in serial hemoglobin or hematocrit determinations may be an important clue to rapid occult hemorrhage, stable hemoglobin or hematocrit determinations over a short period of time do not exclude rapid hemorrhage.

Urine Output

In low-risk routine postoperative surgical patients, urine output is a moderately sensitive indicator of adequate volume status and renal perfusion. Unexpected diminution of urine output may serve as a guide to occult hemorrhage or third spacing of fluids, may serve as a clue to technical problems such as anastomotic leaks, or may herald the onset of sepsis. Decreased urine output in such a patient should prompt a search for causes; this should include careful examination of the patient and hemoglobin determination and often includes assessment with central catheterization if volume status is uncertain. Patients should not be treated with diuretics solely to maintain urine output unless hypovolemia, sepsis, and other possible etiologies have been ruled out.

Reestablishment of normal urine output in a moderately injured patient or in an otherwise healthy postoperative patient can serve as a useful guide to adequacy of volume resuscitation. In the multiply injured trauma patient or other severely ill patient, however, urine output is an unreliable indicator of volume status. Such patients may have low urine output reflecting oliguric acute tubular necrosis despite high filling pressures; may have normal outputs with nonoliguric renal failure, again not reflecting volume status; or may have high urine output secondary to nonoliguric ATN, glucosuria, or diabetes insipidus, regardless of volume status. These patients require invasive monitoring of volume status with a CVP catheter, and often require ascertaining and manipulating of cardiac output, oxygen delivery, and oxygen consumption with a Swan-Ganz catheter. Likewise, renal function in these patients must be assessed with BUN, creatinine, and solute fractional excretion values rather than assuming urine output to reflect renal function.

Electrocardiographic Monitoring

ECG measures voltages at the body surface that reflect electromechanical events of cardiac contraction. The standard 3-lead ECG is recorded from the right arm (RA), left arm (LA), and left leg (LL). The standard limb leads are defined as lead I (LA-RA), lead II (LL-RA), and lead III (LL-LA). Frequently, lead II or other individual leads may be continuously monitored for arrhythmias. The ECG is probably overused and overemphasized in patients with noncardiac general surgical conditions. However, a 12-lead ECG and continuous monitoring are important in patients with known cardiac disease, especially with new onset or history of arrhythmias, and they are useful to rule out cardiac complications in severely injured patients and patients with sepsis. Continuous ECG monitoring is also essential with acute myocardial infarction because arrhythmias are the most common life-threatening complications. Finally, in hypovolemic and traumatic shock, arrhythmias, signs of subendocardial ischemia, and bradycardia may reflect inadequate myocardial oxygen delivery and may portend a precardiac arrest state.

Assessment of Serum Electrolytes and Blood Chemistries

In acute illness, postoperatively, and in trauma patients, serum electrolyte levels are routinely checked. This is particularly important in patients at risk of arrhythmias from hypokalemia, such as from GI losses, alkalosis, or high urine output. Hyperkalemia must be ruled out in patients with acidosis and renal failure, or in patients with massive tissue destruction, such as tumor lysis, burns, crush injuries, or massive hemolysis, or following administration of paralyzing muscle relaxants. Blood glucose should be checked serially in patients with diabetes, severe metabolic stressors, trauma, infections, steroid therapy, or sepsis. Hyperglycemia developing in a previously stable patient may be an important clue to occult infection or worsening sepsis. BUN and creatinine should be checked frequently in patients at risk for developing renal failure. Magnesium levels should be checked particularly in stressed patients with a history of malnutrition, malabsorption, prolonged diarrhea, or chronic alcohol abuse. Calcium levels should be followed closely in patients with severe acute pancreatitis, as well as in patients who have undergone multiple blood transfusions. Hypophosphatemia may develop in patients with acute tubular necrosis or overwhelming sepsis, or during institution of nutritional support in malnourished patients.

In otherwise well, routine postoperative surgical patients without specific risk factors, electrolytes need be checked only once postoperatively and then every other day until the patient resumes oral intake, assuming intravenous therapy in the interim has been appropriate.

Coagulation Factors

Prothrombin time and partial thromboplastin time should be checked in patients in whom a bleeding disorder is suspected, or in patients who have received more than 6 units of packed red blood cells with a risk of ongoing bleeding. If significant derangements exist, treatment with fresh-frozen plasma should be undertaken only if ongoing bleeding is probable. The most frequent causes of coagulation defects after major surgery, trauma, or blood transfusions are hypothermia and thrombocytopenia; these too must be corrected if ongoing bleeding is present. Hypothermia should be anticipated during major surgery and in major trauma, but it can be avoided in large part by use of warming blankets, warming inspired gases, heating the room, and warming intravenous fluids. Fibrinogen, fibrin split products, and platelet counts should be followed closely in patients with or at risk of disseminated intravascular coagulation. Platelet counts should also be followed regularly in patients exposed to heparin, as heparin-induced thrombocytopenia is not uncommon. Therapeutic goals are cessation of ongoing hemorrhage or support of the patient with ongoing intravascular coagulation, not normalization of hematologic values.

Central Venous Pressure

Because of its simplicity and availability, CVP monitoring is routinely used to guide fluid therapy after hemorrhage, surgical trauma, sepsis, and other emergency situations associated with blood volume deficits. It is important to establish a consistent and accurate zeroing to permit meaningful interpretation of values. A point 10 cm above the lowest surface of the back or 10 cm below the sternum in the sixth interspace in a supine position roughly reflects the site of entrance of the SVC into the right atrium. This should always be recalibrated if the bed is raised or lowered.

Average CVP values during normal inspiration in a healthy person are −2 mm Hg to +6 mm Hg. Eight to 10 mm Hg is commonly used as the upper limit of normal for acutely ill patients. However, CVP is affected not only by blood volume but also by venous compliance, right heart chamber compliance, tricuspid valvular disease, right heart failure, and intrathoracic and intra-abdominal pressures. Patients under mechanical ventilation with high mean intrathoracic pressures and positive end-expiratory pressure (PEEP) will have falsely elevated CVP readings. Likewise, patients after major abdominal surgery or trauma with high intra-abdominal pressure can have falsely elevated CVP readings with respect to the true intravascular volume. Thus if patients do not have favorable results with regard to heart rate, blood pressure, urine output, and other assessments after volume replacement using CVP as a guide to therapy, many critically ill patients require placement of a Swan-Ganz catheter to assess left heart filling pressure, cardiac output, and oxygen delivery, as detailed later in this chapter.

Arterial Blood Gases and pH

Measurements of arterial blood gases and pH are useful to screen and assess pulmonary function, in following therapy in patients with ARDS, in weaning patients from the ventilator, and in following metabolic acidosis or base deficits in response to therapy in cardiogenic, hypovolemic, or septic shock and other states of inadequate tissue perfusion. They are also indicated in the initial evaluation and work-up of patients with unexplained tachypnea, dyspnea, tachycardia, burns or smoke inhalation, preoperative evaluation, and postanesthesia surveillance, or of patients with restlessness, anxiety, or mental confusion that may be secondary to hypoxia or hypovolemia. Additionally, intermittent arterial blood gas determinations are useful in following saturation of arterial and venous blood in patients with Swan-Ganz catheters in the determination of oxygen delivery and consumption.

Pulse Oximetry

Pulse oximeters provide a continuous noninvasive estimate of percentage hemoglobin O_2 saturation. Pulse oximetry is designed to measure differences in the SaO_2 waveform; without a good waveform, the instrument will not function accurately. Moreover, it does not distinguish oxyhemoglobin levels from the level of carboxyhemoglobin or that of methemoglobin; assessment of the latter, by cooximetry blood analysis, is needed in patients who have been exposed to carbon monoxide or had prolonged exposure to nitrites or nitroprusside.

Pulse oximetry is particularly useful for titration of FIO_2 and during weaning of patients from mechanical ventilation. Normal SaO_2 values do not, however, rule out CO_2 retention, respiratory acidosis, or impending respiratory arrest. They should not be viewed as a substitute for clinical assessment, or arterial blood gas assessment when indicated.

Blood Volume Measurement

Commonly, blood volume is inferred indirectly from measurements of arterial pressure, heart rate, CVP, urinary output, and hematocrit. These may be useful during resuscitation of patients who are not very ill; however, they are notably unreliable indicators of blood volume in critically ill patients, particularly those in septic shock. Blood volume measurements via dilution of markers or indicators are time consuming and therefore not often clinically useful; a description of these methods is available in the *Textbook*. Clinically, pulmonary artery wedge pressure is the most easily followed assessment of volume status; it should be remembered that this too can falsely overestimate volume status with inappropriately high readings in patients with high mean intrathoracic pressures, or high positive end-expiratory pressure.

Normal blood volume is 2.74 L/m^2 or 7.5 mL/kg for men, and 2.37 L/m^2 or 7 mL/kg for women. The patient in shock due to hemorrhage, trauma, or sepsis may benefit from blood volume levels in excess of these values. Extra volume compensates for maldistribution of blood volume, pooling of blood in the splanchnic bed, blood cell aggregation in the microcirculation, and red blood cell microthrombi. Total intravascular volume secondary to changes in permeability (and hence fluid shift) can occur rapidly in critically ill and especially septic patients, thus demanding constant reassessment of filling pressures and/or volume status, which is best done by means of a PA catheter with continuous measurement displays.

Pulmonary Artery and Precapillary Wedge Pressures Measurement

The balloon-tipped flow-directed PA (Swan-Ganz) catheter is commonly used to measure PA pressures and pulmonary artery wedge pressures, to assess left heart filling pressures, to calculate cardiac output by means of thermodilution, and to draw samples for mixed venous oxygen saturation determinations. From these measurements (along with arterial oxygen saturation and hemoglobin concentration), oxygen delivery and consumption ($\dot{D}O_2$ and $\dot{V}O_2$) can also be calculated. These devices are useful in diagnosis and treatment of volume overload or cardiac failure, and they are also invaluable in the titration of oxygen delivery and oxygen consumption in septic patients and severely injured trauma patients.

In the nonstressed patient without heart disease, left atrial pressure is usually within 2 to 3 mm Hg of right atrial pressure; however, in patients with valvular lesions, with disparity in ventricular compliance due to hypertension or ischemic heart disease, or with chronic or acute increase in pulmonary vascular resistance, there may be marked discrepancy between left- and right-sided filling pressures. In the absence of high pulmonary vascular resistance, pulmonary artery capillary wedge pressure estimates left atrial end-diastolic pressure. In the absence of mitral valvular disease, left atrial end-diastolic pressure is similar to left ventricular end-diastolic pressure, which is an estimate of left ventricular end-diastolic volume, or preload. In patients without increased pulmonary vascular resistance or valvular heart disease, pulmonary artery wedge pressure yields a good first approximation of left-sided heart filling pressure and volume status. Pulmonary artery wedge pressure can, however, also be affected by high mean intrathoracic pressures, positive end-expiratory pressure, abdominal distention, and vasopressors. Pulmonary artery hypertension may also occur in patients after rapid fluid resuscitation and in patients with congenital intra-atrial and intraventricular defects, chronic obstructive pulmonary disease, primary pulmonary hypertension, or acute hypoxemia.

In mitral stenosis, high pulmonary artery wedge pressure cannot be interpreted as adequate left ventricular filling resulting from the increased pressure gradient across the mitral valve. Likewise, when high PEEP and/or high mean intrathoracic pressures are necessary in ARDS patients, PA readings are falsely elevated by high mean intrathoracic pressures; high normal or high PA readings must not be assumed to represent adequate cardiac filling pressures in these circumstances. In these cases, optimal filling pressure can be determined by manipulating PA pressures (increasing with crystalloid or colloid administration, decreasing with nitroglycerin, furosemide, or PGE) and following cardiac output as determined by PA catheter. Another means of establishing volume status in such patients is by use of specialized Swan-Ganz catheters capable of directly estimating right ventricular end-diastolic volume.

Cardiac Output and Hemodynamic Variables

In 1987, Fick postulated that if the oxygen content of arterial (CaO_2) and of mixed venous (CvO_2) blood were known in addition to the oxygen consumption ($\dot{D}O_2$), then blood flow could be calculated using the following equation:

$$\text{Cardiac output} = \frac{CaO_2 - CvO_2}{\dot{D}O_2}$$

The direct Fick method for estimation of cardiac output became the gold standard against which other methods were evaluated. In clinical situations, the direct Fick method required measurement of $\dot{D}O_2$ by spirometry or timed collection of expired gas in a Douglas bag, with simultaneous anaerobic sampling of blood from systemic arterial as well as mixed venous blood.

The indicator dilution technique for estimation of cardiac output was described by Hamilton and coworkers. Originally, an indicator dye dilution technique was utilized. The thermal dilution technique utilized in Swan-Ganz catheters is an application of a modification of the indicator dilution principle.

A low cardiac index may reflect inadequate cardiac filling owing to hemorrhage, pump failure secondary to preexisting left ventricular disease, or acute infarction; can be seen in cases of severe cardiac contusion; and rarely is seen in patients with overwhelming sepsis. Conversely, most patients with septic and traumatic shock are characterized by normal or high blood flow (unless they are also hypovolemic), reflecting physiologic attempts to compensate for greatly increased metabolic demands. The optimal cardiac index for critically ill patients has been stated to be in the range of 4.5 liters/min/m^2, approximately 50% greater than values for an unstressed, healthy volunteer. Patients with severe sepsis, trauma, or burn shock, however, may require more than twice the normal cardiac index. Rather than attempting to assign arbitrary goals for cardiac index or oxygen delivery, it may be best to individualize therapy to demonstrated metabolic demand by the specific patient. Further, it is important to evaluate the ever changing metabolic demands frequently and thus optimally titrate therapy over time.

Oxygen Transport Variables and Other Circulatory Functions

Although cardiac output and pulmonary artery wedge pressure are important hemodynamic variables that reflect cardiac function, the essential overall function of the circulation is to maintain metabolism by tissue perfusion. Shock is a state of inadequate tissue perfusion; persistence of shock may lead to end-organ dysfunction, end-organ failure, or death. The circulatory system exists to transport oxygen, carbon dioxide, nutrients, end-products of metabolism, and metabolites. Of all components of circulation, oxygen has the highest percentage of extraction and is therefore the most flow-dependent blood constituent. Oxygen is essential to efficient energy metabolism and utilization, is the most crucial component in circulatory failure, and is a variable whose arteriovenous gradient is easy to measure. At the present time, it is not possible to measure tissue perfusion directly. Thus, overall circulatory status is best evaluated by observing changes in the temporal patterns of oxygen consumption ($\dot{V}O_2$) in relation to patterns of oxygen delivery ($\dot{D}O_2$).

In the stressed patient, particularly patients with major trauma or sepsis, $\dot{D}O_2$ may be increased above normal values, although it may still be inadequate for the increased metabolic demands of such a patient. A goal in resuscitation of the multiply injured, septic, or otherwise severely ill patient is to establish optimal O_2 delivery, keeping in mind that O_2 requirements in these ill patients may be substantially increased and are continuously changing. This is best accomplished via serial manipulations to augment delivery ($\dot{D}O_2$) until subsequent augmentation of O_2 consumption ($\dot{V}O_2$) no longer occurs, assuming that O_2 consumption will not increase by increasing oxygen delivery unless there was a previously unmet oxygen need or debt, and likewise that further increases in oxygen delivery, once consumption is no longer flow dependent, are of no additional benefit. This concept has been called elimination of "flow dependent" oxygen consumption.

$\dot{D}O_2$ = cardiac output × SaO_2 × hemoglobin (g/dL) × 13.4, and $\dot{V}O_2$ = cardiac output × ($SaO_2 - SvO_2$) × hemoglobin (g/dL) × 13.4. There are several therapeutic options to augment oxygen delivery. First, in patients requiring unusually high oxygen delivery, the saturation of oxygen should be maintained at 95% or better. However, there is little additional benefit by maintaining extremely high SaO_2, and there may be a considerable downside to this if it entails extraordinarily high FiO_2, or extraordinarily high peak/mean airway pressures (barotrauma, decreased cardiac output). Likewise, hemoglobin should be optimized in the range 10 to 11 mg; rheologic flow characteristics are best with a hemoglobin of 9; oxygen-carrying capacity is best at values slightly higher than this. Finally, the major variable available to manipulation when attempting to increase oxygen delivery is the cardiac index.

Optimal filling pressures should first be established as outlined earlier. Thereafter, a variety of inotropes, most commonly dobutamine or dopamine, are available. Phosphodiesterase inhibitors, including amrinone and milrinone, may also have significant beneficial effects in augmenting cardiac index. Additionally, afterload reducing agents such as nitroglycerine or nitroprusside may be of benefit in augmenting cardiac index. With Swan-Ganz catheters capable of a continuous display of cardiac output and SvO_2, serial manipulations of the preceding parameters can be performed rapidly, effects assessed, and delivery and consumption calculated, thus rapidly optimizing oxygen delivery until the patient is no longer flow dependent.

In summary, the low-risk patient may be monitored with routine screening that includes assessment of vital signs and urine output. A CVP catheter is indicated if large fluid shifts are anticipated, particularly in older patients. Serial hemoglobin or hematocrit determinations are useful if bleeding is a possibility. Continuous ECG monitoring is useful in all patients at risk of developing arrhythmias.

More comprehensive hemodynamic monitoring is needed in high-risk surgical patients. Swan-Ganz monitoring may be helpful in high-risk surgical patients with a history of coronary artery disease or left ventricular dysfunction, especially in long, complex abdominal operations in which large fluid shifts can be anticipated. Invasive hemodynamic monitoring may also be useful if routine screening with monitoring of vital signs, CVP, hematocrit, or base deficit by blood gas suggests more extensive hemodynamic problems. Invasive monitoring is also essential when optimizing resuscitation from severe shock.

Continuous mixed venous and cardiac output Swan-Ganz catheters to assess oxygen delivery and consumption are useful for multiply injured trauma patients, septic patients, or severely burned patients, in whom metabolic demands can be exceedingly high and continuously changing, and have disastrous consequences if they remain unmet. Invasive hemodynamic monitoring and oxygen transport monitoring can identify correctable physiologic alterations at the earliest possible time before they become life-threatening or irreversible. Furthermore, such monitoring provides objective circulatory measurements and criteria to titrate therapy. In essence, such monitoring replaces clinical suspicion and guesswork with objective physiologic criteria.

ELECTROCARDIOGRAPHY AND PRESSURE MONITORING: HOW TO OBTAIN OPTIMAL RESULTS

ECG monitoring is useful to detect both arrhythmias and myocardial ischemia. Since a multitude of mechanical factors may yield false information on such monitors, a critical medical strategy to keep in mind is that if there is any doubt regarding the source of unusual information on the monitor, the patient should always be checked first, including the nature and quality of the apical impulse and peripheral pulses.

The electrical signals emitted from the heart, measured at

the skin's surface, have an amplitude of only 2 to 5 millivolts. Proper skin preparation is imperative prior to placing electrodes. Wet or oily skin should be cleansed for 10 seconds with alcohol and dried prior to electrode placement. Likewise, hair should be shaved, dead skin removed, and gel applied prior to placing electrodes. Motion artifact related to placing leads on loose skin, muscle movement, or shivering artifact may be minimized by placing electrodes over bony prominences, such as the sternum or clavicles, if possible. Loosening or corrosion of clips between lead wires and electrode snaps can cause diminution of signal. Poor connections between the lead wires and the patient cable going to the monitor may be improved merely by their disconnection and reconnection. Use of shielded lead wires minimizes the pick-up of alternating current electrical fields from 60 Hz power lines, electrosurgical machines, and radio transmitters. Two ways to minimize the effect of magnetic fields on ECG monitoring are (1) not draping the lead wires over power cords, motors, lights, or other electrically powered instruments, and (2) decreasing the loop area between the patient and the monitoring by keeping the lead wires close together.

Monitors

All monitoring systems contain amplifiers and processors. Low-amplitude ECG signals may be due to low gain on the ECG amplifier. However, if gain is excessive, it may result in false-positive ischemia detection. If QRS amplitude is low despite proper gain settings, this can often be solved by better skin preparation, or changing or moving of electrodes.

The heart rate detector, which is intended to detect QRS complexes, sometimes improperly double-triggers on T waves or pacing spikes. Changing the ECG electrode position or switching to a different monitoring lead may circumvent this problem. More modern monitoring systems have the capability to monitor and display calibrated signals simultaneously from multiple ECG leads.

Optimizing Blood Pressure Monitoring

The Korotkoff auscultatory method for indirect arterial blood pressure measurement has been widely used since it was first described in 1905. The auscultatory measurement of arterial pressure often underestimates systolic pressure. The recently popular automated oscillometric devices also under-read systolic pressures as well as mean pressures at high arterial pressure, and over-read both systolic and mean pressures at low arterial pressures. The most important factor in determining the accuracy of the indirect blood pressure measurement is the selection of the proper cuff size. For overall accuracy, particularly in mean arterial blood pressure, most clinicians prefer the use of invasive arterial catheters when dealing with critically ill patients, especially those in shock.

Although direct blood pressure measurement using arterial catheters represents the most accurate assessment of arterial blood pressure, technical problems with these systems can occur. These include (1) improper system zeroing, and (2) inappropriate dynamic response.

1. Zeroing the pressure monitoring system is the single most important step in setting up a pressure measuring system. Zeroing errors can make a substantial difference in the recording of pressures, particularly those on the right side of the circulatory system such as pulmonary artery pressure and central venous pressure. Pressure monitoring systems should be zeroed frequently and always prior to initiation of treatment changes based on the pressure data. Proper zeroing is done by opening an appropriate stopcock to the atmosphere and aligning the resulting air-fluid interface point at the midaxillary line.

2. The dynamic response of the arterial line monitoring system refers to the natural frequency and damping coefficient of the catheter and tubing used. Systems are designed so as to have the highest natural frequency, which is done by using systems with short tubing, large internal diameter catheters, and transducers and other components that are noncompliant. Dynamic response can be adversely affected by the presence of air bubbles in the system, the use of pressure tubing that is too long or too compliant, or clot formation in the catheter. Of note, the mean arterial pressure is little affected by dynamic response limitations. To rule out an overdamped or underdamped system, fast-flush dynamic response testing should be performed at regular intervals; such testing should always follow a manipulation of the plumbing system, e.g., after drawing a blood sample. The rapid valve closure in the fast-flush dynamic response testing generates a square wave that permits evaluation of the system's frequency and damping coefficient. Examples of both overdamped and underdamped waves are available in the *Textbook.*

INTERPRETATION OF BLOOD GASES

Acid-Base Disturbances

In the normal adult, the 12,000 mEq of hydrogen ions produced each day are a by-product of metabolism. Of this total, approximately 99% of the hydrogen ions are so-called volatile acids—e.g., carbonic acid, which is disposed of by the lungs by means of CO_2. The other 1% of the acid load is composed of nonvolatile acids, which are excreted primarily by the kidney. pH is a measure of the amount of free hydrogen ion exclusive of that bound to buffers in the blood. Free hydrogen ion concentration is related to $PaCO_2$ and HCO_3 via a derivation of the Henderson-Hasselbalch equation as follows:

$$H^+ = 24 \times \frac{PaCO_2}{HCO_3}$$

Human blood contains an enormous buffering capacity, allowing large changes in the amount of hydrogen ions without substantial change in pH. As bicarbonate and other buffers decrease, however, a larger change in pH occurs as a result in change in acid content. With regard to acid-base status, distinctions between metabolic versus respiratory acidosis or alkalosis are important concepts in recognition of the proper course of therapy; ultimately, however, pH (acidemia or alkalemia) and correction of low-flow states (as indicated by metabolic acidosis) are of greater physiologic importance and are the goal of therapy, not correction of pCO_2 or HCO_3 per se.

Evaluation of Metabolic Acid-Base Abnormalities

The concept of base excess or deficit refers to the buffering capacity of blood; an increase in base deficit equals a decrease in buffering capacity, which yields a decrease in pH out of proportion to that which would be expected if normal buffering systems were intact, with any given acid load. This reflects the extent of metabolic acid-base derangement. Base excess or deficit is calculated by comparing measured pH to that predicted by $PaCO_2$ if baseline $PaCO_2$ of 40 mm Hg and baseline pH 7.40 are assumed, in which case an increase in $PaCO_2$ by 10 mm Hg would normally result in a decrease in pH by 0.05; and a decrease in $PaCO_2$ by 10 mm Hg would yield an increase in pH by 0.10. If a base excess or deficit of 10 mmol/L in buffering capacity occurs, this will result in a change in pH beyond that expected of approximately 0.15.

If a patient has abnormal pH but a base excess or deficit of less than 5 mmol/L, this represents a relatively normal metabolic acid-base status; however, a sustained base excess or deficit beyond 5 mmol/L, an increasing excess or deficit, or a base excess or deficit greater than 10 mmol/L represents a clinically significant metabolic acid-base derangement and demands diagnosis and treatment.

METABOLIC ACIDOSIS

Critically ill patients with metabolic acidosis usually have metabolic acidosis secondary to loss of bicarbonate or accumulation of nonvolatile acids (e.g., lactate). Anion gap is a useful concept in delineating the etiology of metabolic acidosis. The anion gap is defined as the sodium concentration minus the sum of chloride and bicarbonate anion concentrations:

$$\text{Anion gap} = Na^{+} - (Cl^{-} + HCO_3^{-})$$

The normal value is 12 ± 4 mEq/liter, plasma albumin normally accounting for 10 mEq/liter of unmeasured anions (anion gap). Patients with lower than expected anion gap usually have values reflecting severe hypoalbuminemia or severe hemodilution.

Anion gap acidosis reflects an increase in minor or unmeasured anions: lactic acidosis, ketoacidosis, renal insufficiency (increased sulfates, increased phosphates), and drugs (salicylates, methanol, ethylene glycol, high-dose penicillin).

Nonanion gap acidosis is often associated with increased chloride replacing depletion of bicarbonate due to gastrointestinal losses of bicarbonate, or renal tubular acidosis wasting of bicarbonate.

Lactate, as an end-product of anaerobic glucose metabolism, has been used to serve as a rough guideline of tissue hypoxia; lactate levels and the area under the curve of total lactate measurement over time have been correlated inversely with patient outcomes. Caution in interpretation is warranted, however. First, anion gap acidosis does not always signify lactic acidosis; conversely, more than half of documented cases of hyperlactatemia in intensive care units manifest nonanion gap acidosis secondary to decreased albumin, increased chloride, or mixed acid-base disturbances. Second, lactate levels do not equate with lactate production, as they may reflect not only production of lactate but also failure of hepatic and renal clearance.

With regard to the administration of bicarbonate, the physiologic goal of management of acid-base status in critically ill patients is maintenance of near-normal pH. Maintenance of pH greater than 7.2 is important with regard to optimal enzyme function, avoiding electrolyte disturbances such as hyperkalemia, proper functioning of autonomic receptors, maintaining cardiac response to endogenous and exogenous catecholamines, maintaining cardiac output, and avoiding arrhythmias. Manipulation of pCO_2 is usually the quickest available means should such dangerously low pH occur; this may necessitate intubation and hyperventilation. The best therapy of lactic acidosis is resuscitation of volume status and cardiac output to eliminate tissue hypoperfusion. Occasionally, when these efforts are unsuccessful, administration of bicarbonate or dialysis may be appropriate.

Administration of bicarbonate is effective only if ventilation is effective; otherwise, the rapid equilibration of bicarbonate and CO_2 within the blood may yield paradoxical worsening of acidosis if the CO_2 thus produced is not eliminated; therefore, bicarbonate administration is not indicated in cardiopulmonary arrest. If the decision to give bicarbonate is made, initial therapy is limited to one third to one half the calculated deficit since it is administered directly to the vascular space, which is significantly less than the volume of distribution used in calculating deficits. Additionally, administration of bicarbonate may be futile in the failing heart, as additional CO_2 load will equilibrate freely by diffusion across cell membranes, thus yielding transient further depression of intracellular pH.

Metabolic Alkalosis

Metabolic alkalosis is the most common acid-base disturbance in hospitalized patients. Metabolic alkalosis is usually due to hydrochloric acid loss (GI, renal), extracellular fluid (ECF) volume contraction, multiple blood transfusions (citrate load), or exogenous administration of bicarbonate. As long as pH is less than 7.6, metabolic alkalosis rarely causes electrophysiologic or enzyme dysfunction, but it may cause hypokalemia, other electrolyte disturbances, or decreased oxygen delivery to the tissues by shifting the oxyhemoglobin dissociation curve to the left.

In determining the etiology of metabolic alkalosis, it is useful to determine the urinary chloride concentration. If urinary chloride is less than 10 mEq/liter, this is usually chloride-responsive alkalosis, usually associated with ECF volume depletion. Therapy is directed toward correction of the underlying disorder and chloride repletion—either with NaCl tablets or with normal saline infusion if volume depletion is present. If the pH is greater than 7.55 or clinically significant systemic effects are present, therapy should include a dilute hydrochloric acid drip.

Chloride-resistant metabolic alkalosis seen with the urinary chloride greater than 20 mEq/liter is less common and is usually not associated with volume depletion. Associated conditions include magnesium depletion, primary aldosteronism, Cushing's syndrome, renal artery stenosis, or severe hypokalemia. Therapy is directed at treatment of the underlying disorder. Whatever the cause of alkalemia, pH greater than 7.7 can lead to cardiovascular collapse. Treatment is by .1 normal HCl drip. H^+ deficit in milliequivalents is calculated as .5 × kg weight × (measured bicarbonate − desired bicarbonate). Replacement is with 20% of the calculated deficit over 30 min, then repeat the arterial blood gas determination. Subsequently, 50% of the calculated deficit is given over the next 12 hours, not exceeding .2 mEq/kg/hour. Alternatively, ammonium chloride drip can be given to correct alkalemia, keeping in mind that this will enhance renal potassium excretion, thus necessitating frequent checks of potassium.

Assessment of Respiratory Acid-Base Imbalance

Respiratory acid-base balance is determined by the effectiveness of the alveolar ventilation. Ventilation is simply the movement of gas in and out of the pulmonary system, and is measured as the volume exhaled in 1 minute (VE). The portion of VE effective in gas exchanges is alveolar ventilation (VA); the ineffective portion of VE is designated as dead space ventilation (VDS). Consequently, VE = VA + VDS and CO_2 is inversely proportional to VA. Manipulation of CO_2, then, results in nearly instantaneous and predictable changes in pH. Assuming normal blood buffers, an acute rise in pCO_2 of 10 mm Hg results in a decrease in pH of 0.05, whereas an acute decrease in pCO_2 of 10 mm Hg results in an increase in pH of 0.1.

ARTERIAL PARTIAL PRESSURE OF CARBON DIOXIDE

Arterial partial pressure of carbon dioxide is determined by the balance of CO_2 excretion by alveolar ventilation as well as CO_2 production, dependent on the metabolic rate. Common circumstances of abnormal CO_2 production are (1) temperature deviation alters CO_2 production approximately 10% per degree centigrade change; (2) excessive muscular activity (shivering, rigors, seizure) can increase CO_2 production three- to tenfold; (3) physiologic stress; (4) sepsis; and (5) parenteral nutrition with glucose providing in excess of 50% of nonprotein calories.

DEAD SPACE VENTILATION

Increases in dead space (VDS) will require an increase in minute ventilation to maintain constant alveolar ventilation. Common circumstances of increased VDS are (1) acutely diminished cardiac output, which enhances the portion of the lung with poor perfusion (high $\dot{V}/\dot{Q}$ ratio); (2) acute pulmonary emboli; (3) ARDS, which creates both zero $\dot{V}/\dot{Q}$ and high $\dot{V}/\dot{Q}$ disease; (4) dead space related to ventilator tubing; (5) increased respiratory rate and decreased tidal volume resulting in ineffective alveolar ventilation.

The clinical observation of increased minute ventilation without an appropriate decrease in $PaCO_2$ then raises the possibility of increased dead space or increased CO_2 production.

MONITORING OF VENTILATORY FAILURE

Ventilatory failure can be a primary event of ineffective ventilation, rising CO_2, and primary respiratory acidemia, or it may represent inadequate respiratory reserve to compensate effectively for a primary metabolic acidemia. Additionally, it may be related to circumstances of abnormally high CO_2 production, and the inability of the pulmonary system to meet the increased demand. When clinically significant acute ventilatory failure occurs, the need for immediate ventilatory assistance and the adequacy of ventilatory assistance must be considered. Often there is concomitant acute metabolic acidosis secondary to inadequate tissue perfusion; metabolic acidosis may also be contributed to by the detrimental work of breathing. Extreme degrees of detrimental work of breathing are clinically recognized as acute respiratory distress with progressive tachypnea, tachycardia, dyspnea, hypertension, intercostal retraction, and use of accessory muscles of ventilation along with diaphoresis and mental status changes.

Clinical recognition of the detrimental work of breathing is important, as initial arterial blood gas may show an acceptable $PaCO_2$; however, if no therapeutic interventions to reduce the work of breathing are instituted, acute ventilatory failure with rising $PaCO_2$ and falling pH will eventually, and perhaps quickly, ensue. The metabolic acidemia and hypoxemia commonly seen in these patients will often rapidly reverse when appropriate ventilatory assistance is instituted.

ACUTE RESPIRATORY ALKALOSIS

The three most common etiologies of acute alveolar hyperventilation in critically ill patients are (1) a homeostatic response to arterial hypoxemia, (2) a homeostatic response to metabolic acidosis, and (3) central nervous system dysfunction. Other causes are pulmonary disease, including pneumonia, pulmonary embolism, or pulmonary edema; the onset of gram-negative sepsis; and severe anemia and/or hypovolemia. CNS etiologies include brain stem bleeds or tumor, CNS infection, or anxiety. When appropriate, carbon monoxide poisoning and methemoglobinemia should also be considered. Treatment is directed toward identification and correction of the cause, not merely normalization of $PaCO_2$.

Increased Peripheral Carbon Dioxide Stores: The "Carbon Dioxide Retainer"

Chronic hypercapnia ($PaCO_2$ greater than 45 mm Hg; arterial pH greater than 7.35) is most commonly seen in patients with chronic obstructive pulmonary disease. However, it can also be seen with chronic restrictive pulmonary disease, morbid obesity (pickwickian syndrome), and rare central nervous system disorders. Chronically hypercapnic patients have a limited capability to increase cardiopulmonary work in response to stress. Although the majority of these patients will not further hypoventilate when given O_2, such therapy must be carefully administered, because some will become significantly more hypercapnic in response to excessive O_2 administration and may develop significant decompensation with acidemia. Too, it is important to recognize that many of these same patients have chronic hypoxia and may have a PO_2 at a baseline of 50 to 60 mm Hg; it is important to keep this in mind when attempting to wean these patients from the ventilator. Proper interpretation of arterial blood gas values depends on recognition and differentiation of acute from chronic factors.

Regardless of the CO_2 level, a pH above 7.30 usually denotes a tolerable change from baseline. If the pH falls below 7.20, evaluation for ventilatory assistance is mandatory.

Oxygenation

Arterial oxygenation is often impaired in critically ill patients. Oxygen consumption is often greatly increased as well, and efforts to optimize oxygen delivery to meet the increased demand may decrease end-organ failure and mortality. Arterial and mixed venous blood gas determinations provide essential information for optimization of therapy, as direct assessment of tissue oxygenation status is not available.

The milliliters of oxygen contained in 100 mL of blood is defined as the oxygen content (mL/dL). The arterial oxygen content (CaO_2) in mL/dL is calculated as $13.4 \times$ Hgb (g/dL) $\times$ (SaO_2) $+ 0.003 \times PaO_2$ (mm Hg). As can be seen in this equation, under normal circumstances less than 5% of the total O_2 content is dissolved in blood, whereas greater than 95% is due to the component bound to hemoglobin. Oxygen delivery is calculated as arterial oxygen content $\times$ cardiac output; oxygen delivery ($\dot{D}O_2$) is then $13.4 \times$ hemoglobin (g/dL) $\times SaO_2 \times$ cardiac output. The small component of oxygen dissolved in plasma is not ordinarily included in these calculations. Oxygen consumption ($\dot{V}O_2$) is calculated as the difference between arterial and mixed venous oxygen contents, or $\dot{D}O_2$ = 13.4 × hemoglobin (g/dL) × (SaO_2 − SvO_2) × cardiac output.

Failure to oxygenate arterial blood adequately can be contributed to by several factors: (1) V/Q mismatch; (2) right to left intrapulmonary shunt; (3) diffusion impairment; (4) alveolar hypoventilation; and (5) low mixed venous oxygenation.

In the acute setting, diffusion impairment or hypoventilation is unlikely to contribute significantly to oxygenation failure. In acute respiratory failure in critically ill patients, both airway and parenchymal disease can contribute to V/Q mismatch, and an increasing portion of the lung with low V/Q ratio, resulting in hypoxemia as ventilation in these alveoli, is inadequate to oxygenate blood flow fully.

Intrapulmonary shunt of flow from the right or left side of the heart without oxygenation exists when pulmonary blood flow occurs through unventilated alveoli. The shunt equation calculates the portion of cardiac output that traverses from the right to left side of the heart without increasing O_2 content. True shunt (Qs/Qt) represents calculation of intrapulmonary shunt with an FiO_2 of 1.0. Physiologic shunt (Qsp/Qt) represents calculation of the intrapulmonary shunt at an FiO_2 of less than 1.0. This calculation then includes both the "true shunt" and V/Q mismatch with shunt effect. The physiologic shunt equation is:

$$QSp/QT = CcO_2 - CaO_2/CcO_2 - CvO_2$$

where CcO_2 is the ideal end-pulmonary capillary O_2 content using the ideal alveolar gas equation, CaO_2 represents the arterial oxygen content, and CvO_2 the mixed venous oxygen content. Although the intrapulmonary shunt equation does not describe regional relationships as well as the V/Q concept does, clinically the concept of shunting is important in understanding why ARDS patients may have hypoxemia refractory to increases in FiO_2. When shunt is a significant factor in hypoxemia, therapy is directed at maintenance and recruitment of alveoli via positive end-expiratory pressure (PEEP), and increased inspiratory times, using reverse I:E ratio ventilation.

Low mixed venous concentration is often seen and can be critically important in critically ill patients. Such patients often have moderate to marked increases in oxygen consumption; if delivery is inadequate to meet increased oxygen demand, low mixed venous O_2 content may result. Additionally, inadequate cardiac output secondary to preexisting or acute cardiac disease may aggravate the imbalance of oxygen delivery to consumption. This not only may reflect inadequate tissue perfusion, but also may adversely affect arterial oxygenation, particularly if severe concomitant pulmonary compromise exists.

In critically ill patients, arterial and mixed venous oxygen saturation values used in the calculation of arterial or mixed venous content delivery and consumption must periodically be established by arterial blood gas determinations. The arterial blood gas utilizes a multiwavelength oximeter that measures oxyhemoglobin and reduced hemoglobin, as well as carboxyhemoglobin and methemoglobin contents. Conversely, pulse oximeters use a dual wavelength spectrophotometer measuring only oxyhemoglobin as a percentage of oxyhemoglobin plus reduced hemoglobin, which may be inaccurate if significant concentrations of carboxyhemoglobin or methemoglobin are present.

When considering oxygen delivery, factors that shift the oxyhemoglobin dissociation curve must also be kept in mind. Factors that shift the curve to the right (decreasing pH, increasing temperature, or increasing 2,3-DPG) augment unloading of O_2 peripherally in excess to the extent that they inhibit loading in the lung; the net effect is increased oxygen delivery peripherally. The opposite holds true for factors that shift the curve to the left (increased pH, decreased temperature, decreased 2,3-DPG).

Whereas an oxygen saturation of 90% or a PAO_2 of 60 mm Hg or greater is generally considered to be adequate in most clinical circumstances, higher arterial oxygen saturation may be required in critically ill patients who manifest extremely high oxygen consumption and therefore demand extremely high oxygen delivery. Higher oxygen saturation, if possible, is also preferable in patients with known coronary artery disease.

Arterial Blood Gases During Cardiopulmonary Resuscitation

In spontaneously breathing patients with poor cardiac output, $P(v\text{-}a)CO_2$ gradient has been observed to increase 50% to 100%; a three- to tenfold increase has been observed in patients receiving CPR. This acute increase in venous PCO_2 results in decreased venous pH with little or no change in plasma bicarbonate concentration. If a patient is unable to unload CO_2 effectively, administration of bicarbonate is contraindicated (administration of sodium bicarbonate intravenously adds H_2CO_3 to blood; HCO_3 is available only after CO_2 load is eliminated by the lungs).

Blood Gas Monitoring

An analyzer is a device that measures fluid, excrement, or tissue permanently removed from the body. In contradistinction, a clinical monitor is generically defined as a patient-dedicated apparatus used to observe or record physiologic phenomena without permanently removing body fluid, excrement, or tissue. The potential clinical advantages of a blood gas monitor versus a blood gas analyzer are (1) analyzers provide only intermittent data with significant delay secondary to transporting of the sample, (2) the frequency of measurement is limited because blood samples are permanently removed from the patient, and (3) the blood gas sample is subject to preanalytic errors. All these disadvantages might be overcome with development of blood gas monitoring that would be providing a continuous readout of information on which to base therapeutic decisions.

Advances in fiberoptic and microprocessor technology, including transmission and fluorescent optodes, have made possible the development of several working models of in-line blood gas monitors. Data from 1989 to the present regarding such systems are reviewed in the *Textbook.* In assessing these systems, it is important to know (1) the accuracy of the device, which is the nearness of a measurement to the actual value of the variable being measured, (2) the bias, which is a consistent difference in the measured value of a known variable, and (3) the precision, which is the closeness of repeated measurements of the same quantity. In addition, these devices must be operable within a 20-gauge arterial catheter and not affect continuous pressure measurement. They must be biocompatible and nonthrombogenic. Their operation must be stable and consistent for at least 72 hours, and they must not be adversely affected by the reduction in local blood flow, temperature, or hemodynamic changes. Additionally, they should be cost effective.

Early systems were fully contained within the intra-arterial catheter; patient-interface problems led to the development of extra-arterial systems with pH, PCO_2, and PO_2 fluorescent optodes within a sensor cassette, inserted in series with the arterial catheter tubing near the patient's wrist. This then is an intermittent extra-arterial blood gas monitor. To measure pH, PCO_2, and PO_2, a stopcock closes the system to the IV fluids source, allowing arterial blood flow into the sensor cassette. When the measurement is complete, the blood in the cassette and tubing is returned to the patient. Bias and precision of the system in a multicenter study was found to be within ± .010 in pH, 1.5 mm Hg PCO_2, and 3.7 mm Hg PO_2.

As these devices are developed, they reduce therapeutic decision time, providing rapid and dependable titration of common therapeutic modalities. Additionally, no blood is removed from the patient, and the risk of nosocomial infection should be reduced because the integrity of the arterial catheter tubing is not interrupted to obtain blood gas values. Finally, it has been suggested that combining a blood gas monitor with capnography may allow observation of trend changes in both cardiac output and intrapulmonary shunting.

Capnography

Capnography is the technique of displaying carbon dioxide (CO_2) concentration changes during the respiratory cycle. A capnogram is a continuous record of CO_2 partial pressure in expired gas. A variety of capnograms in normal and various pathologic conditions are reproduced in the *Textbook.* Figure 3–1 demonstrates a normal capnogram. At the beginning of exhalation, the first gas sampled is the CO_2-free tracheal dead space. Normally, the capnogram should display a segment corresponding to the zero CO_2 concentration of dead space gas. As exhalation continues, CO_2 containing gas from the patient's respiratory tree enters the trachea and then the airway. It appears on the capnograph at point B. As the CO_2 concentration rises, it produces a sharp, smooth upstroke in the capnogram. CO_2 concentration then changes more

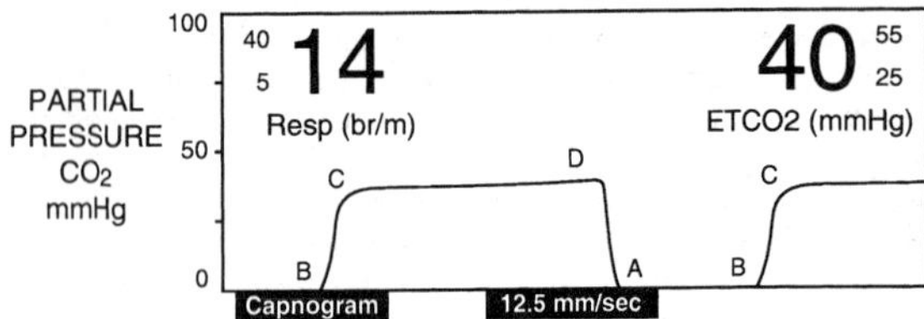

Figure 3–1. A normal capnogram. *Segment A–B* represents the beginning of exhalation, which is free of CO_2 because of the tracheal dead space. *Segment B-C* denotes the detection of CO_2 as exhalation continues. *Segment C–D* is the result of slowly changing CO_2 concentration over time. *Point D* represents end-tidal CO_2, which is the best approximation of arterial P_{CO_2}. Inhalation, which is normally free of CO_2 gas, causes the tracing to return to the zero baseline.

slowly, producing a nearly horizontal alveolar plateau. Near the end of exhalation, the CO_2 concentration approaches a value that is the ventilation-weighted average of ventilating lung units, or $CETCO_2$. In a patient with normal lungs and stable cardiovascular function, end-tidal CO_2 ($PETCO_2$) closely approximates arterial CO_2 ($PaCO_2$); that is, the end-tidal ($PETCO_2$) to arterial ($PaCO_2$) gradient is extremely small. Determination of $PETCO_2$ and capnograms have thus found clinical utility in patients undergoing general anesthesia, in patients requiring hyperventilation for isolated intracranial disease, in neurologically impaired patients requiring ventilatory assistance, and in apnea monitoring.

While the $PETCO_2$-to-$PaCO_2$ gradient is negligible in awake, spontaneously breathing patients with normal cardiovascular function, the gradient becomes substantial in a variety of pathologic circumstances. As dead space increases, $PETCO_2$ reflects to an increasing extent the contribution of CO_2 partial pressure of dead space, which is zero (there is no gas exchange in dead space ventilation, hence no expiration of CO_2). Thus, a decrease in $PETCO_2$ may represent increased alveolar ventilation (decreased $PaCO_2$) or increased dead space ventilation. Since a rapid increase in dead space will lead to a rapid decrease in $PETCO_2$, this system can be used to diagnose rapidly esophageal intubation, massive pulmonary embolus, massive leaks of the breathing circuit or ventilator, or an obstructed endotracheal tube.

$PETCO_2$ also underestimates $PaCO_2$ in patients with pulmonary parenchymal disease (via differing V/Q ratios and emptying times), hypovolemia or decreased cardiac output, or increased PEEP. A slowly progressive drop in $PETCO_2$ with a normal alveolar plateau pattern could be due to decreasing body temperature, decreasing CO_2 production, increasing alveolar ventilation (decreased $PaCO_2$), or slowly decreasing pulmonary or systemic perfusion (with resultant increased dead space). A more rapid progressive drop in $PETCO_2$ over time may portend cardiopulmonary compromise involving increasing physiologic dead space (massive blood loss, circulatory arrest, or pulmonary embolism). If the capnogram loses the normal alveolar plateau, the ventilator system should be checked; possible problems include a loosely fitting endotracheal tube, a leaking or defective tube cuff, partial obstruction of the ventilator, or its partial disconnection.

Analyzing expired gases for CO_2 not only helps with the recognition of esophageal intubation but aids in recognition of disconnection from ventilator systems, airway obstructions, and accidental removal of tracheal tubes. However, in the critically ill patient, distinguishing decreases in $PETCO_2$ and changes in capnograms secondary to increased dead space, increased alveolar ventilation, decreased cardiac output, changes in ventilation perfusion ratios, or changes in CO_2 production is difficult. Thus, while helpful in a variety of clinical circumstances, monitoring $PETCO_2$ alone is not an entirely reliable substitute for arterial blood gas analysis in critically ill patients.

TISSUE OXYGENATION AND HIGH-ENERGY PHOSPHATE METABOLISM

Derangement or failure of cellular energy metabolism results in organ dysfunction and cell death, as control is lost over solute and metabolite exchange across membranes. Following the digestion and metabolism of foodstuffs, energy is stored in high-energy phosphate bonds of adenosine triphosphate (ATP).

Aerobic Energy Production

Generation of ATP occurs in both the presence and absence of oxygen. Significantly more energy is produced when substrate consumption is coupled with the consumption of oxygen. After entry into the cell, glucose and free fatty acids undergo conversion to acetyl coenzyme A (acetyl-CoA); in this process, the constituent hydrogen atoms are transferred to nicotinamide adenine dinucleotide (NAD), producing the reduced form of the pyridine nucleotide (NADH). Oxidation of acetyl CoA to CO_2 in the Krebs cycle generates additional NADH as well as reduced flavin adenine dinucleotide ($FADH_2$). The electron pairs of these reduced dinucleotides then move down the cytochrome chain located in the inner mitochondrial membrane, until the final cytochrome reduces molecular oxygen to water. During this process of oxidative phosphorylation, 3 molecules of ATP are produced per molecule of NADH and 2 of ATP per $FADH_2$.

ATP then diffuses to sites of energy use in the cytosol, such as myofibrils and membrane-associated ionic pumps. ATPase controls the rate of hydrolysis of ATP and subsequent release of the high-energy phosphate bond. The control of ATP production appears to be a function of the concentrations of ATP, ADP, and Pi, which is measured as the phosphate potential:

$$\text{Phosphate potential} = \frac{[\text{ATP}]}{[\text{ADP}][\text{Pi}]}$$

When metabolic rate and energy demands are high, the phosphate potential declines, thus signaling mitochondria to produce more ATP, and O_2 consumption increases. If cellular availability of O_2 is limited, tissues must either lower their energy use or turn to anaerobic sources of energy to supplement aerobic ATP production.

Anaerobic Energy Production

The three sources of anaerobic ATP production are glycolysis, the adenylate kinase reaction, and, in some tissues that require a ready source of energy supply, the creatine kinase reaction.

Glycolysis is a universal cellular reaction to hypoxia, in which glucose or glycogen is metabolized to lactate with a production of ATP. The rate of glycolysis is regulated by several key reactions, the most important being the phosphofructokinase (PFK) reaction. PFK is strongly inhibited by ATP and H^+ and activated by adenine monophosphate (AMP) and Pi.

Production of ATP by glycolysis is an inefficient process. Only 2 mmol of ATP are produced per mole of glucose consumed, compared with 38 ATP when glycolysis is coupled to oxidative phosphorylation. Glycolysis also results in cellular acidosis. When mitochondrial function is limited by O_2 supply, the recycling of protons by oxidative phosphorylation declines and cytosolic H^+ concentration rises. Cellular acidosis also inhibits mitochondrial ATP transport, promoting the loss of adenine nucleotides from the mitochondria. Hypoxia also shifts the distribution of adenine nucleotides, resulting in an increase in the cytosolic pool. The mitochondrial adenylate pool eventually becomes so small that ATP production ceases. Mitochondria may not be capable of renewing aerobic ATP production when O_2 supply returns to normal.

The Adenylate Kinase Reaction

The third anaerobic source of energy is the adenylate kinase reaction, which is present in all cells. The adenylate kinase reaction converts 2 ADP molecules into 1 ATP and 1 AMP. This reaction results in the accumulation of AMP, which is subsequently dephosphorylated to adenosine by 5′ nucleotidase. Because adenosine is a potent vasodilator, the tissues are thus provided with a metabolic feedback loop capable of promoting local increases in blood flow in response to hypoxia. Alternatively, AMP can be deaminated to inosine monophosphate (IMP) by the AMP deaminase reaction that conserves adenine nucleotides, to allow resynthesis of AMP during recovery from exercise or hypoxia. Again, this represents a limited but renewable pool of high-energy phosphates during times of anaerobic metabolism.

The Creatine Kinase Reaction

Organs with high metabolic demand, such as the brain, heart, and skeletal muscle, use the creatine kinase reaction as a ready anaerobic source of ATP in addition to glycolysis. Phosphocreatine (PCr) is metabolized to creatine, transferring its high-energy phosphate bond to ATP. Under physiologic conditions the creatine kinase reaction is in equilibrium. Increases in ADP and H^+ during hypoxia promote the formation of ATP and creatine, whereas the opposite occurs when the supplies of ATP rise. This system provides a renewable but limited source of high-energy phosphates.

Metabolic Indices of Tissue Energy State

Arterial lactate has been proposed as a marker of inadequate tissue oxygenation in critically ill patients. Studies are divided as to whether lactate levels or the total lactate area under the curve over time during shock or sepsis is of value in predicting prognosis. Although elevated blood lactate levels often signify generalized tissue hypoxia, a normal value does not rule out regional lactate production. Arterial or mixed venous lactate concentrations reflect pooling of blood from several tissue beds, thus limiting their usefulness. Venous lactate levels from individual organs may be a more reliable index of anaerobic metabolism. Furthermore, blood lactate levels are heavily influenced by the state of perfusion of the splanchnic bed and liver.

The well-perfused liver clears lactate, via the Cori cycle. As perfusion of the splanchnic bed and liver decreases, often secondary to vasoconstriction related to increased catecholamine levels, the liver can become a net producer of lactate rather than clearing lactate. For these reasons, blood lactate levels may not indicate reliably the extent of anaerobic metabolism nor predict outcome.

Tonometry

Tonometric measurement of intestinal or gastric mucosal pH has recently been developed. By monitoring metabolic events (decreasing pH) from an organ at great risk during periods of hypoxia and low blood flow, tonometry may provide an early assessment of inadequate flow or resuscitation, as well as a response to therapeutic measures undertaken to restore splanchnic flow.

Oxygen Demand

Clearly, oxidative processes are much more efficient than anaerobic processes in the production of high-energy phosphate metabolites. During times of critical illness, major trauma, major burns, or sepsis, tremendous augmentation of the metabolic rate often results in increased oxygen consumption; this can be quantified in patients in whom Swan-Ganz catheters permit measurement of cardiac output, arterial oxygen content, and mixed venous oxygen content, allowing calculation of oxygen consumption. When measured, oxygen consumption varies widely between individuals with similar illnesses and also within a given individual over the course of time. Many of these patients have an unmet oxygen demand unless oxygen delivery is substantially increased.

Central to optimal care of the most critically ill patients is the sequential augmentation of oxygen delivery until oxygen demands are met, as delineated by the point beyond which an increase in oxygen delivery ($\dot{D}O_2$) will no longer increase oxygen consumption ($\dot{V}O_2$). Optimizing O_2 delivery such that O_2 consumption is no longer flow dependent is then continuously reassessed. This allows individualization of therapy to the changing oxygen demands over time. Continuous monitoring of mixed venous oxygen saturation and cardiac output, using the newer pulmonary arterial catheter techniques, allows rapid calculation of oxygen delivery and consumption.

INTRACRANIAL PRESSURE MONITORING

Neurologic examination remains the best clinical assessment of patients with intracranial pathology. Its usefulness, however, diminishes as unconsciousness ensues. Other diagnostic tests such as ICP monitoring, cerebral blood flow, and radiologic imaging then assume increasing importance.

Elevated intracranial pressure (ICP) is always a manifestation of primary intracranial pathology; it may in turn cause secondary injury as well. This may occur as a physical deformation of the brain stem owing to shift of intracranial contents, or from impaired cerebral perfusion. Clinically, the latter can be assessed by what is termed the cerebral perfusion pressure (CPP), defined as the difference between the mean arterial pressure (MAP) and the ICP: CPP = MAP − ICP. In the normal brain, adequate cerebral blood flow (CBF) is maintained for CPP values greater than 50 mm Hg. CBF is governed by multiple autoregulatory mechanisms: metabolism, carbon dioxide, blood viscosity, and perfusion pressure. Depending on the extent of brain injury, one or more of these autoregulatory functions may become impaired. In some clinical situations, both ICP and CPP may play a significant role in the determination of CBF.

The rationale of ICP monitoring is based on the following: (1) identification of subthreshold CPP values, (2) elevated ICP may be causally related to reduced CBF, (3) elevated ICP may cause herniation, (4) changes in ICP dynamics may signify the presence or development of an unexpected mass lesion, and (5) treatment of elevated ICP is not without risks and therefore precise, accurate determination of ICP is mandatory.

ICP has only limited buffering mechanisms because intracranial contents—brain tissue, cerebral spinal fluid, intravascular blood, and mass lesions (if any)—are not compressible. While limited, inherent ICP buffering mechanisms (translocation of CSF to spinal subarachnoid space, or increased absorption of CSF) can maintain a relatively constant ICP in response to slow and limited fluctuations in the volume of any of the intracranial components. Once these limited buffering mechanisms are exhausted, however, ICP may increase dramatically. The rate of change of volume of any of these components can have a significant influence on the rate of pressure change. ICP measurements cannot be interpreted in isolation, as CPP and cerebral capacitance may have a profound clinical impact.

An increase in brain tissue volume often occurs as one of several forms of cerebral edema. Cytotoxic edema is the product of cellular membrane disruption, usually secondary to ischemia or trauma. Vasogenic edema arises from a breakdown in the blood-brain barrier, normally occurring in the presence of neoplasms or cerebral abscesses.

Blockage of the CSF pathways generates elevated pressures because CSF production is independent of pressure, occurring at a constant rate of 20 mL/min. Excessive intravascular intracranial arterial blood volume is not a primary cause of elevated ICP, although loss of cerebrovascular autoregulation may have a significant impact on ICP dynamics.

The most common cerebral mass lesions associated with elevated ICP are hematomas, neoplasms, and infections.

Indications for Intracranial Pressure Monitoring

ICP monitoring is indicated in the treatment of patients in whom intracranial hypertension is suspected and in whom treatment decisions will be influenced by the results. The most common use of ICP monitors is for the treatment of head-injured patients. Approximately two thirds of comatose head-injured patients with a Glasgow Coma Score of 8 or less develop elevated ICP; therefore, ICP monitors are routinely placed in these patients. Exceptions are occasionally made, as in the case of an obviously intoxicated patient with a normal head CT scan. Less common indications for ICP monitoring include illnesses associated with severe brain swelling, such as Reye's syndrome or fulminant hepatitis.

Intracranial Pressure Monitoring Devices

Two fundamental types of ICP monitoring devices are used: those with a fluid-coupled transducer communicating with a ventricular system and those that incorporate a distal transducer subdurally or intraparenchymally. The decision about which type to use is normally based on the ease of ventricular access and whether or not there is need for CSF drainage. With either method, measured ICP values are computed mean values.

The ventriculostomy (ventricular catheter) is a fluid-coupled system. It is normally placed on the right, or nondominant, hemisphere. Placement is desired in the frontal ventricular horn. CSF return and a triphasic waveform usually indicate patency and proper catheter placement. The transducer is zeroed to the level of the external auditory meatus, which serves as an external landmark to the foramen of Monro. Ventriculostomies are managed either by continuously monitoring ICP and intermittent drainage of CSF when pressures exceed 20 mm Hg, or by continuous drainage of CSF, adjusting the level of the collection system to regulate ICP grossly.

Distal pressure transducer devices (such as the Camino monitor) incorporate a counterpressure membrane system. The transducer is zeroed to atmospheric pressure prior to placement. These are typically placed intraparenchymally in the frontal lobe or in the subdural space.

Risks and Pitfalls in Intracranial Pressure Monitoring

Rare complications of ICP monitor placement are subdural or intracerebral hematomas and seizures. Infection is the most common complication, occurring in 3% to 12% of ventriculostomies. There is evidence to suggest that ventriculostomy infection rates increase significantly after 5 days of placement; therefore, some centers place new ventriculostomies every 5 to 7 days. Antibiotic prophylaxis has not been shown to reduce the incidence of ventriculostomy infection.

Inaccurate or misleading measurements are the most common pitfalls encountered in ICP monitoring. A partially obstructed ventricular catheter produces a dampened waveform that underestimates true pressure. Mass lesions in the posterior or middle fossa may produce elevations in ICP that can compress the brain stem, without elevation of ICP measured in the frontal lobe. Neuroimaging studies may help corroborate ICP measurement. Diffusely elevated ICP is suggested by obliteration of the basal cisterns and cerebral sulci.

BRAIN FUNCTION MONITORING

Conceptually, much of the management of acute head injury or other catastrophic brain injuries is intended to maintain adequate cerebral blood flow (CBF); however, CBF is not routinely measured. Most cerebral circulatory information is inferred from knowledge of mean arterial pressure, ICP, and hence cerebral perfusion pressure (CPP). Autoregulation in the normal brain maintains CBF constant over the CPP range of 50 to 130 mm Hg, but after head injury approximately two thirds of the patients maintain autoregulation and in approximately one third autoregulation is impaired or lost. Most patients with mass lesions also have defective autoregulation. Neither ICP nor CPP is equivalent to flow, and maintenance of flow and function are the obvious desired outcomes. Indeed, the mechanism by which decreasing $PaCO_2$ decreases ICP is by decreasing cerebral blood flow in proportion to the decrease in $PaCO_2$. Thus, low ICP may be maintained as well as CPP, at the expense of flow. Other systems have thus been proposed to monitor cerebral blood flow, oxygen consumption, mixed venous cerebral O_2 saturation, metabolic gradients, or brain function.

The first quantitative clinical method of measurement of CBF calculated global CBF from the difference between the arterial and jugular bulb saturation curves of an inhaled inert gas. Later techniques used extracranial gamma detectors to measure regional cortical blood flow via washout curves after intracarotid injection of a radioisotope, such as xenon-133. Carotid puncture was later avoided by techniques that measured cortical blood flow after inhaled or IV administration of xenon-133. Technical difficulties, limiting clinical usefulness, are detailed in the *Textbook.*

In most patients, arterial flow velocity can be measured readily in intracranial vessels, especially the middle cerebral artery, using transcranial Doppler ultrasonography. Since velocity is a function of both flow rate and vessel diameter, there are intersubject differences in flow velocity as compared with CBF. Measurements of jugular venous bulb oxygenation are analogous to measuring systemic mixed venous oxygen saturation: they reflect a global average but may not reflect marked regional hypoperfusion. Conversely, normal or elevated jugular venous saturation does not indicate adequate cerebral perfusion throughout all regions of the brain. In clinical use, trends seen in jugular venous blood sampling for continuous monitoring may detect unexpected cerebral desaturation.

Electrophysiologic Monitoring

The cortical electroencephalogram, altered by mild cerebral ischemia and abolished by profound cerebral ischemia, can be used to indicate potentially damaging hypoperfusion. It may also be useful in patients suspected of having isolated seizures or status epilepticus, in defining the depth or type of coma, and in documenting focal or lateral intracranial abnormalities. Continuous EEG monitoring is cumbersome because of the sheer volume of data produced. Software has been designed to compress the data, which may provide greater clinical utility.

Sensory evoked potentials (EPs), which include somatosensory evoked potentials (SSEPs), brain stem auditory evoked potentials (BAEPs), and visual EPs, can be used as qualitative threshold monitors to detect severe neural ischemia. EPs evaluate the response of the brain to specific stimuli. To record SSEPs, a stimulus is applied peripherally, usually to the median nerve at the wrist. EPs are described in terms of the amplitude at the individual peaks, as well as the delay (latency) from stimulus administration until the appearance of waveforms. SSEPs are unaffected by neuromuscular blocking agents. EPs, especially BAEPs, are modified by sedatives, narcotics, and anesthetics, as well as by trauma, hypoxia, or ischemia. Because obliteration of EPs occurs only under conditions of profound cerebral ischemia or mechanical trauma, EP monitoring can be a specific way of testing neurologic integrity.

EPs have been used to facilitate diagnosis and prognostication in ischemic and hypoxic brain injury. Central conduction time is prolonged in patients who have ischemic complications of subarachnoid hemorrhage (SAH). With impending brain death, cortical SSEPs disappear first; BAEPs disappear only when brain death is imminent. Persistence of the medullary components of SSEP, at a time when the cortical components are no longer present, confirms brain death.

Table 38–4 in the *Textbook* outlines the relative merits and limitations of the various brain function monitoring methods discussed in this section.

PEDIATRIC MONITORING

This section summarizes the major modalities of pediatric monitoring, highlighting aspects that are unique to the pediatric population.

Electrocardiography

Continuous ECG displays are routinely indicated in the pediatric ICU. An infant's ECG normally shows right-sided predominance. By 6 years of age, a child's ECG is similar to an adult's.

Ventricular tachycardia and fibrillation are rare in the pediatric population. The most common pediatric arrhythmias are sinus arrhythmias, bradyarrhythmias, and supraventricular tachycardias. Bradyarrhythmias are defined as heart rates of less than 100 in neonates, 80 in infants, and 70 in older children. This is frequently encountered in critically ill patients and may signal hypoxia in the neonate. Supraventricular arrhythmias are also common. A child's atrioventricular node and His bundle are less refractory to sinus stimulation than those of an adult. Subsequently, children with sinus tachycardias of up to 300 beats per minute may show one-to-one ventricular response. These high rates may sometimes be due to primary conduction disorders, such as Wolff-Parkinson-White syndrome.

Echocardiography

Echocardiography is continuing to replace more invasive monitoring techniques in extremely ill neonates and children, as ultrasonographic technology with the advent of transesophageal ultrasound has increased reliance on this technology, not only for anatomic diagnosis but also to monitor cardiac function intraoperatively and postoperatively. Medical closure of the patent ductus arteriosus (PDA) with indomethacin can be monitored by serial echoes, as can be the response to an infant's heart to digoxin or surgical ductus ligation. Common congenital defects such as aortoseptal override in tetralogy of Fallot can be diagnosed directly from echo. In critically ill neonates, echo can rapidly differentiate low-output states caused by hypoplastic left ventricle from those resulting from remedial heart disease or from sepsis. Additionally, echo is useful in documenting and monitoring shunts: using a rapid bolus of liquid into the circulation, highly echogenic "flurries" are seen in the right side of the heart by dissolution of air microbubbles in the injectate, referred to as microcavitation. These are usually cleared by the pulmonary circulation; a venous injection should not create echoes on the left side of the heart except in patients with right-to-left intracardiac shunt. Echo is also the most sensitive means of detecting pericardial fluid and estimating its volume in children.

Quantitative echocardiography is frequently used for evaluating myocardial performance in infants and children. Left ventricular dimensions are determined from echo, as are ejection fractions and shortening fractions.

Pulsed Doppler Cardiac Output

Further development of ultrasound technology has enabled determination of cardiac output by the application of the Doppler principle. The accuracy of this technique has been validated by some studies, but not all. It appears that Doppler determination of cardiac output may provide a noninvasive, reliable technique, particularly in neonates.

Nuclear Cardiology

Radionuclide imaging techniques can also be used to evaluate both structural and functional aspects of cardiac performance safely and noninvasively in children. These have proved useful in diagnosing congenital heart disease, demonstrating and quantifying shunts, determining ventricular function indices, and monitoring for myocardial ischemia in neonates.

Pulse Oximetry

Pulse oximetry is of great clinical utility in children. Apart from providing respiratory function monitoring, it can also detect changes in hemodynamic shunts. For example, in persistence of fetal circulation, preductal saturation may be 95% to 100% and postductally it may be less, thus reflecting the degree of right-to-left transductal shunting. An increase in peripheral vascular resistance increases the amount of shunting and decreases postductal saturation. Pulse oximetry is also used to assess perfusion distal to arterial catheters. Oximetric catheters are available for pediatric use and are routinely placed in the PA to determine mixed venous saturations and in the jugular bulb as a monitor of cerebral perfusion.

Invasive Monitoring Techniques: Peripheral Artery Catheterization

Although useful for hemodynamically stable children, noninvasive blood pressure monitoring by either oscillometric or ultrasound techniques frequently overestimates blood pressure in children, particularly in shock.

Methods for placing peripheral arterial catheters in larger children are not significantly different from those for adults. In infants and small children, techniques are modified. The radial artery is preferred, but it is extremely small. The first step is a modified Allen's test. While releasing the ulnar artery, perfusion of the entire hand, especially the distal forefinger and thumb, is observed for flushing. Refill should be complete within 10 seconds. Palpation is often inadequate in small infants for localization of the artery. In these cases a Doppler flow detection probe may identify arterial pulsation, or alternatively, a transilluminator can be used to localize the artery. Small Teflon cannulas are used. If the radial artery is not available on either side, dorsalis, pedis, and posterior tibial arteries may be cannulated. The brachial artery is avoided in children since this site has potential for limb loss. When smaller arteries cannot be cannulated, the axillary or femoral arteries may be considered. Axillary cannulation is permissible owing to the rich anastomotic network around the shoulder. When arterial lines are placed in any extremity, circulation in the limb should be constantly monitored by assessing the color, capillary refill, presence of pulses, and temperature. A pulse oximeter probe distal to the insertion site may serve as an early warning to perfusion defects.

Catheter disconnection and bleeding from catheter tubing are probably the most frequent catheter-associated complications in children. Other complications include distal ischemia and infection. Retrograde perfusion and embolization can occur from any site, thus careful flushing techniques are mandatory. This is particularly important in axillary lines in order to avoid retrograde cerebral embolization.

Interpretation of values also merits mention. Attaining normal blood pressure in children may be misleading. Attention to other parameters of tissue perfusion such as skin temperature, capillary refill, blood pH, and serum lactate levels may be important, as blood pressure is the last parameter to decline in decreased perfusion states in children. This is due in part to their less rigid, more responsive vascular beds, and thus compensation in blood pressure despite decreased cardiac output.

Additionally, the presence of vascular left-to-right shunts in children may alter pressure tracings. In children with PDA or aortic incompetence, a wide pulse pressure with rapid diastolic pressure drop is observed. Arterial pressure decay curves have been used to diagnose and monitor response to therapy.

Central Catheterization

Central catheterization insertion is indicated in any child, regardless of size, when the benefit of hemodynamic monitoring outweighs the risks involved. These commonly involve low-output states that are not rapidly responsive to volume loading, uncertain hemodynamic states after cardiothoracic surgery, or situations requiring advanced mechanical ventilatory support.

Central venous catheters can be inserted into the superior vena cava or right atrium via the antecubital, subclavian, jugular, or femoral veins. The femoral vein is generally avoided for long-term use due to risks of thromboembolism and the possibility of line sepsis, but some observers report prospective data documenting few complications with long-term femoral cannulation. Central pressures monitored through femoral lines must be cautiously interpreted in children; if the line is below the diaphragm, it may reflect abdominal pressure and not right atrial pressure. Additionally, with any site, the possibility of paradoxical air embolism across a patent foramen ovale, atrial septal defect, or ventricular septal defect must be considered, which demands rigorous, meticulous nursing care.

Left atrial catheters can be directly inserted into the left atrial appendage during cardiac surgery to monitor LV filling pressures. Although useful in the perioperative period, these represent a potential embolic source in the left side of the heart. They should not be used except for pressure monitoring and a slow, continuous heparin flush to maintain line patency. If blood cannot be freely aspirated, the catheter should be removed rather than flushed. All connections, transducers, and lines that are connected to the left atrial line should be clearly and obviously marked to avoid inadvertent use.

PA catheters can be inserted either operatively or percutaneously. Operatively, catheters are placed directly into the PA or inserted through the RV outflow tract in the RA infundibulum, and from there into the PA. Percutaneously, in children older than 5 years, the selection of site is no different than in adults. In smaller children, the internal jugular or femoral approach is preferred. In the presence of right to left intracardiac atrial or ventricular shunts, the possibility of cerebral embolism demands full aseptic technique and rigorous attention to detail with regard to the possibility of air embolism.

Complications of PA catheters in children during insertion and positioning are most frequently those of atrial or ventricular premature contractions. Constant vigilance of the monitor with prompt withdrawal usually prevents the need for further treatment. A second complication may occur if the cross-sectional area of the inflated balloon significantly obstructs or occludes the RV outflow tract for more than a few seconds. The result is hypoxemia, bradycardia, hypotension, and rapid decompensation. Catheter knotting, pulmonary and tricuspid valve damage, catastrophic PA rupture, and even papillary muscle avulsion are also potential hazards.

Thromboembolic complications may occur from emboli from the catheter tip or in the introducer sheath, which can lead to pulmonary infarction. Leaving the introducer sheath in situ may allow clot formation between the catheter and the sheath wall, with potential for venous embolism. In the presence of a right-to-left intracardiac shunt, this may lead to systemic embolization. This risk may be reduced by using an introducer with a side arm, allowing continuous flushing of the introducer sheath with a heparinized solution, as well as by decreasing the length of time the sheath is left in place.

The risk of infection requires meticulous technique, since changing of sites every 72 hours may not be practical in children with limited sites. Central catheters should be removed as soon as monitoring functions are no longer essential.

Blood loss from the entry wound during or after catheter insertion requires careful monitoring and, if necessary, blood replacement. The absence of a preexisting bleeding diathesis should be confirmed prior to catheter insertion. Platelet consumption coagulopathy may be induced by prolonged PA catheterization; daily platelet monitoring is advisable.

If a child is invasively monitored, pressures and blood samples from all chambers should be studied for abnormal pressure gradients and oxygen saturation variations. Blood samples from the right atrium, RV, and PA demonstrate any significant left-to-right shunts. The techniques for determining cardiac output by dye dilution and thermodilution are essentially the same in children as in adults, unless there is valvular regurgitation or intracardiac shunting, in which case it is not possible to assess cardiac output accurately.

Systemic vascular resistance (SVR) and pulmonary vascular resistance (PVR) may be used to assess the response to cardiovascular therapy. SVR and PVR are expressed as SVRI (index) and PVRI, just as cardiac output is expressed as cardiac index in children. SVRI is expressed in R units, the normal being 15 to 20 R units; PVRI is generally 1/20th that of SVRI; normal is 1 to 3 R units.

Neonatal Catheterization

Catheterization of one of the two umbilical arteries in the neonate is routine for intensive care. In neonates as old as 8 days, umbilical arterial catheters (UACs) can be inserted directly into the cut vessel's lumen, or by cutdown of the umbilical vessels. Catheters may be placed either above the diaphragm or below the third lumbar vertebra. Complication rates appear to be high with either position. Placement below the fourth lumbar vertebra avoids celiac and mesenteric blood supplies as well as that of the renal arteries. Patency is maintained by a slow, continuous infusion of heparinized saline. No other drugs or solutions should ever be infused through these lines. Complications of umbilical artery catheters are increasingly recognized. Septicemia may occur in up to 8% of infants so catheterized, compared with one to three cases per thousand in controls. This is in part attributable to the absence of sterile technique during catheter insertion. Prophylactic antibiotics do not appear to be helpful. Daily cultures may identify early infection or dangerous colonization. The duration of catheterization should be minimized.

Vascular occlusion caused by thrombosis, embolism, or vasospasm has been identified postmortem in 3.5% to 48% of neonates with UACs. Vascular occlusion is generally clinically evident by blanching of limbs, absence of arterial pulses, and discoloration of toes. More severe manifestations may include renal artery thromboembolism. Embolism of spinal arteries causing paraplegia and embolism of the mesenteric blood supply causing gut infarction and large areas of tissue gangrene have also been reported. There is also an increased incidence of necrotizing enterocolitis with the concomitant use of umbilical artery catheters. The current trend is away from UACs and toward noninvasive monitoring of peripheral sites.

As increasingly sophisticated noninvasive means of monitoring are developed, the trend in pediatrics is toward less invasive monitoring, as exemplified by pulse oximetry, echo monitoring, and nuclear cardiography.

CHAPTER 4
Cardiovascular Issues

Michael L. Hess, M.D. • Andrea Hastillo, M.D.

MYOCARDIAL INFARCTION

Diagnosis

Rapid diagnosis and treatment of patients with acute myocardial infarction (MI) are imperative; the sooner thrombolytic therapy is applied, if indicated, the more likely is myocardium to be salvaged. After immediate and rapid clinical evaluation of a patient complaining of chest pain, an electrocardiogram (ECG) should be promptly obtained. Accuracy of the ECG in diagnosis of MI is influenced by the previous medical history. If the ECG was previously normal, sensitivity and specificity approach 80% to 85%; if the ECG was previously abnormal, and especially if the patient has had multiple past MIs, the diagnostic accuracy of the ECG is much reduced and/or indeterminate. Although various enzyme assays have been proposed, analysis of creatine kinase (CK) with measurement of the MB fraction remains the most widely available and reliable diagnostic tool. Both total CK and CKMB rise above normal values within 6 to 8 hours after infarction, reaching a peak at approximately 30 hours (or earlier after successful thrombolysis).

Treatment

Treatment is designed to (1) relieve symptoms, (2) limit the extent of myocardial damage, (3) reduce cardiac work and hence reverse ischemia, and (4) manage complications. About half the mortality of acute MI occurs within the first 4 to 6 hours. Because the major cause of early mortality is primary ventricular fibrillation—ventricular fibrillation occurring without significant premonitory ventricular ectopic beats—access to a monitoring unit as early as possible is essential.

Pain

The initial discomfort of MI may be severe. Morphine, 2 to 4 mg IV, repeated as needed, is highly effective. Morphine has adverse effects, including respiratory depression, some decrease in myocardial contractility, bradycardia, and vasodilatation. The hypotensive effect of morphine often responds to simple elevation of the lower extremities. The ischemic pain of MI may also be relieved by nitroglycerin, which may be administered sublingually (0.4 mg repeated once or twice as necessary), followed by continuous intravenous drip.

Oxygen

Increased left ventricular filling pressure consequent to myocardial dysfunction of acute MI raises pulmonary venous pressure, increases the work of breathing, and reduces pulmonary capillary oxygen tension and partial pressure of arterial oxygen. Hence, treatment with oxygen administered via nasal prongs at a rate of 4 to 6 L/min is reasonable for the first 36 to 48 hours.

Aspirin and Platelet Dysfunction

All patients with suspected MI should receive aspirin in a dose of at least 325 mg immediately, chewed and swallowed for rapid effect, and daily thereafter. Doses less than 162.5 mg take several days to become effective and are probably less useful. Doses higher than 325 mg daily may produce adverse effects.

Restoration of Coronary Flow

See also the later section on thrombolytic therapy.

The following is a reasonable summary of thrombolytic therapy: (1) Effective thrombolysis reduces mortality and salvages myocardium in transmural MI by restoring coronary flow. (2) The sooner a patient is treated, the better the outcome. (3) Thrombolysis appears to be effective until at least 12 hours after onset of infarction. (4) An accelerated dose of tissue plasminogen activator (t-PA) combined with closely monitored intravenous heparin appears to be somewhat more effective than streptokinase with subcutaneous or intravenous heparin. (5) Complications of thrombolysis are mainly bleeding, both cranial and at puncture sites. (6) t-PA has had a slightly higher risk of intracranial bleeds than the other agents, with an incidence averaging less than 1%. (7) Women appear to have a slightly higher risk of intracranial bleed. (8) Allergic reactions to streptokinase are rare, but second courses of treatment with this agent should probably be avoided.

Heparin

Intravenous heparin is clearly effective in the management of unstable angina. Early in the evaluation of thrombolytic agents, it was shown that intravenous heparin maintained a somewhat higher patency rate 24 hours or later after thrombolysis with t-PA. When streptokinase is the agent, no advantage for intravenous heparin can be demonstrated. Thus, despite a strong tradition for use of intravenous heparin in the management of acute MI, especially in the United States, there appears to be no advantage in its combination with streptokinase but modest improvement in survival when combined with t-PA.

Coronary Angiography and Angioplasty

In patients who are considered a good risk, after treatment with a thrombolytic agent, subsequent angiography and associated angioplasty do not contribute to further reduction in mortality when carried out in the first few hours after treatment. Enthusiasts claim that restoration of flow during angiography is quicker, more effective, and potentially cheaper than thrombolysis and has a low rate of complication. In selected patients in certain institutions, immediate angioplasty appears to be a reasonable alternative to noninvasive treatment with thrombolytic agents. The problem is that it is simply not possible to maintain a nationwide network of skilled angiographers to provide this form of treatment to the population in need.

Beta-Adrenergic Blockers

It is reasonable to recommend acute administration of a β-adrenergic blocker in treating acute MI, at least in patients with evidence of heightened sympathetic activity characterized by unexplained tachycardia or hypertension in the absence of contraindications such as heart failure or asthma. A useful regimen is metoprolol, 5 mg IV every 2 to 4 minutes for three doses. If the drug is well tolerated, 50 mg PO is given every 12 hours beginning 15 minutes after the last intravenous dose. The oral medication is continued for 48 hours and then changed to 100 mg daily as a single dose.

Nitrates

Intravenous nitroglycerin is often useful in the early treatment of evolving MI if the dose is carefully monitored and systolic blood pressure is not reduced more than 20 to 30 mm Hg. The possibility of right ventricular infarction should be carefully evaluated before administration of nitroglycerin because the drug's effect on the capacitance system may sharply reduce ventricular flow, resulting in profound hypotension. Nitroglycerin may be administered initially in the emergency department sublingually one to three times in a standard dose of 0.3 mg per tablet. Intravenous nitroglycerin is often initiated at a rate of 5 to 10 μg/min, with the dose increased by 5 to 10 μg every few minutes until the desired response is achieved.

Angiotensin-Converting Enzyme Inhibitors

Several clinical trials have clearly demonstrated that administration of angiotensin-converting enzyme (ACE) inhibitors beginning 12 to 36 hours after onset of infarction can prevent or retard this process with subsequent preservation of ventricular function. Thus, serious consideration should be given to treating patients with a Q wave infarct, especially a large anterior infarct, with an angiotensin-converting enzyme commencing within 1 to 2 days after admission.

Complications

Arrhythmia

Ventricular arrhythmias are extremely common in the first 48 to 72 hours of MI. Within the first few hours of infarction, primary ventricular fibrillation may occur. Although the incidence of primary fibrillation appears to have declined during the past decade, this rhythm is the major immediate cause of the high early mortality in the first few hours after the onset of symptoms. Almost all patients with MI have some ventricular arrhythmia during the first 72 hours of monitoring. A review of clinical trials fails to show an advantage to prophylactic lidocaine. Thus, treatment of ventricular arrhythmia on demand rather than prophylactic therapy is currently recommended.

An initial bolus of lidocaine, 1 mg/kg, may be followed after 3 to 5 minutes by two subsequent doses of 0.5mg/kg. When the arrhythmia responds to the acute dose, an intravenous drip of 3 mg/min is initiated. The infusion rate may be adjusted upward with additional intravenous boluses of drug or downward, depending on the response. Procainamide is also useful for both acute and long-term treatment of ventricular arrhythmia. In recurrent malignant arrhythmia, bretylium or amiodarone may be effective. It should be noted, however, that recurrent ventricular arrhythmia usually reflects ongoing ischemia in an unstable situation.

Right Ventricular Infarction

Right ventricular infarct may be diagnosed with a high degree of certainty by examination of the QRS complex in V_{4R}. In patients who present with inferior infarction and hypotension, measurement of pulmonary artery and pulmonary capillary wedge pressure with the Swan-Ganz technique may be required to distinguish left ventricular forward failure or incipient cardiogenic shock, hypovolemia, or right ventricular infarction. In the presence of low capillary wedge pressure, administration of a volume load is helpful. In hypovolemia, volume administration should increase systemic pressure with maintenance of normal right ventricular hemodynamics. In right ventricular infarction, a high right ventricular filling pressure must be supported by administration of excess volume to maintain adequate left ventricular filling pressures.

Mural Thrombus

Ventricular thrombus develops in about 30% of patients with apical-anterior transmural MI. In patients at risk, it is reasonable to obtain an echocardiogram between the third and fifth day. If thrombus is present, intravenous heparin is given for several days followed by warfarin (Coumadin) therapy for 3 months.

Pericarditis

A transient friction rub is not uncommon in the first few days after transmural MI. Thrombolytic therapy does not increase the incidence of hemorrhagic pericardial effusion. The pericarditis is generally self-limited although the symptoms may be confused with recurrent ischemia or peptic ulcer disease. If rub and pericardial pain are persistent, treatment with a nonsteroidal anti-inflammatory agent may be useful.

Prognosis

Identification and modification of risk factors are major components of postinfarct treatment. Cessation of smoking, management of hypertension, and normalization of cholesterol abnormality improve outcome. Increasing evidence that successful cholesterol reduction retards progress and to some extent influences regression of atherosclerotic obstructive lesions should motivate both patients and doctors to maintain effective lipid-lowering therapy after infarction. Angiotensin-converting enzyme inhibitors reduce ventricular remodeling, especially in patients with large anterior transmural MI. When indicated, these drugs should be continued for at least a year after the initial attack.

Thrombolytic Therapy in Acute Myocardial Infarction

After 30 years of clinical trials with thrombolytic agents, the beneficial effect of this therapy is firmly established. In the majority of patients given t-PA, the infarct-related artery is reperfused. Streptokinase (SK) also produces reperfusion, particularly when given very soon after the acute occlusion. SK and t-PA have been shown to reduce infarct size, improve myocardial performance, and reduce at least immediate and probably late mortality in MI. Successful thrombolysis is achieved with agents or combinations of agents that provide the highest rate of reperfusion with the lowest rate of reocclusion and the lowest rate of bleeding complications.

Time to Reperfusion

The thrombolysis in myocardial infarction (TIMI-I) group demonstrated that when t-PA was given at 100 mg over 3 hours, reperfusion rates of 24% at 30 minutes, 57% at 60 minutes, and 71% at 90 minutes were obtained. When the dose was increased to 150 mg, earlier reperfusion was obtained in more patients (42% at 30 min, 68% at 60 min, and 76% at 90 min). Unfortunately, the incidence of intracranial hemorrhage at this high dose was subsequently observed. TIMI-I also demonstrated that SK given in the currently approved dose of 1.5 million units over 1 hour resulted in substantially lower reperfusion rates compared with t-PA at 30 minutes (8%), 60 minutes (23%), and 90 minutes (31%). In TIMI-I, the interval between onset of symptoms and start of treatment averaged 4.7 hours. Although such delays in therapy do not affect reperfusion rates with t-PA, the efficacy of SK is profoundly reduced. Thus, in TIMI-I, the 90% reperfusion rate for patients treated with SK within 4 hours of the symptoms was twice that for patients treated after more than 4 hours. It is clear that faster reperfusion of the infarct-related artery is beneficial. Both the empiric observation that thrombolytic therapy administered within the first hour of symptoms has marked survival advantages over later therapy and the theoretic concern that 15% of myocardium at risk dies for every 30 minutes of persistent occlusion strongly support the notion that faster reperfusion improves outcome.

REPERFUSION/PATENCY RATE. With t-PA, patency rates ranged from 61% to 79%, and with intravenous SK a 90-minute patency rate of 55% has been documented.

REOCCLUSION. Reocclusion of the infarct-related artery after successful thrombolysis can be documented in angiographic studies. However, it is likely that angiographic reocclusion rates may underestimate the real incidence of this phenomenon. Clinically, reocclusion is taken as recurrent angina and particularly reinfarction in the same myocardial location as that observed on initial presentation. Clinical reocclusion rates are less than those angiographically documented, because many reocclusions are asymptomatic. Angiographic reocclusion rates for native t-PA have been in the 5% to 24% range. The infarction rates after thrombolytic therapy have been documented in numerous studies. In patients receiving t-PA, they range from 2.4% to 13% and for those receiving SK, from 2.8% to 12%.

Bleeding Complications

The rates of bleeding complications with the presumed fibrin-specific t-PA have been surprisingly high. In fact, t-PA caused bleeding complications at a rate that was not statistically different from the incidence of bleeding with SK. The incidence of major bleeding for t-PA ranges from 6.3% to 21% in the six studies listed in Table 4–1, and the incidence of all bleeds, major and minor, ranges from 30% to 45%. Bleeding from puncture sites is extremely common with any thrombolytic agent. It is not clear from the reports cited whether the concomitant administration of heparin or aspirin significantly contributed to bleeding complications.

Mortality Estimates

The first "mega trial," GISSI-I* clearly established that SK significantly reduced the mortality rate as compared with placebo infusion in 12,000 patients. A second trial, the Second International Study of Infarct Survival (ISIS-II), assigned patients at random to placebo, SK, aspirin, and aspirin plus SK therapies. Five-week vascular mortality was reduced by 21% in those taking aspirin versus those taking placebo. SK alone also reduced the mortality by 23% relative to placebo, and when aspirin was given with SK, mortality was reduced by 42% compared with placebo, suggesting additive effects of SK plus aspirin.

The question of the early use of heparin was largely resolved in the heparin-aspirin reperfusion trial (HART). At

---

*Gruppo Italiano per lo Studio della Sopravvivenza nell'Infarto Miocardio.

Table 4–1. INCIDENCE OF BLEEDING COMPLICATIONS IN REPORTED STUDIES

Study	Treatment	*No. of Patients*	Incidence of Bleeding		*Stroke (%)*
			Major (%)	*Minor (%)*	
TIMI-1	SK + H	147	15.6	15.6	0
	rt-PA + H	143	15.4	17.5	0
ECSG-1	SK + H + A	65	7.7	2.3	1.5
	rt-PA + H	64	6.3	26.5	0
ECSG-2	Placebo + H + A	366	2.2	5.2	0
	rt-PA + H + A	355	10.2	29.3	1.7
TAMI-1	rt-PA* + H (± PTCA)	386	21	24	0.5
TAMI-2	rt-PA + H + A (± UK)	147	14	20	0.7
TAMI-3	rt-PA (± H)	175	14	22	1.2

(From Bang NU, Wilhelm OG, Clayman MD: After coronary thrombolysis and reperfusion, what next? J Am Coll Cardiol 1989; 14:837–849.)
*High dose = 150 mg.
Abbreviations: A = aspirin; ECSG = European Cooperative Study Group; H = heparin; PTCA = percutaneous transluminal coronary angioplasty; rt-PA = recombinant tissue type plasminogen activator; SK = streptokinase; TAMI = Thrombolysis and Angioplasty in Myocardial Infarction trial; TIMI = Thrombolysis in Myocardial Infarction trial; UK = urokinase.

the time of the first angiogram, 82% of the infarct-related arteries in the patients assigned to heparin were patent, compared with only 52% in the aspirin group. Of the initially patent vessels, 88% remained patent after 7 days in the heparin group, compared with 95% in the aspirin group. The numbers of hemorrhagic events were similar in the two groups. Later much larger trials confirmed the high incidence of reperfusion and low incidence of reocclusion with early intravenous heparin treatment.

The first study that compared SK and t-PA head to head was GISSI-II, with the main endpoint of mortality rate. The patients were also assigned at random to receive heparin (12,500 units SC twice daily until discharge from the hospital), starting 12 hours after the beginning of t-PA or the SK infusion. The patients were assigned randomly to four treatment groups: SK alone, SK plus heparin, t-PA alone, and t-PA plus heparin. No significant differences between the two thrombolytic agents were detected. Mortality rates were identical in the two groups (8.8% hospital mortality for the study population compared with approximately 13% in the control cohort). The rates of major in-hospital cardiac complications (reinfarction, postinfarction angina) were also similar. The incidence of major bleeds was significantly higher in SK- and heparin-treated patients. The overall incidence of stroke was similar in all four groups.

The second study to examine t-PA versus SK was the Third International Study of Infarct Survival (ISIS-IIIK). There was no significant mortality difference during days 0 to 35 among all randomly assigned patients, and no difference in 6-month survival was apparent. The combined mortalities were exactly identical, 10% for t-PA and 10% for SK. The APSAC (p-anisoyl derivative of streptokinase-plasminogen activator) group was similar in all respects to the SK groups, with no statistically significant differences in treatment outcomes. The only significant differences were found in the rate of reinfarction, 3.26% for SK versus 2.80% for t-PA, and in the frequency of stroke, which was significantly higher among patients receiving t-PA (1.35%) than among patients receiving SK (1.00%). The addition of heparin to either SK, APSAC, or t-PA, as prescribed in the protocol, made no difference in any measured outcomes.

In the GUSTO (Global Utilization of Streptokinase and Tissue Plasminogen Activator to Track Occluded Arteries) trial, 41,021 patients with MI were randomized within 6 hours of symptom onset to one of four treatments: (1) SK (1.5 million IU/60 min + SC heparin), (2) SK (1.5 million IU/60 min + IV heparin), (3) accelerated t-PA + IV heparin, or (4) a combination of SK (1 million IU/60 min) and t-PA (1 mg/kg over 60 min, maximum dose 90 mg, + IV heparin). All patients received aspirin, and 46% received intravenous β-blockade. The combination arm was included because this regimen was believed to be associated with a particularly low reocclusion rate. However, the combination arm did not do well, showing both higher mortality and stroke rates than were seen with t-PA alone. The mortality rates and stroke rates in the different groups are shown in

Table 4–2. GUSTO TRIAL MORTALITY RESULTS

Mortality	SK (SC) (%)	SK (IV) (%)	t-PA (%)	Combination (%)
30-day	7.2	7.4	6.3	7.0
24-hour	2.8	2.9	2.3	2.8

Table 4–2. The difference between the t-PA arm and the SK arms was statistically significant.

As anticipated from the ISIS-III trial, the t-PA arm was associated with a higher incidence of stroke than was SK. Further analysis showed that t-PA remains significantly better than SK even when adverse effects like stroke are included in the assessment of net benefit.

The GUSTO results end the long debate about whether early patency is important or whether the time to reperfusion or patency is irrelevant. The fact that GUSTO showed a correlation between early patency and lower mortality has substantial implications for future research. These include the need to improve early patency further. Even the best group had open arteries in only 53% of patients at 90 minutes. Another issue raised by the GUSTO results is the possible increased role of primary angioplasty in place of thrombolysis. Primary angioplasty is one of the best methods of opening an artery quickly, yielding 90-minute patency rates in the 80% range. It is not likely, however, that primary angioplasty will replace thrombolysis altogether because of the limited numbers of centers and physicians that can conduct the procedure.

Conclusions

The results obtained with thrombolytic therapy in acute MI to date have been impressive. Nevertheless, results can clearly be improved in the area of time to reperfusion, reocclusion, and bleeding complications, with specific reference to intracerebral bleeds. However, it is uncertain whether the incidence of bleeding complications can be reduced. Indeed, it is possible that some of these strategies will result in increased bleeding liability.

Interventional Therapies for Cardiogenic Shock

Acute myocardial infarction complicated by the clinical syndrome of cardiogenic shock (hypotension, oliguria, pulmonary edema, and/or mental obtundation) continues to be a most dreaded and deadly sequel of coronary artery disease. The reported incidence of cardiogenic shock ranged from 5% to 15% of those patients presenting with acute myocardial infarction in the 1950s through 1970. The use of invasive monitoring, pharmacologic inotropic support, and vasodilator therapy has not materially improved patient survival.

Thrombolytic Therapy

See earlier section on thrombolytic therapy.

Intra-Aortic Balloon Counterpulsation

Intra-aortic balloon counterpulsation reduces intrinsic systolic arterial pressure and left ventricular wall tension, correlating with a decrease in myocardial oxygen requirements. Diastolic coronary perfusion pressure and blood flow are augmented not only to the infarct-related artery but importantly to noninfarct-related coronary arteries. Consequently, hemodynamic support may be of secondary benefit by contributing to the maintenance of perfusion pressure and flow in noninfarct arteries containing significant stenoses, thus contributing to global myocardial salvage and function. Because severely ischemic myocardium may not recover immediately with reperfusion, intra-aortic balloon support can "buy time" for recovery within the infarct zone, assuming the occurrence of spontaneous or induced reperfusion within the infarct artery. Unfortunately, the use of intra-aortic balloon pump counterpulsation has not correlated with improved in-hospital or late survival in patients with cardiogenic shock.

Intuitively, one might expect that intra-aortic balloon pump counterpulsation combined with intravenous thrombolytic therapy could lead to improved survival. However, this has not been the case; the combined treatments potentially result in increased bleeding complications. Nevertheless, in the absence of reperfusion, there has been no convincing evidence that intra-aortic balloon pump counterpulsation alone improves survival in patients with cardiogenic shock.

Cardiopulmonary Bypass Support

Percutaneous femoral-femoral cardiopulmonary bypass in the cardiac catheterization laboratory has undergone initial evaluation in several medical centers. Relative to intra-aortic balloon pump counterpulsation, benefits of cardiopulmonary bypass support include the fact that the system's output is independent of the patient's intrinsic cardiac function or rhythm. Consequently, it is entirely possible to maintain a patient's systemic perfusion, noncardiac organ function, and mentation despite ventricular tachycardia, fibrillation, or asystole. Systemic perfusion pressure and blood flow are more effectively maintained than with the intra-aortic balloon pump. Cardiopulmonary bypass does not provide antegrade coronary flow, and regional ventricular dysfunction is not relieved. In general, the use of portable cardiopulmonary bypass is not recommended for longer than 8 hours. Finally, the distinct possibility exists that temporary cardiopulmonary bypass will maintain consciousness and noncardiac organ function in patients who do not have and cannot recover enough left ventricular function to survive without cardiac transplantation.

Coronary Artery Bypass Surgery

Early surgical revascularization of patients presenting with cardiogenic shock has been performed since the 1970s. As indicated by these retrospective reviews of unique experiences from separate medical centers, early surgical revascularization for cardiogenic shock can improve in-hospital and late survival in selected patients. However, the need for 24-hour on-call operating suites with skilled surgeons and support personnel, increasingly limited healthcare resources, and costs have precluded the widespread application of emergency surgery for patients in cardiogenic shock.

Percutaneous Transluminal Coronary Angioplasty

Preliminary reports by several clinician-investigators have implied a survival benefit for those patients in cardiogenic shock who receive emergency cardiac catheterization and coronary angioplasty. The risks of coronary angioplasty for acute myocardial infarction are increased when it is performed in the setting of antecedent intravenous thrombolytic therapy. The systemic lytic state contributes to significantly increased bleeding complications and stroke. Further, there is pathologic evidence that the systemic lytic state may result in intimal, medial, and adventitial coronary artery hemorrhage, in contrast to direct coronary angioplasty without antecedent thrombolytic therapy. Conversion of an otherwise anemic or bland myocardial infarction to a more extensive hemorrhagic myocardial infarction after angioplasty has also been associated with antecedent thrombolytic therapy. Because of the lack of measurable benefit to shock patients treated with thrombolytic therapy alone, the increased risks and compromised results of coronary angioplasty when performed in the setting of systemic lysis, and the clear patient-care advantages derived through catheterization in these critically ill patients, direct coronary angioplasty is considered to be the optimal therapy for patients experiencing acute myocardial infarction and those complicated by cardiogenic shock.

Although no clinical or anatomic factors clearly predict the development of cardiogenic shock, perhaps a "typical" patient is an older man with a history of myocardial infarction, a new acute anterior wall infarction, and underlying multivessel coronary disease. The prompt recognition of patients having this or other high-risk profiles should facilitate immediate triage to a center with the capability for cardiac catheterization and emergency coronary angioplasty. When used, this strategy allows for the possibility of emergency coronary bypass surgery or percutaneous transluminal coronary angioplasty (PTCA). On the basis of limited, nonrandomized data, angioplasty and bypass surgery appear to offer the highest likelihood of in-hospital survival for those patients in cardiogenic shock. Regardless of primary therapy, strategies to decrease long-term mortality in hospital survivors of cardiogenic shock, particularly the subset of shock patients with multivessel disease, await further study.

Conclusions

In the 1990s, cardiogenic shock is an unequivocal indication for immediate transfer to a facility with a catheterization laboratory and personnel and equipment available for emergency coronary angioplasty or bypass surgery. PTCA should be considered as the revascularization therapy of choice. Alternatively, emergency coronary artery bypass grafting, when logistically possible, appears to result in at least comparable patient benefit and improvement in survival. Mechanical hemodynamic support by intra-aortic balloon pump counterpulsation or temporary cardiopulmonary bypass is an integral part of any acute care and revascularization strategy.

CONGESTIVE HEART FAILURE IN INFANTS AND CHILDREN

Signs and Symptoms

In all age groups, CHF implies cardiac enlargement, tachycardia, and tachypnea. In the neonate, because ventricular interdependence makes left- and right-sided heart failure virtually inseparable, hepatomegaly is virtually always present. Exercise tolerance may be manifest as dyspnea on exertion or as undue fatigue in the older child, or it may interfere with feeding in the infant. Hypoxia may be a sign of pulmonary edema, in which case it is generally responsive to oxygen administration, or it may represent an associated aspect of congenital cardiac disease such as right-to-left shunting of blood or admixture of systemic and pulmonary venous return. Radiographic cardiomegaly may represent cardiac dilatation from ventricular volume overload in the patient with an atrial or ventricular septal defect and does not, in itself, establish the presence of CHF.

Poor contractility and reduced ejection fraction, documented by echocardiography or angiography, are often viewed as synonymous with CHF. Their absence, however, cannot be interpreted as a guarantee that cardiac function is normal. The afterload reduction characteristic of mitral regurgitation, ventricular septal defect, or arteriovenous malformation may mask myocardial dysfunction and lend the appearance of normal contractility. Inotropic agents and sympathetic stimulation may also enhance ejection fraction and give the appearance of adequate myocardial function, although intrinsic compensatory mechanisms are no longer capable of supporting normal cardiac output.

Frank cardiogenic shock is a common presentation of congenital cardiac disease. Metabolic acidosis, hypotension, poor perfusion, thready pulses, pallor, and diaphoresis are often presenting findings in ductus-dependent malformations such as coarctation, hypoplastic left-sided heart syndrome, interruption of the aortic arch, and critical aortic stenosis. This presentation is the hallmark of Galen's vein aneurysm. Cardiogenic shock is also an occasional presenting symptom in cardiomyopathy, anomalous origin of the left coronary artery, or myocarditis. In all age groups, sepsis may be accompanied by cardiogenic shock (low cardiac output, hypotension, and impaired cardiac contractility).

Treatment

Of the many components to the treatment of CHF, some are quite specific, such as diuresis in iatrogenic volume overload, control of hypertension in hypertensive cardiomyopathy, transfusion in severe anemia, and balloon atrial septostomy in transposition of the great arteries. The generalities of treatment, however, are readily categorized. Myocardial dysfunction is treated by drug therapy directed at enhancement of contractility. Myocardial dysfunction will occasionally respond to afterload reduction. Cautious vascular volume expansion (preload augmentation of ventricular work using the Frank-Starling mechanism) may improve cardiac output in the patient with cardiogenic shock and is a vital emergency measure.

Reduction of myocardial workload is effective in all categories of CHF. This may be accomplished by bed rest, mechanical ventilation, or afterload reduction. Relief of the underlying cause of ventricular overwork should be immediately planned in the patient with surgically treatable CHF. In certain situations, diuresis may be the mainstay of decongestive therapy. This is most commonly the case when pulmonary dysfunction contributes to symptoms and when edema, especially pulmonary edema, is itself troublesome. Oxygen therapy is effective insofar as it enhances arterial oxygenation, relieves dyspnea, and reduces pulmonary vascular resistance.

Digoxin produces a rise in intracellular calcium that augments contractility. Digoxin is vasomimetic and slows the heart. This may be beneficial because it lengthens diastole, allowing more time for cardiac filling. Digoxin has minimal vasomotor effects but is a modest systemic vasoconstrictor. In the critical care setting, digoxin has seen less use since the introduction of continuous catecholamine infusions because of its relatively long half-life, its predominant renal clearance, and its propensity to cause cardiac arrhythmias. This propensity of digoxin is exaggerated by hypokalemia. Diuretics, which may cause potassium depletion, add to this potential hazard of digoxin therapy.

Catecholamines act through the adrenergic receptor complex. When an inotropic agent causes the heart to pump more blood at constant aortic pressure (a desired effect), cardiac workload is increased. This requires augmentation of oxygen delivery to the myocardium. For this reason, catecholamine use may be associated with myocardial ischemia, even in nonischemic cardiac disease. The commonly used catecholamines—epinephrine, norepinephrine, dopamine, dobutamine, and isoproterenol—all cause tachycardia. As the heart rate increases, diastole shortens proportionally more than systole. This can interfere with cardiac filling, thereby worsening stroke volume. Finally, catecholamines are intrinsically arrhythmogenic.

Methylxanthines (like theophylline) and bipyridines (amrinone and milrinone) augment contractility by elevating intracellular cAMP but using mechanisms independent of the adrenergic receptor. Theophylline inhibits activity of all phosphodiesterases: those that "degrade" cAMP (which augments contractility) and those that "clear" intracellular cyclic guanosine monophosphate (which is thought to decrease contractility). In the aggregate, theophylline is a positive inotropic agent. Amrinone and its milrinone inhibit activity of phosphodiesterase III, which degrades cAMP. Milrinone raises intracellular calcium and is a positive inotropic and a systemic vasodilator. This combination, inotropic activity and afterload reduction, may have special value in low-output states and in situations in which myocardial workload should not be excessively increased.

Treatment of Congestive Heart Failure by Reducing Cardiac Work

The burden of the heart, to meet the needs of the body for systemic oxygen and substrate delivery while supporting its own metabolic requirements, can represent a conflict of interest. In cardiogenic shock, when the heart is unable to bear this burden, forcing it to perform heroics often will cause myocardial necrosis. Other measures that are useful in infants and children focus on reducing cardiac work to allow the pump to recover. This is of special importance after cardiac operations, when the heart has been injured by myocardial incision, put at risk of air embolism by opening the heart, and subjected to coronary ischemia followed by reperfusion with blood. Several of these measures are listed in Table 4–3.

Foremost among them is mechanical ventilation with oxygen, coupled with sedation and, as appropriate, neuromuscular blockade. Mechanical ventilation alleviates the work of breathing, which may be substantial if there is pulmonary edema or lung dysfunction. It protects the patient from risk

Table 4–3. MODALITIES THAT MAY BE USED TO REDUCE MYOCARDIAL WORK

Mechanical ventilation
Sedation
Pain relief
Neuromuscular blockade
Prevention of fever
Pharmacologic afterload reduction
β-blockers
Aortic balloon counterpulsation
ECMO/ECLS, LVAD, RVAD

Abbreviations: ECMO = extracorporeal membrane oxygenation; ECLS = extracorporeal life support; LVAD = left ventricular assist device; RVAD = right ventricular assist device.

of respiratory arrest when narcotics are used. Oxygen should be used to relieve arterial desaturation. PEEP is often used to alleviate arterial desaturation in the patient with pulmonary edema. Sedation, pain relief, and neuromuscular blockade limit endogenous catecholamine secretion, reduce sympathetic vasoconstriction, and prevent patient movement. Prevention of fever reduces the metabolic demand that must be satisfied by activity of the heart. It also reduces heart rate, facilitates cardiac filling in diastole, and prevents or treats junctional ectopic tachycardia. Pharmacologic treatment of excessive afterload may be used to reduce cardiac work to the extent that it does not impair organ perfusion, especially perfusion of the myocardium by the coronary circulation. Agents often used to reduce afterload include nitroprusside, calcium channel blockers, prostaglandin E_1, captopril, and enalapril. Myocardial work may also be limited using β-blockers, because cardiac output need not always be as great as the body appears to demand.

Devices to Support the Failing Heart

Aortic balloon counterpulsation is possible in very small children but becomes increasingly challenging as catheter size declines, heart rate rises, or myocardial function worsens. Arrhythmias interfere with this modality. However, fundamentally, the underlying limitation of aortic counterpulsation is that it pumps no blood. It reduces cardiac afterload and raises diastolic pressure but only by displacing blood that has been ejected by the left ventricle. Infants and children, like adults, can be supported using extracorporeal devices if they suffer temporary or permanent myocardial devastation. Extracorporeal membrane oxygenation (ECMO) has been shown to be useful as a means of cardiac rescue after repair of congenital cardiac malformations. Some postoperative patients are unable to support their circulation despite an adequate repair, and cardiogenic shock develops. Although ECMO raises afterload in this setting by restoring adequate blood pressure, it does relieve the heart of the burden of supporting the entire circulation. At the same time, it raises coronary artery diastolic pressure. ECMO, therefore, "rests" both right and left ventricles. When ECMO is used to "rest" the heart, it must be remembered that the left ventricle may become unable to eject at the higher afterload afforded by the extracorporeal pump. In this setting, left atrial return (flow through the ductus arteriosus, bronchial flow, residual anterograde flow across the pulmonary valve) may pool on the left side of the heart. Pressure could, in theory, rise in the left ventricle and atrium until it equals aortic diastolic pressure.

SPECIFIC CARDIAC RHYTHMS

Normal Sinus Rhythm

In the adult, normal sinus rhythm is due to the SA node depolarizing 60 to 100 times per minute. The P wave is depolarized in a leftward and inferior direction and should be directed to exclude other rhythms at this same rate, notably an accelerated junctional rhythm. Sinus rhythm at a rate of 60 to 100 bpm may be inappropriate in certain circumstances (e.g., in severe hypovolemia or with high fevers).

Junctional Escape Beats

Junctional escape beats may occur with AV block, when the sinus node slows, or when the degree of AV block in atrial fibrillation is high. The junctional escape beat resembles the normal sinus-induced QRS complex and may be associated with an abnormal P wave within or contiguous with the QRS or with an absent P wave. The rate of escape beat is less than 60 bpm. Treatment of the junctional escape beat itself is not indicated. Consideration of increasing the sinus rate or improving AV node conduction may be necessary if cardiac output is jeopardized.

Atrioventricular Nodal Re-Entrant Tachycardia

The arrhythmias grouped together as paroxysmal supraventricular tachycardias (PSVTs) include those resulting from a concealed AV bypass tract (15% to 50%), sinus node re-entry (3%), intra-atrial re-entry (6%), automatic atrial tachycardia, and AV nodal re-entry (50%).

The onset of the arrhythmia is usually abrupt and initiated by a premature complex. Termination is usually abrupt. The QRS is regular and the complex usually narrow in the absence of a preexisting bundle branch block or intraventricular conduction delay. The rate may range from 150 to 200 bpm. P waves may be difficult to visualize and are often within the QRS complex.

Treatment depends on the hemodynamic status, the cause, and the recurrence rate. Severe hemodynamic compromise may require emergency cardioversion using low energy (20 to 50 J). Vagal maneuvers to interrupt the re-entry pathway by slowing conduction, which leads to sudden termination of the arrhythmia, are usually the first line of treatment. Adenosine is a short-lived drug that is very effective in terminating AV nodal re-entry tachyarrhythmias. Although the side effects of adenosine include sinus bradycardia, AV block, and sinus arrest, the effects are transient (less than a minute). It is administered rapidly to maximize its negative dromotropic effect. Verapamil may be used with caution and is quite effective in terminating most AV nodal re-entrant tachyarrhythmias. It is a negative inotrope as well as a negative dromotropic agent, and side effects may include profound cardiovascular and hemodynamic collapse. Other treatment modalities include β-blockers, digitalis, vasopressors, antiarrhythmic agents, edrophonium, and atrial or ventricular pacing.

Concealed Atrioventricular Bypass Tract Tachycardia

This is the second most common cause of paroxysmal supraventricular tachycardia (PSVT). Retrograde conduction down the AV node through the bypass tract may result in a normal QRS complex with the upper rate limited by the AV node. The onset of the tachycardia may be similar to that of AV nodal re-entry tachycardia. The rate may be faster than 200 bpm, and the P wave may be seen after the QRS wave, raising the suspicion of a bypass tract. Termination of this arrhythmia may be due to interruption of the re-entrant loop at a variety of areas but most commonly at the AV node. The AV block results in a dangling retrograde P wave visible after the last QRS of the tachycardia. Treatment may require electrical cardioversion or vagal maneuvers. Drugs used in this situation include adenosine, verapamil, propranolol, and digoxin. Amiodarone has been successful when conventional therapy has failed.

Automatic Atrial Tachycardia

Automatic atrial tachycardia is due to increased automaticity and is often described in persons with cardiac or pulmonary disease, metabolic abnormalities, or digitalis toxicity. When the arrhythmia starts, it often demonstrates a warm-up as the rate of discharge gradually increases for a few beats. The P wave is usually visible and differs somewhat from the sinus-induced P wave because it is shorter in duration and more peaked. The rate of firing ranges from about 150 to 200 bpm. Treatment is difficult. If digitalis or another drug is incriminated as causative, it should be discontinued. Metabolic, cardiac, and pulmonary abnormalities should be treated. If the rhythm is still resistant and not due to digitalis, propranolol or digitalis may be considered if the ventricular rate needs to be slowed.

Atrial Flutter

The usual clinical situation involves an individual with chronic obstructive pulmonary disease or decompensated heart failure. The flutter waves, appearing saw-toothed in leads II, III, and aVF, occur at a regular frequency and with an unvarying height. This characteristic helps differentiate flutter wave from coarse atrial fibrillatory waves. In untreated instances, the flutter waves occur about 300 times per minute but vary between 220 and 350 bpm. In the absence of A-V node disease or agents that slow AV node conduction, the ventricular response will be about 150 bpm.

Severe hemodynamic compromise may require emergency electrical cardioversion at low energy levels (20 to 50 J). Differentiation of type I from type II atrial flutter is important in the decision to attempt overdrive atrial pacing to terminate the atrial flutter. Type I may respond to atrial pacing, whereas type II does not. Pacing starts at a rate just above the native flutter rate and is gradually increased until capture occurs, usually 20% to 30% faster than the native rate. The faster rate should be continued for 20 seconds and abruptly stopped to interrupt the atrial flutter.

Drug therapy is also available for atrial flutter. Digitalis remains the mainstay. Beta-blockers, verapamil, quinidine, and amiodarone may also be used.

Multifocal Atrial Tachycardia (Chaotic Atrial Rhythm)

Multifocal atrial tachycardia (MAT) is most commonly misinterpreted as atrial fibrillation because the RR intervals are so varied. MAT demonstrates an atrial rate greater than 100 bpm. At least three different P waves with three different PR intervals must be present, and no single focus predominates. The presence of P waves may sometimes be misconstrued as fibrillatory waves. MAT is most commonly seen in individuals with severe decompensated lung disease. Treatment is difficult, usually excludes antiarrhythmic medications, and is focused on improving the underlying pulmonary process. Digitalis may worsen the arrhythmia.

Atrial Fibrillation

Atrial fibrillation may occur as an intermittent, paroxysmal phenomenon or as the more typical chronic pattern. Depolarization of the ventricle occurs in a sporadic fashion, with the QRS complexes characteristically occurring at irregular intervals. P waves are not visible because of the disorganized atrial depolarization, although the atrial activity noted on the surface ECG may reach such magnitude that the fibrillatory waves may resemble P waves. Unless aberrancy develops or a bundle branch block was preexisting, the QRS complex is narrow. Aberrancy may occur, and usually the aberrant QRS complex is of a right bundle branch type.

Ventricular Tachycardia

The simplest definition of ventricular tachycardia (VT) is the occurrence of three premature ventricular contractions (PVCs) in a row. The PVCs may be of the same configuration (monomorphic) or may vary (polymorphic), and the RR intervals may be similar or diverse. General terminology assigns the diagnosis of VT to instances in which the ventricular rate is 100 to 120 beats per minute or greater. In instances of VT in which the rate is less than 100 to 120 bpm but greater than 50 to 60 bpm, the term accelerated idioventricular rhythm is used. Rhythm strips may demonstrate that the atrial and ventricular rates are firing independently of one another. The atrial rate is usually slower than the ventricular rate. Should a P wave occur when the AV node and ventricular tissue are not totally refractory, conduction from the supraventricular focus may occur, leading to a normal QRS complex or to a fusion beat. This latter QRS complex often has a configuration that merges supraventricular conduction with ventricular conduction.

It is very important to differentiate supraventricular tachycardia from VT because misdiagnosis may lead to inappropriate treatment with a poor outcome. VT is associated with a number of diseases, commonly atherosclerotic heart disease and cardiomyopathy. Other abnormalities include hypoxia, hypokalemia, hypomagnesemia, digitalis toxicity, right-sided heart catheters, and ventricular pacemakers.

A variety of antiarrhythmic medications are available for

treatment of VT. Selection and route of administration will depend on the patient's hemodynamic status and associated problems. If the patient is hemodynamically unstable, electrical cardioversion may be the first line of therapy. Symptomatic VT is an indication for immediate therapy. Acute situations may require, in addition to possible cardioversion, intravenous treatment with lidocaine, procainamide or bretylium. Intravenous β-blockade and magnesium may also be helpful.

Torsades de Pointes

Torsades de pointes is a specific form of ventricular arrhythmia manifest as a rapid VT with the QRS complex twisting on its axis. The ventricular rate is variable. Initiation is often by a late premature ventricular beat in a person with a long QT interval. Although spontaneous termination occurs frequently, ventricular fibrillation may also develop. Torsades de pointes is often a side effect of Type-I antiarrhythmics or organophosphorus insecticide poisoning and has been associated with liquid protein diets. Isoproterenol infusion may be helpful by increasing the heart rate and shortening repolarization. Either atrial or ventricular pacing may be necessary to suppress the arrhythmia. Correction of magnesium and potassium deficits is warranted.

Ventricular Fibrillation

Ventricular fibrillation is a disorganized "rhythm." P waves are not visible, and QRS complexes are not identifiable because there is no organized ventricular depolarization. Various areas of the ventricle are depolarizing, and subsequently small or even large deflections occurring at various heights and intervals are seen on the surface ECG. Untreated, the deflections become smaller, and all electrical activity ceases or the electrical deflection becomes so small that the tracing demonstrates a flat line. Ventricular fibrillation may occur de novo in acute myocardial infarction, or it may follow an ongoing episode of VT, ventricular flutter, or increased automaticity after treatment for asystole. It is also seen in patients who experience atrial fibrillation with Wolff-Parkinson-White syndrome and anterograde conduction through the accessory pathway.

Defibrillation is the first therapy. If this fails, Advanced Cardiac Life Support (ACLS) guidelines are implemented. Medications include epinephrine followed by lidocaine and then bretylium. If resuscitation is successful, electrophysiologic studies to prevent recurrence of ventricular arrhythmias should be considered.

CONDUCTION ABNORMALITIES

First-Degree Atrioventricular Block

First-degree AV block is characterized by the presence of a prolonged PR interval (more than 0.20 seconds). Each P wave is followed by a conducted QRS complex. First-degree AV block may occur in healthy individuals but may also result from ischemia, high vagal tone, and a variety of drugs, most notably certain calcium channel blockers, β-blockers, and digitalis. Treatment is not needed.

Second-Degree Atrioventricular Block

In second-degree AV block, some but not all P waves are conducted to the ventricles. It is imperative to demonstrate that the nonconducted P waves are not early to avoid confusion with blocked premature atrial contractions (PACs). The failure to conduct may occur at various levels, reflected in the PR interval (for instance, the atrial tissue, the AV node, and the His-Purkinje system) and is not always due to slowing of or failure to conduct solely at the AV node area.

Wenckebach Second-Degree Atrioventricular Block (Mobitz Type I)

This form of second-degree AV block is characterized by regular P wave activity, single P waves not followed by a QRS, and progressive PR prolongation with subsequent failure to conduct while the RR intervals concomitantly shorten. The conduction block most frequently occurs within the AV node. Treatment is usually not needed, but monitoring may be indicated in unstable situations that may progress, such as in acute myocardial infarction.

Mobitz Type II Second-Degree Atrioventricular Block

Mobitz type II second-degree AV block is seen less frequently than Mobitz type I and is viewed as potentially more dangerous. It may be associated with acute anterior wall myocardial infarctions and may be complicated by complete heart block with an unstable escape rhythm. Mobitz type II block demonstrates regular atrial activity with sudden failure to conduct one or more P waves. Often the QRS complex is wider than normal, consistent with the fact that the conduction delay occurs below the bundle of His. Because of this, the PR interval of conducted beats in Mobitz type II is usually normal. Treatment is usually necessary because the conduction abnormality lies in the distal conduction system and is often progressive. A stable and reliable transvenous pacemaker is the usual form of treatment.

Third-Degree Atrioventricular Block

If the basic rhythm is sinus, third-degree AV block is diagnosed by the presence of an atrial rate that is faster than the ventricular rate, a regular ventricular rate that is less than or equal to 60 beats per minute, and the lack of any fixed PR interval. The atria fire independently of the ventricles, and the ventricular rate normally is controlled by an escape rhythm located below the atrium.

Common causes of complete or third-degree AV block

include medications such as digitalis, selective calcium channel blockers and β-blockers, degenerative disease of the conduction system (Lev's disease and Lenegre's disease), and various cardiomyopathies. This may also develop in acute myocardial infarction. If third-degree AV block is due to inferior infarction, it is usually associated with a stable junctional escape rhythm, whereas the third-degree AV block resulting from acute anterior wall myocardial infarction is likely to be associated with an unstable and unreliable ventricular escape rhythm. Endocarditis, especially of the aortic valve, may be complicated by complete heart block as might valve replacement. Lyme disease may cause transient third-degree AV block.

Sinoatrial Exit Block

Similar to AV block, SA exit block may occur, causing pauses on the surface ECG. SA block is presumed to be the cause of a sudden pause if the PP interval surrounding the pause is an exact multiple of the normal sinus PP interval and, of course, no blocked PAC is present. Causes of SA exit block include digitalis, atherosclerotic coronary disease, carotid sinus hypersensitivity, and high vagal tone.

PACEMAKERS AND IMPLANTABLE CARDIOVERTER DEFIBRILLATORS IN THE INTENSIVE CARE UNIT SETTING

Evaluation of pacemaker function requires knowledge of the pacemaker manufacturer and model as well as its programmed settings. Pacemakers may be identified as to manufacturer and type by patient indentification cards issued at implantation, by medical records from implantation, or by appearance and unique identification markings visible on an overpenetrated chest x-ray film. Each manufacturer provides an electronic programmer to interrogate and reprogram the pacemaker. Programming units often display telemetry and marker channels, which are helpful in diagnosing various aspects of pacemaker function and malfunction.

Trouble-Shooting

Failure to Pace with Pacing Stimuli Present

Failure to pace with pacing stimuli present is defined as the presence of pacemaker electrical output without capture of the myocardium. A rise in pacing threshold is seen during the first 4 to 6 weeks after a pacemaker is implanted secondary to tissue reaction at the lead-myocardium interface. In some patients, the rise in threshold observed after implantation can exceed the maximum output of the generator. This is described by the term *exit block*. This may resolve with time (days to weeks), and one may elect to treat patients with steroids in an attempt to hasten this resolution. Pacemaker-dependent patients may require temporary transvenous pacing during this time.

An abrupt rise in threshold or loss of capture within several days to weeks after implantation should arouse suspicion of lead dislodgement. This can also be suggested by a change in the paced QRS complex on 12-lead ECG, indicating the lead has moved, or by the pacing of a different chamber altogether (an atrial lead pacing the ventricle or vice versa). This can be confirmed with a PA and lateral chest x-ray film, noting displacement of the lead compared with the postimplant film.

Another cause of loss of capture is lead perforation of the right ventricle or right atrium. This presents with high pacing threshold or complete loss of capture (or abnormal sensing), or both. Chest x-ray film or echocardiography may reveal the lead outside the cardiac silhouette or a pericardial effusion, or both. Cardiac tamponade, signs of pericarditis, or diaphragmatic pacing may be present.

Other causes of increased thresholds and failure to capture include myocardial infarction near the lead myocardial interface; progressive myocardial fibrosis; electrolyte or metabolic derangements such as hyperkalemia, hyperglycemia, or acidemia; or certain pharmacologic agents, including antiarrhythmic drugs (especially class Ia, Ic, and III agents), mineralocorticoids, glucose with insulin, and hypertonic saline. Thresholds can also increase after direct current (DC) cardioversion. Administration of epinephrine, glucocorticoids, or isoproterenol may reduce pacing thresholds acutely. Elevated thresholds may also be overcome by increasing the energy output of the pacemaker generator or by using temporary pacing modalities.

Primary lead malfunction is another cause of loss of pacing. Leads can malfunction secondary to either an insulation defect or a conductor fracture. An insulation defect effectively shunts current away from the stimulating electrode. Thus, the output must be increased to deliver the same amount of current to the heart. Insulation defects may be associated with pectoral muscle stimulation and low measured impedance on pacemaker interrogation. Generator failure will eventually result in noncapture as the battery is depleted. This usually follows several months of energy-conserving asynchronous pacing and/or slowing of pacing rate below programmed values. Battery depletion may be diagnosed by pacemaker interrogation or response to magnet application.

Failure to Pace with Stimuli Absent

To categorize a pacing system malfunction with stimuli absent, one must first ascertain that pacemaker output is truly absent. A 12-lead ECG is often necessary to confirm a lack of pacing stimuli. With complete lead fractures or dislodgement of the lead from the generator, pacemaker spikes may be absent because of electrical discontinuity between the generator and the body. These conditions should be apparent on a chest x-ray film. Lead problems can result in oversensing with inhibition of output. A break in the inner insulation of an in-line coaxial bipolar lead can lead to large electrical signals because of contact between the inner and outer conductors. These signals are typically extremely large, precluding a decrease in sensitivity as a management option. In the pacemaker-dependent patient, programming the system to the SOO or DOO mode may be the only option until the lead can be replaced.

Temporary Cardiac Pacing

Temporary cardiac pacing is indicated for virtually any symptomatic or hemodynamically compromising bradyarrhythmia, except in the setting of hypothermia (in which refractory ventricular tachyarrhythmias may be induced). Prophylactic temporary pacing is most frequently indicated in the setting of unstable escape rhythms or during acute myocardial infarction. Patients with new onset of two or more first-degree AV blocks, Mobitz type I or II second-degree AV block, left anterior or posterior fascicular block, or right or left bundle branch block have a 25% to 36% risk of complete heart block in the setting of an acute myocardial infarction.

There are several possible modes of temporary pacing, including esophageal, transcutaneous, transvenous, and transthoracic. Esophageal pacing is generally efficacious only for pacing the left atrium and is therefore of limited utility in emergency situations. Transcutaneous pacing is a fast, simple, and effective initial method in bradyasystolic arrest situations. The large pacing electrodes are placed with the negative electrode on the anterior chest wall over the cardiac apex or chest lead, V3 position, and the positive patch over the posterior chest wall between the right or left scapula and spine. The generator uses high current and long pulse widths and obscures unfiltered ECG monitors. Maximum current is recommended initially to ensure ventricular capture in urgent situations. Pacing thresholds are generally in the 40- to 80-mA range and are frequently uncomfortable for the patient. Transcutaneous pacemakers pace the ventricles with hemodynamics similar to that of endocardial VVI pacing.

Transvenous pacing is the most reliable method of temporary pacing but requires more operator skill and time to institute. Temporary pacing leads are best positioned in the right ventricle from a right internal jugular or left subclavian approach. The leads are directed by fluoroscopic or ECG guidance. A defibrillator should always be immediately available during lead manipulation. Ideally, atrial and ventricular capture thresholds should be less than 1 mA and sensing thresholds greater than 1 mV and 6 mV, respectively. Temporary generators are typically VVI or DVI. DDD units have recently become available. Patients suffering an acute myocardial infarction, valvular heart disease, left ventricular systolic dysfunction, or diastolic noncompliance and those recovering from cardiac surgery may benefit hemodynamically from temporary AV sequential pacing. Lead dislodgement is the most common cause of pacing or sensing malfunction or both. Complications include induction of ventricular tachyarrhythmias, vascular damage, myocardial perforation, thrombosis, and infection.

Implantable Cardioverter Defibrillators

General Description

Implantable cardioverter defibrillators (ICDs) are designed to terminate malignant ventricular arrhythmias by delivering an electric shock or antitachycardia pacing to the heart. Shock therapy is delivered through patch electrodes surgically positioned on the epicardium or through transvenous endocardial electrode systems with or without subcutaneous electrodes. Two modes of therapy are used by ICDs to terminate ventricular tachyarrhythmias. The first is delivery of an electric shock to the heart. The energy required to defibrillate the heart is not an absolute value but rather follows a probability function. The programmed energy delivered represents a threshold energy determined at the time of implant plus a safety factor (generally 10 J) to ensure a high likelihood of successful defibrillation. The defibrillation energy requirement at any particular time is influenced by characteristics of the device, impedance to current flow, and presence of ischemia, drugs, myocardial stretch, and other factors. In general, less energy is required to terminate ventricular tachycardia (VT) than ventricular fibrillation (VF). After a maximum of four to seven shocks are delivered without tachycardia termination, no further therapy is available until the device has sensed a heart rate below the tachycardia detection rate for a specified time period.

Evaluation of Recurrent Appropriate Therapy

Appropriate successful ICD shocks can be lifesaving but, if recurrent in a brief time period, are very uncomfortable and contribute to early battery depletion. Additionally, multiple episodes of ventricular tachyarrhythmias and multiple defibrillations can lead to myocardial ischemia, myocardial stunning, and poor cardiac function. Frequent appropriate shocks are best managed by suppression and treatment of the ventricular arrhythmia. Electrolyte abnormalities, especially hypokalemia or hypomagnesemia, should be aggressively treated. New or worsening heart failure can be a cause of more frequent arrhythmias and should be optimally managed. Myocardial ischemia or new infarction must be considered and treated. New antiarrhythmic drug therapy may be proarrhythmic, leading to multiple episodes of polymorphic VT. Treatment with tricyclic drugs, phenothiazines, pentamidine, erythromycin, terfenadine, or astemizole can lead to a prolonged QT interval precipitating torsades de pointes. Discontinuation of previously successful antiarrhythmic drug therapy may result in more frequent tachyarrhythmias.

Some patients will not have an identifiable cause for their multiple episodes of VT/VF. These patients require antiarrhythmic drug therapy to suppress frequent episodes. Specific antiarrhythmic drug therapy is usually empiric. Lidocaine, procainamide, and bretylium are easily administered, rapidly acting, and relatively effective in the short term in the intensive care unit setting. Patients should be monitored during the institution of antiarrhythmic drugs for proarrhythmia (both tachyarrhythmias and bradyarrhythmias). New antiarrhythmic drugs may cause an increase in defibrillation thresholds or slow the tachycardia rate below detection rates. Patients must therefore undergo repeat testing of their ICD after institution of or change in antiarrhythmic drugs.

Inappropriate Therapy

Inappropriate therapy from ICDs may be in response to supraventricular tachyarrhythmias or electronic noise interpreted by the device as a ventricular arrhythmia. Most ICDs use heart rate as the sole criterion to detect ventricular tachyarrhythmias. Any heart rate the device senses above its programmed cutoff rate is treated as VT. Thus, supraventricular tachyarrhythmias exceeding the cutoff rate will also initiate device therapy. Patients may receive inappropriate shocks for atrial fibrillation or flutter, paroxysmal supraventricular tachycardia, or even sinus tachycardia. This is not considered a device malfunction. Raising the cutoff rate for the detection of tachycardia may help prevent this problem. Some patients have overlap between their VT rate and their rates during atrial fibrillation, sinus tachycardia, or supraventricular tachycardia. Medication such as β-blockers, calcium channel blockers, or digoxin may be needed to slow the ventricular rates during these supraventricular rhythms.

Failure to Respond

The time from detection of a ventricular tachyarrhythmia to the response by an ICD varies depending on the device and the programmed therapy. A long detection time or delay with charging for a maximum shock may take 20 seconds or longer to deliver therapy. Telemetry monitoring units may discontinue recording during this delay, leading to a misdiagnosis of failure to respond. Noncommitted devices should not deliver therapy unless the VT persists for that time; failure to respond to nonsustained VT is appropriate.

HYPERTENSIVE CRISES: EMERGENCIES AND URGENCIES

Clinical Manifestations

The clinical assessment of the patient begins with confirmation of the BP measurement in both arms, using an appropriately sized cuff. This is followed by a rapid yet detailed evaluation of the organ systems most susceptible to damage from elevated BP: the central nervous, cardiovascular, and renal systems.

Neurologic Assessment

Central nervous system involvement is suggested by complaints of headache, nausea, vomiting, visual disturbances, confusion, seizures, and focal neurologic deficits. A thorough examination requires inspection of the optic fundi for evidence of hypertensive retinopathy and papilledema. In the absence of other end-organ involvement, the presence of cotton wool exudates or flame-shaped hemorrhages is compatible with a hypertensive urgency. A computed tomographic (CT) scan of the head is often necessary to rule out intracranial hemorrhage, stroke, or other lesions. Focal neurologic findings mandate early CT scan but can be associated with hypertensive encephalopathy.

Cardiovascular Assessment

The cardiovascular consequences of severe hypertension may precipitate symptoms of anginal chest pain, dyspnea, or severe, tearing chest pain associated with acute aortic dissection. Physical findings that suggest acute left ventricular dysfunction include rales, a third heart sound, jugular venous distention, and tachycardia. Findings that may be present with aortic dissection include pulse deficits, a new murmur of aortic insufficiency, and a pericardial friction rub. An electrocardiogram is necessary for evaluating possible ischemia or infarction. A chest radiograph may indicate pulmonary edema or the nonspecific finding of a widened mediastinum suggesting an aortic aneurysm.

Renal System Assessment

Renal involvement resulting from severe hypertension may be clinically silent with nonspecific symptoms of weakness, pedal edema, oliguria, polyuria, or hematuria. A complete assessment involves measurement of blood urea nitrogen and creatinine as well as urinalysis with microscopic examination to detect proteinuria, hematuria, and the presence of cellular casts. The latter two findings are suggestive of glomerulonephritis as a secondary cause of hypertension. A complete blood count and electrolytes should be obtained. A blood smear can be examined for evidence of microangiopathic hemolytic anemia, but this is a rare finding (Table 4–4).

General Principles of Treatment

Although various recommendations for the extent of BP reduction have been proposed, each case must be individualized. A reasonable goal for most hypertensive emergencies is to lower the mean arterial pressure by approximately 25% or to reduce the diastolic BP to 100 to 110 mm Hg over a period of several minutes to hours, depending on the clinical situation. Although BP should be lowered to safer levels, it is not necessary to normalize BP in the first 24 to 48 hours of therapy. After the acute reduction of BP with parenteral agents in hypertensive emergencies, oral medications should

Table 4–4. PRECIPITATING FACTORS FOR HYPERTENSIVE CRISES

Preexisting hypertension	Eclampsia
Progression of disease	Collagen vascular disease
Unrecognized hypertension	Systemic lupus erythematosus
Patient noncompliance	Progressive systemic sclerosus
Renovascular hypertension	Polyarteritis nodosa
Acute glomerulonephritis	Drugs
Parenchymal renal disease	Diet pills
Pheochromocytoma	Cocaine
Antihypertensive withdrawal	Amphetamines
Head injury	Oral contraceptives
Burns	Corticosteroids
MAOI-tyramine interactions	

Abbreviation: MAOI = monoamine oxidase inhibitor.

be instituted within 12 to 24 hours and BP reduced to a normotensive level over the ensuing days to weeks.

Pharmacotherapy for Hypertensive Emergencies

Sodium Nitroprusside

Nitroprusside has been the "gold standard" for treatment of most hypertensive emergencies. Sodium nitroprusside (NTP) causes relaxation of arterial and venous smooth muscle. A controlled reduction of BP is easily achieved because of the rapid onset of the hypotensive effect and the short duration of action. NTP has been used effectively for severe hypertension in encephalopathy, intracranial hemorrhage, myocardial ischemia, left ventricular failure, pheochromocytoma, dissecting aortic aneurysm, and postoperative hypertension. An infusion pump must be used for administration and the BP should be closely monitored. Intra-arterial blood pressure monitoring is preferred.

Infusion of NTP should be initiated at a very low rate (0.3 $\mu g \cdot kg-^{1} \cdot min^{-1}$) and titrated upward every few minutes. If the BP falls below the desired level, discontinuation of NTP results in BP increases within 1 to 10 minutes. Cyanide or thiocyanate toxicity usually does not pose a problem with use of NTP unless the infusion is maintained for more than 72 hours or at doses greater than 3 $\mu g \cdot kg^{-1} \cdot min^{-1}$. The maximum rate of 10 $\mu k \cdot kg^{-1} \cdot min^{-1}$ should not be maintained for more than 10 minutes. Patients with renal insufficiency or hepatic disease are prone to toxicity. Thiocyanate toxicity can manifest as abdominal pain, delirium, headache, nausea, muscle spasms, and restlessness.

Labetalol

Labetalol is an oral and parenteral α- and nonselective β-adrenergic blocker that reduces BP by decreasing systemic vascular resistance (SVR) with little or no change in cardiac output or heart rate. A controlled reduction of BP is possible because of the rapid peak effect with minimal further reduction of BP following an intravenous bolus or discontinuation of an infusion. Hypotension is infrequent provided the total dose remains below the recommended maximum of 300 mg. Selected cases may require prolonged infusions at reduced rates. The β-blocking properties of labetalol contraindicate its use in patients with bronchospasm, severe sinus bradycardia (heart rate less than 50 beats/min), greater than first-degree heart block, or decompensated congestive heart failure. Labetalol is an excellent choice for control of severe hypertension associated with cocaine abuse. An advantage of labetalol is the ability to convert to an oral form of the same drug.

Nitroglycerin

Nitroglycerin is a direct vasodilator, predominantly venous, that also results in coronary artery vasodilatation. Higher doses are capable of producing arterial dilatation. The intravenous form is easily titrated because of the rapid onset of action and short duration of effect, but it is much less potent than other parenteral antihypertensive agents.

Nicardipine Hydrochloride

Nicardipine is a dihydropyridine calcium channel blocker prepared in an oral or intravenous form. The intravenous form may be particularly suited for treatment of hypertensive emergencies because of its potency, rapid onset of action, titratability, and lack of toxic metabolites. It has a direct effect on vascular smooth muscle, resulting in systemic and coronary artery vasodilatation. Nicardipine has minimal or no negative inotropic effects and usually results in increased cardiac output and left ventricular ejection fraction. Heart rate is usually not increased. Caution should be exercised in the elderly or in patients with liver disease who may have decreased hepatic metabolism. Most experience has been with loading infusions followed by maintenance infusions, but bolus administration has also been used. Side effects are similar to those reported for other calcium channel blockers and include headache, flushing, lightheadedness, hypotension, tachycardia, nausea, and vomiting.

Diazoxide

Diazoxide is a potent arterial vasodilator with little or no effect on venous capacitance. The duration of antihypertensive effect is measured in hours, but the short onset of action and short time to peak effect allow for a stepwise reduction of BP with repetitive bolus doses. Current recommendations of minibolus administration or continuous infusion offer greater control and safety. Previous recommendations for a rapid 300-mg bolus to overcome high protein-binding were associated with precipitous drops of BP, leading to myocardial and cerebral ischemia. Diazoxide evokes a reflex tachycardia and, therefore, should not be used in patients with dissecting aortic aneurysm or coronary artery disease. Repetitive doses or prolonged administration may be associated with hyperglycemia, hyperuricemia, displacement of other protein-bound drugs, and salt and water retention, requiring the use of a loop diuretic, The solution is highly alkaline, so great care should be taken to avoid extravasation.

Pharmacotherapy for Hypertensive Urgencies

Nifedipine

Nifedipine is the oral calcium channel blocker used most often in the management of hypertensive urgencies. The reduction in SVR is associated with a mild increase in heart rate. Despite tachycardia, a simultaneous increase in coronary artery blood flow results in reduced myocardial oxygen consumption. These hemodynamic effects make nifedipine potentially advantageous in selected patients with myocardial ischemia or known coronary artery disease. Administration in hypertensive urgencies is best accomplished by having the patient bite the capsule in half before swallowing because absorption is by gastric means rather than the buccal mucosa.

Clonidine

Clonidine is a central α-adrenergic agonist that decreases sympathetic outflow and leads to a reduction in SVR. It has been used extensively in the treatment of hypertensive urgencies. Precipitous drops in BP are less likely with clonidine compared with nifedipine. The sedative properties of clonidine may interfere with neurologic assessment of patients with encephalopathy or cerebrovascular events. Other side effects include dry mouth, orthostasis, and bradycardia. A reduced dose or increase in dosing interval is necessary in the presence of renal insufficiency.

Captopril

Captopril, an oral ACE inhibitor, has been used successfully in hypertensive urgencies. Hypotension after the initial dose may occur, especially in patients with sodium or volume depletion who concurrently use other antihypertensives and in those with renal vascular hypertension. Side effects with short-term use are minimal. Captopril should not be used in patients with suspected bilateral renal artery stenosis.

Specific Clinical Considerations

Hypertensive Encephalopathy

Cerebral dysfunction as a result of severe hypertension mandates rapid reduction of BP with a parenteral agent to prevent progression to coma and death. Severe hypertension can exceed the upper limit of cerebral blood flow autoregulation and result in vasodilatation with cerebral edema. Nitroprusside is the drug of choice with labetalol, nitroglycerin, and diazoxide as potential alternatives.

Acute Aortic Dissection

The initial treatment of a dissecting aortic aneurysm is BP reduction followed by definitive surgical or medical therapy. Proximal aortic dissections or distal dissections complicated by recurrent pain, expansion, vital organ compromise, or falling hematocrit indicate the need for surgical intervention. Distal aortic dissections without complications can be treated medically. The goal of antihypertensive therapy is to lower BP and rescue the shear force or rate of BP rise to prevent extension of injury. Blood pressure should be reduced to the lowest level that relieves pain and allows adequate organ perfusion, usually a systolic BP of 100 to 110 mm Hg. The most commonly used agents are nitroprusside in combination with intravenous propranolol. Alternatives include labetalol and the combination of esmolol and nitroprusside. Trimetaphan is infrequently used because of potential adverse effects, but it may be necessary for patients who are unable to tolerate β-adrenergic blockers.

HYPERTENSIVE EMERGENCIES IN INFANTS AND CHILDREN

Acutely elevated blood pressure in the pediatric patient usually constitutes a medical emergency that can result in significant morbidity or mortality. Several distinct patterns of acute hypertensive crisis have been described. Malignant hypertension is severe BP elevation associated with grade IV Keith-Wagener retinopathy (exudates, hemorrhages, arterial narrowing, and spasm with papilledema). The patient characteristically progresses rapidly to death or renal failure if untreated. Accelerated hypertension is marked BP elevation associated with grade III retinopathy (papilledema is absent). Malignant hypertension and accelerated hypertension usually occur as complications of chronic hypertension. Hypertensive encephalopathy refers to severe hypertension associated with central nervous system (CNS) dysfunction. Malignant hypertension and accelerated hypertension occur much less commonly in children than in adults. Hypertensive encephalopathy is the most common severe manifestation of uncontrolled BP in children.

The clinical manifestations of severe hypertension in pediatric patients are primarily neurologic and cardiovascular. Development of symptoms is directly related to the premorbid BP and the suddenness and degree of BP elevation. Patients in whom hypertension has developed gradually may be asymptomatic in spite of very high sustained BP elevations. In contrast, symptoms may develop in the child who had previously been normotensive when the BP elevation is only modest. In this latter circumstance, the rapidity of BP elevation is more important than the absolute BP value.

The pathogenesis of acute hypertension in children is related to the complex interaction of blood volume, cardiac output, and total peripheral resistance. BP is a function of circulating vascular volume and arteriolar vasoconstriction.

The former is largely determined by sodium balance, whereas the latter is a function of the renin-angiotensin system, catecholamines, and vascular autoregulation. This highly simplistic model provides a framework for etiologic, prognostic, and therapeutic decisions.

Etiology

Severe hypertension is commonly associated with acute nephritis and is particularly evident in acute poststreptococcal nephritis. Hypertension occurs in up to one half of all patients with hemolytic uremic syndrome. Hypertension in chronic glomerulonephritis is related to the severity of glomerular involvement, and its pathogenesis is usually multifactorial. Chronic atrophic pyelonephritis secondary to renal parenchymal infection in children with vesicoureteral reflux may cause severe hypertension. Hypertension may develop if blunt renal trauma produces a hematoma that compresses renal parenchyma or occludes a renal artery or vein. Hypertension is a cardinal feature of coarctation of the aorta. Renal artery stenosis in children is usually due to fibromuscular dysplasia. It may be an isolated finding associated with neurofibromatosis or the result of long-forgotten blunt trauma to the abdomen.

General Principles of Treatment

In the child with acute hypertension, the determination of cause is less important than is immediate BP control. The chronicity of BP elevation indicates both the rapidity and degree by which BP should be reduced. BP reduction should be accomplished within minutes in children with acute hypertensive encephalopathy and within hours to days in children with chronic hypertension and no acute symptoms. Severe acute hypertension usually mandates parenteral or sublingual therapy to reduce BP rapidly and predictably. The effectiveness of therapy in the severely hypertensive child should be monitored serially, ideally by direct intra-arterial measurement of BP. Serial neurologic evaluation is also important in the child with hypertensive encephalopathy.

Pharmacologic Agents

Sodium nitroprusside is an extremely potent vasodilator whose rapid onset and short duration of action allow precise BP titration. This agent should be administered by a constant infusion pump with continuous BP monitoring to ensure safety and efficacy.

Labetalol is an adrenergic-receptor blocking agent that has selective $\alpha 1$- and nonselective β-adrenergic blocking activity in a ratio of 1:7. When given intravenously in gradually increasing miniboluses, a prompt but gradual BP reduction can be achieved without the induction of reflex tachycardia or increased cardiac output, which occurs with the use of direct arteriolar vasodilators. Labetalol should be used with caution in patients with significant left ventricular dysfunction, pheochromocytoma, and bronchial asthma. Because a substantial fall in BP can occur with the assumption of the upright posture, patients should remain supine for at least 3 hours after receiving intravenous labetalol and should assume ambulation gradually.

Diazoxide is a potent vasodilator that promptly reduces BP after rapid bolus intravenous injection. Its effect is more prolonged but less controllable than that of nitroprusside; however, minibolus administration reduces the incidence of hypotension and better controls BP reduction. A diuretic may be used concomitantly with diazoxide to avoid sodium retention.

Phentolamine is used specifically for hypertensive crises caused by catecholamine excess. Trimetaphan, a parenterally administered agent that lowers BP by decreasing peripheral resistance through ganglionic blockade, is not recommended because experience in children is limited, and it offers no advantages over other agents.

Outcome

The exact mortality of children with actual hypertension is unknown. However, the risk of death has been diminished by more widespread recognition of this problem in children and the availability of more efficacious drugs. Hypertension may spontaneously abate with resolution of the underlying condition, as in poststreptococcal glomerulonephritis; may be treated successfully by surgical intervention, as in renal artery stenosis; or may be incurable but controllable, as in chronic glomerulonephritis. Usually, the signs and symptoms of hypertensive encephalopathy or renal failure resolve or improve as BP is controlled; however, residual neurologic abnormalities such as seizure disorders, blindness, cranial nerve palsy, and hemiplegia may persist. In some children with preexisting renal disease, a slightly elevated BP may be necessary for adequate renal perfusion. More commonly, any further deterioration in renal function as BP is lowered will be transient and reversible. The only predictor of transient deterioration is a clinical trial of BP normalization.

VENTRICULAR ASSIST DEVICES AND ARTIFICIAL HEARTS

Indications

Currently, mechanical assistance is indicated in patients with cardiogenic shock refractory to maximal pharmacologic and intra-aortic counterpulsation therapy (Table 4–5). Patients meeting these criteria have an extremely high mortality if mechanical support is not instituted. Subsequent clinical experience with ventricular assist devices (VADs) has confirmed these findings. The metabolic cardiac insult of high doses of inotropic agents contrasts with the favorable decrease in myocardial work and oxygen consumption seen with mechanical assistance. The decrease in myocardial oxygen consumption directly correlates with the degree of ven-

Table 4–5. CRITERIA FOR INSTITUTION OF MECHANICAL SUPPORT

CI <1.8 L · m² · min^{-1}
SBP <90 mm Hg
Atrial pressure(s) >20 mm Hg
Urine output <20 mL/hr (adult)
SVR >2100 dyne · s · cm^{-5}
Metabolic acidosis
Adequate preload, maximum inotropic/IABP support, and inability to tolerate vasodilators without hypotension

(Modified with permission from Pennington DG, Swartz MT: Assisted circulation and mechanical hearts. *In:* Heart Disease: A Textbook of Cardiovascular Medicine. 4th ed. Braunwald E [Ed]. Philadelphia, WB Saunders, 1992, p 537.)

Abbreviations: CI = cardiac index; SBP = systolic blood pressure; SVR = systemic vascular resistance; IABP = intra-aortic balloon pump.

tricular decompression and afterload reduction. Moreover, increased mean intra-aortic pressure, decreased central venous pressure, and decreased ventricular wall tension augment myocardial perfusion and oxygen delivery. The increased myocardial oxygen supply and decreased oxygen demand seen with mechanical assistance promote recovery of stunned myocardium and limit infarct size. Increased extracardiac organ perfusion also prevents systemic organ dysfunction.

Proper patient selection is the most important factor in minimizing the morbidity and mortality associated with mechanical assistance. Mechanical assistance is generally contraindicated for patients meeting any of the exclusion criteria listed in Table 4–6.

Postcardiotomy

When difficulty is encountered while withdrawing patients from cardiopulmonary bypass, the decision to institute mechanical assistance is made routinely. This group of patients represents a preselected population in whom lifesaving support could be easily instituted. Unfortunately, far less than 1% of all cardiotomy patients receive further mechanical support. Device unavailability and pessimism stemming from marginal improvement of patients in early clinical experience have deterred clinicians from instituting support. As a result of this prevailing attitude, morbidity and mortal-

Table 4–6. USUAL CONTRAINDICATIONS TO MECHANICAL ASSISTANCE

Age >70 years
Renal failure
Cerebrovascular insufficiency
Hepatic failure
Coagulopathy
Sepsis
Metastatic cancer

ity in this group of patients are increased because of the coagulation problems associated with long periods of cardiopulmonary bypass. However, improved devices and patient selection markedly decreased morbidity and mortality in later trials of postcardiotomy mechanical ventricular assistance.

Bridge to Transplantation

Transplant candidates are rigorously selected to maximize patient survival and donor organ utilization. Because pretransplant evaluation mostly selects patients with single organ cardiac disease, candidates in whom cardiogenic shock develops are ideally suited for mechanical assistance. Although current mechanical assist devices effectively bridge patients to transplantation, within the decade permanent assist devices could replace cardiac transplantation as the treatment of choice for some patients with end-stage cardiac disease.

Acute Myocardial Infarction

Current medical treatment of acute ischemic cardiogenic shock is associated with an 80% mortality. However, acute revascularization has been shown to improve survival. Unfortunately, early studies of mechanical assistance failed to demonstrate an increase in survival of postinfarction shock patients treated with mechanical assistance. Scheidt and associates demonstrated that the balloon pump improved hemodynamics but did not significantly alter patient survival. Later clinical trials with VADs demonstrated no increase in patient survival when these devices were not used in conjunction with orthotopic heart transplantation. However, these early trials did demonstrate a clear benefit when ventricular support was used as a bridge to cardiac transplantation.

Recently, the percutaneous intravascular Hemopump has been shown experimentally to improve regional myocardial blood flow and to limit infarct size. Preliminary clinical studies of patients with acute ischemic shock have demonstrated that the Hemopump improves the hemodynamics and survival of cardiogenic shock patients. Table 4–7 depicts the suggested algorithm for institution of mechanical support in the postinfarction patient with medically refractory cardiogenic shock.

Orthotopic Heart Transplantation

Without other perioperative complications, patients with cardiogenic shock after heart transplantation remain good candidates for ventricular assistance. Early utilization is the most important factor in post-transplant mechanical assistance because it limits further myocardial insult by preventing distention injury of the acutely denervated heart. Timely support also prevents severe secondary organ injury resulting from prolonged cardiogenic shock. Whereas short-term mechanical assistance decompresses the graft and pro-

Table 4–7. ALGORITHM FOR SUPPORT OF PATIENTS WITH REFRACTORY CARDIOGENIC SHOCK AFTER MYOCARDIAL INFARCTION

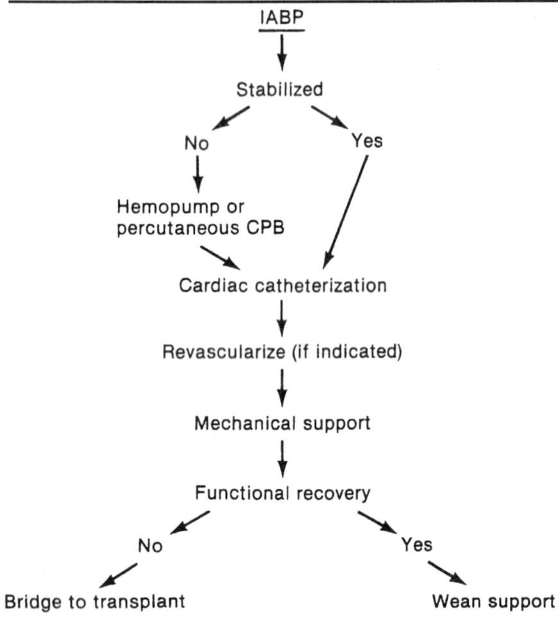

Abbreviations: IABP = intra-aortic balloon pump; CPB = cardiopulmonary bypass.

motes myocardial recovery, longer support can provide a successful bridge to retransplantation.

Resuscitation from Arrest

Recent developments in percutaneous mechanical assist devices have rekindled interest in mechanical resuscitation of patients who have sustained cardiac arrest. Preliminary clinical trials have demonstrated improved survival of such patients treated with percutaneous cardiopulmonary bypass. Moreover, these trials were conducted before the widespread availability of the Carmeda heparin-bonded cardiopulmonary bypass circuit. The biocompatibility of this circuit alleviates the need for full systemic heparinization and may reduce the side effects of extracorporeal membrane oxygenation (ECMO). Although the Hemopump has been experimentally shown to affect resuscitation from ventricular fibrillation favorably, clinical evaluation of its benefit in the treatment of cardiopulmonary arrest is required.

General Considerations

Hematologic Dysfunction

Artificial surfaces provide continual stimulation of the humoral amplification system. Platelet activation, fibrin formation, fibrinolysis, and leukocyte activation continue throughout mechanical assistance. It is not surprising that control of bleeding and thromboembolism remains problematic.

Bleeding is a problem especially in patients requiring high levels of anticoagulation, longer preimplant cardiopulmonary bypass, and treatment with amrinone before institution of mechanical assistance (amrinone-platelet dysfunction). High outflow device pressures and ventricular apex cannulation also predispose to bleeding. Although perioperative mechanical bleeding demands reoperation, coagulopathy related to cardiopulmonary bypass and mechanical assistance can be controlled with judicious use of blood products. As soon as bleeding is under control, anticoagulation should begin. Mediastinal tamponade is a relatively common occurrence that results in obstruction of inflow to the device and low outputs.

Thromboembolism is minimized by standardized anticoagulation. Anticoagulation therapy is device-specific and flow-related. For example, thrombogenic devices such as the Novacor left ventricular assist device (LVAS) require intense anticoagulation with dipyridamole, postoperative heparin, and long-term warfarin. Aspirin is also added if the patient has a transient ischemic attack or other nonhemorrhagic neurologic event. In contrast, the biologic membrane that forms on the Thermocardiosystems LVAS requires minimal anticoagulation with dipyridamole, short-term dextran therapy, and long-term aspirin therapy. Conditions that predispose to thrombus formation require increased anticoagulation. For example, ventricular fibrillation, distention, and hypokinesis promote intracardiac thrombosis during atrioaortic bypass. Kinked cannulas and increased ventricular function decrease device flow and increase intradevice thrombus formation. Most importantly, low device flow during weaning from a device requires heparinization to prevent significant thromboembolism.

Infection

Although infection in these patients is usually at a site distant from the device, treatment of the infrequent device infection requires aggressive operative debridement and antibiotic therapy. It is surprising that current support systems with transcutaneous cannulas do not have a large number of device infections, presumably secondary to the ingrowth of tissue around the cannulas. The newer, totally implantable devices will not have these cannulas as a source of infection.

Secondary Organ Dysfunction

Mechanical assistance commonly affects the renal, hepatic, pulmonary, and central nervous systems. Appropriate patient selection and early institution of mechanical assistance minimize preimplantation organ dysfunction. Intraoperative closure of a patent foramen ovale will prevent postoperative right-to-left shunting and severe peripheral desaturation in patients requiring isolated left ventricular support. After implantation, volume restriction and α-adrenergic agonists remove venous hypertension as a cause of organ dysfunction. As necessary, continuous arteriovenous hemofiltration and albumin administration can control the profound edema that often develops in mechanically assisted patients with organ dysfunction. Most importantly, the intensivist should encourage metabolic recovery of the mechanically assisted patient by minimizing pharmacologic support while maximizing tissue oxygen delivery.

Weaning

Weaning from mechanical assistance should not be attempted earlier than 24 hours after institution of support. Mechanical support is weaned by decreasing the output of the device while evaluating cardiac function with systemic and pulmonary arterial catheters and transesophageal echocardiography. When ventricular function adequately supports the circulation without significant aid from the device, mechanical assistance can be safely discontinued. As previously mentioned, it is necessary to increase anticoagulation while weaning the patient from the device (Table 4–8).

Results

Results of mechanical support are shown in Tables 4–9 and 4–10.

PERICARDIAL TAMPONADE

Pericardial tamponade is a condition caused by accumulation of pericardial fluid that constricts cardiac chambers by acutely increasing pericardial volume and pressure. It is an uncommon clinical condition produced by pericarditis with effusion or hemopericardium from penetrating trauma, central venous catheters, or cardiac instrumentation. The disorder may develop into life-threatening cardiogenic shock if it is not recognized and corrected rapidly.

Table 4–8. GENERAL PRINCIPLES OF CARE FOR MECHANICALLY ASSISTED PATIENTS

Ensure adequate device support.
Extubate and remove indwelling catheters early.
Aggressively mobilize and rehabilitate patient.
Provide adequate nutrition (preferably enteral).
Use device-specific anticoagulation.
Treat infections with organism-specific antibiotics.
Minimize concurrent pharmacologic support.
Maximize oxygen delivery.

Table 4–9. RESULTS OF HEMOPUMP SUPPORT IN THE TREATMENT OF POSTCARDIOTOMY SHOCK

Study	Patients Supported	Patients Discharged
Wampler et al[32]	17	4 (23.5%)
Burnett et al[24]	9	5 (55.5%)
Total	26	9 (34.6%)

For full reference sources, see Chapter 61 in the *Textbook of Critical Care.*

Pericardial Effusion

The volume and significance of effusions vary widely. Effusions may be the cause of cardiogenic shock, a complication of constrictive pericarditis, or an incidental observation in acute pericarditis. Pericardial effusions may occur in a wide spectrum of disorders, including (1) uremia; (2) neoplasms; (3) postmyocardial infarction (Dressler's syndrome); (4) postcardiac surgery; (5) infection, including tuberculosis; and (6) systemic lupus erythematosus (SLE) and other rheumatologic disorders. Tamponade has been an infrequent observation in SLE, malignancies, benign teratoma, myeloid metaplasia, scleroderma, juvenile rheumatoid arthritis, and inflammatory bowel disease. Pericarditis was reported in 75 of 395 (19%) SLE patients.

The physiologic alterations produced by the effusion primarily depend on the volume of the effusion and the rate of its development. For example, small volumes that occur suddenly or large volumes in malignant disorders that take months to form may be well tolerated. In the latter instance,

Table 4–10. RESULTS OF MECHANICAL ASSISTANCE IN TREATING CARDIOGENIC SHOCK IN THE BRIDGE TO TRANSPLANT APPLICATION (FROM ASAIO/ISHT REGISTRY)

Device	Number of Points	Transplantation	Transplantation Points Discharged	Bridge Points Discharged
RVAD	4	1 (25.0%)	1 (100%)	1 (25.0%)
LVAD	122	87 (71.3%)	76 (87.4%)	76 (62.3%)
BVAD	161	105 (65.2%)	73 (69.5%)	73 (45.3%)
TAH	189	135 (71.4%)	67 (49.6%)	67 (35.4%)
Total	476	328 (68.9%)	217 (66.2%)	217 (45.6%)

(With permission from Pae WE: Ventricular assist devices and total artificial hearts: A combined registry experience. Ann Thorac Surg 1993; 55:295–298.)

Abbreviations: ASAIO/ISHT = American Society of Artificial Internal Organs/International Society for Heart Transplantation; RVAD = right ventricular assist device; LVAD = left ventricular assist device; BVAD = biventricular assist device; TAH = total artificial heart.

the relatively elastic pericardium will stretch over time to accommodate as much as 1000 mL of pericardial fluid.

Diagnosis

Symptoms and signs are not specific; they include distant heart sounds, "quiet precordium," increased area of cardiac dullness, or cardiac dullness percussed lateral to the apical impulse. These physical signs are more often seen rather late in the course of the disorder. The diagnosis is often suspected by serial chest radiography or electrocardiography and confirmed by echocardiography, cardiac catheterization, or radionucleotide ventriculography. Early diagnosis is often suspected in patients with cancer of the lung or breast and leukemias, uremic patients on dialysis, patients with unexplained increased central venous pressure (CVP), and patients with enlarged cardiac silhouette.

The ECG may have low voltage and diffuse ST segment elevation in most leads; the ST segments usually retain their normal concave appearance. There may also be PR depression. Chest radiographs that are nonspecific may reveal "water bottle" or globular shapes suggestive of an effusion. Echocardiography is the most sensitive test and can be used in the widest variety of situations. The M mode may show an echo-free space as the site of fluid collection. Two-dimensional echocardiography provides more accurate quantification of the amount of effusion and its distribution, thickening of the pericardium, fibrinous adhesions, and the dimensions of the cardiac chambers. On occasion, ultrasonographic tests may suggest that an apparent cardiac enlargement may be accounted for by an effusion or that both may be present. The computed tomographic scan may demonstrate thickened pericardial sac walls.

PERICARDIOCENTESIS

Pericardiocentesis may be indicated for therapeutic reasons when there is rapid deterioration of hemodynamic function, when there is delay in operative decompression, and for diagnostic reasons in effusions of unknown cause. In the latter instance, the fluid is cultured for bacteria, fungi, and mycobacteria; Gram stained; and analyzed for hematocrit, cell count, cytology, glucose and protein levels, rheumatoid factor, antinuclear antibodies, and complement levels.

Hemopericardium with Tamponade

Clinical Evaluation

The rate of development and severity of pericardial tamponade vary with its cause. Tamponade may abruptly occur after blunt trauma with rupture of the heart, penetrating cardiac injury, and cardiac catheterization or central venous catheterization. A rapidly forming tamponade is often fatal unless immediately corrected by pericardiotomy and decompression. This may be the case in tamponade after instrumentation during cardiac catheterization or placement of a central catheter because there is no route through the pericardium for spontaneous decompression of the pericardial fluid. With penetrating trauma, some of the pericardial blood initially may escape through the pericardial rent until clots obstruct this egress.

It is crucial to suspect tamponade from the clinical setting and to diagnose promptly before shock or arrest occurs. Characteristically, the patient with acute tamponade is anxious, agitated, or even wildly disturbed. In later stages, there may be central nervous system depression, coma, and cardiac arrest. All patients with stab wounds of the chest and epigastrium, not excluding the back and right sides, must be suspected of having possible tamponade. Stab wounds of the right midaxillary line have been known to produce death from tamponade. Similarly, the diagnosis should be entertained in patients with gunshot wounds of the chest, back, or abdomen in which the heart could have been in the direct line of the missile trajectory or could have been injured by the deflected missile. Tamponade should also be suspected in symptomatic patients who have recently undergone cardiac operations, catheterization, and placement of central venous catheters or pacing wires. Finally, tamponade often occurs with significant hypovolemia as a result of blood loss into the pleural cavities from the rent in the pericardial sac; this often produces the typical picture of hypovolemic shock with hypotension, tachycardia, and low CVP. When volume is replaced, the CVP rises, but often hypotension and tachycardia persist.

Rarely, tamponade is also associated with blunt trauma or vigorous cardiopulmonary resuscitation that has fractured ribs. Pericardial tamponade produced by a penetrating chest injury may also occur within minutes, if rapid bleeding from the pierced heart produces clots that block the pericardial laceration and cause blood to accumulate in the pericardial sac. Alternatively, tamponade from a penetrating chest wound may develop over a period of days as blood from the lacerated heart slowly fills the pericardium and then leaks from the torn pericardial sac into the pleural space or mediastinum. This is in contrast to the temporal spectrum of pericardial effusions that produce tamponade slowly over weeks; the pericardial sac distends and may hold large volumes before clinical distress is manifest. In acutely developing tamponade, however, up to 250 mL usually is well tolerated, 250 to 450 mL produces moderately severe hemodynamic alterations, and hemopericardium greater than 450 mL produces severe hemodynamic changes, including shock and cardiac arrest.

Diagnosis

The clinical diagnosis of pericardial tamponade is based on Beck's triad of distant heart sounds, hypotension, and distended neck veins, the last of which reflects an elevated CVP (usually 18 cm H_2O and rising). In addition, there may be an increased area of cardiac dullness outside the apical point of maximum impulse and pulsus paradoxus. The latter is an exaggerated pulse variation with respiration, that is, decreased systolic pressure, pulse pressure, and heart rate during inspiration. It is evaluated as the patient breathes normally; the arm cuff is gradually deflated until the first sound is intermittently heard on auscultation at the brachial artery; this is pressure during expiration. The cuff is again deflated slowly until all beats are heard, especially during inspiration; differences in systolic pressures greater than 15 mm Hg indicate pulsus paradoxus. Although measurable by sphygmomanometer, pulsus paradoxus is best illustrated by a continuous arterial pressure tracing. It is an inconsistent sign in acute tamponade from penetrating chest wounds but is seen more frequently when tamponade slowly develops with pericardial effusions. Conditions that increase intrathoracic pressure, such as chronic obstructive lung disease, obesity, and congestive failure, must be ruled out.

The incidence of tamponade after penetrating chest injury is only 2%. Of those patients with proven cardiac tamponade, only about one third have the entire Beck's triad when first diagnosed. Characteristically, tamponade patients may appear to be stable for varying periods of time, but they may suddenly and rapidly deteriorate. It is most important to make an early diagnosis and give appropriate therapy during the early stage because, if treatment is delayed until all the classic signs of Beck's triad are present, cardiac arrest is likely to intervene. When hypotension occurs, it often leads rapidly to circulatory collapse and arrest. The mortality of patients with tamponade subjected to thoracotomy without delay is 15% to 25%; mortality increases to 60% after cardiac arrest occurs.

Differential Diagnosis

Acute tamponade must be differentiated from other conditions with elevated CVP, including tension pneumothorax, acute right ventricular failure, chronic obstructive lung disease, constrictive pericarditis, acute exacerbation of chronic bronchitis, acute pulmonary embolism, and fat emboli. Also, the increased CVP associated with tamponade must be distinguished from the high CVP resulting from excessive or rapid administration of fluids, abdominal distention from ascites or ileus, acute renal failure, increased intrathoracic pressure from pneumothorax, hemothorax, airway obstruction or mechanical ventilation, administration of vasopressors, and clotted nonfunctioning CVP catheter or a CVP catheter that slipped into the right ventricle.

Therapeutic Management

The major problem is to correct the primary defect, hemopericardium, but a more immediate problem may be to maintain some degree of hemodynamic stability until the patient has definitive correction of the hemopericardium.

Suspected cases of pericardial tamponade should undergo measurements of blood pressure, heart rate, and CVP every 5 to 15 minutes. Rising CVP and an increasing degree of hypotension indicate impending hemodynamic decompensation.

While the patient with suspected cardiac tamponade is being considered for operation, a trial of volume loading may improve hemodynamics and confirms that hypovolemia, myocardial insufficiency, or failure is not the major problem. Volume loading is not contraindicated by high venous pressures because tamponade is produced by inadequate ventricular filling as a result of high atrial pressure, not failure of myocardial performance. Plasma volume expansion in patients with progressive reductions in stroke index improves stroke index, cardiac index, and arterial pressure. Fluid administration despite high venous pressures has a beneficial effect because contractility of the cardiac muscle is not initially impaired. Under these conditions, the heart is able to handle volume loads despite high venous pressures.

When sudden deterioration occurs, emergency thoracotomy may be indicated; if there is delay in operating for any reason, therapeutic pericardiocentesis may be lifesaving. It is not necessary to evacuate the entire pericardial contents; often, withdrawal of as little as 20 to 30 mL of nonclotting blood in acute hemopericardial tamponade may restore hemodynamic stability, because the difference between the amount of blood in compensated and decompensated hemopericardium may be small. Pericardiocentesis improves hemodynamics by reducing intrapericardial pressure; this increases venous return, cardiac output, and coronary perfusion. Additionally, preoperative pericardiocentesis reduces the risk of sudden deterioration and cardiac arrest during anesthesia induction. General anesthesia and positive-pressure ventilation lower cardiac output and blood pressure in tamponade patients, but pericardiocentesis reduces these effects. The goal of optimal therapy is urgently to remove hemodynamically significant pericardial fluid with appropriate expediency (Table 4–11).

Complications

Recovery from tamponade after decompression and pericardial window is usually uneventful unless coronary vessels,

Table 4–11. HEMODYNAMIC CHANGES PRODUCED BY THERAPY

Variable	Pericardiocentesis (n = 3)	Volume Load (n = 5)	Isoproterenol (n = 3)
Stroke index (mL/m^2)	+4	+8	+13
Cardiac index (mL · m^2 · m^{-1})	+0.9	+0.7	+2.3
Mean arterial pressure (mm Hg)	+7.0	+13	+11
Central venous pressure (cm H_2O)	−2.2	+5.7	+3
Heart rate (beat/min)	+14	−1	+18
Mean tension time(s)	−1	−1	−3
Left ventricular stroke work (g · m^2 · m^{-1})	+6	+16	+23

septum, or cardiac valves have been injured by the penetrating injury. The pericardiotomy syndrome, which consists of fever, pain, and pericardial effusion, occurs in a small percentage of patients; this complication may respond to steroids or nonsteroidal anti-inflammatory drugs. Constrictive pericarditis is a rare complication.

PULMONARY HYPERTENSION

Clinical Manifestations

Patients with pulmonary hypertension typically present with nonspecific and nondiagnostic symptoms which include exertional dyspnea, fatigue, chest pain that is often described as a substernal pressure suggestive of angina pectoris, and syncope. The latter complaint is particularly noteworthy because it implies a markedly impaired cardiac output and is a poor prognostic sign. Similarly, edema or anasarca implies the presence of right-sided heart failure and portends a poor prognosis. Raynaud's phenomenon is reported to occur in up to 25% to 30% of patients with primary pulmonary hypertension (PPH), although it is far more common in pulmonary hypertension secondary to connective tissue diseases. Hoarseness may result from compression of the recurrent laryngeal nerve by massively dilated proximal pulmonary arteries. A chronic, nonproductive cough may also be evident and may be due to stimulation of interstitial irritant receptors as a result of vascular enlargement.

The physical examination not only suggests the presence of pulmonary vascular disease but also provides important clues to its cause. Examination of the jugular venous pulse may demonstrate elevation of the venous pressure, suggesting right-sided heart volume overload as well as prominent a or cv waves, indicating altered right ventricular compliance and tricuspid regurgitation. Examination of the chest may disclose abnormalities that point to an underlying specific cause for pulmonary vascular disease, such as obstructive lung disease or restriction resulting from rib cage deformities.

Patients with severe, chronic pulmonary hypertension usually manifest a prominent right ventricular impulse along the parasternal region; a right-sided fourth heart sound and pulmonic component to the second heart sound (P_2) may also be palpable. In contrast, the point of maximal cardiac impulse is frequently displaced to the subxiphoid region in patients with cor pulmonale resulting from severe obstructive lung disease. Auscultation of the heart may disclose an accentuated P_2, right-sided S_4 gallop, or a pulmonic ejection click. An S_3 gallop is indicative of right-sided heart failure and is a serious prognostic finding.

The murmur of tricuspid insufficiency, audible along the lower right sternal border and increasing with inspiration, is a common finding in advanced pulmonary hypertension. On occasion, a murmur of pulmonic insufficiency may be heard at the left second intercostal space and the parasternal area. Fixed splitting of the second heart sound should raise suspicion of an unsuspected atrial septal defect. Short systolic bruits heard while auscultating the lungs may be a clue to the presence of partially occlusive thrombus in the larger pulmonary arteries.

Diagnostic Approach

Chest radiographs may disclose evidence of parenchymal lung disease or demonstrate right ventricular and pulmonary vascular prominence. Electrocardiography may show the characteristic signs of right ventricular hypertrophy, including a QRS axis greater than 110°, RSR complex in V_1 and V_2, and an incomplete right bundle branch block. The presence of an $S_1Q_3T_3$ pattern on the ECG is strongly suggestive of an acute right ventricular pressure overload state, such as massive pulmonary thromboembolism. Prominent, peaked p waves in the inferior and right precordial leads (p pulmonale) are nonspecific findings on ECG and may appear and disappear in patients with acute, reversible airflow obstruction even in the absence of pulmonary hypertension.

Echocardiography may demonstrate right-sided chamber enlargement, flattening of the interventricular septum during systole, or the presence of coexistent left ventricular or mitral valve disease. A pericardial effusion may also be present and is suggestive of either a connective tissue disease or right atrial pressure overload. Doppler studies can be used to determine the presence and estimate the magnitude of tricuspid regurgitation, which may be useful in noninvasively estimating the pulmonary artery systolic pressure.

The severity of pulmonary hypertension correlates closely with the degree of derangement in lung function in patients with chronic parenchymal lung disease. In general, patients with chronic airflow obstruction are likely to have concomitant pulmonary hypertension when the forced expiratory volume in 1 second falls below 1 liter. In chronic restrictive lung disease, pulmonary hypertension is usually present when the vital capacity or the diffusing capacity for carbon monoxide is below 50% of that predicted. Patients whose partial pressure of arterial oxygen is below 55 mm Hg generally will have pulmonary hypertension, and the more severe the hypoxemia, the more severe the pulmonary hypertension is likely to be.

Chronic thrombotic occlusion of the pulmonary vasculature should be considered in any patient with unexplained pulmonary hypertension because it is potentially treatable by thromboendarterectomy. Radioisotope lung scanning is a safe and reliable method to assess the distribution of ventilation and perfusion in the lungs, even in patients with severe pulmonary vascular disease. Patients with PPH usually manifest a homogeneous pattern of perfusion, whereas patients with chronic thromboembolism exhibit multiple perfusion defects of varying sizes. Patients in whom a distinction between PPH and chronic thromboembolic disease cannot be made using noninvasive tests should undergo pulmonary arteriography. Similarly, consideration should be given to acute pulmonary thromboembolism in a patient with chronic cor pulmonale who experiences a sudden clinical deterioration in the absence of clear signs of exacerbation of the underlying parenchymal lung disease. Complete cardiac catheterization should be performed on patients with unexplained, severe pulmonary hypertension to exclude congenital heart diseases, proximal or peripheral pulmonic stenosis, and valvular heart disease.

In most cases, a cause for the pulmonary vascular disease can be ascertained on clinical grounds; however, for a definitive diagnosis to be made, it may be necessary to obtain a specimen of lung tissue from patients with severe pulmonary hypertension who have confusing evidence by physical examination or ancillary laboratory testing. Thoracoscopy-guided biopsy is the preferred approach. Transbronchial biopsy via the fiberoptic bronchoscope is not a suitable alternative to open lung biopsy in the setting of unexplained pulmonary vascular disease.

Approach to Management

The management of pulmonary hypertension should initially be directed at treating the underlying cause. Improving gas exchange and airflow in patients with cor pulmonale resulting from chronic obstructive airways disease usually ameliorates the pulmonary hypertension. Patients with interstitial lung disease and pulmonary hypertension may show marked hemodynamic improvement when lung function is improved with corticosteroid or immunosuppressive therapy. Because hypoxia is a major contributor to both acute and chronic cor pulmonale, correcting hypoxemia is an important component of the therapeutic approach in affected patients. Although the hemodynamic effects of low-flow supplemental oxygen in patients with chronic obstructive lung disease are variable and slow in achieving their maximum, survival is increased substantially when hypoxemia is corrected. Patients with a stable PaO_2 of less than or equal to 55 mm Hg breathing ambient air or a PaO_2 less than or equal to 59 mm Hg and a hematocrit greater than 55%, p pulmonale on ECG or edema should be treated chronically with supplemental oxygen using flow rates sufficient to achieve a PaO_2 greater than 60 mm Hg.

Polycythemia, resulting from the effects of chronic hypoxia in patients with severe parenchymal lung disease or congenital heart disease, may contribute to elevations in pulmonary vascular resistance by increasing blood viscosity. Isovolemic phlebotomy to a hematocrit of 50% to 55% may reduce the degree of hyperviscosity without compromising tissue oxygen delivery.

Other Therapeutic Alternatives

A variety of systemic vasodilators have been shown to reduce pulmonary artery pressure in experimentally induced pulmonary hypertension, including hydralazine, calcium channel blockers (nifedipine, diltiazem, and verapamil), prostaglandins E_1 and I_2 (prostacyclin), adenosine, and nitrates (nitroglycerin and nitroprusside). These agents have also been used to treat selected patients with either primary or secondary pulmonary hypertension. A report from the National Institutes of Health–sponsored Registry on PPH suggests that approximately two thirds of patients manifest acute responses to vasodilator administration, which, if sustained, may be beneficial.

The goal of vasodilator therapy is to reduce right ventricular afterload and increase cardiac output and systemic oxygen delivery. A substantial reduction in pulmonary arterial pressure concomitant with an increased stroke volume and an unchanged or minimally reduced systemic arterial pressure constitutes the optimal hemodynamic response to vasodilator administration and is frequently associated with evidence of regression of right-sided heart abnormalities and improved survival. This "ideal" response is seen in only 25% to 30% of patients with PPH. In the remaining 30% to 40% of "responders," cardiac output is increased in the absence of any significant change in pulmonary artery or systemic blood pressures. The decision to institute long-term vasodilator therapy in these patients should be based on individual assessment.

The major adverse effects that may result from vasodilator administration include (1) systemic hypotension, which may result either from systemic vasodilation in the absence of any pulmonary vascular effect or from a reduced cardiac output caused by the negative inotropic properties of some drugs, (2) worsening pulmonary hypertension, which is due to an increased cardiac output flowing through a vascular bed with a fixed resistance, and (3) worsening hypoxemia caused by either an increased perfusion to poorly ventilated lung units (decreased ventilation:perfusion ratio) or increased right-to-left shunting if the systemic vascular effect predominates. Patients with right-sided heart failure appear to be at the greatest risk for experiencing adverse effects with vasodilator administration.

Because the risk of sustained adverse effects is greatest with long-acting agents, the use of potent, short-acting, titratable vasodilators to test vasoreactivity has been advocated. Prostacyclin (prostaglandin I_2), prostaglandin E_1, adenosine, acetylcholine, nitroglycerin, and nitric oxide have all been used in this manner and appear to be well tolerated. The acute responses to prostacyclin have been useful in predicting responsiveness to orally active drugs. Accordingly, prophylactic anticoagulation has been advocated for patients with severe, nonthrombotic pulmonary hypertension, and survival may be improved in patients receiving anticoagulants. However, anticoagulant therapy is not without risk in this setting, and life-threatening side effects, including hemoptysis from spontaneously ruptured pulmonary vessels, may occur.

If therapy with warfarin is contemplated, the prothrombin time should be monitored frequently and maintained at a level of 3 to 5 seconds above control. Adjusted-dose subcutaneous heparin may be a suitable alternative to warfarin, although it is more cumbersome to administer and its use should be reserved for patients who have a greater risk for complications with warfarin therapy. Acutely ill patients with nonthrombotic pulmonary hypertension should receive low-dose heparin subcutaneously during the acute illness.

Diuretics can be helpful in treating right-sided heart failure but should be used cautiously in this setting because decreasing right ventricular preload may result in a reduction in cardiac output. There is little role for cardiac glycosides in the acute or chronic management of pulmonary vascular disease, with the exception of supraventricular tachyarrhythmias or biventricular failure.

Combined heart-lung transplantation has been considered the surgical treatment of choice for severe pulmonary hypertension that is refractory to medical management. However, the dearth of suitable organ donors and the limited number of centers with the expertise to perform this procedure have limited its availability. Early experience suggests that single lung transplantation may result in marked hemodynamic improvement in patients with isolated pulmonary vascular disease. The greater availability of donor organs for lung transplantation may enable a larger number of seriously ill patients to undergo transplantation.

The treatment of choice for chronic thrombotic pulmonary hypertension is pulmonary thromboendarterectomy. However, only organized thrombus in the proximal vessels is approachable by this technique. Preoperative evaluation should include complete pulmonary angiography to determine the site and extent of thrombosis. Marked hemodynamic improvement frequently results from successful removal of organized thrombus. Patients with acute cor pulmonale caused by massive pulmonary embolism should be evaluated for emergency embolectomy if death is imminent and there is insufficient time for thrombolytic therapy to effect enough clot lysis to restore the integrity of the pulmonary vascular bed.

Prognosis

In the settings of both chronic obstructive pulmonary disease and adult respiratory distress syndrome (ARDS), the presence of cor pulmonale contributes significantly to a shortened survival. The 3-year survival in patients with severe airflow obstruction and a pulmonary vascular resistance three to four times normal is less than 10% to 15%. Survival is similarly influenced by the presence of pulmonary hypertension in chronic restrictive lung diseases and connective tissue diseases.

Mortality from PPH is, in large part, dependent on the state of the right ventricle. Patients with symptoms of severe right-sided heart dysfunction, such as syncope, and hemodynamic evidence of impaired right ventricular function, such as a reduced cardiac output or mixed venous saturation and an elevated right atrial pressure, usually succumb to the disease within 1 to 2 years. Patients with milder symptoms and relatively well-preserved right-sided heart function survive longer, although the course is highly variable. The impact of therapy on survival has not been addressed in large-scale, prospective studies.

DIAGNOSIS AND TREATMENT OF MASSIVE PULMONARY EMBOLISM

Patients with acute massive pulmonary embolism usually have a dramatic presentation: sudden onset of severe shortness of breath, hypoxemia, and right ventricular failure. Symptoms include central chest pain, often identical to angina; severe dyspnea; and frequently syncope and confusion; or tachypnea, cyanosis, and hypotension. The marked increase in pulmonary vascular resistance leads to acute right ventricular failure, with the presence of large a waves in the jugular veins and a right ventricular diastolic gallop. With pulmonary hypertension, there is marked right ventricular dilatation with a shift of the intraventricular septum, decreasing cardiac output, and further decreasing coronary perfusion; this frequently results in cardiorespiratory arrest. If patients with a massive pulmonary embolus survive, they are acutely threatened by any further pulmonary thromboembolism.

The emergency management of massive pulmonary embolism includes the use of intravenous heparin; the use of oxygen with or without mechanical ventilation, which may include positive end-expiratory pressure; volume resuscitation; and the use of inotropic agents and vasodilators. In addition to these supportive measures, specific treatment options for massive pulmonary embolism include (1) thrombolysis; (2) pulmonary thrombectomy with or without cardiopulmonary bypass support, (3) transvenous catheter embolectomy or clot dissolution, and (4) insertion of an inferior vena caval filter.

Thrombolytic Treatment for Massive Pulmonary Embolism

Random clinical trials have demonstrated that the mortality rate from venous thromboembolism can be decreased by anticoagulant treatment. A mortality rate of less than 5% should be achieved with intravenous heparin and oral anticoagulants, and this can be further reduced with the use of low-molecular-weight heparin. However, patients who present with acute massive pulmonary embolism and hypotension have a mortality rate of approximately 20% despite the use of anticoagulants and other supportive measures. For such patients, the appropriate use of thrombolytic agents has a role. A high percentage of acute pulmonary emboli occur within 10 to 14 days of surgery; therefore, they are excluded from treatment protocols using thrombolytic agents. These patients may be candidates for local infusion of low-dose thrombolytic agents.

Pulmonary Embolectomy in Massive Pulmonary Embolism

Pulmonary embolectomy is occasionally indicated in the management of massive pulmonary embolism. This is defined as a sudden occurrence of a massive embolus producing severe cardiovascular decompensation with severe hypotension, oliguria, and hypoxia refractory to aggressive treatment. A somewhat more generous indication would be an obstruction of more than 50% of the pulmonary vasculature, arterial oxygen saturation of less than 60 mm Hg, systolic blood pressure of less than 90 mm Hg, and urine output of less than 20 mL per hour. In some centers, patients who have contraindications to thrombolytic therapy or who have failed a trial of thrombolytic therapy are considered candidates for thrombectomy. On the other hand, others argue that a patient who survives the first 2 hours after an acute massive pulmonary embolus will probably survive with adequate medical management if no further pulmonary emboli occur. It is unlikely that it will be possible to perform a randomized trial comparing thrombolytic therapy with pulmonary embolectomy, and it is difficult to compare one case series of pulmonary thrombectomy with another because the case material is often not comparable.

Percutaneous Clot Extraction or Disruption in Treatment

Pulmonary embolectomy via a catheter suction device inserted into the jugular or femoral vein under local anesthetic has been used in the treatment of patients with acute massive pulmonary embolism who have contraindications to anticoagulants or thrombolysis. Mortality rates of 27% and 28% were observed. The most common cause of death is cardiac arrest from ventricular arrhythmia, right-sided heart failure, and pulmonary hemorrhage. Some patients in whom clot extraction was not possible have gone on to successful pulmonary embolectomy on bypass. Inferior vena caval filters are used in conjunction with catheter embolectomy.

Inferior Vena Caval Interruption in Treatment of Pulmonary Thromboembolism

Characteristics of an ideal filter include one that is easily and safely placed percutaneously, is biocompatible and mechanically stable, is able to trap emboli without causing occlusion of the vena cava, does not require anticoagulation, and is not ferromagnetic (does not cause artifacts on magnetic resonance images). Although there is as yet no ideal filter, several of the available devices have proved useful. These include the Greenfield stainless steel filter, titanium Greenfield filter, bird's nest filter, Vena Tech filter, and the Simon-Nitinol filter. In experienced hands, these devices can be quickly and safely inserted under fluoroscopic control. One novel filter can be inserted temporarily when needed, used in conjunction with thrombolytic therapy, and then removed. With the available follow-up to date, the Greenfield filter has had the best performance record, and any future comparative studies should use this filter as the standard.

The main indications for vena caval filters are when contraindications to anticoagulants exist, or there is recurrent thromboembolism despite adequate anticoagulation, and as prophylactic placement in high-risk patients. In the latter category are patients with cor pulmonale or a history of thromboembolism who are in high-risk situations (e.g., they have an acetabular fracture or have cancer). Patients who have had pulmonary embolectomy either surgically or via percutaneous catheters should have inferior vena caval filters inserted. As the filters have become safer and easier to implant, the indications have expanded somewhat. Their use in young individuals with a long life expectancy has been discouraged because it is unknown how well they will last in vivo. Complications of inferior vena caval filter placement include misplacement and tilting and occasional migration and perforation, but these complications are rare.

DIAGNOSIS AND THERAPY OF EMERGENT VASCULAR DISEASES

Acute Arterial Insufficiency

Acute arterial occlusion from trauma, embolus, or thrombosis frequently requires emergency surgery to prevent irreversible tissue loss. Symptoms are pain, analgesia or anesthesia, and discoloration of the ischemic tissue. Embolic arterial occlusion produces symptoms that vary with the origin of the embolus. Emboli originating in the heart or ascending aorta cause central nervous system, visceral, or upper/lower extremity symptoms, whereas emboli from the abdominal aorta and from iliofemoral or popliteal lesions affect only the lower extremities. The blue toe syndrome describes multiple bilateral ischemic areas in the lower leg caused by atheromatous debris showered distally from disease in aortoiliac vessels. Ischemic paralysis and hypalgesia may develop in acutely ischemic limbs as a result of neurovascular compression from increased fascial compartment pressure. Compartmental compression syndromes require expedient decompression by fasciotomy to prevent irreversible neurovascular damage. Embolic occlusion of visceral arteries may be insidious; pain, indigestion, or hematuria is often the only symptom.

Thrombotic arterial occlusion usually occurs as a result of decreased blood flow in progressively narrowed, atherosclerotic vessels. Acute thrombosis of diseased arteries may be due to hypovolemia or a sudden decrease in cardiac output. Frequently, elderly patients with cardiac failure or intraperitoneal disease have ischemic lower extremities, which simulates an aortic occlusion or a dissecting aneurysm. Appropriate attention to cardiac or intra-abdominal disease and restoration of blood volume often alleviate the ischemic symptoms. Axillary arterial thrombosis subsequent to intimal damage produced by repeated strain or trauma occurs in athletes, particularly baseball pitchers, and in individuals using crutches. Rarely, acute arterial thrombosis occurs in severely dehydrated children or in patients with hematologic disorders.

Chronic Arterial Insufficiency

Because chronically ischemic limbs are easily ulcerated by local irritation, patients (especially diabetics) must be instructed in meticulous foot care, and any lesions should be aggressively treated. All patients with arterial insufficiency should be encouraged to quit smoking, control their diet, and immediately visit their physician if foot problems develop. Approximately 50% of patients with claudication will experience less pain on activity if they follow these recommendations and start a supervised exercise program. The onset of rest pain heralds complications and limb loss unless surgical intervention can restore adequate oxygenation.

Diseases of the Aorta

Thoracic aortic aneurysms frequently can be visualized by chest radiograph, ultrasonography, or CT; however, arteriography is the most reliable method of defining the extent of the lesions. Aneurysms may affect speech by irritating the recurrent laryngeal nerve, or they may cause dysphagia by compressing the esophagus. Pain from a dissecting thoracic aneurysm may be substernal or referred to the intravascular area. Migration of excruciating pain suggests extension of a dissection. Major arterial branches of the thoracic aorta may be occluded by extension of a subintimal dissection, causing a cerebrovascular accident or diminishing pulses in the upper extremity. Control of hypertension will frequently prevent further dissection. In unstable patients, immediate surgery occasionally may be the only chance for survival.

Upper Extremity Ischemia

Vascular ischemia of the upper extremity is caused by atherosclerosis, thoracic-outlet compression, trauma, and systemic or local inflammatory diseases. Upper extremity ischemia from acute arterial occlusions causes limb loss in 10% of lesions in the subclavian artery, 15% in the axillary artery, and less than 5% in the proximal brachial artery. Most acute arterial obstructions in the upper extremity are caused by trauma. Upper extremity digital gangrene is infrequent but not rare. Approximately 50% of patients with digital ischemia have a correctable aneurysm, traumatic lesion, or embolic source proximal to the hand. Digital ischemia may also appear as a symptom of vasospastic or obliterative arterial disease in patients with systemic inflammatory processes. Connective tissue disorders, particularly scleroderma, are associated with progressive occlusion of medium- and small-diameter arteries.

Cerebrovascular Insufficiency

Transient ischemic attacks (TIAs), visual disturbances, and contralateral weakness can often be relieved by carotid endarterectomy. Patients with less specific symptoms such as headaches, dizziness, or unusual distribution of sensory or motor abnormalities require extensive evaluation to document the relationship of neurologic symptoms to carotid stenosis. Patients with asymptomatic carotid lesions can be treated with antiplatelet medications instead of carotid endarterectomy; however, data suggest that endarterectomy reduces the incidence of subsequent stroke despite an initial elevation in morbidity and mortality related to surgery.

Mesenteric Arterial Insufficiency

Visceral ischemia may be acute or chronic. Acute insufficiency can cause nonspecific colicky pain and guaiac-positive stools, or it may produce sepsis, acidosis, and rapid hemodynamic deterioration. The symptoms of chronic intestinal ischemia are postprandial pain and weight loss. Approximately 40% of acute ischemic events are caused by emboli, 50% are associated with low-flow states and arterial thrombosis, and 10% or less are due to venous occlusion. In general, at least two of three mesenteric vessels must be significantly obstructed for occlusion of any one vessel to impair mesenteric blood flow markedly. Occasionally, acute occlusion of the inferior mesenteric artery by thrombosis or surgical ligation causes an ischemic colitis that is characterized by severe abdominal pain in the lower left quadrant, abdominal tenderness, and bloody stools.

Although the superior mesenteric artery is subject to acute ischemia from either a thrombotic or embolic event, thrombosis usually results in more extensive ischemia because it occurs in severely diseased arteries and frequently involves the entire vessel. By contrast, emboli tend to lodge distal to the origin of the middle colic artery and may be found in otherwise normal intestinal vasculature. Mesenteric arterial emboli may require only embolectomy, whereas mesenteric thrombosis often requires resection of a large segment of devitalized intestine.

Thrombosis of the superior mesenteric veins is associated with low blood flow, hypercoagulation, and portal vein thrombosis from compression or invasion by malignancy, particularly pancreatic tumors. Splanchnic venous engorgement with edematous thickening of bowel loops produces a thumbprint pattern of gut folds, evident on upper gastrointestinal contrast radiography. Mesenteric venous thrombosis results in gut necrosis in 20% to 70% of patients. Mortality increases rapidly if therapy is delayed longer than 12 hours after the onset of symptoms and approaches 100% by 48 hours. Frequently, acute mesenteric venous occlusion requires thrombectomy, resection of devitalized bowel, and anticoagulation.

Venous Disease

Thrombophlebitis is venous thrombosis that follows inflammation of the vein wall and causes severe pain and swelling of the extremity. The three apparent causes of venous thrombosis are stasis, injury to the vessel wall, and increased coagulability of the blood (i.e., Virchow's triad). Fibrinogen radionuclide studies performed on hospitalized patients demonstrate that thrombi develop in areas of stasis and turbulent blood flow near venous valves. Continued thrombosis occludes the vessel lumen and produces distal venous hypertension. Frequently, blood flow through the vein is restored by resorption and organization or embolization of the thrombus. However, organization of venous thrombosis destroys the valves, and recanalized veins are prone to subsequent thrombosis.

Chronic venous obstruction and valvular insufficiency are characterized by discoloration and induration of the overlying skin. If venous hypertension is greater than capillary diffusion pressure, edema develops. Tissue ischemia and venous gangrene develop if venous pressures exceed capillary perfusion pressure. Venous thrombosis of the upper extremity requires therapy if the deep veins are involved. Exertion, intravenous catheters, trauma, intravenous drug abuse, neoplastic disease, and congenital venous malformations have been described as causes of axillary–subclavian vein thromboses. Intermittent subclavian vein obstruction and thrombosis can follow compression of the vein between the first rib and clavicle. Axillary–subclavian vein thromboses cause severe pain and swelling of the arm and hand, and frequently there is percussion tenderness over the clavicle and axillary vein. These thromboses can be a source of hemodynamically significant pulmonary emboli, particularly when associated with causes other than exertion.

A venous thrombosis may become infected, or it may be caused by infection. Infected thromboses are usually seen in intravenous drug abusers and in debilitated patients who have had multiple intravenous catheters. Infected thromboses may be the source of systemic sepsis, endocarditis, or septic emboli. Immediate excision of the entire vein is required to prevent complication.

Diagnosis and Therapy

Venography is the most accurate method for diagnosing significant venous thromboses, although a combination of Doppler ultrasound and impedance plethysmography has a 95% accuracy in detecting deep venous thrombosis of the leg. A difference of 1.5 cm in diameter between a swollen leg and the contralateral leg offers corroborative physical evidence of venous thrombosis. Calf tenderness and Homans' sign are less reliable diagnostic signs. Therapy for venous thrombosis ideally prevents propagation of the thrombosis, late sequelae related to destruction of venous anatomy, secondary infection, and pulmonary emboli. Destruction of the valves by the organizing thrombus increases venous pressures and ultimately leads to the postphlebotic syndrome, which is a debilitating and irreversible venous disease.

There are a few surgical alternatives, and therapy relies primarily on custom-fitted support stockings and meticulous skin care. Tortuous varicose veins can be removed if they are painful or unsightly, but varicosities frequently recur from persistent venous hypertension or primary venous degenerative disease. The superficial venous system should not be removed if there is deep vein occlusion, because in this instance the superficial veins are the only route for egress of blood from the extremity. Excision of varicose veins near stasis ulcers improves wound healing. In certain cases, valvuloplasty or crossover venous reconstructions can reestablish venous flow and reduce venous hypertension.

SEVERE HEART FAILURE IN CARDIOMYOPATHY

Dilated cardiomyopathy is characterized by ventricular dilatation, impairment of systolic function as evidenced by a markedly reduced left ventricular ejection fraction, and a clinical picture of congestive heart failure. Distinguishing features of restrictive cardiomyopathy include normal left ventricular cavity dimensions, normal or only mildly reduced systolic function, and markedly reduced ventricular compliance often leading to signs and symptoms of biventricular heart failure. Restrictive cardiomyopathy exhibits many similarities to pericardial constriction. The third category of cardiomyopathy is the hypertrophic form, which is due to inappropriate left ventricular hypertrophy. The hypertrophic form often involves the interventricular septum, leading to decreased compliance and impaired diastolic function. Table 4–12 classifies these cardiomyopathies.

Dilated Cardiomyopathy

It is thought that dilated cardiomyopathy may represent the final common pathway as a consequence of chronic recurrent myocardial damage from a wide variety of insults.

Patients presenting with heart failure usually complain of symptoms related to low cardiac output, such as weakness, fatigue, and decreasing exercise tolerance. Shortness of breath, dyspnea on exertion, and orthopnea appear as pulmonary vascular congestion develops. Symptoms related to right heart failure, such as increasing abdominal girth and peripheral edema, generally appear late and connote a poor prognosis. Chest pain is observed in 25% to 50% of patients with idiopathic dilated cardiomyopathy. It is believed that decreased coronary blood flow reserve leading to subendocardial ischemia may be partly responsible for angina-type chest pain.

On physical examination, patients may demonstrate generalized wasting and pallor. The systolic blood pressure may be low, with a narrow pulse pressure and pulsus alternans. Wheezing due to bronchospasm and engorgement of the bronchial vessels, as well as moist rales, is often noted on pulmonary examination. Pleural effusion on the right side may be detected. The apical impulse is displaced laterally. Heart sounds are often diminished, with an S3 gallop noted at the apex. A murmur of mitral regurgitation due to left ventricular dilatation leading to nonapposition of mitral leaflets is frequently audible. With right heart dilation and failure, jugular venous distention with prominent a and v waves is present. The liver may be tender, enlarged, and pulsatile, with demonstrable hepatojugular reflux. Ascites and peripheral edema are usually found.

A chest radiograph reveals generalized cardiomegaly and signs of pulmonary vascular hypertension. Kerley's lines,

Table 4–12. CLASSIFICATION OF THE CARDIOMYOPATHIES

	Dilated	Restrictive	Hypertrophic	
			Nonobstructive	*Obstructive*
Left ventricular end-diastolic pressure	↑ ↑	↑ ↑	↑ ↑	↑ ↑
Left ventricular end-diastolic volume	↑ ↑	nl or ↓	nl or ↓	nl or ↓
Diastolic compliance	↑	↓ ↓	↓ ↓	↓ ↓
Left ventricular ejection fraction	↓ ↓	nl or ↑ ↓ late	nl or ↑ ↓ late	nl, ↓, ↑
Echocardiography	↑ ↑ LV dimension ↓ ↓ ventricular systolic function	nl or ↓ LV dimension nl ventricular systolic function	nl or ↓ LV dimension nl or ↑ ventricular systolic function	LV outflow tract obstruction Systolic anterior motion of mitral valve
	AV valve regurgitation	↑ LV wall thickness and mass	Localized ↑ LV wall thickness (septum)	Mitral regurgitation

Abbreviations: AV = atrioventricular; nl = normal; LV = left ventricle; ↑ = slightly increased; ↓ = slightly decreased; ↑ ↑ = greatly increased; ↓ ↓ = greatly decreased.

peribronchial cuffing, and interstitial and alveolar edema can also be seen. Pleural effusions are often present.

The ECG may demonstrate sinus tachycardia as well as atrial or ventricular tachyarrhythmias. Conduction disturbances, including atrioventricular block and bundle branch block, are associated findings. Loss of anterior R wave forces and the presence of Q waves may resemble ischemic heart disease. ST segment and T wave abnormalities are the rule, and P wave changes consistent with left atrial enlargement may be noted. Twenty-four-hour Holter monitoring reveals ventricular arrhythmias, with approximately 50% of patients demonstrating nonsustained ventricular tachycardia.

Two-dimensional and Doppler echocardiography is extremely useful. Ventricular chamber dilatation is always present with a left ventricular end-diastolic diameter exceeding 2.7 cm/m^2. Ventricular wall thickness is normal or thin with global hypokinesis, with or without regional variation, and associated with fractional shortening of less than 30%. Intracavitary thrombi may be present. Involvement of the right ventricle is considered common in dilated cardiomyopathy.

Heart failure is commonly diagnosed hemodynamically by finding elevated filling pressure by placement of a flow-directed pulmonary artery catheter. Dilated cardiomyopathy produces a decreased stroke volume and increased left ventricular end-diastolic pressure. Mean left arterial pressure and pulmonary capillary wedge pressure (PCWP) are elevated to a degree corresponding to the extent of impairment of left ventricular systolic performance. Chronic elevation of left heart pressures may lead to moderate pulmonary vascular hypertension. Elevation of right ventricular end-diastolic and right atrial pressures signals the presence of right ventricular failure. Large V waves may be noted in the pulmonary capillary wedge tracing in patients with mitral regurgitation. Coronary angiography reveals no evidence of significant coronary artery disease. Contrast left ventriculography demonstrates global hypokinesis, sometimes with segmental wall-motion abnormalities, chamber enlargement, decreased ejection fraction, and often mitral regurgitation.

Treatment (Table 4–13)

In patients with dilated cardiomyopathy, irreversible myocardial injury leading to impairment of systolic performance, with resultant decrease in ejection fraction and mean arterial blood pressure, sets into motion a series of compensatory mechanisms directed at maintaining cardiac output and tissue perfusion. A cardiac index of less than 2.5 L • min • m^2 and a left ventricular end-diastolic pressure of greater than 27 mm Hg herald severe impairment of left ventricular function.

Diuretics and digitalis preparations together represent the most common agents used in the treatment of heart failure. Diuretics inhibit renal tubular solute reabsorption and induce salt and water excretion. The result is decreased intravascular volume. Patients with significant decompensated heart failure usually require a loop diuretic. Metolazone, a

Table 4–13. THERAPEUTIC MODALITIES IN DILATED CARDIOMYOPATHY

Diuretics
Digitalis glycosides
Vasodilators
Direct-acting
Angiotensin-converting enzyme inhibitors
Inotropic agents
Beta-adrenergic blocking agents
Immunosuppressive agents
Anticoagulants
Antiarrhythmic therapy, including implantable defibrillators
Cardiomyoplasty
Mechanical circulatory support devices
Heart transplantation

thiazide diuretic, may exert a synergistic diuretic effect when combined with a loop diuretic. Potassium and magnesium losses with such therapy can be substantial, and care must be taken to avoid hypokalemia and hypomagnesemia, which may contribute to digitalis toxicity and ventricular dysrhythmias. Water restriction, particularly in the presence of hyponatremia, remains an important adjunct to diuretic therapy.

Vasodilators, both venous and arterial, can produce significant improvement in hemodynamics as well as in signs and symptoms of congestive heart failure. Critically ill patients with severe congestive heart failure refractory to conventional oral medications may be treated with intravenous nitroprusside or nitroglycerin with improvement in clinical and hemodynamic parameters but without altering survival. Angiotensin-converting enzyme inhibitors have now become an essential part of all medical regimens for the treatment of chronic congestive heart failure. These drugs inhibit formation of angiotensin II and aldosterone and result in decreased systemic vascular resistance. Prospective randomized trials of the addition of enalapril to conventional therapy for heart failure have demonstrated improvement in signs and symptoms of heart failure as well as prolonged survival. Newer vasodilators, such as dihydropyridine and the calcium channel blocker amlodipine, have been shown to exert beneficial effects in patients with refractory heart failure.

Short-term administration of inotropic agents can produce sustained improvement in hemodynamic and clinical parameters in patients with dilated cardiomyopathy in severe congestive heart failure. Dobutamine, a β_1-selective sympathomimetic agent, has positive inotropic and vasodilating properties and is widely used for severely decompensated heart failure. The phosphodiesterase inhibitors amrinone and milrinone have hemodynamic effects similar to those of dobutamine. In addition, chronic long-term intermittent infusion of intravenous inotropic agents may be of value in treating patients with severe congestive heart failure despite maximum medical therapy.

Restrictive Cardiomyopathy

Of the different forms of cardiomyopathy, restrictive cardiomyopathy is the least common. As depicted in Table 4–12, patients with restrictive cardiomyopathy frequently present with congestive heart failure, a small or only mildly enlarged heart, and relatively preserved left ventricular systolic function. The mechanism of heart failure in restrictive cardiomyopathy is related to reduced ventricular compliance and impaired diastolic relaxation, resulting in restricted ventricular filling, high ventricular filling pressures, and reduced stroke volume despite normal systolic contractile function. The pathophysiologic mechanism leading to impaired diastolic function is related to decreased ventricular distensibility limiting diastolic filling as a result of morphologic alterations in the myocardium.

Hypertrophic Cardiomyopathy

Therapy in hypertrophic cardiomyopathy is aimed at improving symptoms and decreasing the risk of death. Pharmacologic agents that decrease filling pressure, improve left ventricular diastolic relaxation, or reduce the magnitude of the left ventricular outflow tract pressure gradient improve symptoms in this disorder. Beta-adrenergic blocking agents are the mainstay of therapy in patients with hypertrophic cardiomyopathy. Such drugs slow heart rate and lengthen the diastolic filling period, thus improving the diastolic filling abnormality associated with this condition. Beta-adrenergic blocking agents also decrease myocardial oxygen consumption and improve ischemia. In patients with pulmonary congestion, careful use of diuretics may be beneficial. Calcium channel antagonists such as verapamil and to a lesser extent nifedipine and diltiazem have been postulated to improve left ventricular relaxation and ventricular diastolic filling in patients with hypertrophic cardiomyopathy with or without left ventricular outflow tract obstruction. Disopyramide, presumably because of its negative inotropic effect, has also been shown to improve symptoms and exercise tolerance. These agents all must be used with caution, because the potential for serious side effects such as bradycardia and hypotension is a genuine concern.

Cardiomyopathies and the Critical Care Environment

Management of Cardiomyopathy Using Invasive Hemodynamic Monitoring

A first step to improving hemodynamics is to optimize preload in a way that obtains maximum cardiac index without exacerbating pulmonary edema. By using the pulmonary capillary wedge pressure (PCWP), one can administer fluids until a PCWP of 15 to 20 mm Hg is achieved. When PCWP exceeds this level, pulmonary edema tends to occur. It should be emphasized that PCWP is a measurement of left ventricular diastolic pressure and does not necessarily reflect left ventricular volume. This is particularly true of patients with impaired diastolic relaxation or decreased compliance, such as in restrictive or hypertrophic cardiomyopathy. In such patients, a small change in intravascular volume may produce a small change in ventricular volume but a large increase in ventricular filling pressure, leading to worsening pulmonary edema. Patients with restrictive or hypertrophic cardiomyopathy exhibit reduced compliance and abnormal ventricular diastolic relaxation. Such patients may generally achieve a PCWP of 20 mm Hg with very little fluid supplementation. In addition, echocardiography is also helpful in assessing left ventricular systolic function and valvular regurgitation and the ruling out of pericardial effusion and tamponade.

Important Rhythm Disturbances

Rhythm disturbances are another special problem encountered when treating patients with severe heart failure and cardiomyopathy. For example, patients with restrictive or hypertrophic cardiomyopathy may exhibit hemodynamic deterioration in the presence of atrial fibrillation, owing to loss of the active atrial contribution to cardiac output. In such cases, aggressive measures to restore and maintain normal sinus rhythm should be implemented, including electrical cardioversion and use of antiarrhythmic agents. Recurrent ventricular arrhythmias also represent a serious problem for patients with cardiomyopathy. Type 1 antiarrhythmic agents are often poorly tolerated because of their negative inotropic and proarrhythmic effects. Care should be taken to avoid electrolyte derangements, myocardial ischemia, and drug toxicity, all of which can exacerbate ventricular arrhythmias in these patients. Amiodarone can be effective in treating both supraventricular and ventricular arrhythmias in patients with dilated cardiomyopathy.

THE HEART IN SEPSIS

Hemodynamic Changes

From the earliest clinical studies, it was reported that the ability to maintain a normal or increased cardiac output was associated with a higher survival rate. Several studies, however, have documented that the initial hemodynamic profile does not differ between survivors and nonsurvivors. It is clear that septic shock is most commonly associated with a decrease in peripheral vascular resistance, which results in hypotension despite a normal or increased cardiac index. Most nonsurvivors of septic shock demonstrate persistent vasodilation and hence refractory hypotension. Failure of the peripheral vasculature may be one of the major determinants of mortality in septic shock.

Myocardial Depression

Despite the hemodynamic state found by measuring conventional hemodynamic parameters in patients with septic shock, significant reversible myocardial depression has been demonstrated using radionuclide heart scanning with simultaneous thermodilution hemodynamic studies. The survivors have an initially depressed ejection fraction with an increased end-diastolic volume index. These changes return toward normal as a patient recovers from septic shock (normal ejection fraction, .50; normal end-diastolic volume index, 90 mL/m^2). The nonsurvivors have a minimally decreased ejection fraction that is not associated with ventricular dilation.

Management

The initial treatment of patients with septic shock is fluid resuscitation. Although many studies have addressed the benefits of colloid versus crystalloid fluid resuscitation, clear advantage of one type of fluid over the other has not been demonstrated. Accordingly, many clinicians and investigators have used increases in oxygen delivery or oxygen consumption as therapeutic goals in the management of patients with septic shock. Although one can clearly increase oxygen delivery and often oxygen consumption, it is not yet clear that therapy designed to meet specific hemodynamic endpoints will improve survival from septic shock. It does appear that patients who are able to reach a high oxygen delivery have a better prognosis.

If fluid resuscitation fails to reverse hypotension and inadequate organ perfusion, then treatment with inotropes or vasopressors must be considered. Dopamine is the most commonly used initial catecholamine. In low doses (1 to 5 $\mu g \cdot kg^{-1} \cdot min^{-1}$), it has positive inotropic effects as well as effects on the dopaminergic receptors in the kidneys. The latter improves renal blood flow, with the hope of decreasing the risk of renal failure, which is a common complication of septic shock. At higher doses (10 $\mu g \cdot kg^{-1} \cdot min^{-1}$ or more), dopamine becomes an α-adrenergic agonist and loses its dopaminergic renal effects. The α-adrenergic effects of dopamine may be useful in supporting blood pressure and perhaps organ blood flow in patients with septic shock who have a low systemic vascular resistance.

Dobutamine is a β-adrenergic agent with potent inotropic effects as well as vasodilating effects. The inotropic effects may be beneficial in patients with septic shock because of the myocardial depression that is present, and dobutamine is commonly used for that reason. In patients with high filling pressures or a relatively low cardiac index, dobutamine may be of particular value; however, it must be used with caution to insure that the vasodilating effects do not worsen hypotension. Dobutamine increases oxygen delivery, and this may be a benefit in some patients with sepsis.

Norepinephrine is a potent vasoconstricting agent that is frequently used in treating patients with septic shock that has not responded to fluid resuscitation and low-dose dopamine. Many clinicians have been reluctant to use norepinephrine because of fear of reducing renal blood flow and precipitating acute renal failure. However, the addition of low-dose dopamine to norepinephrine results in significantly higher renal blood flow and lower renal vascular resistance. This observation provides a rationale for the use of low-dose dopamine plus norepinephrine for the treatment of patients with septic shock and persistent hypotension related to decreased systemic vascular resistance.

Epinephrine has also been used in the management of septic shock. The hemodynamic effects of epinephrine are to increase heart rate, blood pressure, stroke volume index, cardiac index, and oxygen delivery and consumption, without changing systemic vascular resistance. Some clinicians have reservations about using epinephrine because of the concern about precipitating myocardial ischemia by increasing myocardial oxygen demand. Nonetheless, epinephrine is a potentially useful drug in the treatment of patients with septic shock, especially younger patients.

Patients with septic shock may have highly variable courses and unpredictable responses to therapeutic maneuvers. Although one can set general therapeutic goals of supporting blood pressure, improving oxygen delivery, and improving tissue perfusion, no single management approach can be expected to work most of the time. Each patient must be closely monitored, and if the response to a therapeutic change is not the expected one or if a patient's condition changes, a change in therapeutic interventions should be made. By close monitoring and frequent reassessment, a physician has the greatest chance of a successful outcome in the management of septic shock.

AIR EMBOLIZATION

Venous Air Embolism

Etiology and Occurrence

Neurosurgical procedures and head and neck surgical procedures performed on patients in the sitting position and insufflation of air or other gases into the peritoneum are situations in which venous air embolism (VAE) frequently has been described. In total hip arthroplasty, VAE is more frequent than was previously thought. Hepatic surgery, including both liver resection and transplantation with venovenous bypass, has also resulted in VAE. Use of the neodymium:yttrium-aluminum-garnet laser in uterine surgery has resulted in several deaths attributed to air embolism. VAE is known to occur in prostate surgery and in as many as 97% of cesarean sections. It may occur in any surgical procedure in which a plexus of veins is opened. Both positive-pressure ventilation in infants with hyaline membrane disease and high peak airway pressure in mechanically ventilated adults have been reported to cause VAE. In the intensive care unit, VAE is most likely encountered during or after insertion of a central venous catheter (CVC). The occurrence rate of this problem is variable, reported as 1 in 47 CVC insertions to none in 355. However, the mortality rate of VAE is significant. By 1987, only 79 cases related to CVC had been described in the world literature, but 25 (32%) of these cases had a fatal outcome.

Pulmonary artery catheter introducers have been implicated as causes of VAE. Soon after these catheters came into widespread use, anesthesiologists noted a potential for air embolism through the introducers that were left in place for vascular access after removal of the catheter. However, changes made by manufacturers followed, and self-sealing valves in introducers became standard. Nonetheless, it is recommended that the introducer be removed along with the pulmonary artery catheter or that an obturator be used to occlude the introducer if it is left in situ.

Clinical Manifestations

A "gasp" has been reported to follow the initial infusion of air into the pulmonary circulation, possibly a reflex response. Intrathoracic pressure is thereby decreased, facilitating greater air entry into the venous system. Patients often complain of breathlessness, lightheadedness, chest pain, or a feeling of impending doom. In one series of 14 cases, all patients had sudden onset of dyspnea.

Signs of air embolism are seldom specific. Significant embolism results in tachypnea, tachycardia, and frequently hypotension. The only sign specific for air embolism, the rare "mill-wheel" murmur, occurs late and is dependent on the presence of a large collection of air in the right ventricle. In a large proportion of patients, neurologic signs predominate. These manifestations include altered mental status, frank coma, and focal deficits. Whether hypoxia, hypotension, paradoxic embolism, or some combination of these factors is responsible for this neurologic compromise is uncertain. In some individuals, rales or wheezing can be detected on auscultation of the lung fields minutes to hours after air embolism occurs, indicating pulmonary edema. The coexistence of increased pulmonary arterial pressure and pulmonary edema protein content with normal pulmonary artery occlusion pressures suggests that increased vascular permeability underlies the development of abnormal extravascular lung water.

Differential Diagnosis

When respiratory complaints and signs are evident, VAE must be differentiated from other causes of sudden pulmonary compromise, such as pulmonary clot embolism, pneumothorax, acute bronchospasm, and pulmonary edema. If signs of CNS compromise predominate, the clinician must consider focal or global brain ischemia, hemorrhage into the parenchyma or subarachnoid spaces, hypoxia, trauma, intoxication, and hypoglycemia. In many cases, cardiovascular compromise dominates the clinical picture. This is usually in the form of hypotension, in which case VAE must be considered, along with other causes of obstructive shock, hypovolemia, primary cardiac dysfunction, and acute vasodilator states such as septic shock. VAE has also been reported to manifest as electromechanical dissociation, probably a result of right ventricular outflow obstruction, which reduces the cardiac output without initially disturbing cardiac electric activity.

Management

Closed-chest cardiac massage has been recommended as a means to force air out of the right ventricular outflow tract and into small pulmonary vessels. A more direct approach to the treatment of air embolism is withdrawal of air from the right side of the heart. To reduce the size of embolized bubbles, all patients with suspected VAE should receive 100% oxygen, because this favors nitrogen diffusion out of the bubbles and into the alveoli (nitrogen "washout"). For patients under general anesthesia, it is imperative that nitrous oxide be discontinued because it diffuses rapidly into all air-containing cavities in the body, including intravascular bubbles, significantly increasing their size and the obstruction they present to the circulation.

For those patients not responding to these measures, hyperbaric oxygen (HBO) therapy should be considered. This modality has long been used in the treatment of arterial gas emboli resulting from barotrauma in scuba divers.

Prophylaxis

Most hospital episodes of VAE are related to CVCs, making preventive measures particularly important when these catheters are used. Adequate hydration should be ensured before catheter insertion to militate against the low venous pressure of hypovolemia that encourages air entry. All connections to the central venous line should be tightly sealed using LuerLok adapters. Placing an occlusive dressing over the catheter when in place and over the tract for 24 hours after removal also helps prevent air emboli.

As with insertion, removal of the catheter in a head-down position is recommended. In the operating room, monitoring for air embolism during high-risk procedures using precordial Doppler and capnography has become standard. Avoiding procedures performed in the seated position should reduce the incidence of VAE. In particular, preoperative screening by echocardiography for the presence of a patent foramen ovale may alert the surgeon and anesthesiologists to those patients who are at risk for the severe consequences of paradoxic air embolism (PAE). Gas insufflation for diagnostic purposes should be accomplished with CO_2, not air, because CO_2 has a low surface tension, is absorbed quickly, and causes less obstruction if embolism occurs.

Finally, if a patient experiencing air embolism can be ventilated with positive pressure, this procedure is preferable to spontaneous breathing because it reduces unfavorable pressure gradients, permitting air entry. However, high peak inspiratory pressure causing barotrauma may itself be a reason for VAE and must be avoided.

Arterial Air Embolization

Etiology and Occurrence

The two most common iatrogenic causes of arterial air embolization (AAE) are the use of cardiopulmonary bypass (CPB) and neurosurgical procedures performed with patients in the sitting position. CPB offers ample opportunity for entrainment of air into the arterial circulation. The most common source of air entry is the oxygenator itself. Other sources of potential air entry during cardiac surgical procedures include cardiotomy suction blood return, cannulation of the ascending aorta, entrapment of air when closing the left ventricular or atrial chamber, the cavitation effect from the roller pump, and inadvertent direct injection of air through vascular catheters. During coronary artery bypass grafting (CABG), air also may be introduced directly into the coronary arteries. It is interesting that when the left ventricle is vented during CABG, negative intracavitary pressures encourage retrograde air entry into the aortic root from the open coronary arteriotomy sites, and from here it may embolize elsewhere after release of the aortic crossclamp.

Scuba divers experience the majority of cases of noniatrogenic AAE treated in hyperbaric chambers. Although inexperienced divers are more susceptible to AAE, this unpredictable occurrence strikes seasoned divers as well. Mechanical positive-pressure ventilation also places patients at risk for entry of air into the arterial system. Particularly in patients with inhomogeneous lung injury or chronic obstructive pulmonary disease, much of the positive-pressure inflation is directed away from the affected, poorly compliant alveoli into those that are more compliant. These may rapidly overexpand, rupture, and release air into the interstitium, predisposing to pneumothorax and entry of air into pulmonary capillaries or veins. This may occur with ventilator insufflations, spontaneous breaths from a positive-pressure circuit, or manual bag ventilation.

Clinical Manifestations

In dysbaric diving accidents, the end-organ most commonly affected is the CNS. The most common sign reported in submarine escape training and among scuba divers is an abrupt loss of consciousness and collapse within seconds or minutes of surfacing.

The great majority of episodes of loss of consciousness occur within 10 minutes of surfacing. Other evidence of CNS injury includes asymmetric multiple limb weakness, sensory loss, and frequent neuropsychiatric deficits. Patients may present with cognitive abnormalities alone, and a thorough mental status examination is imperative. Severe headache is common among divers sustaining AAE. The manifestations of AAE are diverse and may overlap considerably with the neurologic signs and symptoms of decompression sickness, which may be expressed by spinal cord injury with symmetric limb weakness or sensory loss.

CPB may cause focal, obvious neurologic deficits as a result of air bubbles or cellular debris acting as emboli, but it is much more likely to result in subtle cognitive deficits. This occurs in up to 70% of patients. In penetrating chest trauma, the creation of a bronchopulmonary venous fistula may be manifested by sudden cardiovascular collapse, hemoptysis, bloody foam emanating from a hole in the lung or great vessel, seizures, or direct visualization of air in the coronary arteries at thoracotomy. Four signs of AAE have been described as pathognomonic of this entity: skin marbling, reduced perfusion of all or part of the tongue, bloody froth emanating from a wound or a needle-stick site, and air bubbles in the retinal vessels.

Management

The management of AAE varies somewhat with the setting. In CPB procedures, the sequence of interventions should begin immediately on detection of air embolism, including placing patients in the head-down position, stopping air entry, compressing the carotid arteries, discontinuing administration of nitrous oxide, starting inhalation of 100% oxygen, and venting the aorta. Limited data support the use of retrograde (venoarterial) circulation through the superior vena cava to help clear cerebral arterial air. When penetrating chest trauma is complicated by AAE, the head-down position and 100% oxygen administration should be accompanied by emergency thoracotomy and clamping of the entire hilum of the involved lung, vigorous open-chest cardiac massage, and aspirating the left ventricular apex for air or foam. Emergency CPB may be indicated, but no data exist to support use of this technique. Coronary artery air embolism occurring during percutaneous transluminal coronary angioplasty is generally managed with supportive care alone.

Data supporting the use of HBO therapy in AAE and VAE are largely anecdotal. Still, available clinical and experimental evidence supports use of HBO, and it is considered the standard of care in circumstances in which a patient can be safely transported to a hyperbaric chamber. When AAE is suspected, the clinician should ensure that no secondary brain injury complicates the primary insult. Seizures, hyperthermia, hypoxia, and hypotension or hypertension must be carefully avoided.

CHAPTER 5

Respiratory Function

Kang H. Lee, MA, MB BChir, MRCP(UK) • Barbara A. Kerwin, MD • Adelaida M. Miro, MD

STRUCTURAL BASIS OF PULMONARY FUNCTION

The lungs perform a multitude of functions above and beyond the exchange of oxygen (O_2) and carbon dioxide (CO_2), including vascular autoregulation to optimize ventilation-perfusion (V/Q) matching, filtration of systemic venous blood, metabolism of vasoactive substances, and removal or neutralization of foreign material (dust, inorganic material, microorganisms).

Respiratory Pump

Ventilation

Ventilation is the movement of air through the upper airways, trachea, and conducting airways that terminates in the gas-exchanging units of the lungs followed by flow in the reverse direction during exhalation. The pressure gradient necessary to move air during inspiration is generated by contraction of respiratory muscles of inspiration, which produces a negative alveolar pressure, relative to the pressure at the mouth. During a passive exhalation, the elastic fibers and collagen generate a recoil pressure that increases alveolar pressure, resulting in gas movement from the alveoli to the mouth. At end-exhalation, the pressures within the lungs and thoracic cavity are balanced, so there is no net gas movement. The lung volume at this balanced end-expiratory state is referred to as the *functional residual capacity* (FRC). The FRC is altered with intrinsic lung diseases and is usually increased during obstructive airway disease and decreased during restrictive lung diseases.

Thoracic Cage and Respiratory Muscles

Tidal inspiration is achieved through coordinated contraction of the inspiratory muscles—the diaphragm (primarily) and the external intercostals (secondarily). The diaphragm is innervated by the phrenic nerves arising from cervical nerve roots C-3 through C-5. The diaphragm contracts in a craniocaudal direction, increasing the intrathoracic volume by forcing abdominal contents downward. The change in abdominal volume is greater than that in rib cage volume because of diaphragmatic contraction. The diaphragm is composed primarily of slow, fatigue-resistant type I fibers, which permit significant repetitive work without fatiguing. The external intercostal muscles are innervated by intercostal nerves T-1 through T-12. Contraction of these muscles elevates the ribs and increases the anteroposterior diameter of the chest. Accessory muscles of inspiration activated during high minute ventilation ($\dot{V}_E$) requirements include the scalene and sternocleidomastoid muscles. Active expiration is achieved through contraction of the internal intercostal and abdominal muscles. With lung disease of neuromuscular dysfunction, paradoxical movement of the rib cage and abdomen occurs and decreases the efficiency of respiration while increasing the inspiratory work of breathing.

Airways and Airflow

Tracheobronchial Tree

Air is filtered, warmed, and humidified by the upper airways during inspiration. The conducting airways then transport the gas into the terminal bronchioles and finally into the gas-exchanging airways. The anatomic dead space includes the upper airways and conducting airways that do not participate in gas exchange. This anatomic dead space accounts for 25% to 30% of the normal tidal breath. Airway resistance is affected primarily by the radius of the airway and also by the airway geometry, flow rate, and flow characteristics. The highest airway resistance is found in large, proximal bronchi, where airflow velocity is highest and most turbulent.

Airway Structure

The composition of the airways (and thus their function) depends on the airway generation. Bronchial ciliated epithelium is found in the conducting airways until they disappear in the terminal or respiratory bronchioles. The rhythmically beating cilia propel mucus-embedded foreign material proximally toward the pharynx until expectoration or swallowing occurs. The goblet cells within the bronchial epithelium secrete the mucus that covers the luminal surface of the conducting airways. This mucus layer prevents desiccation of the epithelium, clears inhaled particles, and performs antimicrobial functions. Structural support of the airways is provided by the cartilaginous plates in the bronchi, the concentric smooth muscle layer, and the tethering action of radially arranged elastic fibers. Airway smooth muscle and mucus glands are controlled by the parasympathetic nervous system supplied by the vagus nerves. The conducting airways receive their blood from the bronchial arteries. The lungs also contain cells associated with the neuroendocrine system, which consists of neurons and amine precursor uptake and decarboxylation (APUD) cells. These APUD cells contain vesicles with serotonin, dopamine, norepinephrine, vasoactive intestinal peptide, substance P, and so forth. The exact function of these hormones are unknown, however.

Surfactant System

Surfactant Structure and Synthesis

Surfactant is secreted into the alveoli by type II alveolar pneumocytes. Once in the alveoli, the surfactant proteins undergo a refinement process necessary to promote adsorption and spreading of a thin layer across the alveolar surface. In adults, about half of the synthesized surfactant is recycled, but the turnover process remains poorly defined.

Surfactant Failure

Following acute lung injury (adult respiratory distress syndrome [ARDS], widespread pneumonia), surfactant failure leads to (1) widespread collapse of lung units, leading to microatelectases; (2) V/Q mismatch with arterial hypoxemia; and (3) increased work of breathing. These effects necessitate significantly higher pressure to distend the lungs.

Pulmonary Circulation

The pulmonary circulation is a low-pressure, high-volume system, with pulmonary vascular resistance only one tenth of the systemic vascular resistance. Pulmonary vascular tone can be altered by a wide variety of vasoactive substances. Potent pulmonary vasoconstrictors include histamine, serotonin, angiotensin II, prostaglandin $F_2\alpha$, and prostaglandin E_2. Alveolar hypoxia is also a common, potent stimulus for pulmonary vasoconstriction, permitting a redistribution of blood flow away from hypoxic areas and preserving V/Q matching. In contrast to alveolar hypoxia, arterial blood hypoxemia does not provoke pulmonary vasoconstriction. Pulmonary vasodilators include bradykinin, endothelium-derived relaxing factor, and prostacyclin. Alveolar pressure and lung volume may have a significant impact on pulmonary vascular resistance. Increases in pulmonary vascular resistance are observed not only at low lung volumes but also after inflation to high lung volumes. Positive end-expiratory pressure (PEEP) can compress the alveolar capillaries and increase the physiologic dead space.

Pulmonary Interstitium

The interstitial space separates the alveoli from the vascular space. Fluid and protein exchange between the microvasculature and the alveolar air spaces occurs in this region. Interstitial fluid may increase when left ventricular end-diastolic pressure is increased (cardiogenic pulmonary edema) or when primary injury occurs to the lung's microvascular surfaces (ARDS).

Pulmonary Gas Exchange

The transfer of O_2 and CO_2 across the alveolocapillary membrane is a passive process accomplished by diffusion. Diffusion of O_2 can triple as pulmonary blood volume and pulmonary capillary recruitment increases. Diffusion can be decreased by (1) thickened alveolocapillary membrane (pulmonary fibrosis), (2) decreased driving pressure (alveolar hypoxia), or (3) reduced equilibration time (increased blood velocity due to decreased number of capillaries).

The V/Q ratio is a major determinant of gas exchange.

Low V/Q most commonly develops as a result of reduced ventilation of the airways but may also result from overperfusion of normally ventilated lung units as can occur following pulmonary embolism. High V/Q can be artificially created by mechanical ventilation with PEEP, which can result in both hypoxemia and hypercapnia. When the V/Q inequality is mild, Pa_{O_2} increases almost linearly as F_{IO_2} is increased. As the degree of V/Q inequality worsens, improving Pa_{O_2} by O_2 administration becomes more difficult. Correction of hypercapnia requires an increase in alveolar ventilation. The term *shunt* refers to blood entering the systemic arteries without first flowing through ventilated lung units. Most commonly, shunt results from passage of blood through pulmonary capillaries in contact with atelectatic or fluid-filled alveoli. With large shunt fractions, administration of O_2 in concentrations as high as 100% has minimal impact on the Pa_{O_2}.

Control of Ventilation

The arterial Pa_{O_2} and Pa_{CO_2} are regulated by a network of feedback controls. Pa_{CO_2} is the single most important factor in the control of ventilation under normal conditions. The effects of hypoxic ventilatory drive become important only in patients with severe lung disease and chronic hypercapnia.

Sensors

CHEMORECEPTORS

Central chemoreceptors in the medulla respond to changes in the hydrogen ion (H^+) concentration of the surrounding brain and extracellular fluid. In conscious humans, central chemoreceptors account for 70% to 80% of the ventilatory response to hypercapnia. Increases in blood Pa_{CO_2} cause a virtually linear increase in ventilation. Tidal volume (V_T) increases first, and elevation in respiratory frequency follows.

Peripheral chemoreceptors are located in the carotid bodies at the bifurcation of the common carotid arteries and in the aortic bodies near the aortic arch. Peripheral chemoreceptors respond primarily to hypoxemia, with the maximal response occurring at Pa_{O_2} below 50 mm Hg. Patients undergoing bilateral carotid body resection have complete loss of hypoxic ventilatory drive.

MECHANORECEPTORS

The three types of respiratory mechanoreceptors are (1) stretch receptors in the airway smooth muscles, which respond to lung distention; (2) irritant receptors in the airway epithelium, which are stimulated by noxious gases, mechanical traction such as atelectasis, or reduced lung compliance; and (3) juxtacapillary (J) receptors within the lung interstitium responding to distention of pulmonary capillaries, increased interstitial fluid, and exposure to chemical agents such as histamine. Some investigators believe that J receptors play a significant role in the sensation of dyspnea associated with pulmonary edema and interstitial lung disease. The intercostal muscles, diaphragm, joints, and tendons within the chest wall are also involved in the sensation of dyspnea.

Central Controller

The central controller is located in the pons and medulla. Inherent rhythmicity and respiratory rate are controlled by the interaction of these cells. Breathing is under voluntary control to a considerable extent, however, and the cortex can override the function of the brain stem within limits (i.e., breath holding).

Controlled System

The complex system of checks and balances serves to maintain smooth, efficient ventilation, and gas exchange not only during health but also in response to sudden stresses and the crisis of disease.

Lung Defense

Particles deposited on the central or mainstem airways are subject to removal by sneeze or cough mechanisms. Secondarily, particles are subject to mucociliary clearance. Particulate material beyond these areas to the terminal airways of the lung are cleared by lung phagocytes (macrophages and neutrophils).

Macrophages constitute the main phagocytic defense of the lung. Macrophages are mobile scavengers that are attracted to an infected focus. Polymorphonuclear neutrophils are recruited into the lungs from the circulation to boost host defenses. Plasma cells or B cells can secrete IgG and IgA into the airways. After an infectious (bacterial, viral) or antigen challenge, T cells capable of nonspecific cytotoxic activity represent the first line of defense killing in a specific fashion.

Metabolic Function of the Lung

Pulmonary endothelial surfaces metabolize a number of biogenic blood-borne substances, including prostaglandins of the E and F series, amines (norepinephrine and serotonin), peptides (angiotensin I, bradykinin), and adenine nucleotides and adenosine. Furthermore, uptake and metabolism of drugs and also of surfactant are important in both health and disease.

RESPIRATORY MUSCLE FAILURE IN CRITICAL ILLNESS

Types of Respiratory Muscle Dysfunction

Weakness

Respiratory muscles are striated skeletal muscles. The force of contraction varies with the strength and frequency of stimulation. Muscle weakness (lower contractile force than expected) can result from denervation, faulty transmission across the neuromuscular junction, and impairment of contractile apparatus in the muscle. Unlike fatigue, muscle weakness is not reversed by rest alone.

Respiratory Muscle Fatigue

Respiratory muscle fatigue is a particular form of weakness that is brought on by excessive work. Contractile force can return to normal by resting the muscle.

Low-Frequency and High-Frequency Fatigue

Low-frequency (10 to 20 Hz) fatigue may be related to muscle injury caused by O_2 free radicals. Recovery time is measured in hours. High-frequency (50 to 100 Hz) fatigue probably results from electrolyte shifts secondary to membrane depolarization, and recovery occurs within minutes. The diaphragm can suffer from both low- and high-frequency fatigue when the resistive load of breathing is increased.

Fatigue Threshold

The fatigue threshold for static contractions (e.g., weight lifting) is 15% of maximum contractile force. In rhythmically contracting muscles, both force and duration contribute to the fatigue threshold. The inspiratory pressure-time index includes both these factors, and diaphragmatic fatigue develops when this index exceeds 0.15. The fatigue threshold can be exceeded by an increase in the pressure needed to take a breath, an increase in the duration of inspiration, or a combination of the two. The time to overt fatigue varies inversely with the pressure-time index.

Respiratory failure is thus defined as an inability of the inspiratory muscles to maintain the patient's ventilatory demands, resulting in ventilatory failure with the attendant hypercapnia.

Clinical Manifestations

Prevalence in Critical Illness

Respiratory muscle weakness is fairly common in critically ill patients. It is the primary factor leading to the need for mechanical ventilation, and its prevalence may contribute to prolonged mechanical ventilation from failure to wean. In one study, when maximal inspiratory pressure (PImax) was measured at the onset of ventilator weaning, about 40% of patients had inspiratory muscle weakness.

Pattern of Breathing

Rapid, Shallow Breathing and Dyspnea

Rapid, shallow breathing and dyspnea are considered markers of respiratory muscle failure. These symptoms are not specific for respiratory muscle failure, however, and occur in other conditions. This type of breathing pattern is probably a defense mechanism to minimize dyspnea.

Recruitment of the Upper Airway, Neck, and Abdominal Muscles

Flaring of the nostrils and enhanced use of the neck accessory inspiratory muscles are often seen in patients with respiratory muscle failure. Rib cage–abdominal asynchrony is seen during respiratory muscle fatigue, but this is also manifest during increased respiratory load without the presence of fatigue. When the diaphragm is weak or paralyzed, patients experience orthopnea and have paradoxical inward displacement of the abdomen during inspiration. Central ventilatory drive is usually increased in patients with ventilatory failure as they try to compensate for the muscle weakness.

Diagnosis of Respiratory Muscle Failure

Clinical clues such as dyspnea; rapid, shallow breathing; use of accessory inspiratory muscles; and paradoxical breathing help identify the presence of respiratory muscle failure. Relief of these signs and symptoms by mechanical ventilation is supportive of the diagnosis. Performance of pulmonary function testing to aid diagnosis is difficult in critically ill patients. Vital capacity may be a useful marker, especially in patients with neuromuscular disorder. The best measure of weakness is the maximum static respiratory pressures, and thus the use of negative inspiratory pressure is a commonly measured parameter before weaning. This test, however, often depends on the patient's effort and level of cooperation.

Complications

Cough, Aspiration, and Pneumonia

Coughing is dependent on adequate respiratory muscle function. With muscle weakness, coughing ability is impaired and patients are at risk of aspiration, pneumonia, and atelectasis. In addition, mucociliary clearance is impaired in respiratory muscle weakness.

Ventilatory Failure

Respiratory muscle weakness ultimately leads to hypercapnic ventilatory failure. In pure respiratory muscle weakness without concomitant lung disease, hypercapnia does not develop until the strength is less than 30% of predicted. When coexisting lung disease is present, such as chronic obstructive pulmonary disease (COPD), however, ventilatory failure can develop with loss of less respiratory strength. Hypercapnia develops secondary to decreased CO_2 elimination due to low V_T respirations.

Causes of Respiratory Muscle Weakness

Hypoxia and Hypercapnia, Acidosis, and Electrolyte Imbalance

Hypoxia reduces the endurance of respiratory muscles for sustaining a contractile effort. Hypercapnia reduces both the strength and endurance of respiratory muscle. Metabolic acidosis has a lesser effect on diaphragmatic contractility than does respiratory acidosis. Hypokalemia, hypomagnesemia, and hypophosphatemia all lead to muscle weakness and can precipitate acute ventilatory failure.

Shock and Sepsis

In animal studies, sepsis causes a reduction in muscle strength, which can be prevented by oxygen radical scavengers and N-acetylcysteine. For humans, an entity called *polyneuropathy of the critically ill* is an axonal neuropathy leading to muscle weakness. This condition can contribute to weaning failure from mechanical ventilation.

Malnutrition and Cachexia

Many patients with respiratory failure, especially those with COPD, are malnourished. This leads to atrophy of the diaphragm and other respiratory muscles.

Heart Failure, Renal Disease, and Diabetes

In congestive heart failure, generalized muscle weakness, including of the respiratory muscles, is common. It is hypothesized that cachexia or diminished muscle blood flow is responsible for the generalized muscle weakness. Patients with renal disease also have respiratory muscle weakness, which may be a result of electrolyte imbalance or acidosis, in addition to protein loss. Diabetic patients tend to have a less severe weakness.

Corticosteroids and Paralytic Agents

The combination of steroids and muscle paralytic agents has been implicated in prolonged muscle weakness. The mechanism is unknown but has a profound impact when present. It affects many muscle groups and leads to difficulty weaning from the ventilator. Steroids alone can induce a proximal myopathy that leads to loss of respiratory muscle strength, but it is distinguished from the former type by a slower form of onset and less notable muscle weakness.

Mechanical Disadvantage

The diaphragm is the respiratory muscle most affected by mechanical disadvantage leading to a reduction in PImax. Hyperinflation of the lung, as with obstructive airway disease, causes the diaphragm to be shorter than normal and, conversely, abdominal distention may overstretch the diaphragm. These alterations affect the diaphragm's tension–length relation and reduce its ability to generate an inspiratory force.

Treatment

Respiratory Muscle Rest

Mechanical ventilation with full ventilatory support provides a recuperation period for the respiratory muscles. Patients feel better and their sense of dyspnea is relieved, allowing them to rest and sleep. Full ventilatory support allows for adequate oxygenation while correcting any respiratory acidosis. It also reduces the O_2 consumption ($\dot{V}O_2$) of the respiratory muscles.

Restoration of Normal Environment

By supporting the respiratory system with mechanical ventilation, other problems that may take several days to reverse can be addressed (e.g., treating infection, congestive heart failure). If the lungs themselves are the root of the problem, specific therapy should be directed to them (e.g., bronchodilators and steroids for asthma, thoracentesis for pleural effusion). Weaning from mechanical ventilation should not be attempted until the cause of respiratory failure has fully resolved. It must be ensured that the endotracheal tube and mechanical ventilator are not the cause of increased work of breathing, resulting in muscle fatigue and unsuccessful weaning.

Rebuilding the Contractile Apparatus

Nutritional Repletion

Nutritional repletion improves respiratory muscle function. Therefore, it is important to ensure adequate nutritional support for critically ill patients. Debate has surrounded whether overfeeding with carbohydrates relative to fat can lead to respiratory failure in patients with COPD by increasing CO_2 production. Total calorie intake itself may be more important than the relative distribution of the calories between fat and carbohydrate.

Respiratory Muscle Training

Some investigators have used inspiratory flow-resistive devices and voluntary hyperventilation to enhance respiratory muscle strength and endurance. These are not uniform practices and have yet to be subject to large controlled trials.

Summary

Respiratory muscle weakness is both an important factor for ventilatory failure that necessitates mechanical ventilation and a hindrance to weaning from mechanical ventilation. It is an important factor in prolonging intensive care and hospital stay, with attendant increases in respiratory complications and costs. Respiratory muscle weakness has many causes and may be part of a multiorgan dysfunction state. It is usually characterized by rapid, shallow breathing with complaints of dyspnea. Prominent use of accessory muscles of breathing and rib cage–abdominal asynchrony are common. Treatment relies on treating the underlying cause and, if needed, the supportive intervention of mechanical ventilation. The work of breathing should be reduced if this is the cause of failure (e.g., through bronchodilation and relief of abdominal distention). Once the cause of respiratory failure has been resolved, the patient can be weaned from mechanical ventilatory support. It is important that adequate nutrition is provided during the course of illness. If muscle paralytic agents are used, close monitoring is required.

THE WORK OF BREATHING

Measures of Respiratory Muscle Activity

The measures of respiratory muscle activity can be considered under three headings:

1. Work of breathing
2. O_2 consumption
3. Pressure-time product

The respiratory muscles normally provide the force for inspiration. Expiration is usually passive, with expiratory flow driven by the elastic recoil of the respiratory system. In conditions of increased expiratory flow resistance, however, expiration is frequently an active process.

Work of Breathing

The physical definition of work is the product of force and the distance moved. For the respiratory system, this is represented by the product of pressure and the change in volume (the integral of PdV). This is expressed most commonly in joules (J), where 1 J = 10 cm $H_2O \cdot L$. Values are then listed as either work per liter of ventilation or work per minute (power). Thus, the work of the respiratory system can be calculated from the following equations using esophageal pressure as a surrogate for pleural pressure:

$$W_L = \int (Paw - Pes)dV$$

$$W_{CW} = \int (Pes - Patm)dV$$

where W_L is the work to inflate the lung; W_{CW} is the work to expand the chest wall, and Paw, Pes, and Patm are central airway, esophageal, and atmospheric pressure, respectively. The main limitation of using work as the expression of respiratory muscle activity is the failure to account for the energy expanded during conditions of isometric muscle contraction in which there is no change in volume. The actual methods of calculating the work of breathing for spontaneous and assisted mechanical breathing are discussed further in the textbook.

Respiratory muscle efficiency is the ratio of work performed to energy expended. As mentioned, isometric muscle contraction is an example of reduced muscle efficiency, since the energy expended in contraction is not manifested in work. Other measures, such as $\dot{V}O_2$ and the pressure-time product, have therefore been used to assess the activity of the respiratory muscles.

Oxygen Consumption

Respiratory muscle, unlike other skeletal muscles, functions primarily under aerobic metabolism. Hence, measurement of respiratory muscle $\dot{V}O_2$ provides an accurate measurement of the muscle's energy expenditure. In the clinical setting, only indirect measures of respiratory muscle oxygen consumption are available. The difference in $\dot{V}O_2$ during controlled mechanical ventilation and during assisted mechanical ventilation or spontaneous ventilation is assumed to represent the respiratory muscle $\dot{V}O_2$. This approach has many technical problems, however. Measurement of $\dot{V}O_2$ is limited by high fraction of inspired oxygen (FIO_2), as well as the changes in $\dot{V}O_2$ over time that is not reflected by a short period of measurement. In addition, during active breathing, the increased $\dot{V}O_2$ may not be due solely to respiratory muscle activity. For instance, any patient unable to sustain life with spontaneous breathing will have high catecholamine production during trials of spontaneous breathing, causing a strong increase in $\dot{V}O_2$ (as high as 50%) in addition to that caused by the need of respiratory muscles.

Pressure-Time Product

Isometric respiratory muscle contraction is accounted for by the pressure-time product, which is calculated by the integral of esophageal pressure over time ($\int$ Pes ΔT). Certain studies have shown a correlation between the pressure-time product and $\dot{V}O_2$ measurements, but others have shown otherwise.

Respiratory Muscle Activity in Patients with Acute Respiratory Failure

Spontaneous Ventilation

The $\dot{V}O_2$ of respiratory muscles in normal humans during quiet spontaneous breathing is approximately 0.25 to 0.50 mL of O_2 per liter of ventilation, or about 1% to 2% of total body $\dot{V}O_2$. In intubated postoperative patients who are breathing spontaneously with normal lungs, the mean O_2 cost of breathing is between 11% and 13% of total $\dot{V}O_2$. During weaning, values of 16% to 27% have been measured.

Patients with lung disease have abnormal respiratory mechanics that lead to decreased muscle efficiency and hence increased energy expenditure. Intubated patients have increased workload imposed by the presence of the endotracheal tube, which acts as resistance. Both the diameter of the tube and the flow rate influence the amount of resistance. Furthermore, ventilator tubing and both exhalation and inhalation valves increase the respiratory load.

The time lag from the patient's inspiratory effort to the delivery of gas flow from the ventilator results in continued patient muscle effort despite the initiation of ventilator gas flow. Efforts to reduce this time lag have focused on providing a continuous flow system as well as to ensure that the demand valve sensitivity is set appropriately with adequate gas flow delivery.

Assisted Mechanical Ventilation

Pressure support ventilation allows the patient to exert control over the inspiratory flow rate, inspiratory time, and VT. This can be used as total ventilatory support at high levels of assistance; at lower levels of support (e.g., 5 to 10 cm H_2O), it is used to compensate for the increased respiratory workload caused by the endotracheal tube, ventilator tubing, and the mechanical ventilator.

It is commonly believed that the work of breathing of the assisted breaths is provided entirely by the ventilator during assisted ventilation. This is not true, however, as the level of support is reduced. Surprisingly, the patient's work of breathing may be similar for both assisted and nonassisted breaths. The work during assisted breaths may be the result of a low ventilator trigger sensitivity, a lower preset machine inspiratory flow rate below a patient's spontaneous flow rate, a high minute ventilation ($\dot{V}E$), or the time lag from the patient's inspiratory effort to the actual delivery of gas flow. Thus, the possibility of fatiguing patients even on assisted mechanical ventilation has to be recognized.

Effects of Intrinsic Positive End-Expiratory Pressure

Intrinsic PEEP (PEEPI) indicates the presence of PEEP at the onset of inspiration. This is the result of inadequate expiration time for a given minute ventilation from increased expiratory airflow resistance or an excessively high minute ventilation. The presence of PEEPI increases respiratory muscle work needed to provide a given level of ventilation. In mechanically ventilated patients, additional pressure has to be generated to overcome PEEPI before the sensitivity threshold of the demand valve is triggered.

It is important to ensure adequate expiration time by increasing inspiratory flow rate and reducing expiratory flow resistance (e.g., with bronchodilators, clearance of secretions, and the use of large diameter endotracheal tubes). The application of extrinsic PEEP (PEEPE) to counterbalance the PEEPI can be beneficial but has to be done carefully. It can reduce dynamic hyperinflation by splinting open the airways and reducing the effort needed to trigger the ventilator. PEEPE has been shown to reduce the pressure-time product and respiratory work in patients with expiratory flow limitation. The level of PEEPE should be less than that of PEEPI and should not increase the overall PEEP or produce any adverse hemodynamic effect. If PEEPE is applied indiscriminately, especially in patients without expiratory flow limitation, it could lead to increases in end-expiratory lung volumes, total PEEP, and airway pressures, and can have detrimental hemodynamic consequences.

Clinical Considerations

Because mechanical ventilation is commenced for respiratory failure, it is assumed that the initial objective is to rest the respiratory muscles. This can be achieved with high levels of assisted ventilation plus sedation to blunt the respiratory drive. As the patients recover from respiratory failure and efforts are begun to wean them from mechanical ventilator support, it is important to be cognizant of the external factors that lead to increased respiratory load. Thus, (1) sensitivity thresholds should be at a high level ($\leq$2 cm H_2O); (2) the inspiratory flow rate should exceed the patient's spontaneous inspiratory flow rate; (3) adequate levels of pressure support should be provided; (4) continuous flow systems can be considered; and (4) if PEEPI is present, efforts to reduce it should be sought and the utility of providing the appropriate level of PEEPE should be explored.

ASSESSMENT OF PULMONARY FUNCTION IN CRITICALLY ILL PATIENTS

The role of pulmonary function testing in critically ill patients is assuming more importance and has expanded to include other measures besides arterial blood gas analysis. Pulmonary function testing helps determine whether mechanical ventilation is indicated, assesses response to therapy, optimizes ventilator management, and assists in deciding on the timing for weaning, as well as predicting likely weaning success.

Clinical Assessment

Much information can be gained from a careful observation of patients as they breathe. Signs such as respiratory rate, use of accessory muscles for respiration along with suprasternal and intercostal space recession, and paradoxical breathing (rib cage–abdominal asynchrony) provide useful information on the patient's work of breathing.

Vital Capacity

The vital capacity is the greatest volume of gas a person is able to exhale after maximum inspiration. The vital capacity indicates a patient's ability to inspire deeply and cough. Normal vital capacity is between 65 and 75 mL/kg, and a vital capacity of at least 10 mL/kg is needed for spontaneous ventilation. Therefore, in neuromuscular conditions (e.g., Guillain-Barré syndrome), elective intubation for mechanical ventilation should be considered for those with measurements below 10 mL/kg. Vital capacity is also reduced in obstructive and restrictive lung diseases. A vital capacity above 10 mL/kg has been proposed as an outcome predictor of weaning success.

Functional Residual Capacity

The FRC is the volume of gas remaining in the lungs when the respiratory muscles relax at the end of a normal expiration. It represents the equilibrium point between elastic recoil of the lung and that of the chest wall; it is the major reservoir of O_2, minimizing fluctuations in arterial O_2 tension during breathing; and it determines the resting length of the respiratory muscles and thus their force-generating ability. FRC measurements are difficult to perform at bedside. Changes in FRC can be inferred from changes in end-expiratory level from an inductive plethysmography signal, but this requires special equipment (refer to the textbook for details).

Bedside Measurement of Thoracic Compliance

To achieve ventilation, elasticity (defined in terms of compliance) of both lungs and the chest wall has to be overcome. Compliance is calculated as the change in volume for a given change in distending transthoracic pressure. In mechanically ventilated patients, compliance calculated at zero gas flow is termed *static compliance* and is defined by the tidal volume divided by the end-inspiratory plateau airway pressure minus total PEEP. This compliance measurement includes both lung and chest wall compliances. If airway pressure is high, there may be distention of the ventilator tubing (compression volume) with volume loss or air leaks that would lead to an erroneously high compliance value unless corrections are made. Other errors result from inaccurate volume measurements at extremes of flow rate and patient effort. If the patient is not completely relaxed and is actively inspiring, the pressure developed by the ventilator is less than the total pressure required for thoracic inflation, and a falsely high compliance is obtained.

A decrease in thoracic compliance occurs in disorders of the thoracic cage and with a reduction in the number of functioning lung units (e.g., lung resection, bronchial intubation, pneumothorax, pneumonia, atelectasis, or pulmonary edema).

Dynamic compliance employs peak airway pressure instead of the plateau pressure. This includes a resistive component. Therefore, if dynamic compliance is much lower than the static compliance, an increase in airway resistance can occur (e.g., bronchospasm, mucus plugging, kinking of endotracheal tube).

If a patient develops hypoxemia without any change in compliance, pulmonary embolism should be suspected.

Respiratory Center Function

An abnormality of the respiratory control system should be suspected when hypercapnia exists in the following settings:

(1) FEV_1 exceeds 1.3 L; (2) the alveolar-arterial O_2 gradient is normal; (3) correction to normocapnia is possible after voluntary hyperventilation; and (4) respiratory muscle weakness is absent. Occlusion pressure is the airway pressure measured 0.1 second ($P_{0.1}$) after initiation of an inspiratory effort by abruptly occluding the airway (without warning to patient). This is taken to reflect respiratory neural drive. Although this is a negative pressure, it is customary to report it in positive units. The normal range is 0.93 ± 0.48 cm H_2O. The ability of $P_{0.1}$ to predict weaning outcome is still under investigation.

Maximum Respiratory Pressures

Respiratory muscle fatigue is now considered an important contributor to ventilatory failure. No good clinical measure of respiratory muscle fatigue has been developed, however, and assessment of respiratory muscle function is limited to measurements of maximum respiratory pressures. Respiratory muscle strength is assessed by measuring the maximum inspiratory and maximum expiratory pressure (PImax and PEmax) generated against an occluded airway. PImax is measured after expiration to residual volume, and PEmax is measured after inspiration to total lung capacity.

Considerable variations in maximal inspiratory pressures are obtained with different techniques and patient effort. Marini and colleagues attempted to standardize the measurement of PImax by using a one-way expiratory valve to ensure that inspiration begins at a low lung volume and also by standardizing the period of occlusion to 20 seconds. Three measurements are made and the highest (most negative) value is taken. When PImax is reduced to one third of the normal predicted value, hypercapnia is likely to develop. Traditionally, PImax values more negative than −30 cm H_2O are reported to predict weaning success, whereas values no lower than −20 cm H_2O predict weaning failure. More recent studies, however, have cast doubt on PImax for predicting weaning outcomes.

PImax is a measure of muscle strength and not endurance. The converse of endurance is fatigue, which is defined as the inability of a muscle to generate and sustain a required contractile force. A number of techniques have attempted to measure respiratory muscle fatigue, such as phrenic nerve stimulation, power spectral analysis of the electromyogram, and calculation of the pressure-time product. Their utility in the intensive care unit remains to be determined, however.

Minute Ventilation

Minute ventilation (VE) and $PaCO_2$ provide a good measure of the demands placed on the respiratory system. A VE below 10 L/min is considered a requirement for weaning. Because $PaCO_2$ is determined by the relation between alveolar ventilation and CO_2 production, a high VE in the presence of hypercapnia indicates the presence of either increased CO_2 production or increased dead space ventilation. Conversely, hypercapnia associated with a low VE should make one suspicious of the presence of decreased respiratory drive, structural abnormality of the thoracic cage, or respiratory muscle dysfunction. It is always important to partition the V_E measurement into V_T and respiratory frequency. A ratio of frequency to tidal volume (f/V_T) less than 100 is used as a predictor of weaning success. Measurement of ventilatory volumes in spontaneously breathing patients is difficult with mouthpieces or masks, and inductive plethysmography is used instead. This method also allows the measurement of the degree of paradoxical breathing. Mean inspiratory flow rate (V_T/T_I, where T_I is inspiratory time) can be calculated as a measure of respiratory center drive and respiratory asynchrony. These parameters have been also been used to predict weaning outcome.

Maximum Voluntary Ventilation

Maximum voluntary ventilation is the volume of air that can be inhaled and exhaled with maximum effort over 1 minute. It is usually measured for 15 seconds and then multiplied by four. Normal values range from 50 to 200 L/min. The relation between resting V_E and maximum voluntary ventilation indicates the degree of reserve available for increased respiratory demands. The ability to achieve maximum voluntary ventilation at least double resting V_E has been used as a predictor of weaning success.

Work of Breathing

Work of breathing is increased in situations in which airway resistance is increased or lung compliance is decreased. Work-of-breathing measurements are difficult in clinical practice, however, and are largely restricted to research studies.

Assessment of the Surgical Patient

Patients with abdominal or thoracic incisions have compromised lung function that leads to increased pulmonary complications. The presence of preexisting lung disease increases the risk for pulmonary complications. Preoperative lung function testing allows patients at risk to be identified and perioperative respiratory care to be optimized.

Lung resection demands a preoperative assessment of lung function to determine whether the patient is able to tolerate the loss of lung volume proposed by the surgery. For a pneumonectomy, a forced expiratory lung volume in 1 second (FEV_1) of 2 L or greater is considered adequate. If it is below 2 L, split lung function studies are required. If the predicted postoperative FEV_1 is 0.8 L or more, the patient is suitable for pneumonectomy.

Summary

Pulmonary function in the intensive care unit differs from that in the lung function laboratory. It is useful as a trend monitor and provides some guide to weaning outcomes.

The information derived from the tests, in combination with the clinical assessment, can provide a useful insight into the pathophysiologic nature of a patient's disease.

REGULATION OF CAPILLARY EXCHANGE OF FLUID AND PROTEIN

Structure of the Capillary Wall

Continuous capillaries have a dense and continuous basement membrane. They are highly permeable to small solutes such as sodium chloride, glucose, and water.

Fenestrated capillaries have diaphragms that cover the fenestrae. They are found in organs in which large amounts of small solutes and fluid move into or out of the microcirculation (e.g., glomeruli, gastrointestinal tract).

Discontinuous capillaries have huge gaps between endothelial cells and no basement membranes. They are highly permeable to plasma proteins and exchange freely all constituents of plasma. They are found in the liver, spleen, and some glands.

Tissue Fluid Pressure, the Effective Osmotic Pressure, and Lymph Flow

When the capillaries filter fluid into the interstitium, tissue pressure increases, retarding interstitial fluid accumulation. When the tissues swell to some critical value, however, only small increases in tissue pressure cause fluid to accumulate in the tissues. In most capillary beds, lymph flow increases with net capillary filtration and reaches a plateau as the lymphatic system saturates. The importance of lymph flow in removing excess capillary filtration fluid is not well understood and certainly varies from tissue to tissue. The lymphatics represent the only means by which plasma proteins can re-enter the plasma once they have leaked into the interstitium.

Relevance to Critical Care Medicine

Understanding capillary fluid and protein exchange is important in managing edema, especially pulmonary edema. If the capillaries are leaky to proteins, albumin administration is not an effective treatment for the reduction of edema. Normally, colloids and plasma proteins expand blood volume and increase pulmonary capillary pressure. If the lung capillary permeability is increased, the effective osmotic pressure gradient acting across the capillaries is small, and the use of colloids actually accelerates interstitial fluid accumulation as Ppc increases. This occurs because pulmonary capillary pressure is increased by the removal of interstitial fluid from the large muscle and subcutaneous tissue spaces secondary to an increase in protein osmotic pressure in plasma. When the lungs are more permeable to plasma proteins, accurate estimate of pulmonary capillary pressure becomes an important measure in the critically ill patients, since even slight elevations in pulmonary capillary pressure can cause severe pulmonary edema.

Measure of Pulmonary Capillary Pressure

It is extremely important to measure the pulmonary capillary pressure in critically ill patients, since this pressure is the most important determinant of lung water accumulation, even in patients with "leaky capillaries." The pulmonary capillary pressure can be measured using a pulmonary artery catheter and analysis of the wedged pressure tracing. The pulmonary capillary pressure is *not* identical to pulmonary arterial wedge pressure. When the balloon catheter is inflated, the catheter tip pressure rapidly decreases to the pulmonary capillary pressure and then slowly approaches the wedge pressure (left atrial pressure). The pulmonary capillary pressure can be estimated by simply identifying the inflection point at which the pressure changes from a rapid to the slow component of the wedge tracing (Fig. 5–1). If, after balloon inflation, pulmonary artery pressure drops rapidly toward the pulmonary wedge pressure, the resistance is precapillary; if it decreases slowly to the wedge pressure, the resistance is mostly postcapillary. Since the pulmonary capillary pressure is such an important determinant of transcapillary fluid flux, it should be routinely measured when the pulmonary arterial wedge pressure is monitored in critically ill patients.

Plasma Volume Expansion with Albumin

For both normal and increased vascular pressures, addition of protein could be beneficial in removing extravascular water, but the effect lasts only a short time. Increasing plasma proteins when capillary endothelium is damaged provides almost no absorptive effects. In fact, edema can become more severe after colloid usage. Crystalloid volume replacement causes fewer lung problems because pulmonary capillary pressure values do not remain elevated and lymph flow can increase to extremely high levels. Colloid therapy can elevate pulmonary capillary pressure for several hours

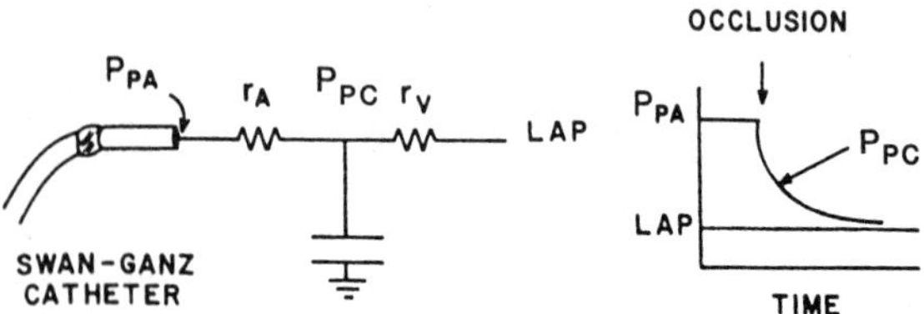

Figure 5–1. Schematic representation of the pulmonary arterial occlusion method for determining capillary pressure. A simple two-resistance, single-capacitance electrical model is shown on the right, and a pressure tracing observed after balloon occlusion of the pulmonary artery is shown on the left.

because of retention of fluid absorbed from large tissue spaces in skin and muscles, and it can actually promote rather than resolve pulmonary edema.

INCREASED LUNG VASCULAR PERMEABILITY: MEDIATORS AND THERAPIES

Basic Pathophysiology of Lung Fluid Balance

The forces affecting the movement of fluid and solutes across the walls of microvessels into the lung interstitium are described by the Starling equation. It was initially believed that under normal conditions, the net Starling forces should be in the direction of absorption. In fact, the difference between pulmonary arterial wedge pressure and plasma oncotic pressure is still often used as an index toward the development of pulmonary edema. Recent work has demonstrated, however, that transvascular filtration is present under normal conditions, but this does not lead to pulmonary edema. Instead, several features act as safety factors against pulmonary edema—increased lung lymph flow, decreased perimicrovascular oncotic pressure, and increased interstitial hydrostatic pressure.

For pulmonary edema to occur, there are two possible scenarios. The first involves the so-called high-pressure or cardiogenic pulmonary edema that results from an increase in capillary pressure. Abnormalities are therefore extrinsic to the lung itself. Second, an increase in capillary permeability leads to excessive fluid and protein leakage. This phenomenon is called *increased permeability edema* or *noncardiogenic pulmonary edema* and results from an intrinsic abnormality of the lung. Clinically, this is referred to as ARDS.

Role of Metabolites of Arachidonic Acid and Granulocytes in Lung Edema Caused by Increased Microvascular Permeability

Lung injury causes the release of phospholipids containing arachidonic acid from cell membranes. Through the action of phospholipases, free arachidonate is formed, which can be metabolized either into prostaglandins and thromboxanes through a cyclo-oxygenase enzyme or into leukotrienes by means of the lipoxygenase enzymes. Prostaglandins E_2 and F_2 are pulmonary vasoconstrictors, which, along with thromboxane, also act as a bronchoconstrictor. In contrast, prostacyclin is a pulmonary vasodilator, and leukotrienes are chemoattractive for granulocytes.

Cyclo-oxygenase inhibitors (e.g., indomethacin, ibuprofen, and meclofenamate) appear to have beneficial effects on the lungs in animal models of ARDS. This may be related to the maintenance of the hypoxic pulmonary vasoconstrictor response, which is impaired with the release of prostacyclin. High doses of corticosteroids are also beneficial in animal models of gram-negative endotoxemia causing lung injury by preventing the increased generation of both cyclo-oxygenase and lipoxygenase products. The precise mechanism of steroid-induced effect on acute lung injury is not known, however.

Granulocytes can lead to lung injury with increased capillary permeability through the release of proteolytic enzymes, as well as the generation of superoxide and other free radicals that damage the pulmonary endothelial cells. Granulocytes may also have a role in amplifying the lung injury and may also participate in lung repair.

Therapeutic Implications in Humans

Hypoxemia in ARDS is a result of pulmonary edema, abnormal airway function, and impaired hypoxic pulmonary vasoconstriction. Therefore, management based solely on minimizing fluid administration may be inappropriate in patients without excessively high pulmonary arterial wedge pressures and may even be harmful by decreasing O_2 delivery as a result of a lower cardiac output.

No pharmacologic treatment for ARDS has been shown to improve mortality. Steroids have not been shown to be superior to placebo in the treatment of ARDS. There are several promising agents, however. Cyclo-oxygenase inhibitors may be useful for restoring hypoxic pulmonary vasoconstriction and improving oxygenation. Other drugs for the future include free radical scavengers to reduce lung injury.

The current therapy for ARDS remains largely supportive. Supplemental oxygenation and mechanical ventilation with PEEP improves oxygenation. Most patients benefit from invasive monitoring with a pulmonary artery catheter to evaluate pulmonary arterial wedge pressure and cardiac output measurements for the calculation of O_2 delivery. It would be prudent to maintain a modest level of filling pressure and a reasonable level of O_2 delivery. The type of fluid resuscitation (colloids or crystalloids) is still being debated, and no clear answer is in sight.

Prognosis

The mortality related to ARDS ranges from 50% to 70% in different studies. The cause of ARDS is an important determinant of mortality rates, as is the way ARDS is defined. The severity of ARDS measured either by oxygenation indices or the amount of extravascular lung water did not predict the prognosis associated with ARDS. Finding the source of the problem (e.g., an abdominal abscess), however, and treating it aggressively are crucial for a successful outcome. Pulmonary abnormalities may persist for several months in survivors of ARDS. These take the form of mild to moderate restriction defects with mild hypoxemia. Normalization of oxygenation and chest radiographs may occur over several months.

APPROACH TO THE PATIENT WITH ACUTE RESPIRATORY FAILURE

Respiratory failure can be defined as impairment in gas exchange with resultant arterial hypoxemia or hypercapnia.

On the basis of the duration of impaired gas exchange, respiratory failure is classified as either *acute* or *chronic.*

Mechanisms of Abnormal Gas Exchange

The effectiveness of the lungs in exchanging O_2 and CO_2 is determined by three factors: alveolar ventilation, V/Q matching, and the extent of equilibration between alveolar gas and pulmonary blood. Because the equilibration of O_2 and CO_2 across the alveolocapillary interface occurs rapidly, diffusion impairment leading to hypoxemia or hypercapnia is rare, except with severe parenchyma and pulmonary capillary destruction. Therefore, V/Q mismatching and alveolar hypoventilation are the major mechanisms of abnormal gas exchange. Other factors influencing PaO_2 and $PaCO_2$ include the FIO_2, and mixed venous O_2 and CO_2 concentrations.

Ventilation–Perfusion Imbalance

The V/Q ratio of the alveolus determines the PO_2 and PCO_2 of the capillary blood that leaves it. In the ideal situation, there is a close to perfect matching of V/Q, with a value of 1.0. Effects of posture (through gravity effects) and disease states, however, lead to an imbalance of V/Q. An increase of the V/Q ratio to infinity is called *dead-space ventilation,* whereas the opposite to zero V/Q ratio is called *a right-to-left intrapulmonary shunt.*

The effect of an intrapulmonary shunt is to increase venous admixture as mixed venous blood is shunted unaltered into the systemic circulation. The shunt fraction (Qs/Qt) can be calculated ($Qs/Qt = [CcO_2 - CaO_2]/[CcO_2 - CvO_2]$), although this assumes the absence of any lung VO_2. Changes in VE, cardiac output, and FIO_2 can all affect venous admixture. Thus, a better overall descriptor of V/Q relations is the alveolar-arterial PO_2 difference ($[A - a]PO_2 = PAO_2 - PaO_2$, where $PAO_2 = [PB - PH_2O] \times FIO_2 - PaCO_2/RQ$, where PB is the barometric pressure, PH_2O is the partial pressure of water in the alveoli [47 mm Hg at body temperature], and RQ is the respiratory quotient [normally 0.8]). Unfortunately, this is not ideal either, since it is influenced by FIO_2, age, and the presence of severe hypercarbia.

Dead space ventilation is the total volume of air entering the respiratory tract that does not contribute to gas exchange. The presence of dead space ventilation reduces the efficiency of CO_2 elimination. Thus, to maintain the same $PaCO_2$, VE has to be increased if dead space ventilation increases. If this cannot be sustained as the work of breathing becomes excessive, respiratory failure ensues. Physiologic dead space to VT ratio (VDS/VT) can be calculated from the Bohr equation ($VDS/VT = [PaCO_2 - PECO_2]/PaCO_2$, where $PECO_2$ is mixed expired PCO_2 and VDS is dead space ventilation.) This represents anatomic and alveolar dead space plus apparatus dead space if present. Anatomic dead space can be estimated as 1 mL per pound of (ideal) body weight.

Table 5–1. CLASSIFICATION OF RESPIRATORY FAILURE

Type		Pa_{O_2}	Pa_{CO_2}	$PA_{O_2} - Pa_{O_2}$
1	Oxygenation failure	↓	NL-↓	↑
2	Ventilation failure	↓	↑	NL
3	Combined failure	↓	↑	↑

Alveolar Hypoventilation

The presence of hypercapnia indicates alveolar hypoventilation assuming that CO_2 production is constant and dead space has not increased. As predicted by the alveolar gas equation, an increase in the Pa_{CO_2} in turn leads to a fall in Pa_{O_2}, but alveolar–arterial P_{O_2} remains constant.

Classification of Respiratory Failure

There are three types of respiratory failure based on the underlying mechanism, and each has a characteristic Pa_{O_2} and Pa_{CO_2} pattern (Table 5–1):

Type 1 (oxygenation failure): There is V/Q imbalance and shunt leading to an increased alveolar–arterial P_{O_2}
Type 2 (ventilation failure): There is alveolar hypoventilation and thus normal alveolar–arterial P_{O_2}
Type 3 (combined hypoxemia and hypercapnia)

The most common cause of all these types of respiratory failure are given in Tables 5–2 to 5–4.

Diagnosis

Respiratory failure is diagnosed in the presence of hypoxemia ($Pa_{O_2} < 60$ mm Hg) or hypercapnia ($Pa_{CO_2} > 45$ mm Hg). Clinical symptoms and signs of respiratory failure are determined by the underlying cause and the effects of hypoxemia or hypercapnia. Hypoxemia may be accompanied by tachypnea, tachycardia, hypertension, and the presence of cyanosis. Pulse oximetry measuring arterial O_2 satu-

Table 5–2. CAUSES OF TYPE 1 (OXYGENATION) FAILURE

Adult respiratory distress syndrome
Asthma
Atelectasis
Cardiogenic pulmonary edema
Chronic obstructive pulmonary disease (including bronchiectasis and cystic fibrosis)
Interstitial fibrosis
Pneumonia (infectious or chemical)
Pneumothorax
Pulmonary embolism
Pulmonary hypertension

Table 5–3. CAUSES OF TYPE 2 (VENTILATION) FAILURE

Disorders Affecting Central Respiratory Drive
Brain stem infarction or hemorrhage
Brain stem compression from supratentorial mass
Drug overdose (e.g., narcotics, benzodiazepines, tricyclics)
Disorders Affecting Signal Transmission to the Respiratory Muscles
Amyotrophic lateral sclerosis
Guillain-Barré syndrome
Multiple sclerosis
Myasthenia gravis
Spinal cord injury
Disorders of the Respiratory Muscles of Chest Wall
Muscular dystrophy
Polymyositis or dermatomyositis
Flail chest

ration may be a useful noninvasive method of detecting hypoxemia. Various technical factors (jaundice, skin pigmentation, and levels of carboxyhemoglobin) may affect its accuracy, however. Furthermore, it provides no information on $Pa{CO_2}$. Cerebral effects of hypoxemia vary from mild confusion to delirium. The primary effects of hypercapnia is on the central nervous system, and it can cause coma at very high levels of $Pa{CO_2}$.

All the features described here may not become manifest until a dangerous level of respiratory failure is reached. Thus, arterial blood gas measurements should be obtained periodically if progressive respiratory insufficiency is suspected.

Evaluation

Once respiratory failure is suspected, the evaluation process should include a history and physical examination to elicit the underlying cause, followed by an arterial blood gas and a chest radiograph.

Management

There are four essential components to the management of respiratory failure:

1. Establish a patent airway.
2. Maintain sufficient ventilation.

Table 5–4. CAUSES OF TYPE 3 (COMBINED OXYGENATION–VENTILATION) FAILURE

Adult respiratory distress syndrome
Asthma
Chronic obstructive pulmonary disease (including bronchiectasis and cystic fibrosis)

3. Ensure adequate O_2 delivery to the tissues.
4. Treat the underlying cause of respiratory failure.

Airway Management

First, the patency of the upper airways should be assessed and the presence of upper airway obstruction excluded. Placing the head in the sniffing position and providing an oropharyngeal airway may alleviate the obstruction from a floppy tongue. Indications for tracheal intubation include the presence of upper airway obstruction that is not easily remediable, inability to protect the airway from aspiration, inability to adequately clear secretions, and respiratory failure (inadequate oxygenation or ventilation) that is not rapidly correctable.

Ventilation

Hypercapnia may result from decreased alveolar ventilation or increased dead space and low V/Q lung units. The traditional treatment is endotracheal intubation and mechanical ventilation. Noninvasive ventilation can also be considered if airway patency is not at stake.

The decision to initiate mechanical ventilation should be based on the overall assessment of the patient. Clinical signs of respiratory muscle fatigue or decreased mentation, abnormal and worsening arterial blood gas values, and decreasing vital capacity (<15 mL/kg in a patient with neuromuscular disease) are factors to consider. There is no absolute level for intubation based on arterial $PaCO_2$. It is important to consider arterial pH as well to determine the chronicity of the hypercapnia (compensated or noncompensated). It is also safer to perform a planned elective intubation, however, rather than undertake intubation as an emergency procedure.

Once the patient is intubated, several modes of mechanical ventilation are available. The ventilator should provide adequate ventilatory assistance for the patient and allow the respiratory muscles to rest. The ventilator mode should also provide a minimum safe or a back-up minute ventilation. The assist-control and synchronized intermittent ventilation modes are the most frequently used in this situation. Pressure-set modes (pressure support and pressure control) should be used only with great caution, since the V_T delivered with each mechanical breath depends on the resistance and compliance of the respiratory system. The ventilator mode, V_T (8–12 mL/kg), respiratory rate, and FIO_2 have to be selected. Different modes offer different advantages, discussed more fully in the textbook. Arterial blood gas analysis and pulse oximetry are used to guide further changes in ventilator settings.

Oxygenation

The fundamental principle of the management of respiratory failure is to provide adequate O_2 to all tissues. O_2 delivery depends on more than adequate arterial O_2 saturation and includes adequate hemoglobin concentration and cardiac output.

Supplemental O_2 should be provided to achieve a target PaO_2 between about 60 and 70 mm Hg. This range is chosen based on the shape of the O_2-hemoglobin dissociation curve. Below 60 mm Hg, relatively small decreases in PaO_2 result in a significant fall in arterial O_2 saturation, and increases in PaO_2 above this level have a lesser impact on arterial O_2 saturation.

Initial levels of supplemental O_2 should be based on the underlying mechanism of hypoxemia. V/Q mismatches can be treated with lower inspired O_2 concentrations as compared with conditions with significant intrapulmonary shunts, which require higher levels to correct arterial hypoxemia. Patients with preexisting COPD and hypercapnia should have controlled administration of O_2 to prevent excessive worsening of hypercapnia. The primary emphasis is always to provide adequate oxygenation, and the fear of potentiating hypercapnia is of secondary importance. Other potential causes of hypercapnia must always be considered, particularly sedative agents. Mechanical ventilation should be considered if adequate oxygenation cannot be achieved without a marked worsening of hypercapnia and respiratory acidosis.

Patients who have significant intrapulmonary shunting (e.g., pneumonia, pulmonary edema, ARDS) should initially receive the highest possible concentration of oxygen through a high-flow aerosol mask or a nonrebreather mask. Patients with refractory hypoxemia should be mechanically ventilated to allow delivery of a higher concentration of O_2, to permit application of PEEP to recruit atelectatic alveoli, and to reduce O_2 consumption by resting the respiratory muscles. Although PEEP may improve PaO_2, it can worsen O_2 delivery if cardiac output is reduced by a decrease in venous return. Thus, monitoring of O_2 delivery is recommended at high levels of PEEP.

PRINCIPLES OF RESPIRATORY CARE

Oxygen Therapy

High-Flow Systems

High-flow systems can provide a precise and consistent FIO_2 independent of alterations in patient ventilatory pattern. These systems must provide a flow of gas exceeding patient demand (system flow greater than peak inspiratory flow rate or four times the patient's VE). In adults, a high-flow system must be capable of delivering at least 40 L/min of conditioned gas.

Low-Flow Systems

Most common O_2 delivery systems are classified as low flow, including the nasal cannula, simple mask, and mask with a reservoir. With these devices, the FIO_2 depends on several

Table 5–5. ESTIMATED FIO_2 WITH LOW-FLOW SYSTEMS*

System	Flow (L/Min)	FIO_2
Nasal cannula	1	0.24
	2	0.28
	3	0.32
	4	0.36
	5	0.40
	6	0.44
Mask		
Simple	≥5	0.40–0.60
Partial rebreathing	≥8	≥0.60
Nonbreathing	≥10	≥0.80

*Values are estimated based on a tidal volume of 500 mL, respiratory rate of 20 breaths/min; inspiratory time of 1 second, and an anatomic reservoir of 50 mL.

factors and does not remain constant. Approximate FIO_2 ranges for these various systems are listed in Table 5–5.

Humidification of Inhaled Gas

Spontaneous Breathing

With low-flow O_2 therapy delivered through a mask, a simple bubble-through humidifier is always used. During nasal cannula therapy, a humidifier is needed only when gas flow exceeds 4 L/min.

Artificial Airways

All patients with artificial airways require the addition of water to the gases they inspire because the gas-conditioning portion of the respiratory tract is largely bypassed.

Mechanical Ventilation

During mechanical ventilation, gas is inspired exclusively from the ventilator circuit and must be fully conditioned before entering the patient's airway. Gas conditioning is usually performed using heated humidifiers or artificial noses.

Heated Humidifiers

High-flow heated humidifiers can provide relative humidity of 100% at body temperature. The temperature in the humidifier reservoir is typically greater than that of the gas delivered to the patient. Cooling of the gas between the humidifier and the patient causes condensation ("rain out"). Water that collects in the tubing can serve as a source of nosocomial infection or can produce accidental lavage of the patient's airway. Water that condenses in the tubing should be collected in a water trap. This water should be considered contaminated and should not be drained into the humidifier reservoir. Cascade-type (bubble-through) humidifiers can also markedly increase the effort required to trigger the ventilator.

Artificial Noses

The artificial nose passively humidifies inspired gas and is ideally suited for transport and during anesthesia. If these devices are used for prolonged periods, the patient should be assessed for signs of inadequate humidification. The artificial nose may also increase inspiratory resistance to gas flow and may not be tolerated in patients with a poor ventilatory drive or marginal respiratory reserve.

Aerosolized Pharmacologic Agents

Small-Volume Nebulizers

The efficacy of drug delivery with small-volume nebulizer is influenced by the following:

Solution Volume: Large volume of solution (4 mL) maximizes delivery.
Nebulizer flow rate: Six to 8 L/min is optimal.
Intermittent versus continuous nebulization: Intermittent activation increases the quantity of drug actually delivered to the respiratory tract but requires patient coordination and prolongs treatment time, which may adversely affect compliance.

In spontaneously breathing patients, the aerosol should be inhaled through the mouth rather than the nose to minimize deposition of the drug in the nose and nasopharynx. A slow inspiratory flow rate (0.5 L/min) at normal V_T with an occasional inspiration to total lung capacity and inspiratory hold, is recommended. These techniques are summarized on Table 5–6.

Metered-Dose Inhalers

A summary of the techniques that should be employed for metered dose inhaler use is summarized on Table 5–7. In the intensive care unit, the use of a spacer is recommended for nonintubated patients unless the patient has prior experience with a metered-dose inhaler. In the intensive care unit, it is particularly difficult to teach proper metered-dose inhaler technique and to ensure that this technique is always used. Table 5–8 summarizes the advantages and disadvantages between small-volume nebulizers and metered-dose inhalers in spontaneously breathing patients.

Delivering Aerosolized Drugs During Mechanical Ventilation

Factors that affect delivery during mechanical ventilation differ greatly from those that affect delivery during spontaneous breathing.

Table 5–6. TECHNIQUE FOR USE OF A SMALL-VOLUME NEBULIZER (SVN) DURING SPONTANEOUS BREATHING

1. Place drug in nebulizer.
2. Dilute with physiologic saline (0.9%) to 4 mL total volume.
3. Incorporate a finger port into the driving gas system to provide intermittent nebulization during inspiration only.
4. Set driving gas flow at 6–8 L/min.
5. Connect patient to SVN by a mouthpiece or mask (in some patients, a nose clip may be necessary).
6. Instruct patient to inspire through open mouth if using a mask or to close lips around mouthpiece.
7. Have patient inhale slowly (0.5 L/s) at normal tidal volume.
8. Have patient occasionally inspire to total lung capacity and incorporate a 4 to 10-s breath hold.
9. Tap sides of nebulizer to minimize dead volume.
10. Continue treatment until no aerosol is produced.
11. Monitor patient for presence of side effects (e.g., tachycardia or tremor) and beneficial effects (e.g., improved breath sounds, peak flow, and FEV_1).

(Modified with permission from Kacmarek RM, Hess D: The interface between patient and aerosol generator. Respir Care 1991; 36:952–976.)

Small-Volume Nebulizers

During mechanical ventilation administration, only 2.9% to 4.8% of the aerosolized drug reaches the lower respiratory tract. Factors affecting this decreased delivery include the following:

Endotracheal tube size: The amount of drug reaching the lower respiratory tract is directly related to the diameter of the tube (e.g., less drug reaches the lower airways with smaller size endotracheal tube).

Table 5–7. TECHNIQUE FOR USE OF METERED-DOSE INHALER (MDI) WITH SPACER DURING SPONTANEOUS BREATHING

1. Warm MDI to body temperature.
2. Shake canister vigorously.
3. Hold canister upright.
4. Actuate MDI.
5. Place mouthpiece in patient's mouth.
6. Close patient's lips about mouthpiece.
7. Instruct patient to inspire slowly ($\leq$0.5 L/s) from spacer.
8. Instruct patient to continue to inspire to total lung capacity.
9. Have patient hold breath 4–10 seconds.
10. Have patient repeat inspiration with breath hold if indicated by spacer manufacturer.
11. Wait 3–10 min between subsequent actuations.
12. Monitor patient for presence of side effects (e.g., tachycardia or tremor) and beneficial effects (e.g., improved breath sounds, peak flow, and FEV_1).

(Modified with permission from Kacmarek RM, Hess D: The interface between patient and aerosol generator. Respir Care 1991; 36:952–976.)

Table 5–8. ADVANTAGES AND DISADVANTAGES OF THE USE OF SMALL-VOLUME NEBULIZERS (SVNs) AND METERED-DOSE INHALERS (MDIs)

Advantages	Disadvantages
SVN	
Less patient coordination required	Expensive
High doses possible (even continuous)	Wasteful
No chlorofluorocarbon release	Not all medications available
	Pressurized gas source required
	More time required
MDI	
Convenient	Patient coordination required
Inexpensive	Patient activation required
	Results in pharyngeal deposition
	Has potential for abuse
	Difficult to deliver high doses
	Not all medications available
	Dependent on ozone-depleting chlorofluorocarbons
MDI With Auxillary Device	
Less patient coordination required	More complex process for patients who can use MDI alone
	More expensive than MDI alone
	Less portable than MDI alone

(Modified with permission from Kacmarek RM, Hess D: The interface between patient and aerosol generator. Respir Care 1991; 36:952–976.)

Continuous versus intermittent nebulization: Intermittent inhalation is preferred over continuous nebulization.

Location of nebulizer placement in the ventilator circuit: This is the single most important factor affecting the volume of drug deposited beyond the endotracheal tube. Ideally, the small-volume nebulizer should be placed at least 18 inches from the endotracheal tube.

Table 5–9 summarizes the guidelines for using small-volume nebulizers in ventilator circuits.

METERED-DOSE INHALERS

During O_2 delivery by metered-dose inhalers in mechanically ventilated patients, only 4% to 6% of the actuated aerosol (about 50% less than during spontaneous breathing) reaches the patient's respiratory system. Studies have also shown that more aerosol exits the endotracheal tube if actuation occurs just after the start of a mechanical tidal volume delivery than if actuation begins before the onset of the mechanical breath. Table 5–10 summarizes the guidelines for drug administration by metered-dose inhalers during mechanical ventilation.

On the basis of data on lung deposition, standard drug doses should be doubled to deliver a dose equivalent to that

Table 5–9. TECHNIQUE FOR USE OF A SMALL-VOLUME NEBULIZER DURING MECHANICAL VENTILATION

1. Place drug in nebulizer.
2. Dilute with physiologic saline (0.9%) to 4 mL total volume.
3. Insert nebulizer into inspiratory limb of ventilator circuit at least 18 inches from Y.
4. Use intermittent nebulizer flow from ventilator if available.
5. If continuous flow is used, set at 6–8 L/min.
6. Set ventilator rate at 4–8/min or higher if not contraindicated.
7. Lengthen inspiratory time if tolerated and not contraindicated.
8. Set tidal volume at 12 mL/kg or more unless contraindicated. If PSV rate drops, add back-up SIMV rate.
9. With children, adjust ventilator flow to ensure that total flow is unchanged during pressure-limited ventilation.
10. With children (and some adults), readjust tidal volume during continuous-flow nebulization to maintain constant tidal volume and peak airway pressure.
11. Tap sides of nebulizer to minimize dead volume.
12. Continue treatment until no aerosol is produced.
13. Remove equipment from ventilator circuit.
14. Return ventilator to pretreatment settings.
15. Monitor patient for presence of side effects (e.g., tachycardia or tremor) and beneficial effects (e.g., improved breath sounds, peak flow, and FEV_1).

(Modified with permission from Kacmarek RM, Hess D: The interface between patient and aerosol generator. Respir Car 1991; 36:952–976.)

Abbreviations: PSV = pressure support ventilation; SIMV = synchronized intermittent mandatory ventilation; FEV_1 = forced expiratory volume in 1 second.

during spontaneous breathing. More importantly, dosing should be tailored to patient response. Many patients require doses that are three or four times higher than standard doses.

Airway Suctioning

In general, suctioning should not be performed on a scheduled basis but only when physical examination reveals the presence of secretions in the airway.

Complications of Suctioning

Hypoxemia: This is the most likely complication and is best avoided by hyperoxygenating with 100% oxygen before the procedure.

Atelectasis: Ideally, the amount of time that the catheter is within the airway should be limited and suctioning should be used only during removal of the catheter.

Cardiac arrhythmia: Bradyarrhythmias are the most common arrhythmias and usually are due to hypoxemia or vagal stimulation.

Airway trauma: Appropriately sized catheters, appropriate vacuum setting (intermittent rather than continuous), and an overall gentle approach are helpful in avoiding trauma to the airway.

Table 5–10. TECHNIQUES FOR USE OF METERED-DOSE INHALER (MDI) DURING MECHANICAL VENTILATION

1. Place MDI adapter into circuit.
2. Adjust ventilator to deliver volume-limited breaths or use a manual ventilator.
3. Warm MDI to body temperature.
4. Shake MDI vigorously.
5. Place MDI in circuit.
6. Actuate MDI immediately after the beginning of a mechanical breath; if spacer is used, actuate 1–2 seconds before mechanical breath or near end-exhalation, depending on the rate.
7. Apply a 2–3 second inflation hold, if not contraindicated.
8. Wait 1 minute between actuations.
9. Return ventilator to pretreatment settings.
10. Monitor patient for presence of side effects (e.g., tachycardia or tremor) and beneficial effects (e.g., improved breath sounds, peak flow, and FEV_1).

(Modified with permission from Kacmarek RM, Hess D: The interface between patient and aerosol generator. Respir Care 1991; 36:952–976.)

Increased intracranial pressure: This usually occurs in patients who cough excessively or who become markedly agitated during the procedure.

Off- Versus On-Ventilator Techniques

Studies that have compared open- with closed-system suctioning suggest that oxygenation during suctioning was similar with the two systems. We continue to recommend a closed suctioning technique, however, when oxygenation is tenuous and when momentary disconnection of PEEP or mechanical ventilation is poorly tolerated.

CONVENTIONAL AIRWAY ACCESS

Airway Assessment

A rapid assessment of the airway should be performed when management decisions involve the maintenance of airway patency and gas exchange. This evaluation should include the following:

Underlying disease: This involves knowledge of patient disease that may alter airway anatomy (e.g., acromegaly, tumors, immobility).

Mallampati airway classification: This depends on the structures visible to the observer when the patient is sitting upright, with the head in a neutral position, the mouth maximally open, and the tongue protruded maximally.

- *Class I:* soft palate, fauces, uvula, anterior and posterior tonsillar pillars
- *Class II:* soft palate, fauces, uvula
- *Class III:* soft palate, base of uvula

Class IV: soft palate only

The ease or difficulty of laryngoscopy and subsequent intubation has been correlated with the Mallampati classification, with class I representing the easiest and class IV the most difficult for successful intubation.

Evaluation of atlanto-occipital extension: This is contraindicated with suspected or confirmed cervical spine injury.

Thyromental distance: This is measured as the number of fingerbreadths (or centimeters) between the thyroid cartilage and the point of the chin, determining the acuity of the laryngopharyngeal axis. The more acute the angle, the greater the difficulty in alignment of these axes.

Special Considerations

- In patients with obvious or potentially diffficult airways, equipment for alternative means of airway control and intubation should always be assembled.
- Obstetric patients are often difficult to ventilate by mask and to intubate because of physiologic changes of pregnancy, such as airway mucosal edema. Inability to intubate the trachea of these patients is a leading cause of maternal death. These patients also are at greater risk for gastric aspiration, since gastric emptying is delayed and intragastric pressure increases.
- Obesity and pregnancy decrease FRC, which leads to rapid development of hypoxia with apnea of even short duration.

Airway Control

Triple Airway Maneuver

Maintaining airway patency with the triple airway maneuver (head tilt, anterior displacement of the mandible, and jaw thrust) should be initiated immediately in an unconscious patient. The exception to this rule is in patients with suspected or documented cervical spine injury.

Oropharyngeal and Nasopharyngeal Airways

Oropharyngeal and nasopharyngeal airways are important adjuncts to airway control and are designed to hold the tongue away. In general, oropharyngeal airways should be not be used in patients with intact upper airway reflexes because they may provoke laryngospasm, vomiting, coughing, and bronchospasm. Nasal airways are softer and better tolerated by conscious patients. Contraindications for nasal airways are identical to those for nasal intubation. Insertion should be preceded by application of topical vasoconstrictors.

Bag-Mask-Valve Units

A clear mask allows early visualization of regurgitation. The bag-mask-valve units can deliver 100% O_2 and can be used with a mask, endotracheal tube, tracheostomy tube, esophageal obturator airway, and so forth.

Equipment

Once an indication has been met for endotracheal intubation, special equipment considerations include those listed in Table 5–11.

Awake Intubations

Awake intubation should be considered in unfasted (full-stomach) patients and in anticipated difficult airways. Various approaches of awake intubations can be used, including the following:

Orotracheal intubation: This should be used in patients who have an absolute or relative contraindication to nasal intubation. Oral tubes are usually larger than those used nasally and are advantageous in patients with excessive secretions.

- *Blind orotracheal intubation:* This is best reserved for experienced personnel. It may be helpful in victims of facial trauma and when anatomic landmarks are obscured.
- *Orotracheal intubation under direct laryngoscopy*
- *Orotracheal intubation with fiberoptic bronchoscopy:* The oral route is usually more difficult than the nasotracheal route and is chosen only when necessary to avoid the nasal route.

Nasotracheal intubation: The decision to place a nasotracheal

Table 5–11. EQUIPMENT FOR INTUBATION

Mandatory Equipment
Suction
Yankauer tip (large-bore tonsil tip)
Suction catheters (sized to permit passage through ETT)
Oxygen source
Bag-valve device
Masks (at least two sizes)
Oral and nasal airways
ETTs (include sizes smaller than anticipated)
Laryngoscope handle and blade (various sizes)
Syringe for cuff inflation
Stylet
Method for securing ETT (i.e., tape)
Monitors on electrocardiogram, pulse oximetry, blood pressure cuff or device (manual or automated)
Resuscitation drugs
Stethoscope
Highly Suggested Equipment
Tongue depressors
Local anesthetics (for topical application)
Topical vasoconstrictors
Lubricants
Intravenous access
End-tidal CO_2 monitoring

Abbreviations: ETT = endotracheal tube.

tube is based on traumatic or surgical deformities or personal bias. Blind nasotracheal intubation is performed through the larger naris. A tube 1 mm (internal diameter) smaller than that used for an orotracheal intubation is selected.

Retrograde intubation: This requires preparation and time and is not usually suitable for emergency airway access.

Confirmation of endotracheal tube placement

Clinical methods: Direct visualization of the endotracheal tube passing between the cords followed by inspection, palpation, and auscultation of the chest. Auscultation of bilateral breath sounds is mandatory. Auscultation over the epigastrium to confirm no air movement is also indicated.

Verification of exhaled carbon dioxide: This can be assessed with capnography, capnometry, or disposable calorimetric indicators that change color when exposed to CO_2.

Fiberoptic bronchoscopy

Lighted stylet

LARYNGOTRACHEAL INJURY FROM PROLONGED INTUBATION

Frequency and Types of Complications

Common and rare complications associated with prolonged intubation are listed in Table 5–12. The complication rate is related to the duration of intubation. Other predisposing factors include the presence of diabetes mellitus, atherosclerotic heart disease, and immunosuppression.

Tracheal Tube Problems

Complications resulting from tracheal tubes are due to factors such as size, tip design, rigidity, position, and shape. A tracheal tube injury is localized primarily to the posterior glottis. Although a smaller tube lessens the laryngeal wall pressure, the sealing cuff pressure required for effective

Table 5–12. COMPLICATIONS ASSOCIATED WITH PROLONGED INTUBATION

Common	*Rare*
Infection	Cricoarytenoid subluxation
Hemorrhage	Cricoarytenoid fixation and scarring
Aspiration	Vocal cord paralysis
Air leak	Tracheal necrosis
Subcutaneous emphysema	Tracheal rupture
Pneumomediastinum	Paratracheal abscess
Pneumothorax	Tracheoinnominate artery fistula
Atelectasis	Tracheoesophageal fistula
Laryngeal edema	
Laryngeal ulceration	
Laryngeal granuloma	
Laryngotracheostenosis	
Tracheomalacia	

ventilation may increase as the tube diameter decreases. This occurs because smaller tubes have a smaller cuff resting diameter and may fail to act as large-diameter, high-volume cuffs. Thus, the most effective regimen is to use an appropriately sized tube that obtains an effective seal at approximately 25 cm H_2O of intracuff pressure.

The issue of the oral versus the nasal route for tracheal intubation is widely debated. The most common complication of nasotracheal intubation is bleeding, which occurs in about 45% of patients. Iatrogenic sinusitis also occurs more frequently with nasal (43%) than with oral (2%) tubes. Nasal tubes appear to be more comfortable to patients, however, and they also show a lower incidence of laryngeal damage and so may be more suitable for long-term intubation.

Cuff Problems

Cuff problems have decreased in both frequency and severity with the almost exclusive use of large-diameter, large-volume cuffs. The cuff should be inflated to no more than 25 cm H_2O at the end of exhalation. Intracuff pressure should be monitored frequently to avoid tracheal mucosal injury. Cuff damage usually presents initially as tracheal dilatation. Another significant cuff-related complication is aspiration. Secretions pooled above the cuff may slowly leak into the trachea, causing subsequent infection. In intubated patients, mechanical ventilation is associated with less aspiration than is spontaneous breathing. The addition of PEEP further decreases aspiration.

Assessment of Injuries and Therapeutic Intervention

The radiographic appearance of an overdistended cuff often precedes tracheal dilation, subcutaneous emphysema, or pneumomediastinum. Computed tomography is capable of detecting a variety of conditions, including fracture or dislocation of laryngeal cartilages and subcutaneous emphysema.

The management of immediate postextubation tracheal stenosis includes both medical and surgical approaches. Medical therapy includes inhaled, intralesional, and systemic corticosteroids. Large granulomas can be removed by endoscopic laser surgery. More severe and extensive stenosis can require surgical resection.

Timing of Tracheostomy

The timing of tracheostomy for patients requiring prolonged mechanical ventilation remains one of the most controversial issues in intensive care medicine. Recommendations suggesting a specific duration of tracheal intubation with the least traumatizing tube followed by tracheostomy should be individualized according to patient diagnosis, condition, predicted clinical outcome, and laryngeal appearance at repeated examinations.

SURGICAL AIRWAY, CRICOTHYROIDOTOMY, AND TRACHEOTOMY: PROCEDURES, COMPLICATIONS, AND OUTCOME

A surgical airway is needed for emergency laryngotracheal intubation in only 3% of such emergencies. The most common indications for an emergent surgical airway are suspected cervical spine fracture, oromaxillofacial trauma, and laryngeal trauma. When an emergency surgical airway is required, cricothyroidotomy is the procedure of choice, except in patients with laryngeal trauma. The clinical presentation of severe laryngeal trauma includes stridor, dyspnea, subcutaneous emphysema, pneumomediastinum, and hemoptysis. Laryngeal injury is a relative contraindication to crycothyroidotomy. This situation remains the only indication for emergency tracheostomy. A summary of indications and contraindications for choice of surgical airway access is presented in Table 5–13.

Cricothyroidotomy

The indications for cricothyroidotomy vary, but the technique is useful in any condition in which conventional intubation is not immediately successful. This technique is suitable for both emergent and elective situations. With proper training, the procedure is easily and rapidly performed and is the emergency airway procedure of choice, especially for patients with life-threatening airway obstruction. The elective indications for cricothyroidotomy include the need for secretion clearance and prolonged mechanical ventilation. Because of the high risk of mediastinitis, cricothyroidotomy has been recommended instead of tracheostomy after recent cardiac surgery through a midline sternotomy.

Complications

Complications of emergent cricothyroidotomy include hemorrhage, tube occlusion from debris, tube misplacement, and late subglottic stenosis. Elective cricothyroidotomy usually has only minor sequelae, such as voice changes and subglottic stenosis. Risk factors for complications include cricothyroidotomy for longer than 30 days, preceding intubation for more than 7 days, diabetes mellitus, advanced age, and stomal infection causing subglottic granulation tissue.

Percutaneous Cricothyroidotomy

Percutaneous cricothyroidotomy can be performed with a variety of commercially available kits. This technique allows practitioners of all specialties to place a definitive airway in routine and emergency settings. Some kits provide dangerously traumatic equipment, however. Furthermore, there can

Table 5–13. ARTIFICIAL AIRWAY CATEGORIES

Intubation	Surgical Cricothyroidotomy	Percutaneous Catheter Cricothyroidotomy or Tracheotomy	Surgical Tracheotomy
Indications			
General anesthesia	Failed intubation	Failed intubation	Failed cricothyroidotomy
Respiratory arrest	Upper airway obstruction	Cervical fracture	Upper airway obstruction
Airway obstruction	Secretion retention	Partial airway obstruction	Long-term mechanical ventilation
Respiratory distress	Medium-term mechanical ventilation	Pharyngeal foreign body	Difficult weaning
Hemorrhage	Respiratory failure after recent sternotomy		Endotracheal tube laryngeal injury
Secretion retention	Cervical fracture		Speech capability
Pulmonary contusion	Facial trauma (severe)		Need for oral intake
Facial trauma (moderate)	Emergency airway		Psychosocial benefit
Penetrating neck trauma			Oromaxillofacial trauma
Cardiac instability			Pharyngeal or glottic edema
Cardiac arrest			Nasal, oral, or laryngeal hemorrhage
Coma			Neurologic deficit
Contraindications			
Anatomic difficulty	Laryngeal infection	Complete airway obstruction	Recent sternotomy
Coagulopathy (nasal)	Laryngeal trauma	Pediatric patients (relative)	Emergency airway
Facial fracture (nasal)	Intubation (>3 days)	Laryngeal trauma (relative)	
Cervical spine fracture (relative)	Pediatric patients (relative)		
	Coagulopathy		

be serious complications when placed by an inexperienced operator.

Surgical Tracheotomy

The indications for surgical tracheostomy are diverse. The only contraindication is the necessity for an emergency airway, because this procedure is time-consuming and requires significant expertise. The emergency indications for tracheostomy are few (high-grade upper airway obstruction, massive neck swelling, and laryngeal injury).

Complications

Most initial perioperative tracheostomy complications, including hemorrhage and subcutaneous emphysema, are minor. Major early complications include the loss of airway control, obstruction, excessive blood loss, mediastinal emphysema, and pneumothorax. The most often discussed complication is tracheal stenosis, which is usually due to excessive cuff pressure. Stenosis at the stoma may be due to excessive movement of the tracheostomy tube or removal of too much of the tracheal wall. The most common complication is infection, leading to tracheobronchitis or necrotizing tracheitis. Life-threatening hemorrhage can result from a trachea–inominate artery fistula or an extratracheal inominate artery erosion. Tracheoesophageal fistula occasionally occurs and is difficult to treat; it has an associated poor prognosis.

Percutaneous Transtracheal Catheterization

With this technique, a catheter-over-needle assembly is percutaneously inserted into the upper trachea. The most critical issue about the efficacy of the ventilation is the diameter of the catheter. The minimum catheter size should be 14 gauge. Exhalation must take place through the patient's natural airway. The flow delivery system is next in importance when determining ventilatory efficiency. The pressure gradient required to achieve adequate ventilation through a catheter of such small diameter is provided by a 50-psi source (not by manual bag-valve). The indications for emergency use include partial airway obstruction. Complete airway obstruction does not provide for adequate exhalation, however, and results in hyperinflation and potential barotrauma. Complications include catheter displacement, total expiratory obstruction, and barotrauma.

Percutaneous Dilatational Tracheostomy

Several percutaneous dilatational tracheostomy kits are commercially available. The procedure can be performed electively, urgently, or as an emergency procedure. The complication rate of hemorrhage is minimal. Occasional cases of life-threatening hemorrhage or pneumothorax have been reported, however.

LIFE-THREATENING ASTHMA

Pathophysiology of Asthma

Asthma is an inflammatory syndrome precipitated by numerous stimuli, which often go unidentified. Airway inflammation is present even in patients with mild asthma; the degree of inflammation parallels the clinical severity of asthma.

Inflammation in asthma has three airway components—alterations in constitutive cells, infiltration by inflammatory cells, and thickening of the basement membrane. The surface secretory cells and mucous glands become hyperplastic and experience hypertrophy, and airway smooth muscle layer thickens. Mast cells increase in numbers, along with a proinflammatory phenotype of T lymphocytes (TH_2). These cells release cytokines, leading to several effects, including the promotion of the synthesis of immunoglobulin E, enhancement of mast cell differentiation, and the differentiation and recruitment of eosinophils into the airway. The airway wall becomes thickened as a result of both the increased cellular components and alterations in the collagen component of the basement membrane.

Activated mast cells and eosinophils then elaborate inflammatory mediators—histamine, leukotrienes, platelet-activating factor, prostaglandins, thromboxane-A_2, and various proteases. These primary effector molecules stimulate airway smooth muscle, increase microvascular permeability, and cause release of mucin. They are also potent chemoattractants for eosinophils and can stimulate sensory nerve fibers within the airway. Nerve stimulation leads to the elaboration of secondary effector molecules (substance P and neurokinin A) and of secondary inhibitor molecules (vasoactive intestinal peptide and nitric oxide). Degranulation of eosinophils can release toxic substances that cause further injury.

Clinical Presentation

History

PRECIPITANTS. The most common stimulus of life-threatening asthma is an upper respiratory tract infection, commonly viral in origin. Other infectious causes include *Chlamydia pneumoniae* and tracheobronchitis due to herpes simplex. Various allergens or certain drugs can also precipitate an asthma attack. Environmental and occupational factors, along with exercise and emotional stress, can be responsible for an asthma attack.

DURATION. Several days to weeks of deteriorating symptoms may occur and be associated with increased usage of β-agonist therapy. A small subgroup of patients may have sudden asphyxic asthma with an abrupt onset, resulting in respiratory failure in minutes to hours.

SYMPTOMS. These consist of a triad of dyspnea, cough, and wheezing. There may be increased nocturnal awakenings, as well as more profound wheezing on less exertion.

Physical Examination

During an acute exacerbation, the patient is in respiratory distress and prefers to sit upright. The inability to talk is a sign of severe asthma. Patients become tachypneic and tachycardic and use their accessory muscles of breathing (sternocleidomastoid, intercostal, and abdominal muscles). With more severe attacks, retractions of these muscle groups and abdominal paradox may signal incipient respiratory failure. The degree of pulsus paradoxus correlates with the severity of the attack, which, because of increased intrathoracic pressure, also causes cardiac tamponade with reduced venous return and cardiac output. The chest is hyperinflated, and diffuse expiratory and inspiratory wheezes are heard on auscultation. With increasing airflow obstruction, the chest may become silent.

Laboratory Findings

BLOOD TESTS. Peripheral eosinophilia is common. Hypokalemia and hypophosphatemia may occur from β-agonist usage. Hyponatremia has also been reported from inappropriate antidiuretic hormone release.

PULMONARY FUNCTION TESTS. Peak expiratory flows are depressed, and marked diurnal variation may have been present. Spirometry is abnormal with a low FEV_1 and an obstructive picture with a low FEV_1/FVC ratio.

ARTERIAL BLOOD GASES. Mild hypoxemia (PaO_2 65–85 mm Hg) is common, resulting from $\dot{V}/Q$ mismatching caused by mucus plugging and bronchospasm. Beta-agonists may aggravate the hypoxemia by reversing hypoxic vasoconstriction and worsening V/Q mismatching. Most patients experience mild hypocapnia from the tachypnea. The presence of eucapnia or, especially, hypercapnia portends the onset of respiratory failure and the need for mechanical ventilation. In these patients, close observation in an intensive care unit is mandatory.

SPUTUM EXAMINATION. The sputum may be thick and contain tenacious plugs. Gram staining is useful to exclude a concomitant bacterial infection. *Aspergillus* species may occasionally be seen with allergic bronchopulmonary aspergillosis. The mucus may take the form of casts of the distal airways (Curschmann spirals) and often shows eosinophils and Charcot-Leyden crystals when examined.

CHEST RADIOGRAPHS. The lungs are commonly hyperinflated. Pneumothorax, atelectasis, pneumonia, and congestive heart failure should be excluded.

ELECTROCARDIOGRAM. Sinus tachycardia is the most common electrocardiographic finding. In older patients, myocardial ischemia should be excluded.

Management

General Principles

Bronchodilators are needed to reverse the bronchoconstriction, and anti-inflammatory agents (corticosteroids) are given to control the underlying inflammatory process. The rest of management is supportive, and close monitoring is required, because the situation can be highly labile.

Primary Therapies

BETA-ADRENERGIC AGONISTS. Nebulized or metered-dose inhalers can be used to deliver β-adrenergic agonists, with nebulizers employed more commonly for patients with severe asthma. The most commonly used β-agonist for adults is albuterol, 0.5 mL diluted in 2.5 mL normal saline, given at intervals of 20 to 30 minutes, or continuously for patients in extremis, until the condition begins to improve. It is useful to watch patients as they are receiving the nebulizer to evaluate whether the aerosol is actually being inspired or whether the airflow obstruction is so severe that all the aerosol is wasted around the patient's face. If this is the case, one can consider other routes of delivery, like subcutaneous injections of epinephrine or terbutaline or even intravenous β-agonists. These agents have significant cardiac side effects, and patients require close monitoring. Metered-dose inhalers with a spacer device can be used if the patient can cooperate.

CORTICOSTEROIDS. These are given as soon as possible to treat the underlying inflammatory process. They should be given intravenously in severely asthma patients to ensure reliable delivery. Both hydrocortisone and methylprednisolone are efficacious. Methylprednisolone has the theoretic advantage of fewer mineralocorticoid side effects. The dose is still a matter of debate. A regimen consisting of methylprednisolone, 80 to 125 mg intravenously every 8 hours, or hydrocortisone, 6 mg/kg/d, is acceptable. The effects of steroids for asthma may not be immediate, and a delay of 6 hours or longer is common. Thus, vigorous bronchodilator therapy is needed in the interim. Once patients are stable with improving peak expiratory flows, consideration can be made to switch them over to oral prednisone therapy, 0.5 to 1 mg/kg/d). Inhaled steroids of high topical potency can be additional therapy.

OXYGEN THERAPY. O_2 is administered to keep arterial O_2 saturation above 90%. Patients with hypercapnia should be considered for mechanical ventilator support.

Adjunctive Therapies

METHYLXANTHINES. These are at best modest bronchodilators. Methylxanthines can also have other salutary effects, however, including inhibition of spasmogenic mediator release, improved diaphragmatic contractility, increased mucociliary transport and clearance of mucus plugs, and decreased pulmonary arterial pressures. The therapeutic range for theophylline is 10 to 20 μg/mL. Toxicity may be a problem, with gastrointestinal, central nervous system, and cardiac side effects. If a patient has not previously taken theophylline, a loading dose of 5 to 6 mg/kg/h can be given as a slow bolus, followed by a continuous infusion of 0.5 to 0.9 mg/kg/h. Patients already receiving theophylline should not be given the loading dose, and levels should be measured. Theophylline is metabolized in the liver. In nonsmoking elderly patients and patients with liver disease or heart failure, the infusion dose should be reduced to 0.1 to 0.5 mg/kg/h. Factors known to increase theophylline clearance include use of tobacco or marijuana, and treatment with rifampin, barbiturates, phenytoin, cimetidine, fluoroquinolone antibiotics, erythromycin, propranolol, or antiepileptic agents. Disease states that decrease theophylline clearance include liver disease and heart failure. The elderly also have decreased clearance.

ANTICHOLINERGIC AGENTS. Inhaled atropine can produce bronchodilation and may be useful to reduce mucus hypersecretion or an overtly neurogenic component of their bronchoconstriction, but it is limited by systemic side effects. Inhaled ipratropium bromide is an alternative. These agents contribute little to the benefits of aggressive β-agonist therapy, however.

MAGNESIUM SULFATE. Intravenous magnesium may have a benefit to β-agonists, but a randomized trial has suggested minimal if any benefits.

OTHER TREATMENT. Inhalational anesthetics such as halothane and intravenous thiopental have been reported to have efficacy in severely asthmatic patients, but their role has yet to be fully defined. Ketamine may be an alternative anesthetic agent. Routine antibiotics are not recommended unless the patient has evidence of bacterial pneumonia. Mucolytic agents such as N-acetylcysteine can cause bronchoconstriction and should not be used. Adequate hydration and humidification of inspired air are important. Bronchoscopic lavage to remove mucous plugs carries a significant risk of worsening bronchospasm, airway obstruction, and barotrauma. Other agents with bronchodilator effects have been investigated in the laboratory but have yet to be used in clinical practice.

RESPIRATORY FAILURE: INTUBATION AND MECHANICAL VENTILATION

Epidemiology

Even though less than 5% of patients with acute asthma require intubation and mechanical ventilation, this group has the greatest risk of morbidity and mortality.

General Principles of Management

Intubation ideally should be performed electively instead of emergently. A transoral route is preferred, and the largest endotracheal tube tolerated should be used to reduce expiratory resistance.

Mechanical ventilation is supportive and undertaken to allow the primary therapies to work. It is important to avoid the adverse effects of mechanical ventilation. One is barotrauma, and the second is auto-PEEP. The high airway resistance leads to high peak airway pressures if conventional V_Ts are delivered (although peak airway pressures poorly reflect alveolar pressure when high airflow resistance is present). This may lead to barotrauma and the possibility of death due to tension pneumothorax. Lower V_Ts (7 to 10 mL/kg) are now favored, with the policy of permissive hypercapnia. The prolonged expiratory phase in asthma leads to auto-PEEP. This has several adverse effects, especially if they go unrecognized, including depression of cardiac output from decreased venous return (even to the extent of cardiac arrest), increased dead space ventilation, and the possibility of barotrauma from lung overdistention. If a patient suddenly becomes hypotensive after intubation, it may be a result of auto-PEEP. A bolus of fluid should be given, and one can temporarily discontinue positive-pressure ventilation and observe for an improvement in arterial blood pressure. Initial ventilator settings of 7 to 10 mL/kg for V_T, frequencies of 10 to 15 breaths per minute, and peak inspiratory flow rates of 80 to 100 L/min can be used. Applied PEEP should not be used, although it can be beneficial if expiratory flow is limited.

Sedation is often required to minimize the patient's discomfort and anxiety. Furthermore, muscle paralysis is often used to reduce patient–ventilator dyssynchrony. Concerns have been expressed, however, about neuromuscular blocker overdosage with potential for prolonged paralysis and a drug-induced myopathy, especially when given in combination with high-dose corticosteroids. If neuromuscular blockers are used, it is incumbent to employ a peripheral nerve stimulator for train-of-four monitoring. Dosing of neuromuscular blockers should be titrated to maintain two of four twitches.

Monitoring

The mechanics of the respiratory system can be measured if the patient is not breathing spontaneously. Airway resistance and dynamic compliance are useful measures to follow for the resolution of severe asthma. It is common to have an indwelling radial arterial line for the monitoring of blood pressure and arterial blood gas analyses. Pulse oximetry is a useful for titrating supplemental O_2 and maintaining an arterial saturation above 92%. Serum electrolytes, especially phosphorus, and potassium levels should be monitored closely. Theophylline levels should be closely monitored. Chest radiographs are required to check the positioning of the endotracheal tube and to monitor for barotrauma, atelectasis due to mucus plugging, and pneumonia.

Course and Prognosis

Most patients improve within 24 to 48 hours after intubation. Once respiratory mechanics have improved on intermittent bronchodilator therapy and secretions are minimal, patients can be weaned with a view to extubation when sedation and neuromuscular blockade have been reversed. Mortality rates of 0% to 22% have been reported. It is important to provide close outpatient follow-up, since these patients are at high risk for death due to asthma.

PULMONARY ASPIRATION OF STOMACH CONTENTS

Acid is the main cause of severe pulmonary injury after aspiration of stomach contents. After aspiration, acid rapidly spreads throughout the lungs and produces diffuse damage. In general, the more acidic the aspirated fluid and the greater its volume, the greater the lung damage caused. The chemical burn induced by the acid aspiration appears to be the most severe problem. It causes a loss of alveolocapillary integrity and an exudation of fluid and protein into the interstitial spaces, the alveoli, and the bronchi. The most immediate and severe physiologic problem is the hypoxemia that occurs within minutes of acid aspiration. The mechanism for this hypoxemia include reflex airway closure, destruction or alteration of the normal surfactant activity, and migration of fluid and protein into the damaged tissue leading to pulmonary edema.

The aspiration of acid may also affect the pulmonary vasculature and cause pulmonary hypertension. Increases in pulmonary vascular resistance may be due to hypoxemia, hypercarbia, and loss of lung volume. Acute increases may precipitate right ventricular failure.

Large particulate aspirates obstruct major airways. Small, nonobstructing food particles can produce prolonged inflammatory response similar to that caused by acid.

Therapy

Prophylaxis

The risk of aspiration in an unconscious patient can be reduced by careful observation and by positioning the patients in a semiprone position with the head down. Several drugs are useful in altering residual gastric volume and pH. Histamine$_2$ receptor antagonists reduce gastric volume and increase pH. Metoclopramide facilitates gastric emptying and has a central antiemetic effect. Proton pump inhibitors prevent secretion of hydrogen ion into the stomach, lessen gastric acidity, and raise the pH. Particulate antacids reduce gastric acidity but can lead to persistent pulmonary lesions if aspirated. A nonparticulate oral antacid can effectively buffer the stomach acid without risking severe pulmonary insufficiency if the solution is aspirated.

Endotracheal Suctioning

If aspiration has occurred, the trachea should be suctioned, if possible. Liquid and small particulate aspirates disperse rapidly, however, and damage the lungs almost instantaneously. Suctioning can remove only a portion of the aspirate and is only the first step in therapy.

Mechanical Ventilatory Support

Positive pressure ventilation with PEEP or the administration of continuous positive airway pressure (CPAP) reduces the blood gas abnormalities and increases the rate of survival after acid aspiration. If the patient is alert and further aspiration is not a risk, CPAP by mask may reinflate alveoli, increase FRC, and decrease intrapulmonary shunt. If the patient is obtunded, cannot maintain a patent airway, or is at risk for further aspiration, intubation of the trachea with a cuffed endotracheal tube and mechanical ventilation are indicated. Optimal PEEP or CPAP minimizes the intrapulmonary venous admixture without compromising the circulation. A patient with severe ARDS due to gastric aspiration may require extracorporeal circulation with CO_2 removal through a venovenous bypass system.

Bronchoscopy and Lavage

Bronchoscopy should be performed if a patient is suspected of having aspirated large particulate matter, particularly if clinical and radiographic signs of lung volume loss are present. Bronchoscopy is potentially hazardous in patients with severe respiratory distress, however, and should be undertaken with extreme care. Only small amounts of saline should be used to clear the airway of secretions or aspirated material. Pulmonary lavage with neutral or alkaline solutions to neutralize the acid is not useful and actually further compromises pulmonary function.

Corticosteroids

No conclusive clinical or experimental data document that corticosteroids are useful for patients with aspiration pneumonitis. In fact, corticosteroid administration may interfere with normal healing, and we do not recommend corticosteroid use.

Antibiotics

Infection in patients who have aspirated frequently is difficult to document. Antibiotics should be withheld until clinical evidence of infection can be produced. Treatment can then be based on analysis of well-controlled smear and culture preparations.

Fluids

Proper use of fluids is clinically important in patients with severe aspiration. Intravascular volume lost through pulmonary edema must be restored. Patients must be monitored carefully, and a pulmonary artery catheter or transesophageal echocardiography or both are frequently indicated.

Summary

The simplest and most efficient therapy for aspiration of stomach contents is prevention. If aspiration does occur, the following steps are recommended:

1. Suction the trachea.
2. Analyze arterial blood for gas tensions and pH.
3. Apply aggressive mechanical ventilatory support.
4. Ensure adequate fluid replacement.
5. Perform bronchoscopy if large particulate aspirates obstruct airways.

We do not recommend corticosteroids, prophylatic antibiotics, or pulmonary lavage with a large volume of neutral or alkaline solutions.

FIBEROPTIC BRONCHOSCOPY IN CRITICAL CARE MEDICINE

Technique

Intubation is recommended in most critically ill patients undergoing fiberoptic bronchoscopy, since the procedure may worsen oxygenation and ventilation. An 8-mm or larger endotracheal tube should be used to ensure that ventilation is not compromised during bronchoscopy. Intubation can be accomplished over the fiberoptic bronchoscope at the time of the procedure through either an orotracheal or nasotracheal route. Swivel adapters allow insertion of the fiberoptic bronchoscope into the endotracheal or tracheostomy tube and maintain an adequate seal during mechanical ventilation. Clear gel or silicone spray can be used to facilitate the passage of the bronchoscope through the artificial airway. Premedication usually includes parenteral analgesics, intramuscular atropine (to decrease secretions and avoid vasovagal reflexes), anxiolytics, and topical lidocaine. Monitoring during the procedure should consist of continuous pulse oximetry to detect any significant hypoxemia, electrocardiogram to monitor cardiac rhythm, and intermittent or continuous arterial blood pressure measurements. During fiberoptic bronchoscopy, the inspired O_2 concentration should be increased to higher levels to avoid potential hypoxemia.

Use With Endotracheal and Tracheostomy Tubes

Intubation

The flexible fiberoptic bronchoscope can be used to overcome intubation difficulties in many patients. Intubation with the flexible fiberoptic bronchoscope is contraindicated in patients who are apneic or who have extreme ventilatory difficulty. In these circumstances, laryngoscopic intubation is more appropriate. The fiberoptic bronchoscope can also be used to change endotracheal tubes in critically ill patients. Once the endotracheal tube is in the trachea, the fiberoptic bronchoscope can be used to position the tube in its desired location above the carina.

Diagnostic Applications

Fiberoptic bronchoscopy is an excellent tool for airway inspection before extubation or to document complications of prolonged or difficult intubations such as muscosal damage, hematoma, or tracheomalacia. It can also be used to document aspiration around the endotracheal tube cuff.

Atelectasis

The value of fiberoptic bronchoscopy over vigorous conventional pulmonary toilet for acute lobar collapse is controversial. Suction through the bronchoscope is performed in attempts to extract the mucus. Saline or 10% N-acetylcysteine may be required to extract tenacious mucus. When air bronchograms are seen on the chest roentgenogram, neither aggressive respiratory therapy nor fiberoptic bronchoscopy is successful in reversing the volume loss. Fiberoptic bronchoscopy is most effective if there is central mucus plugging. A practical approach to a patient with acute lobar collapse follows:

1. Air bronchograms should make one reluctant to approach volume loss with fiberoptic bronchoscopy.
2. The initial treatment for lobar atelectasis in most cases should be intensive respiratory therapy.
3. If respiratory therapy fails to clear atelectases, fiberoptic bronchoscopy is a reasonable next step.

When fiberoptic bronchoscopy is done for therapy of atelectases, the bronchoscope with the largest suction channel is preferred. The inability to perform intensive respiratory therapy may be encountered in patients with multiple rib fractures, cervical spine injuries, multiple plaster casts, or traction devices.

Upper Airway Obstruction

Causes of upper airway obstruction in adults include epiglottitis, bilateral vocal cord paralysis, laryngeal edema, and foreign body aspiration. Fiberoptic bronchoscopy should be diagnostic in all of these conditions, and fiberoptic bronchoscopy intubation should be therapeutic in all except foreign body aspiration, in which condition rigid bronchoscopy or tracheostomy may be more appropriate.

Acute Inhalation Injury

Both upper and lower airway injuries can be diagnosed with fiberoptic bronchoscopy. Regardless of the symptoms at the time of evaluation, if any of the risk factors depicted in Table 5–14 are present, fiberoptic bronchoscopy should be performed to rule out upper airway damage. If fiberoptic bronchoscopy reveals evidence of significant glottic or tracheal edema or mucosal damage, intubation should be prophylactically performed over the fiberoptic bronchoscope.

Diagnosis of Bacterial Pneumonia with Fiberoptic Bronchoscopy

Sputum cultures and routine bronchial washings from the suction channel are unreliable for a specific diagnosis of

Table 5–14. CONSIDERATIONS FOR FIBEROPTIC BRONCHOSCOPY IN ACUTE INHALATION INJURY

Singed nasal hairs
Facial burns about nose or mouth
Oral or nasopharyngeal burns
Carbonaceous sputum
Physical examination or review of systems results suggestive of upper airway obstruction (wheezing, sore throat, hoarseness)
Steam inhalation

bacterial pneumonia because of their poor specificity. Two techniques that use quantitative cultures of lower airway tract secretion obtained by fiberoptic bronchoscopy are the protected brush catheter and bronchoalveolar lavage. These sampling techniques are more reliable for identifying a specific causative organism for bacterial pneumonia and for differentiating between infectious and noninfectious infiltrates. With a protected brush catheter, concentrations of 10^3 colonies/μL or higher is more likely to identify the causative agent, whereas those growing in colonies with counts lower than this are more likely to be contaminants. With bronchoalveolar lavage, a count of 10^4 to 10^5 colonies/mL is used to differentiate between contaminants and causative agents. Sensitivity of these diagnostic techniques is decreased by the prior administration of antibiotics and by the presence of diffuse infiltrates (sampling error).

Pulmonary Infection in the Immunocompromised Host

The value of fiberoptic bronchoscopy in the diagnosis of opportunistic pulmonary infection is of major importance in critically ill patients, including transplant patients receiving immunosuppressive drugs; patients receiving long-term, high-dose steroid therapy; patients undergoing chemotherapy for malignancies; and patients with acquired immunodeficiency syndrome. Although many different bronchoscopic sampling techniques can be performed, bronchoalveolar lavage has become the standard because of its sensitivity and risk-benefit ratio. It is particularly helpful in identifying organisms that do not colonize the tracheobronchial tree in the absence of infection, including *Pneumocystis, Histoplasma, Blastomyces, Mycobacterium tuberculosis, Coccidiodes, Nocardia,* and *Mucor* species. Transbronchial biopsy is of value if it shows tissue invasion of such organisms as *Aspergillus,* atypical *Mycobacterium, Candida,* and *Cryptococcus* species.

Hemoptysis

Fiberoptic bronchoscopy is indicated in the diagnosis of nonmassive hemoptysis (less than 200–600 mL in 24 hours). In massive hemoptysis, however, its use is controversial. Traditionally, the rigid bronchoscope is preferred in this circumstance. The therapeutic approach of patients with life-threatening hemoptysis is described separately.

Complications

Hypoxemia

Arterial desaturation may occur during fiberoptic bronchoscopy because of the removal of oxygen-rich tracheal gas by suction or irrigation or administration of anesthetic solutions. Patients should be monitored with pulse oximetry, the FIO_2 should be increased, and suctioning should be minimized during the procedure. A chest radiograph should be obtained after the procedure to rule out pneumothorax.

Arrhythmias

Hypoxemia with PaO_2 below 60 mm Hg correlates with cardiac arrhythmias. Hemodynamic changes such as increased mean arterial pressure, heart rate, and cardiac index have been observed and are attributed to reflex sympathetic discharge caused by mechanical irritation of the airways.

Complications Secondary to Fiberoptic Bronchoscopy, Transbronchial Brushing, and Biopsy

Minimal data have been published about transbronchial biopsy in ventilator-dependent patients. Data suggest that indicated transbronchial biopsy may be performed on mechanically ventilated patients, although the use of PEEP is a relative contraindication. Although no studies have addressed hemorrhagic complications in critically ill patients undergoing transbronchial biopsy, previous work shows an extremely low rate of life-threatening hemoptysis.

Fever and Pneumonia

Fever higher than 101°F (38.3°C) and parenchymal infiltrates have been reported within 72 hours after fiberoptic bronchoscopy. Data do not support pneumonia as the cause of these infiltrates.

Topical Anesthesia

The most commonly used topical anesthetic is lidocaine, which is less toxic than tetracaine or cocaine. Anesthetics applied locally are rapidly absorbed, with peak blood levels in 10 to 15 minutes. The maximal topical lidocaine dose should be limited to 200 to 300 mg.

LIFE-THREATENING HEMOPTYSIS

Definitions

LIFE-THREATENING HEMOPTYSIS. In a subpopulation of patients, hemoptysis is a potentially fatal occurrence. Blood in the airways rapidly coagulates and obstructs the main branches of the bronchial tree, leading to death by asphyxiation. Death by exsanguination is a rare occurrence.

MASSIVE HEMOPTYSIS. This is an expectorated volume of blood greater than 200 to 500 mL during a 24-hour period. This amount of blood is generally considered life-threatening in any patient.

EXSANGUINATING HEMOPTYSIS. Patients who lose more than 600 mL in 16 hours or more than 1000 mL at a rate greater than 150 mL/h are experiencing exsanguinating hemoptysis. This group has a 75% mortality rate if aggressive surgical intervention is not undertaken.

Etiology

Bronchial Artery

The bronchial arteries are visceral branches of the descending thoracic aorta and are distributed through the lung along the major bronchi. Life-threatening hemoptysis has its source in the bronchial artery in 95% of patients. The most common precipitating factor for bronchial artery bleeding is inflammatory lung disease, particularly tuberculosis. It is postulated that mural disruption of a dilated, thin-walled bronchial vessel by cough, direct inflammatory involvement, or aneurysmal rupture is the precipitating event in most cases of life-threatening hemoptysis.

Pulmonary Circulation

The pulmonary circulation is the origin of massive hemoptysis in less than 5% of patients. The most common cause of bleeding from this site is flow-directed pulmonary artery (Swan-Ganz) catheterization. Injuries to the pulmonary artery by these catheters is due to either perforation by the tip of the catheter or balloon overinflation in relation to the involved pulmonary artery branch. Techniques to avoid potential pulmonary artery rupture include limiting advancement from the insertion site, judicious observation of waveforms during balloon inflation, and verification of deflation between wedge pressure measurements.

Other causes of hemoptysis are listed in Table 5–15. A reasonable index of suspicion for the pulmonary circulation as a source of bleeding should be maintained, particularly when therapeutic measures directed at bronchial bleeding sites are ineffective.

Systemic Artery (Nonbronchial)

The most infrequent cause of life-threatening hemoptysis is fistulization of the bronchial tree with a nonbronchial systemic artery. In most cases, hemorrhage in the airways is likely to be massive and acute, with the patient at risk for both asphyxiation and exanguination. Many patients have a premonitory, self-limited, "herald" hemorrhage, which may alert the clinician to the need for intervention before the potential manifestation of massive hemoptysis. Therapy at

Table 5–15. ETIOLOGY OF LIFE-THREATENING HEMOPTYSIS

Bronchial Artery (95%)
Inflammatory lung disease
Tuberculosis, cavitary (70%) or acute (30%)
Histoplasmosis
Aspergillosis
Bronchiectasis
Lung abscess
Necrotizing pneumonia
Broncholithiasis
Pneumoconiosis
Neoplasm
Bronchogenic carcinoma
Endobronchial carcinoid tumor
Endobronchial metastases
Cryptogenic hemoptysis
Pulmonary Circulation (<5%)
Flow-directed pulmonary artery catheterization
Pulmonary infarction
Pulmonary embolism
Postresectional bronchovascular fistula
Pulmonary arteriovenous fistula
Rasmussen's aneurysm
Nonbronchial Systemic Artery (<1%)
Penetrating trauma
Tracheoinnominate artery fistula
Thoracic aortic aneurysm
Post-traumatic aortic pseudoaneurysm
Subclavian artery aneurysm

this juncture has a greater likelihood of success compared with therapy at the time of massive bleeding.

Diagnosis

The most significant factor in the treatment of life-threatening hemoptysis is the ability to localize the site of bleeding. Diagnostic modalities are therefore the initial steps in the management of massive hemoptysis.

History and Physical Examination

HISTORY

Previous episodes of hemoptysis
Previous history of tuberculosis or exposure to tuberculosis
Risk factors for bronchogenic carcinoma
Familial disorder (cystic fibrosis)
Medication (anticoagulants)

PHYSICAL EXAMINATION

Gurgling sensation on the side of bleeding
Character of blood
Quantity of blood
Appearance of blood

Radiographic Studies

A chest radiograph should be obtained for all patients with massive hemoptysis. The aim of radiography is to identify whether the bleeding site can be lateralized to one lung. A diffuse abnormality may be present if there is aspiration of blood throughout the bronchial tree. Computed tomography of the chest has a limited role but can assist in identifying regions of bronchiectasis, cavitation, and calcification (broncholithiasis).

Bronchoscopy

Bronchoscopic evaluation is the pivotal examination in patients with life-threatening hemoptysis. Bronchoscopy allows evaluation of both the cause and the site of bleeding and also provides information about the most appropriate form of definitive management. Rigid and flexible bronchoscopy are useful in evaluating such patients. The advantages of each procedure are outlined here:

Rigid Bronchoscopy

ADVANTAGES

Rapid aspiration of blood and clots
Stable field of vision
Passage of various interventional devices (e.g., balloon catheters)
Ventilation of nonbleeding lung

DISADVANTAGES

Requires general anesthesia and operating room environment
Limited maneuverability

Flexible Bronchoscopy

ADVANTAGES

Segmental bronchus visualization
Visualization of upper lobes
Ease of insertion with local anesthesia

DISADVANTAGES

No ventilatory assistance
Limitations of suction channels
Frequent loss of visual field by blood

Management

Management of life-threatening hemoptysis follows several basic principles:

- Securing the airway and ventilation of nonbleeding lung tissue
- Specific localization of bleeding site

- Isolation of bleeding site from other portions of the tracheobronchial tree
- Control of the source of bleeding

Initial Intervention

- Rapid assessment of the rate and amount of bleeding
- Assess respiratory status (determine need for intubation)
- Sputum for Gram stain, acid-fast bacillus analysis, fungal smears, cytologic evaluation
- Typing and crossmatching for blood transfusion needs
- Coagulation studies
- Arterial blood gas analysis
- Large-bore intravenous line
- Initial placement of patient in semi-Fowler's position; placement of the bleeding lung dependently once site is identified to prevent soilage into the nonbleeding lung
- Humidified O_2 to maintain hydration of the tracheobronchial secretions
- Mild antitussive medications to prevent or treat intractable coughing
- Low-level sedation with anxiolytic
- Careful monitoring of vital signs (electrocardiography, pulse oximetry, blood pressure)
- Urgent thoracic surgery evaluation
- Early bronchoscopy after initial evaluation and stabilization

Endobronchial Control Measures

Selective Bronchial Intubation

Selective bronchial intubation is achieved by advancing an uncut endotracheal tube into the appropriate bronchus of the nonbleeding lung, which isolates the bleeding and directs all ventilation to the nonbleeding lung. A double-lumen endotracheal tube offers the advantage of isolation and independent lung ventilation, but its placement demands skill, the lumina are relatively small, and pulmonary separation is not always maintained.

Endobronchial Balloon Tamponade

A Fogarty-type embolectomy catheter can be positioned in the mainstem, lobar, or segmental bronchi to isolate the bleeding site. When used in intubated patients, the catheter is placed intratracheally outside the endotracheal tube. The inflated cuff of the endotracheal tube helps to maintain the position of the catheter. The balloon should be inflated under direct vision with a bronchoscope. Once in position, the catheter should not be deflated for at least 12 hours. It is a temporizing measure that may allow achievement of normal hemostasis, further diagnostic evaluation, and optimization of the function of the nonbleeding lung. Without subsequent definitive intervention, recurrent bleeding occurs in more than 35% of patients.

Endobronchial Iced Saline Lavage

Endobronchial iced saline lavage can temporarily control bleeding by the induction of hypothermic vasospasm of the likely bronchial artery source. It is not appropriate for patients with very rapid bleeding, in whom bronchial isolation or balloon tamponade is more appropriate.

Endobronchial Packing

Endobronchial packing with tamponade material soaked in vasoactive substances has an extremely limited role in the management of life-threatening hemoptysis. The tamponade material has the potential for subsequent dislodgment, migration, and airway obstruction.

Surgery

Surgical resection of the site of bleeding is the primary form of definitive therapy in patients with life-threatening hemoptysis. Surgical resection is performed after the bleeding site has been identified as specifically as possible by bronchoscopic and radiographic evaluation. In most cases, resection is carried out after the patient has been stabilized. Exanguinating hemoptysis or bleeding from a nonbronchial artery source, however, requires emergent surgical intervention. Surgery is usually indicated in patients with nonterminal diseases and those with sufficient pulmonary reserve to enable a functional lifestyle postoperatively. Typically, resection involves a lobectomy or occasionally a segmentectomy. Pneumonectomy is rarely necessary.

Transcatheter Vessel Embolization

Occlusion of the bleeding vessels by transcatheter embolization can be applied from either the involved bronchial or pulmonary artery. Typically, this technique can be used as an alternative to surgery in patients who are poor candidates for lung resection. The angiographer is directed to the bleeding vessel by the bronchoscopic findings. Extravasation of the contrast medium is rarely seen angiographically. A major risk of bronchial artery embolization is related to the proximity of the spinal cord vasculature. The risk of spinal cord injury is less than 5% following this procedure.

PULMONARY GAS EXCHANGE, TRANSPORT, AND DELIVERY

The lungs play a central role as a site for gas exchange, thereby providing O_2 for the whole body, as well as CO_2 elimination.

Gas Exchange in the Lung

The determinants of alveolar O_2 tension (P_{AO_2}) is F_{IO_2}, the barometric pressure, P_{ACO_2} and the respiratory quotient:

$$P_{AO_2} = (F_{IO_2} \times 713) - P_{ACO_2}.$$

This equation assumes barometric pressure at sea level and respiratory quotient of 1, and that Pa_{CO_2} (arterial CO_2) can be used instead of P_{ACO_2} (alveolar CO_2).

P_{AO_2} determines Pa_{O_2} based on the diffusion gradient and the solubility coefficient of O_2. Thus, the effective way to increase the O_2 diffusion gradient is to increase F_{IO_2}.

Hemoglobin is responsible for most of the carriage of O_2, and the amount of O_2 dissolved in plasma is very low under normal conditions. The solubility of O_2 in blood at 37°C is 0.003 mL/dL/mm Hg. A person breathing room air carries little more than 0.3 mL/dL of O_2 in solution. During breathing of 100% O_2, the dissolved arterial O_2 content increases to about 2 mL/dL.

The position of the oxyhemoglobin dissociation curve and the factors (hydrogen ions, CO_2, 2,3-diphosphoglycerate, and temperature) that influence it affect the rate of O_2 uptake in the lungs. A leftward shift decreases and a rightward shift increases O_2 transfer rates in the tissues, but the opposite occurs in the lungs.

Alveolar CO_2 tension (P_{ACO_2}) is determined by CO_2 production ($\dot{V}_{CO_2}$) and alveolar ventilation (V_A) as follows:

$$P_{ACO_2} = (\dot{V}_{CO_2}/V_A) \times 713 \text{ mm Hg}$$

where 713 mm Hg is barometric pressure (normally 760 mm Hg) minus water vapor pressure (47 mm Hg at 37°C). Thus, a modest increase in ventilation could double the diffusion gradient between the pulmonary arterial and alveolar tensions of CO_2. If V_A is increased, the elimination of CO_2 is also increased, leading to a lower P_{ACO_2}. Because the alveolus has a rapid turnover, a new stable Pa_{CO_2} is reached in 9 to 12 minutes. On the other hand, if V_A is decreased, P_{ACO_2} rises much slower as the whole-body content (about 120 L as CO_2 and bicarbonate ions) is replenished at a metabolic production rate of 200 mL/min. Thus, the establishment of a new steady-state may take well over an hour. The implication for respiratory care is that when blood for an arterial blood gas measurement is drawn, most changes resulting from increases in the ventilation or from alteration of the F_{IO_2} can be assessed in a few minutes, whereas the Pa_{CO_2} may continue to increase for more than an hour after a reduction in V_E.

CO_2 is transported in the blood in solution and as bicarbonate and is combined with amino groups (particularly on hemoglobin) as carbamino compound. The normal resting venoarterial CO_2 tension difference is 4 to 6 mm Hg. This difference becomes greater in conditions of low-flow states, especially during cardiac arrest.

Carbon Monoxide

Carbon monoxide (CO) has a 200-fold greater affinity for hemoglobin than does O_2. At carboxyhemoglobin (COHb) saturations over 40%, heme–heme interactions are far more pronounced in COHb than in oxyhemoglobin. Thus, with

COHb saturations over 40%, the oxyhemoglobin dissociation curve is shifted to the left, leading to increased affinity. CO also combines to the heme of cytochrome oxidase and cytochrome P_{450} systems.

Chronic exposure of CO can cause compensatory polycythemia, decreased exercise tolerance, angina, and possibly even myocardial infarction. Acute CO poisoning results in severe metabolic acidosis as a result of anaerobic metabolism.

The primary treatment for CO poisoning is to provide 100% O_2 so that there is a competitive release of CO from hemoglobin. With room air breathing, the COHb reduction takes 4 hours; it takes only 40 minutes with pure O_2 breathing. Administration of hyperbaric O_2 reduces the time for COHb reduction even further (20 minutes at three atmospheres).

Tissue Oxygenation

To achieve adequate tissue oxygenation, O_2 has to diffuse across the alveolocapillary membrane into erythrocytes binding to hemoglobin, which is then transported to the tissues as a function of cardiac output, where it then dissociates from hemoglobin and diffuses across the endothelium into the cell mitochondria for oxidative phosphorylation. Besides adequate cardiac output, the distribution of blood flow is important in determining tissue oxygenation. This depends on tissue pH and the release of endothelial-derived factors (nitric oxide and adenosine).

Systemic O_2 transport (Do_2) is assumed to reflect O_2 delivery and is defined as:

$$Do_2 = Q \times Cao_2,$$

where Q is cardiac output and Cao_2 (arterial O_2 content) is calculated as:

$$Cao_2 = 1.34 \times (\text{hemoglobin}) \times Sao_2 + 0.003 \times Pao_2$$

Systemic oxygenation consumption ($\dot{V}o_2$), as an estimate of tissue oxygenation demand, is defined as:

$$\dot{V}o_2 = Q \times (Cao_2 - Cvo_2),$$

using the Fick equation, in which Cvo_2 is the mixed venous O_2 content. When cellular O_2 is compromised, however, anaerobic metabolism is needed for the generation of adenosine triphosphate, and $\dot{V}o_2$ no longer reflects total energy utilization. Furthermore, calculating $\dot{V}o_2$ by the Fick equation assumes there is no significant lung O_2 consumption (O_2 consumed directly from the alveoli). Obtaining systemic $\dot{V}o_2$ by direct analysis of inspired and expired gases is preferable. This method includes lung $\dot{V}o_2$, which can be substantial with acute lung injury. However, this technique is generally unreliable when Fio_2 is greater than 0.6, although there are newer metabolic monitors in which this limitation is no longer a problem.

The relationship of Do_2 to $\dot{V}o_2$ in normal conditions is dictated by $\dot{V}o_2$. Thus, Do_2 increases as $\dot{V}o_2$ increases, such as in exercise. Alternatively, if Do_2 is decreased, $\dot{V}o_2$ remains constant until a critical level of Do_2 (Do_2 crit) is exceeded. $\dot{V}o_2$ then falls with Do_2, and anaerobic metabolism is thought to exist with the expression of lactic acidosis. This is termed *pathologic O_2 supply dependency*. Early studies claimed that it existed in patients with ARDS and sepsis and recommended increasing Do_2 in an attempt to improve survival. These studies were flawed, however, by methodologic errors that resulted from mathematical coupling and that lead to the erroneous conclusion of pathologic supply dependency. The mathematical coupling was due to thermodilution cardiac output measurements being used for both Do_2 and $\dot{V}o_2$ calculations. When the studies were repeated with respiratory gas analysis for $\dot{V}o_2$ measurement, pathologic O_2 supply dependency was not demonstrated even in patients with lactic acidosis. Furthermore, attempts to increase Do_2 in critically ill patients by administering dobutamine have led to an increased mortality. This area remains highly controversial and has its detractors.

Regional Oxygenation

Systemic measurements provide little information about the adequacy of O_2 supply to individual organs. Gastric tonometry was developed to measure the adequacy of O_2 delivery to the splanchnic circulation. This technique assumes the equilibration of CO_2 between the gastric mucosa and the saline in the silastic balloon of the tonometer. The gastric pH_i (tissue pH) is then calculated from the Henderson-Hasselbach equation. A low gastric pH_i is predictive of morbidity and mortality in critically ill patients. Attempts made to correct a fall in gastric pH_i have been associated with an improvement in survival. Gastric pH_i may be falsely low if the arterial bicarbonate is lowered for other causes besides hypoperfusion (e.g., renal failure). Thus, the tonometer–arterial Pco_2 difference should probably be examined instead of the pH_i.

Summary

The lungs play the crucial role in gas exchange for O_2 and CO_2. This allows the delivery of adequate O_2 and elimination of CO_2 to and from the tissues respectively. Global measures of Do_2 and $\dot{V}o_2$ may be insufficient to assess the adequacy of tissue oxygenation. Regional measurements of oxygenation are needed, and gastric tonometry is a promising prospect.

OXYGEN THERAPY AND TOXICITY

With the advent of methods to measure arterial O_2 saturation and the partial pressure of O_2 (Pao_2) in plasma, it became recognized that supplemental O_2 could increase the level of both O_2 content and PaO_2, leading to increased delivery to the tissues.

Effects of Oxygen in Disordered Gas Exchange

Oxygen delivery to the tissues is depends on the O_2 content of blood, binding to hemoglobin, cardiac output, and distribution and diffusion from capillary blood. Increasing FIO_2 increases PAO_2, which increases PaO_2 as predicted by the alveolar gas equation if V/Q relationships remain normal. In disordered gas exchange, the response to O_2 therapy is determined by the pattern of breathing and V/Q mismatching. For instance, in patients with chronic bronchitis and hypoxemic respiratory failure, supplemental O_2 easily corrects the hypoxemia, although hypercapnia may worsen despite constant VE and respiratory drive. Similarly, diffusion impairments can be overcome by having a higher PAO_2. With shunts or extreme V/Q mismatching, however, supplemental O_2 is less effective in increasing PaO_2. In certain states of decreased O_2 delivery (e.g., hemorrhagic or cardiogenic shock), supplemental O_2 may increase O_2 delivery by increasing the amount of dissolved O_2 in the plasma.

Oxygen Delivery Equipment

Oxygen therapy equipment for nonintubated patients and the indications for their use are shown in Table 5–16. Mechanical ventilation allows a choice of FIO_2 of 0.21 to 1.00.

Mechanisms of Oxygen Toxicity

Normal cellular respiration in the mitochondria produces partially reduced, reactive O_2 metabolites. The production of incompletely reduced O_2 increases as intracellular PO_2 rises. This leads to the generation of O_2 free radicals ($O_2H\cdot$ and $OH\cdot$) and hydrogen peroxide (H_2O_2), which are toxic for cell components through destructive oxidation and reduction reactions.

Table 5–16. OXYGEN DELIVERY EQUIPMENT FOR SPONTANEOUS BREATHING

Target FIO_2*	Device	O_2 Flow (L/min)
0.21–0.40	Nasal cannula	1–6
0.35–0.50	Facemask	5–10
0.50–0.90	Reservoir mask (rebreathing)	5–15
0.50–0.90	Reservoir mask (nonrebreathing)	5–15
0.24–0.40	Venturi mask	4–10
0.50–1.00	Continuous positive airway pressure†	10–15

*FIO_2 is approximate and depends on mask fit and ventilatory pattern.
†Tight mask seal, high gas flow rate, and expiratory resistance are required to maintain positive airway pressure.

Antioxidant Systems

The antioxidant systems neutralizes toxic O_2 free radicals. The prototypes are metalloproteins termed *superoxide dismutases*. They convert superoxide anion (O_2^-) to H_2O_2. Catalase and glutathione peroxidase sequentially degrade H_2O_2 to water and O_2. Glutathione is the primary, nonprotein sulfhydryl intracellular antioxidant. Other nonenzymatic antioxidants include vitamin A, α-tocopherol, ascorbate, cysteine, ceruloplasmin, urate, and hemoglobin.

Physiologic Responses to Oxygen

Physiologic responses to O_2 are defined as completely reversible changes on discontinuation of supplemental O_2 therapy. The cardiovascular response is inconsistent. There is a decrease in pulse rate and blood pressure, a decrease in cardiac index, and an increase in peripheral vascular resistance.

Clinical Effects of Oxygen Toxicity

Oxygen toxicity causes symptoms of chest pain that may be pleuritic in nature and coughing with nasal congestion. Neurologic symptoms of paresthesia and anorexia may also be present. Vital capacity decreases because of decreased lung compliance or absorption atelectases. The symptoms appear reversible over days to weeks in studies involving normal human subjects.

Several human studies examining the effect of 100% O_2 in normal subjects have shown that within 48 hours there is no detectable damage on the physiologic functioning of the lungs. After 6 hours of O_2 breathing, however, there may be a decrease in tracheal mucus velocity followed by tracheobronchitis in 12 hours.

The pathology of O_2 toxicity appears similar to other causes of alveolar injury, it is difficult to be certain that the pathologic changes seen in these patients are due solely to O_2 toxicity. The pathologic changes have a characteristic time course. The earliest detectable injury is endothelial injury, followed by neutrophil aggregation and thickening of the alveolar interstitium. In the later phases, loss of alveolar type I cells, denudation of basement membranes, and proliferation of alveolar type II cells are seen. After about 10 days, deposition of interstitial collagen, elastin, and fibrosis occurs.

Drug Interactions

Many drugs make O_2 toxicity worse by several mechanisms, including increased O_2 consumption, increased free radical production during their metabolism, and effects on the antioxidant systems. A summary of these interactions are listed in Table 5–17.

Pharmacologic Modulation of Oxygen Toxicity

No effective therapy is available to ameliorate the effects of O_2 toxicity, although many animal studies show promising

Table 5–17. POTENTIAL OXYGEN–DRUG INTERACTIONS

Drug	Effect
Catecholamines	
Epinephrine	Decreased survival
Norepinephrine	
Corticosteroids	
Methylprednisolone	Increased lung injury
Dexamethasone	Decreased survival
Chemotherapeutics	
Bleomycin	Increased lung injury
Cyclophosphamide	
1,3-Bis(2-chloroethyl)-1-nitrosourea	
Antibiotics	
Nitrofurantoin	Increased lung injury

results. Pretreatment with low doses of endotoxin and interleukin-1 increases lung antioxidant enzymes and protects the lung against O_2 toxicity. Other therapeutic interventions include exogenous administration of antioxidants encapsulated in lipid vesicles and surfactant replacement therapy.

PULMONARY EDEMA

Pulmonary Edema of Mixed or Incompletely Understood Pathogenesis

Clinical and pathophysiologic overlap often exists between hydrostatic and permeability pulmonary edema. Several other types of pulmonary edema exist and are discussed here.

High-Altitude Pulmonary Edema

High-altitude pulmonary edema results from rapid ascent to altitudes above 2500 m (7644 ft) followed by strenuous exercise with individual susceptibility. The pathogenesis is unknown. Hypoxemia increases pulmonary vascular resistance, and increased pulmonary artery pressure is seen with a normal pulmonary artery wedge pressure (PAWP). Edema fluid is protein rich, with increased alveolar macrophages. Ideal treatment is rapid descent and supplemental O_2. This condition can be fatal if treatment is not available. Nifedipine, acetazolamide, and dexamethasone can be used prophylactically.

Neurogenic Pulmonary Edema

Pulmonary edema has been described with various neurologic catastrophes (e.g., head trauma, central nervous system bleeding, seizures). It can be acute or insidious. The pathogenesis is not fully understood. There may be an increased centrally mediated sympathetic discharge leading to generalized vasoconstriction and resulting in an elevated PAWP.

This is usually transient, but most patients have persistent edema even after the PAWP normalized. There may also be a direct toxic effect on the myocardium from the massive sympathetic discharge, since myocardial necrosis has been described in such cases. The edema fluid usually has an increased protein concentration, however, suggesting that there may be a role for both hydrostatic and permeability pulmonary edemas.

Re-expansion Pulmonary Edema

Pulmonary edema occasionally occurs after rapid re-expansion of a collapsed lung. This is usually unilateral but can be contralateral. External suctioning, creating a negative intrathoracic pressure, can lead to pulmonary edema. PAWP is normal and edema fluid protein is elevated. Animal studies suggest that this may be a form of reperfusion injury.

Pulmonary Edema Associated with Narcotic Overdose

Narcotic overdoses can lead to pulmonary edema. There may be a component of neurogenic pulmonary edema from opiate-mediated hypothalamic dysfunction and cerebral edema. Hypoxemia from the respiratory depressant effect can lead to left ventricular dysfunction, although PAWP is usually normal and edema fluid protein concentration is increased. Impurities in the illicit drugs have been implicated to have a direct toxic effect, but pure pharmacologic preparations can cause pulmonary edema as well.

Pulmonary Edema Associated with Tocolytic Therapy

Up to 4% of pregnant women develop pulmonary edema from β-sympathomimetic agents given to inhibit preterm labor. It is thought that a combination of volume overload, decreased colloid oncotic pressure, and physiologic alterations caused by pregnancy and tocolysis produce pulmonary edema.

Resolution of Pulmonary Edema

Resolution of pulmonary edema is still not completely understood. Fluid has to be actively transported by the epithelial cells from the alveoli into the interstitium. From here, the pulmonary lymphatics return the fluid to the intravascular compartment. The pleural space is also an important route for clearing interstitial edema.

Diagnosis

History and Physical Examination

Acute pulmonary edema is associated with complaints of severe dyspnea, orthopnea, and cough. Sputum may be frothy and tinged with blood. Apprehension, cyanosis, tachypnea, and tachycardia may be found on examination, along with crackles and wheezes on chest auscultation. Chronic pulmonary edema, on the other hand, can present with fatigue and nonproductive cough.

The cause of pulmonary edema should be actively sought in the history, examination, and investigations. Clinical signs are poorly correlated with actual invasive hemodynamic monitoring.

Chest Roentgenograms

In hydrostatic pulmonary edema, there is equalization of apical and basilar pulmonary vessel size (upper lobe diversion). With increasing interstitial fluid, the interlobular septa become radiographically visible as septal lines or Kerley lines. Kerley B lines are horizontal lines adjacent to the pleural surface. Peribronchial cuffing appears. As fluid gathers in the alveolar air spaces, the acinar shadows become confluent. These opacities are poorly defined, bilateral, symmetric, and more prominent in dependent areas of the lung. Cardiomegaly, bilateral pleural effusions, and increased pulmonary vascular pedicle width are common associated findings.

Permeability pulmonary edema, as in ARDS, can be characterized by three radiologic stages. In the acute stage, no radiographic abnormality is seen. This is followed by alveolar flooding and a radiographic appearance similar to that of hydrostatic pulmonary edema, except the distribution tends to be more peripheral. As ARDS evolves into the chronic fibrotic stage, diffuse reticular infiltrates predominate.

Hemodynamic Measurements

Pulmonary artery catheters allow the measurement of pulmonary artery occlusion pressure, also referred to as PAWP, and can help to distinguish between cardiogenic and noncardiogenic pulmonary edema and to guide therapy. No controlled studies have ever documented any increase in survival with its use, however.

Pulmonary Edema Fluid Protein Concentration

There is an increased ratio of edema fluid to plasma protein concentration for those with permeability pulmonary edema. Furthermore, patients with hydrostatic pulmonary edema have been found to have a higher fractional content of small proteins and a lower fractional content of large proteins in edema fluids than patients with permeability pulmonary edema. Despite several enthusiastic reports, analysis of pulmonary edema fluid protein concentration is of little value in the clinical assessment of individual patients with pulmonary edema.

Other Methods of Quantifying Pulmonary Edema or Evaluating Permeability

Extravascular lung water can be measured by double-indicator techniques such as the cold/indocyanine green method.

Permeability leak can be evaluated with tracer protein equilibration, magnetic resonance imaging, position emission tomography, and clearance of aerosolized technetium 99m–labeled diethylenetriamine penta-acetate. These techniques are used for research purposes and are not routine for patient management.

Therapy

Acute pulmonary edema is a medical emergency. While supportive measures are being provided, the cause of pulmonary edema should be determined quickly and definitive therapy given.

Hypoxemia is common, and supplemental O_2 should be provided. Non-invasive respiratory support such as CPAP by mask may be helpful; in severe cases, however, intubation and mechanical ventilation are needed. Reduction of extravascular lung water by diuresis is especially important in hydrostatic pulmonary edema. Even in permeability pulmonary edema, there is an emerging consensus to keep the lung as dry as possible, since this may decrease the length of mechanical ventilation and improve outcome. If needed, ultrafiltration should be considered as another mode for fluid removal, especially in patients with renal failure.

The treatment of the underlying cause is important and can aid the resolution of the pulmonary edema. For example, myocardial ischemia treated with vasodilating agents can improve myocardial function, relieving pulmonary edema.

Prognosis

Outcome from pulmonary edema depends on the underlying cause. For instance, in hydrostatic pulmonary edema resulting from myocardial infarction, the prognosis depends on residual myocardial function and attempts at revascularization. For patients with ARDS, the overall mortality rate is high, although different causes have different prognoses. Patients with trauma-related ARDS have a better prognosis than those with sepsis-related ARDS. Elderly patients with ARDS do worse than their younger counterparts. Most late deaths of patients with ARDS are from sepsis and multiorgan failure.

PATHOPHYSIOLOGIC FEATURES OF INFANT AND ADULT RESPIRATORY DISTRESS

Hyaline Membrane Disease

Hyaline membrane disease is seen in infants and is characterized by widespread atelectasis, hyaline membranes at the respiratory bronchiolar, alveolar duct, and air saccular levels; pulmonary edema; and lymphatic dilatation. Hyaline membrane disease is initiated by a deficiency in surfactant, resulting in high surface tension forces at the alveolar level and failure of airspace expansion. *Bronchopulmonary dysplasia* includes alveolar and bronchiolar necrosis, bronchial epithelial metaplasia, and interstitial fibrosis. In "healed" stages of bronchopulmonary dysplasia, alveolar septal fibrosis is the main residual feature.

In addition to the lack of surfactant, a lack of collateral ventilation in the human lungs predisposes to atelectasis distal to obstructed airways, to a decrease in elastic recoil, and to an increase in airway resistance, and promotes pulmonary interdependence to produce the overdistended, emphysematous lung regions in bronchopulmonary dysplasia. Second, the extraordinarily compliant neonatal chest wall distorts the chest wall during inspiration and allows the surfactant-depleted lung to collapse on expiration. Increases in pulmonary vascular resistance may be seen with hyaline membrane disease, but it is unclear whether this is a primary cause of bronchopulmonary dysplasia or a secondary reflection of the pulmonary hypertension from arterial hypoxemia.

Chronic interstitial emphysema, a manifestation of barotrauma, is much more severe in infants than adults. Affected infants usually have bronchopulmonary dysplasia and concomitantly exhibit numerous air-filled, interstitial cysts.

Diffuse Alveolar Damage

Diffuse alveolar damage is characterized by an increased permeability lesion that gives rise to pulmonary edema and hyaline membrane formation. Suspected mediators of the pulmonary microvascular injury include the following:

CELLULAR

Polymorphonuclear leukocytes
Platelets
Lymphocytes
Macrophages

HUMORAL

Complement activation factors
Lipid mediators
Coagulation and fibrinolytic factors
Kallikrein-kinin agents
Cytokines
Histamines

The histopathologic features of diffuse alveolar damage are separated into the exudative and reparative (proliferative) phases. The main histologic features in each of these phases are as follows:

EXUDATIVE PHASE (<6 days)

Degeneration or necrosis of alveolar lining cells
Degeneration or necrosis of endothelium
Increased permeability of blood vessels
Proteinaceous exudates
Hyaline membranes
Alveolar wall edema
PMN infiltration of alveolar walls and spaces
Microatelectases

REPARATIVE PHASE (>6 days)

Hyperplasia of type II epithelial cells
Interstitial mononuclear infiltrate
Aggregation of hyaline membranes
Increased fibroblasts in alveolar walls and in organizing alveolar exudates

If the reparative phase persists, these patients can eventually develop widespread fibrosis.

Factors Affecting Both Hyaline Membrane Disease–Bronchopulmonary Dysplasia and Diffuse Alveolar Damage

Oxygen

Susceptibility to O_2 injury varies with development and species. O_2 toxicity in infants and adults is due to the recruitment of white blood cells from the vascular stream into the alveolar space through the release of chemotactic factors, especially from alveolar macrophages. There is no well-defined safe concentration of inspired O_2 that does not interfere with reparative regeneration or that retards the development of lung fibrosis.

Infection

A lung injured by diffuse alveolar damage has a diminished capacity for antimicrobial defense. Colonization of pathogenic bacteria is seen first in the upper respiratory tract followed by colonization of the trachea. In adults, gram-negative bacteria dominate the colonizing and infective microbes. In infants, coagulase-negative staphylococci are seen first and gram-negatives are acquired later in the hospital course. The exact role of infection in the evolution of bronchopulmonary dysplasia or development of pulmonary fibrosis is not yet known.

Mechanical Ventilation

An emerging consensus is that any ventilatory modality that induces any form of overinflation is the underlying genesis of ventilator-induced lung injury. Finding ways to monitor lung volumes rather than just airway pressure may be the key to preventing damage to healthy lungs and to avoiding further damage to diseased lungs.

Outcomes of Hyaline Membrane Disease, Bronchopulmonary Dysplasia, and Diffuse Alveolar Damage

Children who have had hyaline membrane disease and have lived for 5 to 10 years after their disease experience nearly complete recovery. Low-birth-weight infants who survive the respiratory distress syndrome have low maximum expiratory flow rates at 8 to 10 years of age. In adults who survive ARDS, lung function usually shows little or no long-term impairment.

ADULT RESPIRATORY DISTRESS SYNDROME

Definition

Adult respiratory distress syndrome is a pathophysiologic syndrome and not a single disease. It is commonly associated with sepsis and multiple organ failure, and is associated with a high mortality rate. There is diffuse alveolar damage with lung inflammation, along with pulmonary microvascular thrombosis. This leads to increased pulmonary capillary permeability and extravascular lung water. The pathophysiologic mechanism of ARDS is still incompletely understood and may vary according to the cause. Patients with pulmonary capillary hypertension leading to "cardiogenic" pulmonary edema and patients with chronic lung disease are usually excluded from the definition of ARDS, although these conditions can coexist with ARDS.

The usual clinical definitions include the presence of severe arterial hypoxemia (PaO_2/FIO_2 ratio below 200 mm Hg), bilateral alveolar infiltrates compatible with pulmonary edema on chest radiographs, decreased lung compliance, and the presence of a known etiologic factor. The newer American-European Consensus definition recognizes that ARDS is a severe form of acute lung injury and requires a PaO_2/FIO_2 ratio below 200 mm Hg regardless of the level of PEEP, chest radiographic changes of bilateral alveolar infiltrates, and no evidence of pulmonary capillary hypertension. Four parameters have been identified to define the lung injury score (Table 5–18) as a measure of severity, although this score has not been correlated with outcome.

Incidence

Because of the lack of a uniform definition of ARDS, its true incidence is unknown. One 1972 estimate from the National Heart and Lung Institute suggested that there were 72 cases per 100,000 population. A more recent study from the Canary Islands found a lower incidence of 3.5 cases per 100,000 population.

Etiology

Numerous risk factors are associated with ARDS and commonly include sepsis (especially gram-negative sepsis), aspiration, severe trauma, and multiple transfusions. The risk of ARDS development increases in a stepwise fashion with the additional presence of other risk factors. It is important to search for the underlying cause of ARDS, since cause-targeted treatment is essential.

Pathophysiology

Inflammatory Response

Although ARDS has multiple causes, the end result is remarkably uniform—an intense inflammatory response re-

Table 5–18. COMPONENTS AND INDIVIDUAL VALUES OF THE LUNG INJURY SCORE

Component		Value
Chest Roentgenogram Score		
No alveolar consolidation		0
Alveolar consolidation confined to 1 quadrant		1
Alveolar consolidation confined to 2 quadrants		2
Alveolar consolidation confined to 3 quadrants		3
Alveolar consolidation in all 4 quadrants		4
Hypoxemia Score		
PaO_2/FIO_2	>300	0
PaO_2/FIO_2	225–299	1
PaO_2/FIO_2	175–224	2
PaO_2/FIO_2	100–174	3
PaO_2/FIO_2	<100	4
PEEP Score (When Ventilated)		
PEEP	≥5 cm H_2O	0
PEEP	6–8 cm H_2O	1
PEEP	9–11 cm H_2O	2
PEEP	12–14 cm H_2O	3
PEEP	≥19 mL/cm H_2O	4
The final value is obtained by dividing the aggregate sum by the number of components that were used		
	Score	
No lung injury	0	
Mild to moderate lung injury	0.1–2.5	
Severe lung injury (ARDS)	>2.5	

(From Murray JF, Matthay MA, Luce JM, et al: An expanded definition of the adult respiratory distress syndrome. Am Rev Respir Dis 1988; 138:720.)

sulting in alveolar and endothelial damage. There are cellular and humoral inflammatory responses that are currently being studied. Macrophages have an important role in recognizing initiating factors such as endotoxin, which responds by expressing cytokines with a role in modulating the inflammatory response. Neutrophils are recruited to the pulmonary microcirculation in the early stages of ARDS by various chemoattractants, causing damage through the release of various proteolytic enzymes and the generation of free O_2 radicals.

Histologic Changes

The endothelium becomes increasingly permeable to fluid and protein, leading to interstitial edema and alveolar flooding. Alveolar surface cells (type I) are destroyed, leaving exposed alveolar basement membrane, which is covered with alveolar type II cells within several days. Plasma proteins, cellular debris, fibrin, and surfactant remnants aggregrate to form the characteristic hyaline membranes covering the basement membranes of alveoli and alveolar ducts. Once the acute exudative phase is over, fibroproliferation occurs. Depending on various factors, fibrosis or resolution can result.

Surfactant

Surfactant is secreted by alveolar type II cells and reduces surface tension. In ARDS, the amount and composition of surfactant is altered. Furthermore, serum proteins that have leaked into the alveolar spaces inactivate surfactant. This leads to increased surface tension, promoting alveolar collapse.

Lung Mechanics and Gas Exchange

Lung compliance is reduced in ARDS as a result of widespread atelectases from alveolar flooding and surfactant abnormalities. Airway resistance is also increased. The severe hypoxemia in ARDS is due to intrapulmonary shunting and areas of low V/Q.

Extrapulmonary Organ Failure

Adult respiratory distress syndrome is often part of multiple organ failure. It can be considered the pulmonary response to the systemic inflammatory response syndrome. Inflammatory mediators involved in ARDS are probably operative in other types of organ failure as well.

Clinical Features

The underlying cause of ARDS obviously has an impact on the clinical features. High-pitched end-expiratory crackles are present on auscultation. Chest radiographs typically have diffuse infiltrates that become more dense as alveolar flooding occurs. Computed tomography has shown that despite the diffuse picture apparent on the chest radiographs, there is a patchy distribution of abnormalities, especially atelectasis, in the dependent lung portions. The application of PEEP increases FRC and improves the appearance of the chest radiograph with increased aeration. It is unclear whether ventilation is correspondingly increased. When viewing the chest radiograph, signs of barotrauma (i.e., mediastinal emphysema, subcutaneous emphysema, and pneumothorax) should be sought.

Management

The cause for ARDS has to be identified and treated. In the interim, supportive measures are required.

Mechanical Ventilation

Most patients with ARDS require support of positive-pressure ventilation for their hypoxemia. The goals of positive-pressure ventilation are to restore arterial oxygenation, to maintain systemic O_2 delivery, and to avoid complications associated with mechanical ventilation. These patients require full ventilatory support either with assist-control or synchronized intermittent ventilation. Because there is regional inhomogeneity from lung injury, the use of conventional VT values may overdistend areas of normal alveoli. Therefore, low VT settings of 7 to 10 mL/kg may be appropriate.

Using pulse oximetry, F_{IO_2} should be titrated below 0.5 to avoid pulmonary toxicity. PEEP can be added to improve oxygenation. PEEP decreases intrapulmonary shunting and improves V/Q matching. As more PEEP is applied, however, hemodynamic complications may become apparent. PEEP can reduce venous return, leading to an overall decrease in O_2 delivery from a decreased cardiac output. Alternatively, it can overdistend the alveoli with consequent increase in pulmonary vascular resistance and right ventricular failure. Therefore, as high levels of PEEP are employed, a pulmonary artery catheter should be inserted to monitor O_2 delivery.

If there is persistent hypoxemia, sedation and pharmacologic paralysis should be employed to reduce O_2 consumption. Efforts to increase O_2 delivery should include the optimization of hemoglobin concentration and the maintenance of adequate cardiac output.

Other means of ventilation can be used in patients who fail on conventional ventilation. These include pressure control–inverse ratio ventilation, high-frequency jet ventilation, and airway pressure release ventilation. These modalities are associated with a reduction of peak airway pressure. Outcomes or complications, however, are not altered. Tracheal gas insufflation can be considered at low flows to aid in CO_2 elimination.

Hemodynamic Monitoring and Fluid Balance

A pulmonary artery catheter in patients with ARDS is useful for fluid management and the measurement of O_2 delivery. The relation of O_2 consumption to O_2 delivery in ARDS has been studied extensively. New data suggest that the earlier reports of pathologic supply dependency may have been due to mathematical coupling. Furthermore, it is unclear whether manipulations to increase O_2 delivery above the normal range will have a beneficial outcome.

Fluid management has to be balanced between the adequacy of O_2 delivery and the need to keep the lung "dry" because of the increased capillary permeability. Whether crytalloids or colloids should be used remains controversial. It is clear, however, that crytalloids are less expensive than colloids.

Nutrition

Patients with ARDS are hypermetabolic. It is important to provide adequate nutrition, preferably by the enteral route. This can reduce the presence of bacterial translocation from disrupted mucosal integrity and potentially alleviate the persistent systemic inflammatory response that would otherwise continue to fuel the ARDS and lead to multiple organ failure.

Extracorporeal Membrane Oxygenation

The initial study on extracorporeal membrane oxygenation reported in 1979 showed it had no benefit over conventional mechanical ventilation, and patients had a survival rate of less than 10%. A modification by Gattinoni using low-frequency positive-pressure ventilation and extracorporeal CO_2 removal with apneic oxygenation showed an improvement in survival rate (49%). Their study had no contemperaneous control group, however. Preliminary reports from a controlled study from Salt Lake City showed no benefit of this form of extracoporeal support over pressure control–inverse ratio ventilation when a computerized ventilator management protocol was used.

Controversies

The optimal approach to mechanical ventilation in patients with ARDS remains unclear. There is general agreement that pressure-limited therapy can reduce lung overdistention and therefore ventilator-associated lung injuries. This pressure-limited approach employs lower $V_{T}s$ (6–8 mL/kg) than conventional practice to maintain a low transalveolar pressure (<35 cm H_2O). This can result in hypercapnia, which is tolerated (permissive hypercapnia) unless severe adverse effects are present. Mean airway pressure can be increased with alterations in the inspiratory pressure waveform, increases in PEEP, or increases in the inspiratory time fraction.

Pneumonia is a dreaded complication of ARDS. It is unclear whether selective gastrointestinal decontamination has any impact on this problem.

No pharmacologic agent has been proved to be effective for the treatment of ARDS. Corticosteroids may be useful in the fibroproliferative phase of ARDS, but further trials are needed. Inhaled nitric oxide may improve V/Q matching and alleviate hypoxemia, as well as treating pulmonary hypertension. No outcome data are available, however, and its effects are unpredictable.

Surfactant replacement is indicated in neonatal respiratory distress syndrome, but its utility for ARDS has yet to be proved. Furthermore, which preparation of surfactant to give and the mode of delivery have yet to be finalized.

Complications

The potential for complications exists in any critically ill patient, and a number of these possibilities are given in Table 5–19.

Outcome

The mortality rate of ARDS remains about 50% despite modern intensive care, although it appears that overall the outcome has improved. Initial studies suggested that patients with ARDS died early of their underlying illness, and late deaths are due to sepsis and multiple organ failure. A more recent report, however, emphasized the increased

Table 5–19. COMPLICATIONS ASSOCIATED WITH ADULT RESPIRATORY DISTRESS SYNDROME

Pulmonary
- Pulmonary emboli
- Pulmonary barotrauma
- Pulmonary fibrosis
- Oxygen toxicity

Gastrointestinal
- Gastrointestinal hemorrhage
- Ileus
- Gastric distention
- Pneumoperitoneum

Renal
- Renal failure
- Fluid retention

Cardiovascular
- Invasive catheters
- Arrhythmia
- Hypotension
- Low cardiac output

Infection
- Sepsis
- Nosocomial pneumonia

Hematologic
- Anemia
- Thrombocytopenia
- Disseminated intravascular coagulation

Other
- Hepatic
- Endocrine
- Neurologic
- Psychiatric
- Malnutrition

Complications Attributable to Intubation and Extubation
- Prolonged attempt at intubation
- Intubation of a mainstem bronchus
- Premature extubation
- Self-extubation

Complications Associated with Endotracheal or Tracheostomy Tubes
- Tube malfunction
- Nasal necrosis
- Paranasal sinus infection
- Tracheal stenosis
- Tracheomalacia
- Polyps
- Erosion
- Fistulas
- Airway obstruction
- Hoarseness

Complications Attributable to Operation of the Ventilator
- Machine failure
- Alarm failure
- Alarms silenced
- Inadequate nebulization or humidification

Complications Occurring During Positive Airway Pressure Therapy
- Alveolar hypoventilation
- Alveolar hyperventilation
- Massive gastric distention
- Barotrauma
- Atelectasis
- Pneumonia
- Hypotension

(From Taylor RW: The adult respiratory distress syndrome. *In:* Respiratory Failure. Kirby RR, Taylor RW [Eds]. Chicago, Year Book Medical Publishers, 1986, pp 208–244.)

incidence of patients dying of respiratory failure. Patients who do survive may continue to have improvements in their pulmonary function up to 1 year after ARDS.

PATHOPHYSIOLOGY AND MANAGEMENT OF ADULT RESPIRATORY DISTRESS SYNDROME

This section summarizes the temporal relation among blood volume, hemodynamics, oxygen transport (DO_2), and cytokine patterns before and after the onset of ARDS. Therapeutic options are also described.

Diagnosis and Conventional Therapy

Adult respiratory distress syndrome is clinically defined as hypoxemia ($PaO_2 < 55$) on room air, requiring mechanical ventilation with increased FIO_2 for more than 24 hours. Chest radiographs can show bilateral infiltrates. The PaO_2/FIO_2 ratio is less than 200, shunt is less than 20%, and there is decreased chest compliance. ARDS occurs most often postoperatively or after trauma in hemodynamically unstable patients.

Conventional therapy is to achieve normal vital signs, hematocrit, urine output, and arterial blood gas values. After normal vital signs are achieved, the goal of the therapy of ARDS consists of fluid restriction and diuretic administration, which prevent or minimize pulmonary edema, maintaining low pulmonary artery occlusion pressure. Therefore, the conventional approach maintains the patient on the dry side. This is more a philosophical statement of intent, however, rather than a useful operational therapeutic rule. Data suggest that trauma patients who are resuscitated with greater amounts of fluid to achieve supranormal DO_2 and $\dot{V}O_2$ have improved survival with fewer lung and other organ complications. Finally, pulmonary edema can be produced by many conditions, and, in postoperative patients, it is more often the effect than the cause of ARDS.

Therapy

Based on previous studies, high-risk patients undergoing major surgical operations had improved survival if the following hemodynamic parameters could be achieved with the first 8 to 12 hours postoperatively:

1. Cardiac index greater than 4.5 L/min/m^2
2. DO_2 over 600 mL/min/m^2
3. $\dot{V}O_2$ above 170 mL/min/m^2
4. Blood volume higher than normal (i.e., 3.2 L/m^2 for men, and 2.7 L/m^2 for women)

Optimal goals may be higher for patients with severe trauma and sepsis. It has generally been observed that survivors of ARDS demonstrated supranormal values for cardiac index, DO_2 and $\dot{V}O_2$ postinsult (surgery, trauma), which may have been compensatory for "peri-insult" reduced circulatory function. Basically, O_2 debt is greater in patients with organ failure and in nonsurvivors. Several trials have shown that reaching empiric supranormal (cardiac index, Do_2, $\dot{V}o_2$) values in survivors significantly reduced O_2 debt, organ failure, and death in high-risk surgical patients. It may be possible to increase $\dot{V}o_2$ by augmenting cardiac index or Do_2 (optimize hematocrit, arterial O_2 saturation, and cardiac pump function) at some lower levels of Do_2 and $\dot{V}o_2$, when $\dot{V}o_2$ may be Do_2 dependent. Data also show, however, that increasing Do_2 does not necessarily increase $\dot{V}o_2$ (which actually reaches a plateau).

Goals for high-risk postoperative patients and those with severe trauma should therefore include prevention of tissue hypoxia and O_2 debt, which can lead to ARDS. In addition to ventilatory and hemodynamic support (inotropes, vasopressors), plasma volume must be adequate. Recent studies show that albumin solutions (25%) expanded the plasma volume more than crystalloids and did not "leak" into the extravascular space. Colloid, therefore, limited the overexpansion of the pulmonary interstitium and the resultant interference with oxygenation. The benefits of colloids were maximal in the first 48 hours and were insignificant after 6 days or in the last 48 hours of life in nonsurvivors.

Summary

Hypoxia to the lung per se increases pulmonary arterial pressure, pulmonary vascular resistance, and shunting. These events occur prior to ARDS and are not the result of ARDS. Therapy should include measures to correct early circulatory deficiencies, to reverse O_2 debt, and to limit overexpansion of the interstitium.

ACUTE RESPIRATORY FAILURE IN CHRONIC OBSTRUCTIVE PULMONARY DISEASE

Chronic obstructive pulmonary disease is a process characterized by chronic bronchitis or emphysema, which can lead to the development of variably reversible airway obstruction. Conventional criteria for respiratory failure include Pao_2 below 60 mm Hg and $Paco_2$ above 50 mm Hg. For patients with COPD, however, acute respiratory failure occurs when the Pao_2 is less than or the $Paco_2$ greater than the individual's baseline arterial blood gas value. COPD accounts for a significant number of all cases of acute respiratory failure, although most patients do not require mechanical ventilation. Mortality rates are 5% to 38%, with reduced premorbid clinical status, reduced albumin, and severe acidemia boding the worst prognosis.

Precipitating Factors for Exacerbations

Tables 5–20 and 5–21 outline factors that can exacerbate COPD.

Table 5–20. PRECIPITATING FACTORS FOR CHRONIC OBSTRUCTIVE PULMONARY DISEASE EXACERBATIONS

- Infection
  - Bacterial
  - Viral
- Cardiac disease
  - Cardiac arrhythmia
  - Coronary artery disease
  - Cor pulmonale
- Environmental
  - Allergens
  - Occupational irritants
  - Humidity
  - Air pollution
  - Primary or secondary smoke exposure
- Medications
  - Beta agonists
  - Narcotics or sedatives
- Oxygen therapy
- Pneumothorax
- Pulmonary thromboembolic disease
- Respiratory muscle fatigue

Pathophysiology of Respiratory Failure

The primary mechanism of hypoxemia in patients with COPD results from a dispersion of V/Q units, leading to a higher ventilatory requirement to maintain PaO_2 and $PaCO_2$ than in normal subjects. Faced with expiratory airflow obstruction, the patient with COPD must increase inspiratory flow rate or lung volume to meet heightened ventilatory demands (to allow adequate time for expiration). Both adaptations place a significant burden on the inspiratory muscles.

Table 5–21. NONMECHANICAL FACTORS THAT CONTRIBUTE TO RESPIRATORY MUSCLE FAILURE IN PATIENTS WITH CHRONIC OBSTRUCTIVE PULMONARY DISEASE

- Drug therapy
  - Sedatives
  - Paralytics
- Electrolyte abnormalities
  - Hypocalcemia
  - Hypokalemia
  - Hypophosphatemia
  - Hypomagnesemia
- Endocrine disorders
  - Hypothyroidism and hyperthyroidism
  - Glucocorticoid excess (include exogenous administration)
- Gas exchange abnormalities
  - Hypoxia
  - Hypercapnia
- Nutritional status
- Oxygen delivery

Hyperinflation in the setting of dynamic airway collapse increases the end-expiratory elastic recoil pressure of the respiratory system. This PEEP is called auto-PEEP or $PEEP_I$. It places an additional load on the inspiratory muscles, since the patient must generate a negative inspiratory force equal (and opposite) to the level of auto-PEEP for inspiratory airflow to begin. Hyperinflation leads to structural and biochemical changes in the muscle fibers, and it predisposes the patient to cardiovascular compromise (due to elevated intrathoracic pressures) and to barotrauma.

To maintain adequate alveolar ventilation in the face of these mechanical changes, efferent neural drive to the respiratory muscles must be increased. Patients with COPD tend to breathe using higher respiratory rates and smaller V_T. The reduced V_T and increased dead space of each breath (V_D/V_T) effectively reduce alveolar ventilation.

Clinical Presentation

The primary symptoms of acute respiratory failure in COPD include progressive dyspnea and cough or sputum that is changed from baseline. Symptoms of diaphoresis, mental status changes, headache, asterixis, and tremor are usually secondary to the associated gas exchange defect. Early physical findings are tachypnea, tachycardia, and a reduced resting V_T. More progressive signs are asynchronous respiratory movements, use of accessory muscles, and paradoxical motion.

Distinctive presentations include "pink puffers" and "blue bloaters." The former have predominant dyspnea, marked hyperinflation, body wasting, mild hypoxemia, and only late hypercapnia. The latter show early hypercapnia and hypoxemia with chronic sputum production, signs of right-sided heart failure, and recurrent bouts of bronchitis.

Treatment

Correction of Gas Exchange Defects

The initial step in the management of acute COPD is correction of the gas exchange abnormalities, especially hypoxemia. O_2 administration must achieve two simultaneous goals—correcting hypoxemia while minimizing O_2-induced hypercapnia. The administration method is less critical (i.e., Venturi mask versus nasal cannula) than careful monitoring to keep arterial O_2 saturation at approximately 90%. Pulse oximetry must be used with caution in patients with COPD because of issues concerning the shape of the O_2–hemoglobin dissociation curve, inability to assess the adequacy of ventilation, and loss of accuracy in the presence of significant carboxyhemoglobin (patients who continue to smoke).

Examination of the relation between the arterial pH and Pa_{CO_2} can help to distinguish between acute and chronic ventilatory failure. In acute conditions, an increase in Pa_{CO_2} by 10 mm Hg decreases the pH by 0.08 units. Under chronic conditions, an increase in $Paco_2$ by 10 mm Hg decreases the pH by only 0.03 units.

Respiratory stimulants (e.g., methylxanthines, narcotic antagonists, progesterone, acetazolamide, doxapram, almitrine) have been used to correct the gas exchange defects, but their use is controversial.

Minimize Expiratory Airflow Obstruction

Bronchodilators, specifically $beta_2$ agonists, are the main therapy to reduce airway resistance. Medications available in the United States include metaproterenol, salbutamol, terbutaline, pirbuterol, and biltolterol. The inhaled route is preferable over oral or subcutaneous administration because of more rapid onset and reduced toxicity. In general, the onset of action is within 3 to 6 minutes and the duration of action is 4 to 6 hours. Nebulizers or metered-dose inhalers are similar in their therapeutic effectiveness. For spontaneously breathing patients, however, the correct technique for metered dose inhalation is essential. A spacer device can assist in proper drug administration. During acute exacerbations, $beta_2$ agonist can be given every 15 to 20 minutes, depending on tolerance, for three or four doses. After acute stabilization, the dosing frequency is usually every 2 to 4 hours.

Anticholinergics act to inhibit parasympathetic activity and promote bronchodilation. Atropin and glycopyrrolate are available by aerosol but ipratropium bromide is available only by metered dose inhaler. Ipratropium is preferred because of less systemic absorption, which minimizes systemic anticholinergic side effects. The time to maximal effect is 30 to 60 minutes. In contrast to $beta_2$ agonists, ipratropium bromide administration does not exhibit tachyphylaxis or paroxysmal lowering of the Pao_2.

The use of theophylline for acute and chronic therapy remains controversial. Although theophylline appears to be only a mild bronchodilator, other proposed benefits include improvements in respiratory muscle strength, ventricular contractility, and mucociliary clearance. The optimal therapeutic range remains undefined, but toxicity is increased with higher serum levels.

Corticosteroids are frequently administered, although the mechanism of action remains unknown. They can reduce the airway inflammation and enhance responsiveness to catecholamine bronchodilators. A randomized trial of methylpredinisolone, 0.5 mg/kg every 6 hours suggested a benefit as assessed by measurement of FEV_1. If corticosteroids are necessary, they should be started early because they have delayed onset. Conversion to oral therapy (prednisone, 40–60 mg/d) and rapid tapering (<2 weeks) should be the goal.

For secretion clearance, coughing is the most effective method. Dehydration should be avoided, although overhydration to loosen secretions is not advised. Mucolytic agents such as N-acetylcysteine can provoke bronchospasm when administered by aerosol.

Treatment of the Precipitating Cause

A carefully obtained history and physical examination are necessary to identify precipitating factors. Drug toxicities must be identified and corrected. If tachyarrhythmias are present, theophylline is best withheld. Beta-blockers and sedatives should be withdrawn.

Antibiotics are definitely indicated for bacterial pneumonia. It is not clear whether patients with acute bronchitis should receive antibiotics. Data suggest, however, that patients with acute bronchitis who received antibiotics had a more prompt resolution of symptoms, earlier improvement in peak flow measurements, and reduced rate of hospitalizations. Therefore, the benefit-risk ratio for antibiotic use in acute bronchitis seems favorable.

Respiratory muscle function should be optimized by correction of electrolyte imbalances, hypoxemia, and hypercapnia, and optimization of cardiac performance.

Enteral nutritional support should provide maintainance of caloric balance and correction of any deficiencies. Caloric requirements are estimated by use of conventional formulas. Protein requirements are between 1.2 and 1.5 g/kg/d. Aggressive attempts at overfeeding should be avoided, since this can increase CO_2 production and increase ventilatory requirements.

Mechanical Ventilation

One must consider both the mechanical ventilatory mode and the method of delivery. Noninvasive ventilatory support is appropriate for patients who are awake, oriented, and without secretion problems. These patients must be able to tolerate a tight-fitting facemask. The exact criteria for selecting patients for noninvasive ventilation is not yet well defined. For patients requiring intubation and mechanical ventilation, a wide range of ventilatory options is available.

ACUTE PHASE

In the initial ventilatory management, the selected mode should adequately "unload" the work of the respiratory muscles. In general, this is accomplished using either the assist control or synchronized intermittent ventilation mode. General guidelines for mechanical ventilator settings include the following:

VT and VE: 7 to 10 mL/kg/breath. Machine-supported VE adjusted to approximately two thirds of the spontaneous VE. Normalization of the $PaCO_2$ should be avoided because this can lead a posthypercapnic respiratory alkalosis with cardiac arrhythmias, seizures, and prolonged ventilator weaning.

Inspired oxygen concentration: FIO_2 0.8 to 0.9 until patient is stabilized. Further adjustments are guided by arterial blood gas data or pulse oximetry results (titrate to maintain arterial O_2 saturation at 92% to 95%).

Peak inspiratory flow rate: Set to five or six times the resting

VE to meet demands without generating high peak airway pressures.

External PEEP settings: These are used only in patients with an inability to trigger the ventilator that cannot be addressed by reducing VE and airflow obstruction. If used, the external PEEP should be set below the level of auto-PEEP to avoid further hyperinflation and hemodynamic embarrassment.

CHRONIC PHASE

The focus for patients with COPD on long-term mechanical ventilation must be to minimize the risk of complications. Peak airway pressures should be less than 40 cm H_2O to avoid barotrauma. Anxiety management with pharmacologic interventions or specific biofeedback techniques can be beneficial to the weaning process. Minimizing "external" workload from the ventilator system can be accomplished by using an endotracheal tube of adequate diameter, low levels of pressure support on spontaneous breaths, and matching ventilator sensitivities and flow settings to patients demand.

Prognosis

The mortality rate for respiratory failure in patients with COPD ranges from 5% to 38%. Adverse prognostic variables include reduced premorbid clinical status, reduced serum albumin, and the severity of acidosis on presentation.

PULMONARY HOST DEFENSE AND INFLAMMATORY LUNG DISEASE

Normal pulmonary function depends on the ability of the lungs to maintain a sterile subglottic environment. The first level of host defense consists of physical mechanisms (cough and sneeze reflexes, mucociliary clearance, immunoglobulins) to prevent colonization. Beyond the bronchioles, the alveolar macrophages are especially effective against gram-

Table 5–22. POSSIBLE PATHOPHYSIOLOGIC SEQUENCE INVOLVED IN THE DEVELOPMENT OF NOSOCOMIAL PNEUMONIA

Gastric colonization
Oropharyngeal colonization
Aspiration
Depressed cough and sneeze reflexes
Inactive mucociliary escalation
Tracheobronchial colonization
Sufficient bacterial burden and virulence
Overwhelmed resident and recruited phagocytic defense
Pneumonia

Table 5–23. RISK FACTORS FOR THE DEVELOPMENT OF NOSOCOMIAL PNEUMONIA

Endotracheal intubation
Altered consciousness or coma
Nasogastric tube
Gram-negative pharyngeal colonization
Advanced age
Poor nutrition
Witnessed aspiration
Treatment with antacids or histamine$_2$ blockers
Upper abdominal or thoracic surgery
Multiple trauma
Barbiturate treatment

positive bacteria. They are sometimes augmented by recruitment of granulocytic phagocytes. Neutrophils are essential for containment of gram-negative bacteria. Cytokines (chemokines, interleukin-8) are important in regulating neutrophilic inflammation in both infectious and noninfectious inflammatory lung disease.

Nosocomial pneumonia is defined as a lower respiratory tract infection that develops in hospitalized patients in whom the infection either was not present or was not incubating at the time of admission and occurs beyond 72 hours of hospitalization. The pathophysiologic sequence, risk factors, and bacterial species involved in the development of nosocomial pneumonia are summarized in Tables 5–22 to 5–24. The incidence outside of the intensive care unit is 0.5% to 5%, but it is 11% to 21% in mechanically ventilated patients and at least 50% to 70% in long-term ventilated patients. The mortality rate is 25% to 55%, making pneumonia the leading cause of death from nosocomial infection.

Diagnosis of Nosocomial Pneumonia

The diagnostic specificity of fever, leukocytosis, radiographic infiltrates, purulent sputum, and the presence of a bacteria on sputum Gram stain is decreased in the intubated popula-

Table 5–24. BACTERIAL SPECIES COMMONLY ASSOCIATED WITH NOSOCOMIAL PNEUMONIA

Pseudomonas aeruginosa
Staphylococcus aureus
Klebsiella pneumoniae
Legionella pneumophila
Acinetobacter calcoaceticus
Streptococcus pneumoniae
Haemophilus influenzae
Enterobacter cloacae
Serratia marcescens
Escherichia coli

tion. Fever and leukocytosis can result from extrapulmonary infections, and a wide variety of radiologic changes can occur in the absence of infection. Recent data indicate that a threshold exists in the number of airway organisms that separates colonization from infection. Bronchoscopic techniques such as protected specimen brushing and bronchoalveolar lavage, with quantitative cultures ($>10^3$ colony-forming units) are the most accurate for diagnosis of nosocomial pneumonia. Future studies are necessary to make more specific recommendations about the diagnostic utility of these techniques for nosocomial pneumonia.

Airway Defense Barrier

Passive Upper Airway Defense Mechanisms

Bacteria reach the lungs by one of four routes: inhalation of infectious droplets, hematogeneous seeding from a distant site, direct contiguous spread, and aspiration of contaminated secretions from a colonized upper airway. In mechanically ventilated patients, bacteria usually penetrate the lung by either aspiration or inhalation of contaminated droplets. Hospitalized patients have their pharyngeal flora colonized by potentially pathologic gram-negative bacteria. Endotracheal intubation and mechanical ventilation allow all sizes of droplets to have unimpeded access to the distal lung.

Reflexes

Sneezing and coughing clear foreign particles from the nose, pharynx, and large airways. Endotracheal intubation blocks effectual cough reflexes by decreasing the peak attainable intrathoracic pressure.

Mechanical Lower Airway Mechanisms

Mucociliary clearance moves mucus-embedded particles toward the pharynx, where they can be swallowed or expectorated.

Immunologic Lower Airway Mechanisms

Bronchoalveolar lavage specimens from normal individuals contain 45% albumin and 17% immunoglobulins. The role of airspace immunoglobulins in lung defense is not fully understood.

Mechanical Ventilation, Airway Colonization, and the Development of Nosocomial Pneumonia

Colonization of the Oropharynx

Bacterial colonization of the oropharynx routinely precedes the occurrence of lower respiratory tract infections. The incidence of oropharyngeal colonization appears to be related to the severity and duration of illness. Because endotracheal intubation bypasses all the host defenses proximal to the vocal cords, this predisposes to bacterial colonization and subsequent infection. The inflated cuff of an endotracheal tube is also a physical barrier to mucociliary transport. Although endotracheal intubation prevents massive aspiration, it can facilitate microaspiration of infected upper airway secretions.

Bacterial Factors That Predispose to Colonization

Bacterial factors are related to the size of the inoculum and virulence of the organism. *Pseudomonas aeruginosa* is notoriously virulent and accounts for 20% to 15% of all nosocomial pneumonias, with a 70% to 90% mortality rate. About 40% of patients who are colonized with *Pseudomonas* ultimately acquire nosocomial infections.

Host Factors That Predispose to Colonization

The rate of colonization with gram-negative species appears to parallel the extent and duration of systemic illness. The incidence of colonization is related to the underlying disease, nutritional status, prior antibiotic therapy, endotracheal intubation, gastric intubation, gastric colonization, advanced age, altered consciousness, hemodynamic instability, presence of lung disease, and incidence of renal failure.

Role of Gastric Colonization in the Development of Nosocomial Pneumonia

The gastrointestinal tract can serve as a reservoir for bacterial and retrograde pharyngeal colonization by organisms. When gastric acid is absent (histamine blockers), the risk of infection and gastric colonization is increased. Migration occurs from the stomach to the oropharynx and subsequent pulmonary aspiration. Factors that facilitate this process include the presence of a nasogastric tube, the method of nutrient delivery, patient position, and gastric motility. Selective decontamination of the gastrointestinal tract by nonabsorbable antibiotics can decrease the incidence of nosocomial pneumonia, but conclusive evidence is lacking.

Noninfectious Inflammatory Lung Disease

Idiopathic pulmonary fibrosis is an interstitial lung disease of unknown cause with a prevalence of 5 per 10^5 population. It occurs in the fifth decade and has a slight male predominance. The mean length of survival after diagnosis is 3 to 5 years. Clinical findings include symmetric coarse basilar crackles, clubbing, restrictive volumes on pulmonary function tests, decreased diffusion capacity, widened alveolar-arterial O_2 gradient with stress, resting hypoxemia refractory to O_2 administration, late hypercapnia, and progressive basilar infiltrates with eventual honeycomb pattern at end stage. Diagnosis is obtained by open lung biopsy, showing intra-alveolar and interstitial inflammation and fibrosis. Attempts to reverse the inflammation with corticosteroids, cyclophosphamide, and azathioprine have not been successful.

The best current hope for prolonged survival after diagnosis is lung transplantation.

PRINCIPLES OF MECHANICAL VENTILATION

Modern mechanical ventilation is capable of providing full or partial ventilatory support. This section describes operator-controlled variables of positive-pressure ventilators, which enable clinicians to balance the detrimental effects of mechanical ventilation with the achievement of desired physiologic goals.

Operator Control of Mechanical Insufflation

Insufflation mechanism uses two electromechanical valves to proportion air and O_2 to achieve selected FIO_2 (range, 0.21–1.0) with a precision of 0.04 to 0.07. Inspiratory valves are used to modulate gas flow rates according to the selected control panel variables. Gas from the inspiratory valve passes through a bacterial filter and humidifier into the breathing circuit. These devices do not add significant resistance to the gas flow.

Volume Control Mechanical Insufflation

The operator-selected variables available in the volume control ventilatory mode include the following:

Initiation and termination mechanism: Each volume-controlled breath can be initiated automatically (controlled or intermittent mandatory ventilation) or can be synchronized with spontaneous inspiration (assist control or synchronized intermittent mandatory ventilation). A threshold pressure change to begin mechanical insufflation is selected as the least possible value that avoids autoinitiation. The mechanical insufflation is terminated after a selected time (time cycled) or volume (volume cycled) has been delivered.

V_T: This can be selected directly or indirectly by setting the ventilator rate and V_E.

Flow characteristics: During volume-controlled mechanical insufflation, the flow can be constant, sinusoidal, or decelerating. Available data suggest that at the same V_T and inspiratory time, alveolar ventilation is unchanged by different inspiratory flow patterns. The selected gas flow should equal to or slightly above the patient's intrinsic flow requirements.

Postinsufflation pause mechanism: Activation of this parameter delays opening of the expiratory valve after a normal volume- or time-cycled mechanical breath. A postinsuflation pause can improve alveolar gas mixing and enhance CO_2 elimination. It is also used to estimate quasistatic recoil pressure of the respiratory system (quasistatic compliance). This parameter should be titrated in increments, because patient–ventilator asynchrony may limit its use.

Pressure Control Mechanical Ventilation

Operator or selected variables for pressure control ventilation include the following:

Initiation and termination mechanisms: Mechanical insufflation can be initiated automatically (pressure control) or can be synchronized with spontaneous inspiration (pressure support). Insufflation termination can be time-cycled (see earlier) or can occur when inspiratory flow declines to a factory-selected level. For additional safety, insufflation also terminates if an upper limit of pressure is reached. Pressure support can be used alone or combined with volume control ventilation (synchronized intermittent mandatory ventilation).

Mechanical insufflation pressure: Because the volume delivered during pressure control depends on the resistance and compliance of the respiratory system, V_T fluctuates with alterations of respiratory system impedance. When insufflation pressure is constant, inspiratory flow is initially maximal and then declines as Pi approaches alveolar pressure. Some ventilators allow a gradual increase of pressure toward the selected insufflation pressure.

Automatic Pressure-Regulated Ventilation

A selected V_T or V_E can be achieved with automatic regulation of insufflation pressure. With this technique, the insufflation pressure is automatically titrated based on the respiratory mechanics to achieve a desired inspired V_T. The insufflation pressure can be automatically increased or decreased depending on the selected V_T or V_E. The selected V_T is sustained even when respiratory rate increases and the actual V_E is greater than the selected V_E. If the spontaneous breathing rate is less than anticipated, the electronic logic automatically calculates a new target V_T to sustain selected minimum V_E.

Operator Control After Completed Mechanical Insufflation

When mechanical insufflation is terminated, expired gas is vented to the environment through an electromechanical or pneumatic balloon valve. Ideally, an expiratory valve should permit rapid reduction of breathing circuit pressure to atmospheric pressure or selected level of PEEP. The expiratory time is determined by the inspiratory time and total cycle time.

Some ventilators allow an expiratory pause hold to determine end-expiratory lung pressure. When the end-expiratory pressure is increased above atmospheric pressure or the selected PEEP level, this is termed *dynamic hyperinflation* or *auto-PEEP* and implies an inadequate expiratory time. Increasing expiratory time while preserving optimized V_T can be accomplished by decreasing cycle frequency or decreasing inspiratory time (directly or by increasing gas flow rate).

PEEP can be used during spontaneous breathing and is usually administered as CPAP. As the patient breathes, CPAP is regulated by modulation of gas flow and tension of the expiratory valve.

Technical Considerations of Mechanical Ventilator Monitoring

Electronic Source

In the event of inadvertent power cord disconnection, a fully charged battery or capacitor should provide sufficient audible tone for at least 5 minutes.

Pneumatic Source

If either the O_2 or the air gas source decreases below a critical pressure, it should activate an audible alarm and visual pressure indicator.

Oxygen Concentration

Most O_2 monitoring systems in mechanical ventilators activate an alarm when the delivered O_2 concentration deviates from the selected threshold.

Gas Flow and Volume Monitoring

Continuous monitoring of inspired and expired gas flow is performed to rapidly detect hypoventilation caused by ventilator failure or leaks in the patient–ventilator system.

Alarms

An audible alarm can be adjusted to indicate a low or high V_E or V_T. Alarms are also available to detect a preset peak airway pressure limit, low inspiratory pressure, and loss of PEEP or CPAP. An acute decrease in peak airway pressure should prompt evaluation of exhalation valve malfunction or hypoventilation. An acute increase in peak airway pressure should prompt evaluation for airway secretions, H_2O condensate in tubing, bronchospasm, kinked endotracheal tube, tension pneumothorax, patient–ventilator phasing problems, and improper valve function.

AIRWAY PRESSURE THERAPY

Classification

The goals of airway pressure therapy are (1) static alteration in transpulmonary pressure to change resting lung volume and (2) dynamic, cyclic alteration to augment alveolar ventilation.

The interfacing of spontaneous and mechanical ventilation is done by modulating V_E or V_T. V_E is modulated by adding mechanical breaths to spontaneous breathing such as with intermittent mandatory ventilation. This ventilatory technique provides a minimum $\dot{V}_E$ regardless of spontaneous drive, but it leaves some or all additional spontaneous respiratory efforts unsupported and does not respond to an increase in ventilatory demand. Pressure support ventilation provides support of each spontaneous breath, and the mechanical ventilatory support increases in response to an increased ventilatory demand. It requires sensitive synchronizing mechanisms and reliable spontaneous respiratory efforts.

Static Airway Pressure Therapy: Positive End-Expiratory Pressure and Continuous Positive Airway Pressure

Sustained elevation in lung volume can be accomplished by applying PEEP when patients are receiving mechanical ventilation and CPAP with patients are breathing spontaneously. The goals of increasing end-expiratory lung volume include improvement of V/Q matching to alleviate hypoxemia and to decrease the work of breathing.

Ventilation, Perfusion, and Positive End-Expiratory Pressure

Most gas exchange between the lungs and blood occurs during the expiratory phase. PEEP augments ventilation in poorly aerated alveoli and by recruiting previously collapsed alveoli into effective gas exchange. Thus, it alleviates V/Q mismatching and intrapulmonary shunting of blood. PEEP can also lead to overinflation and can increase physiologic dead space, however, and thereby can decrease effective alveolar ventilation. Therefore, to minimize V/Q mismatching in all lung regions, it is important to allow spontaneous ventilation to persist at a level comfortable to the patient, while mechanical ventilation is used to prevent respiratory acidemia and excessive work of breathing. The lowest possible F_{IO_2} to maintain an acceptable Sa_{O_2} maximizes alveolar nitrogen concentration, minimizes absorption atelectasis and right-to-left intrapulmonary shunting, and may decrease the need for PEEP. The optimal PEEP level must take into account pulmonary gas exchange, lung mechanics, and circulatory function.

Work of Breathing

When the distending pressure of the lung–thorax system is zero, as occurs when airway pressure is ambient, the lung volume is the FRC. In patients with acute lung injury, a shift in the volume–pressure curve not only decreases FRC but can increase the work of breathing by requiring a greater pressure change for the same V_T. By applying PEEP to increase distending pressure, the FRC is restored and the pressure change required to produce V_T is smaller. Thus, lung compliance is improved and the work of breathing is reduced. The application of CPAP or PEEP can also reduce respiratory work related to increased upper airway resistance.

In patients with obstructive airway disease and expiratory airflow limitation, low levels of PEEP can improve the efficiency of ventilation and reduce the dyspnea. In these cases, PEEP can decrease the inspiratory muscle work required to overcome the resting pressure gradient between the alveoli and airway opening (equal to the amount of auto-PEEP). If excess PEEP is applied, however, it can lead to further hyperinflation and circulatory compromise.

Continuous Positive Airway Pressure

Spontaneous respiration with elevated airway pressure has been used for more than six decades. In patients with low end-expiratory lung volumes, CPAP can improve compliance, improve V/Q matching, increase oxygenation, and reduce the work of breathing. CPAP can be delivered by means of a tight-fitting facemask without endotracheal intubation in patients with intact protective reflexes.

Adverse Effects of Sustained Positive Airway Pressure

Excessive PEEP can overinflate the lungs, increase physiologic dead space, and impair pulmonary and systemic blood flow. Spontaneous respiratory work increases because of the low compliance of the distended lungs, and the respiratory muscles are forced to operate at an unfavorable length–tension range. Patients who have high lung compliance and low chest wall compliance are particularly susceptible to circulatory impairment from elevated airway pressure.

Complications such a pneumothorax, pneumomediastinum, and interstitial pulmonary emphysema, which are seen in patients receiving mechanical ventilatory support, are rare in patients who breathe spontaneously with positive airway pressure. With appropriate PEEP level, improvement in lung mechanics should allow a reduction in mechanical ventilatory support with fewer positive-pressure breaths, minimizing the risk of barotrauma.

Mechanical Ventilatory Support

Partial and Total Ventilatory Support

The goals of mechanical ventilation in patients with acute respiratory failure are to provide treatment of the symptoms of alveolar hypoventilation and to reduce the respiratory work of breathing. Complete control of ventilation in patients with an intrinsic respiratory drive is difficult. Sedatives can be used to raise the apneic threshold, but deep sedation and prolonged neuromuscular blockade are not without significant risks. Controlled mechanical ventilation for prolonged periods can result in a reduced respiratory muscle strength and uncoordinated breathing when spontaneous ventilation is resumed. Maintenance of some spontaneous breathing activity during the course of ventilator therapy is desirable.

Ventilation by Increase in Airway Pressure

The following techniques use an increase in airway pressure to generate V_T. They differ from one another in the method of interfacing spontaneous breathing and mechanical ventilation.

Intermittent Mandatory Ventilation

Intermittent mandatory ventilation is one of the most widely used ventilatory techniques in critically ill patients. During intermittent mandatory ventilation, positive-pressure breaths are delivered with an operator-adjusted rate, and unassisted spontaneously breathing is allowed to occur simultaneously. The degree of mechanical ventilatory support can vary from 0% to 100%.

Mandatory Minute Ventilation

Mandatory V_E provides positive-pressure ventilatory support similar to the function of a demand cardiac pacemaker. If a patient's spontaneous V_E is less than a preset level, the ventilator provides the difference. If the patient's V_E matches the desired level, no ventilatory support is provided.

Inverse Ratio Ventilation

Inverse ratio ventilation has an inspiratory-to-expiratory ratio greater than 1. The prolonged inspiratory phase maintains a higher mean alveolar pressure to maximally recruit alveolar units. Inverse ration ventilation can be used with either volume control or pressure control ventilation.

Assisted Mechanical Ventilation

With assisted mechanical ventilation, the ventilator responds to each spontaneous breathing effort with a positive-pressure mechanical breath. The V_T depends on the ventilator setting and not on the patient's effort.

Pressure Support Ventilation

Pressure support ventilation augments spontaneous breathing by providing a variable airflow that increases until the airway pressure reaches the preselected level above baseline. The level is adjusted to achieve a desired V_T, ventilatory rate, and patient comfort.

Proportional Assist Ventilation

Proportional assist ventilation provides breath-to-breath ventilatory assistance with positive airway pressure that is determined by the degree of patient effort. The amount of positive airway pressure support is proportional to the instantaneous inspiratory flow and volume generated by the patients. The potential advantage results from the patient's control of the ventilator throughout the ventilatory cycle.

Ventilation by Decrease in Airway Pressure

Airway Pressure Release Ventilation

With airway pressure release ventilation, a CPAP circuit maintains baseline airway pressure above ambient pressure. There is subsequent release of positive airway pressure through a release valve in the expiratory limb. The release valve is controlled by a time that adjusts the duration and frequency of pressure release. Airway pressure release ventilation augments alveolar ventilation as an adjunct to spontaneous breathing with CPAP.

Intermittent Mandatory Pressure Release Ventilation

Intermittent mandatory pressure release ventilation combines pressure support ventilation with CPAP and airway pressure release ventilation. The respiratory cycle begins with a pressure support breath, followed by airway pressure release below the CPAP level. This requires a microprocessor-controlled ventilator and is not routinely available.

HIGH-FREQUENCY VENTILATION AND OSCILLATION

High-frequency ventilation delivers 3000 breaths per minute (1–50 Hz) with VTs that are near or less than anatomic dead space. The goals of high-frequency ventillation and oscillation are to improve gas exchange while minimizing barotrauma, decreasing adverse hemodynamic effects of mechanical ventilation, and facilitating ventilation during certain procedures, such as laryngoscopy and bronchoscopy.

Types of High-Frequency Ventilation

High-Frequency Positive-Pressure Ventilation

High-frequency positive-pressure ventilation (HFPPV) is basically intermittent positive-pressure ventilation at increased rates with low VT. However, standard ventilators cannot effectively provide HFPPV because of high internal and circuit compliance. HFPPV uses frequencies of 60 to 100 breaths per minute, VT of 3 to 5 mL/kg, and inspiratory–expiratory ratios of less than 0.3. Expiration is passive.

High-Frequency Jet Ventilation

With high-frequency jet ventilation (HFJV) small VT is delivered through a catheter placed in the trachea. Because of entrainment of additional gas, the actual VT may be greater than the volume delivered from the jet catheter. An ancillary circuit provides continuous flow of humidified gas. The V_T is proportional to the size of the jet catheter, driving pressure and inspiratory time. Generally, frequencies of 100 to 150 breaths per minute at driving pressures of 10 to 40 psi are used with a resultant V_T of 2 to 5 mL/kg. Inspiratory–expiratory ratios range from 0.1 to 0.5, and exhalation is passive.

When switching a patient from conventional ventilation to HFJV, the following general guidelines should be followed:

1. Set frequency of 100 to 150 breaths per minute
2. Inspiratory to expiratory ratio (I/E) set at 1/10–1/2
3. F_{IO_2} and PEEP levels equal to the pre-HFJV level
4. Driving pressure adjusted to produce a mean airway pressure equal to that on conventional positive-pressure ventilation

Arterial oxygenation can be altered by changing F_{IO_2}, mean airway pressure (driving pressure), and FRC (PEEP level). Increasing CO_2 elimination (increasing alveolar ventilation) can be accomplished by increasing driving pressure or inspiratory time.

High-Frequency Oscillation

High-frequency oscillation differs from the other modes of high-frequency ventilation in that both inspiratory and expiratory phases are active, V_Ts are smaller, and frequencies are higher. Typically, frequencies of 4 to 15 Hz are used with the oscillatory amplitude, and the rate of bias flow is adjusted as needed to target appropriate Pa_{CO_2} levels. Oxygenation is determined by lung volume and F_{IO_2}.

Clinical Uses of High-Frequency Ventilation

Management of the Difficult Airway

Percutaneous transtracheal HFJV can be used emergently in patients who cannot be intubated or ventilated by mask ventilation. HFJV is achieved by puncturing the cricothyroid membrane with a 14- to 16-gauge catheter that is connected to a high-pressure gas source.

Ventilation During a Diagnostic or Surgical Procedure

Both HFJV and HFPPV have been used during laryngoscopy, bronchoscopy, endoscopic laser surgery, upper airway and tracheal surgery, extracorporeal shock wave lithotripsy, and anterior thoracic spinal fusion. High-frequency ventilation is beneficial for any procedure in which it is advantageous to minimize lung or diaphragmatic movement.

Infant and Adult Respiratory Distress Syndrome

In infants, high-frequency ventilation can reduce the complications associated with conventional positive-pressure ventilation, such as bronchopulmonary dysplasia, although this is not universally accepted. Often, it is used to manage severe respiratory failure that might otherwise require treatment with extracorporeal membrane oxygenation. In adults, despite theoretic advantages, studies have failed to show any advantage of high-frequency ventilation over conventional positive-pressure ventilation.

Bronchopleural Fistula and Airway Disruption

High-frequency ventilation can provide superior oxygenation and ventilation in the presence of a bronchopleural fistula with a large air leak. Not all published studies support this conclusion, however.

Hemodynamic Instability

When high-frequency ventilation is synchronized to the cardiac cycle during systole, there is an increase in cardiac output in conditions of hypovolemia, cardiac tamponade, acute mitral regurgitation, and heart failure.

Enhanced Mucus Clearance

During asymmetric high-frequency oscillation (expiratory greater than inspiratory flow), an increased volume of sputum appears in the central airways. This ventilatory technique may prove useful as an adjunct to physiotherapy.

Weaning from Assisted to Spontaneous Ventilation

There is no clear agreement on the role of high-frequency ventilation for weaning from mechanical ventilation. The use of high-frequency ventilation alone or superimposed on conventional positive-pressure ventilation warrants further investigation.

Potential Complications and Limitations

The following complications are relatively unique to high-frequency ventilation:

Necrotizing tracheobronchitis: secondary to "jackhammer" effect of high-velocity gas flows and difficulty in humidifying inspired gas adequately

Airway obstruction: due to inadequate humidification, which leads to desiccated, inspissated airway secretions and epithelium

Dynamic hyperinflation: can lead to barotrauma and have deleterious hemodynamic effects

Lack of familiarity with high-frequency ventilation: ventilatory parameters are very different form conventional positive-pressure ventilation, and adjustments are largely empiric.

INDEPENDENT LUNG VENTILATION

Independent lung ventilation is justified when conventional pulmonary support fails in patients with any kind of acute, asymmetric lung injury. It has been used most commonly for the following conditions:

1. Selective airway protection: lavage for alveolar proteinosis, purulent secretions, massive unilateral hemoptysis
2. Correction of severe, life-threatening hypoxemia due to V/Q mismatching: pneumonia, pulmonary contusion, pulmonary hemorrhage or refractory atelectasis
3. Management of bronchopleural fistula (uses hypoventilation and less PEEP)
4. Single- and double-lung transplants

Criteria and Methods for Institution of Independent Lung Ventilation

The evaluation and management of potential candidates for independent lung ventilation should proceed in an orderly sequence in the application of mechanical ventilation. A trial of combined gravitational maneuvers (i.e., positioning) and aggressive respiratory therapy is initiated to reverse the primary disorder. During mechanical ventilation with a conventional single-lumen tube, specific maneuvers designed to recruit collapsed alveoli include lateral decubitus positioning (with the affected lung uppermost) and periodic hyperoxic hyperinflations.

Patients with asymmetric lung disease have a maldistribution of PEEP, V_T, and pulmonary blood flow. Pathologic conditions that are amenable to the benefits independent lung ventilation are those in which bulk gas flow is affected because of unilateral differences in airway resistance or compliance. When a paradoxical decrease in PaO_2 is seen in response to PEEP, it strongly suggests inhomogeneous lung disease. Besides physically separating the lungs to prevent contamination of blood, purulent matter, or fluid, independent lung ventilation is useful primarily in redistributing the delivery of positive-pressure ventilation to match pulmonary blood flow and enhance oxygenation and ventilation.

Synchronous Versus Asynchronous Independent Lung Ventilation

In studies on patients undergoing thoracic surgery, only minor alterations have been reported in heart rate, systemic blood pressure, cardiac output, intracardiac pressures, venous admixture, and arterial blood gases with the more cumbersome technique of synchronizing two independent ventilators when performing independent lung ventilation.

Intubating Technique

Left-sided double-lumen endobronchial tubes are indicated in most situations except for left bronchial mainstem stenosis or obstruction and some thoracic aortic aneurysms. Left-sided bronchial intubation is preferred to avoid occluding the right upper lobe bronchial orifice. A stylet is used to position the distal curved angle anteriorly when passing the tube tip between the vocal cords. Once past the cords, the stylet is removed and the tube is rotated 90° to the left and advanced toward the intended left mainstem bronchus until slight resistance in encountered. The cuffs are then inflated using minimum occluding volume to stop leakage (if more than 3 mL is required, the distal cuff is probably dislodged above the carina). Confirmation of tube placement can be done "blindly" or, preferably, with fiberoptic bronchoscopy visualization. The tube can be secured by combining neck stabilization (rigid collar) with tube fixation.

Once independent lung ventilation is started, monitoring must be compulsive to ensure proper separation of ventilation and to troubleshoot for arterial hypoxemia (Tables 5–25 and 5–26).

Complications Associated with Double-Lumen Endobronchial Tubes

A rare and disastrous potential complication of the double-lumen endobronchial tube is tracheobronchial rupture after insertion. Risk factors for this complication include placement by an inexperienced operator, stylet use, multiple placement attempts, tracheal abnormalities, overdistention of tracheal or bronchial cuffs, and advanced patient age. Patient movement can result in bronchial laceration.

Table 5–25. DIFFERENTIAL DIAGNOSIS OF ARTERIAL HYPOXEMIA DURING INDEPENDENT LUNG VENTILATION

Mechanical Tube Obstruction
Distal migration of either right or left DLEB tube, which impairs ventilation
Distal migration of the tracheal cuff into the unintubated mainstem bronchus
Proximal migration of the DLEB tube cuff with herniation into the trachea or opposing mainstem bronchus
Inadvertent intubation of the opposing mainstem bronchus
Intraluminal obstruction caused by secretions or blood
Extraluminal obstruction caused by kinking, mediastinal mass, or cuff overinflation
Nondependent Lung Factors (Shunt Physiology)
Pulmonary: altered HPV
Cardiac: pulmonary hypertension with a patent foramen ovale or atrial septal defect
Dependent Lung Factors (Gravitational Effects of Qpa)
Worsening of $\dot{V}/\dot{Q}$ matching due to mediastinal and diaphragmatic shifts in decubitus positions
Cardiac Output-Related Factors (Cardiopulmonary Interactions)
Auto-PEEP limiting venous return with elevation in right ventricular afterload and reduced cardiac output
DLEB tube cuff inflation obstructing pulmonary artery outflow and limiting cardiac output

Abbreviations: DLEB = double lumen endobronchial; HPV = hypoxic pulmonary vasoconstriction; Qpa = pulmonary artery blood flow.

Table 5–26. MONITORING OF EFFECTIVE LUNG SEPARATION DURING INDEPENDENT LUNG VENTILATION*

Chest auscultation
- Clamping and declamping of tracheal and endobronchial lumens sequentially

Serial analysis of differential pulmonary parameters
- Exhaled tidal volume
- Peak-airway pressure
- Auto-PEEP
- Varying FIO_2
- Comparison of dual capnograms
- Pressure-volume hysteresis loops

Chest radiographs

Flexible fiberoptic bronchoscopy

*Serial documentation in establishing a baseline for comparison is more helpful than any one parameter alone.

Weaning from Independent Lung Ventilation

Weaning should commence when the physiologic differences between the two lungs have resolved or diminished sufficiently to allow conventional ventilation. Criteria to predict success in converting from independent lung ventilation to conventional ventilation are described in Table 5–27. To test the feasibility of whole-lung ventilation and the termination of independent lung ventilation, the endobronchial cuff can be deflated and a Y-adapter inserted to allow single ventilatory support through the double-lumen endobronchial tube. If hemodynamics and gas exchange remain stable (2–4 hours), exchange of endotracheal tubes is accomplished, and the patient is placed onto a conventional mode of ventilation.

Table 5–27. WEANING CRITERIA TO SINGLE-LUMEN VENTILATION FROM INDEPENDENT LUNG VENTILATION

- PEEP differential < 5 cm H_2O
- Compliance differential < 10 mL/cm H_2O
- Raw < 3 cm $H_2O \cdot L^{-1} \cdot S^{-1}$
- Stability of PaO_2 on equalizing selective PEEP*
- Stability of left-sided and right-sided heart function on equalizing selective PEEP*
- Chest radiographic resolution of asymmetry after equalizing selective PEEP*
- Combined differential minute ventilation < 12 L/min
- Bronchopleural fistula closure

*Deflation of endobronchial cuff with Y-adapter linking the tube to a single mechanical ventilator.

Abbreviation: Raw = airway resistance.

COMPUTERIZED MANAGEMENT OF MECHANICAL VENTILATION

The primary areas of computer application in the management of mechanical ventilation are operation of mechanical ventilators, charting and information systems, and decision support.

Computers in the Operation of Mechanical Ventilators

Microprocessors can provide rapid and precise control of gas delivery while simultaneously collecting data and monitoring ventilator performance. For example, to produce pressure support ventilation, the ventilator monitors airway pressure and opens or closes valves as needed to maintain the desired pressure level.

Charting and Informational System

Respiratory care information systems have not received widespread acceptance, most likely because of an inability to justify the cost. Studies have demonstrated that data management systems can increase productivity, reduce the number of errors, and improve quality, accuracy, and timely capture and retrieval of data. There is no documentation of decrease in the staffing requirements or improvement in the quality of patient care, however.

Fully Integrated Data Base

An effective system needs to interface with other sources of data outside the intensive care unit such as admissions, discharges, and transfers, laboratories, radiology department, operating rooms, and outpatient clinics.

Automated Charting of Data from Mechanical Ventilators

Only custom interfaces that are specifically matched to a particular ventilator are available. Future systems need to incorporate standards for artifact rejection and significant event identification. Little or no data are available on how automated charting of mechanical ventilation data can affect patient outcome.

Tools for Decision-Making Support

These tools must provide decision-making support that includes the following: (1) access to information systems (e.g., MEDLINE), (2) alarms and alerts, (3) expert systems, and (4) closed-loop control

ON-LINE ACCESS TO REFERENCE AND TRAINING MATERIALS

On-line access would provide the ability to have immediate access to further information on any clinical scenario.

For example, if a clinician is reviewing a flow-volume loop and wants more information on interpretation, the computer could retrieve the latest journal articles on the subject.

Integrated Alarms and Alerts

Automated alarms and alerts can generate a wide variety of data, such as drug allergies, drug–drug interactions, drug selection and dosing, blood ordering, infectious disease surveillance, organ dysfunction, and critical changes of laboratory or physiologic parameters. Respiratory care alerts can be triggered in response to elevated endotracheal cuff pressures, high PEEP, high inspired O_2 concentration, or carboxyhemoglobin.

Expert Systems

Expert systems can be used for either diagnostic or therapeutic purposes. Most are traditional rule-based expert systems ("if A is greater than two, do B"). Pulmonary diagnostic expert systems include interpretation of blood gas data, ventilator management, and weaning from mechanical ventilation.

Closed-Loop Control

Closed-loop control is similar to an expert system except that the computer directly adjusts the mechanical ventilator. Despite the development of several clever and sophisticated systems, none of the closed-loop systems have had a major impact on clinical care.

HEMODYNAMIC EFFECTS OF MECHANICAL VENTILATION

Cardiopulmonary interactions can occur that significantly alter cardiac output and thus O_2 delivery to the tissues. Accordingly, the critical care physician must understand the hemodynamic effects of mechanical ventilation to optimize cardiorespiratory support (Table 5–28).

Table 5–28. FACTORS THAT DETERMINE HEART–LUNG INTERACTIONS

- Lung volume
- Pulmonary vascular resistance
- Ventricular interdependence
- Mechanical heart–lung interactions
- Pressure gradient for systemic venous return, modified by:
  - Circulating blood volume
  - Peripheral vasomotor tone
  - Intra-abdominal pressure
- Pressure gradient for left ventricular ejection, modified by:
  - Ventricular contractility
  - Mitral valve function

Effects of Ventilation on Lung Volume and Intrathoracic Pressure

Ventilation can affect hemodynamics by changing lung volume or intrathoracic pressure. The hemodynamic alterations can be mediated by mechanical factors, neuroreflex mechanisms (autonomic tone), and humoral cardiodepressant substances.

Because intrathoracic pressure increases during positive-pressure inspiration and decreases during spontaneous inspiration (whereas lung volume increases during both), the effects of positive-pressure ventilation on cardiovascular performance are not the same as those of spontaneous respiration, despite similar changes in lung volume.

Right Ventricular Performance

Right ventricular (RV) systolic performance is determined by preload, afterload, contractility, interdependence with the left ventricle (LV), and its own conformational changes. The *unstressed volume* refers to RV filling that occurs without changes in RV wall stress. Thus, it is difficult to assess RV preload from measures of RV filling pressures.

During spontaneous inspiration, right atrial pressure decreases, increasing the pressure gradient between the systemic veins and the right atrium, and augmenting systemic venous return. This results in an increase in RV preload and augments RV stroke volume. Conversely, positive-pressure inspiration increases right atrial pressure, so that venous return, RV preload, and RV stroke volume are lower, and so, ultimately, is cardiac output.

RV afterload is a function of RV end-diastolic volume and systolic RV pressure (related to pulmonary vascular resistance). Overdistention of the lungs—as in obstructive lung disease, ventilation with large V_T and high levels of PEEP—increases pulmonary vascular resistance. Mechanical ventilation can decrease pulmonary vascular resistance if it increases alveolar O_2 concentration and re-expands collapsed alveoli.

The effects of positive-pressure ventilation on RV performance depend on the degree to which venous return (preload) is reduced and pulmonary vascular resistance (afterload) is increased. In most patients, it serves to decrease cardiac output compared with spontaneous breathing.

Left Ventricular Performance

Left ventricular performance is determined by preload, contractility, afterload, and heart rate. Artificial ventilation can decrease LV end-diastolic volume by decreasing systemic venous return, leftward shift of interventricular septum when RV dilates because of increased pulmonary vascular resistance (ventricular interdependence), and limitations imposed by the semirigid pericardium.

Although septal shift, pericardial constraints, and mechanical heart–lung interactions (compression of heart by expanding lungs) function by different means, all three mechanisms decrease the "effective" LV diastolic compliance and respond to volume challenges with an increased cardiac output.

Overestimation of LV end-diastolic pressure can be minimized by measuring at its nadir immediately after airway disconnection (known as getting a "pop-off" wedge pressure). Artificial ventilation can improve LV performance for a given LV preload by eliminating the negative pressure fluctuations in intrathoracic pressure seen during spontaneous ventilation. This works by decreasing afterload LV ejection pressure. The net hemodynamic effect is determined by the balance between preload and afterload.

Cardiac Performance During the Ventilatory Cycle

With decreased lung compliance, or increased resistance to inspiration, spontaneous inspiratory efforts may be associated with profound negative fluctuations in intrathoracic pressure that increase venous return and reduce LV output, resulting in pulmonary edema. This is a postulated mechanism of pulmonary edema in patients with asthma and upper airway obstruction.

In addition, artificial ventilation minimizes the work of breathing and decreases O_2 consumption, thereby increasing the mixed venous O_2 content. Under these conditions, artificial ventilation can increase the arterial O_2 content without primarily affecting either gas exchange or cardiac output.

WEANING FROM MECHANICAL VENTILATION

Prolonged mechanical ventilation increases the risk for nosocomial pneumonia and the cost of care. Most patients, especially postoperative surgical patients, do not have a problem with discontinuation of ventilatory support. A significant minority, however, require a longer period before this can be achieved. The transition between mechanical ventilation and spontaneous breathing is referred to as *weaning*.

Determinants of Weaning Outcome

Adequacy of Pulmonary Gas Exchange

Hypoxemia may result with a return to spontaneous ventilation from impaired pulmonary gas exchange, hypoventilation, or decreased mixed venous saturation.

Respiratory Muscle Performance

Inadequacy of respiratory muscle function is the most common cause of failure to wean. It can result from decreased neuromuscular capacity, increased demand or load, or a combination of both.

Decreased Neuromuscular Capacity

Decreased respiratory center function can result in a failure to wean. In most patients who fail to wean, however, respiratory drive is actually increased.

The phrenic nerve may be dysfunctional after cardiac surgery, from hypothermic injury or stretching of the nerve. In some patients with sepsis and multiple organ failure, an entity called *polyneuropathy of critically ill* leads to axonal neuropathy.

Respiratory muscle function itself can be impaired by several factors. Dynamic hyperinflation, malnutrition, electrolyte imbalance (potassium, calcium, phosphate, and magnesium), and endocrine abnormalities (hypothyroidism and hyperthyroidism) reduce respiratory muscle function. Other factors include decreased O_2 supply to the respiratory muscles from LV dysfunction, possible respiratory muscle atrophy from prolonged mechanical ventilation, and respiratory muscle fatigue. Fatigue is difficult to define. Electromyographic power shifts, clinical observations of abdominal paradox, and respiratory alternans have been suggested as markers for fatigue. This area remains controversial, however. Abdominal–respiratory muscle paradox may represent increased respiratory loading conditions rather than fatigue.

Increased Respiratory Load

Respiratory load can be increased from either increased ventilatory requirements or increased work of breathing. Increased ventilatory requirements result from increased $\dot{V}CO_2$, increased dead space ventilation, or an inappropriately elevated respiratory drive. If $\dot{V}CO_2$ is high, a physiologic dead space to tidal volume ratio above 0.6 is considered to preclude weaning because of the excessively high ventilatory requirements.

Excessive work of breathing (joules per liter of ventilation or joules per minute) often leads to failure to wean, but the threshold value for successful weaning varies among studies. In healthy humans at rest, the O_2 cost of breathing is less than 5% of total body O_2 consumption, but this may become excessively high (>50%) for some patients as they are weaned because of involvement of other factors (e.g., catecholamine release) adding to the increased $\dot{V}O_2$ of spontaneous breathing.

Psychologic Factors

Feelings of insecurity, anxiety, fear, agony, and panic have been associated with problems of weaning. There are few data, however, on the degree to which they contribute to ventilator dependency.

Predicting Weaning Outcome

Various indices are available to predict weaning outcome ("science" of weaning) with varying reported success. The physician's bedside assessment probably remains the most valuable indicator for success ("art" of weaning).

Gas Exchange

Different indices of oxygenation have been used ($Pa{O_2}/FI{O_2}$ ratio, alveolar-arterial $P{O_2}$ gradient), but prospective evaluation has yielded poor predictive values, although the oxygenation criteria given in Table 5–29 are widely accepted.

Maximum Inspiratory Pressure

Respiratory muscle function is an important factor in determining weaning outcome. Global information on respiratory muscle strength can be obtained by measuring PI_{max}. Recent prospective studies, however, have failed to confirm the predictive value of this test. This may be a reflection of poor patient cooperation.

Vital Capacity

A normal vital capacity is between 65 and 75 mL/kg. A value of 10 mL/kg or more has been suggested as vital for sustaining spontaneous ventilation, but again prospective studies have failed to confirm its utility.

Respiratory System Compliance

The compliance of the respiratory system is a direct determinant of the amount of work performed by the respiratory muscle. Yang and Tobin, in their prospective study, found that a value of at least 33 mL/cm H_2O had a positive predictive value of 0.6 and a negative predictive value of 0.53 for a successful weaning outcome.

Minute Ventilation and Maximum Voluntary Ventilation

The relation between resting V_E and maximum voluntary ventilation identifies the degree of reserve available for further respiratory demands. A V_E below 10 L/min with the

Table 5–29. VARIABLES USED TO PREDICT WEANING SUCCESS

Gas Exchange
$Pa{O_2} \geq 60$ mm Hg with $FI{O_2} \leq 0.35$
Alveolar-arterial $P{O_2}$ gradient < 350 mm Hg
$Pa{O_2}/FI{O_2}$ ratio > 200
Ventilator Pump
Vital capacity >10–15 mL/kg
Maximum negative inspiratory pressure < -30 cm H_2O
Minute ventilation < 10 L/min
Maximum voluntary ventilation more than twice resting minute ventilation

ability to double this value formed the basis for predicting successful weaning. Again, results conflict when this index has been prospectively tested.

Airway Occlusion Pressure

Airway occlusion pressure is a measure of respiratory drive. Pressures generated are negative, but $P_{0.1}$ values are reported in positive units. Values are usually less than 2 cm H_2O in healthy subjects. In patients who fail weaning, $P_{0.1}$ values are usually elevated. Others have added a hypercapnic challenge to discriminate further the predictive value of this measure for weaning outcome.

Rapid Shallow Breathing

Tachypnea is usually present with a decrease in V_T in patients who fail weaning. A high f/V_T ratio means rapid shallow breathing and is easily determined at the bedside. Yang and Tobin evaluated this ratio prospectively in spontaneously breathing patients and found that a f/V_T threshold value of less than 105 had the best predictive power in identifying patients who were successfully weaned.

Rib Cage–Abdominal Motion

Marked asynchrony and paradoxical motion of both the rib cage and abdomen have distinguished weaning success from failure. Likewise marked variability in breath-by-breath contribution of the rib cage to V_T (percentage of rib cage involvement) distinguished the failures. The degree of paradoxical breathing and the percentage of rib cage involvement are measured by respiratory inductive plethysmography.

Integrative Indices

Because weaning failure is usually a multifactorial problem, it is not surprising that using a single index has a poor predictive value. An index such as CROP (compliance, rate, oxygenation, and pressure) integrates a number of physiologic functions:

$$\text{CROP index} = (\text{Cdyn} \times \text{P}_{\text{I}}\text{max} \times [\text{PaO}_2/\text{PAO}_2]/\text{rate})$$

Yang and Tobin evaluated this index prospectively and found positive and negative predictive values of 0.71 and 0.70, respectively, for a successful weaning outcome.

Methods of Discontinuing Mechanical Ventilation

Abrupt Discontinuation

Patients who receive short periods of ventilator support, especially postoperative patients, can be extubated rapidly when the effects of anesthetics and muscle-relaxing drugs have worn off or are reversed.

Spontaneous Breathing Trials

A spontaneous breathing trial using a T-piece trial is the traditional method of weaning. Respiratory gas flow to the inspiratory limb of at least twice the patient's spontaneous VE is provided to meet the patient's peak inspiratory flow rate. An extension piece should be added to the expiratory limb to prevent entrainment of room air. Such T-piece trials can be used for short periods at regular intervals, providing for rest between trials with gradual prolongation of the trials if the patient tolerates them well. Once a patient can undertake a T-piece trial for 30 to 60 minutes, he or she usually can be extubated successfully if there are no other concerns about upper airway control or obstruction. Alternatively, T-piece trials can be used for 30 minutes at the start if one believes that the patient can be rapidly weaned. During these trials, the patient should be closely monitored for signs of hemodynamic or respiratory distress and should receive continuous psychologic support.

Intermittent Mandatory Ventilation

When a patient is deemed ready for weaning, the intermittent mandatory ventilation rate can be reduced in stages while arterial blood gases are monitored. Proponents have cited the benefits of intermittent mandatory ventilation weaning as preventing the patients from fighting the ventilator, reducing the need for sedation and muscle paralysis, and decreasing respiratory alkalemia. The work of breathing during both spontaneous and assisted breaths is increased, however, as support is reduced with demand valve circuits. This can lead to the development of fatigue and actually prolong the weaning process. No advantage of intermittent mandatory ventilation weaning has been demonstrated over T-piece weaning.

Pressure Support Ventilation

Pressure support ventilation is considered a more comfortable mode of weaning, because the patient can control the depth, length, and flow profile of each breath. Appropriate levels of pressure support ventilation can also counteract the increased work from the resistive load of the endotracheal tubes and ventilator circuits. The level of pressure support ventilation is usually set to match the VTs and frequency of the patient on full ventilatory support. The pressure support ventilation is then gradually reduced as tolerated by the patient. Respiratory muscle rest can be provided at night with full ventilatory support. Once a pressure support ventilation level of approximately 5 cm H_2O is reached, the patient is usually ready for extubation. Despite theoretic benefits, pressure support ventilation has not been demonstrated to be superior to any other techniques of weaning.

Summary

Most patients have no trouble with weaning from mechanical ventilation. The major respiratory determinants are respiratory muscle performance, adequacy of gas exchange, and psychologic factors. Cardiac dysfunction can also have a significant impact. The rapid shallow breathing index is a useful bedside aid for predicting successful weaning outcome. Although several techniques for weaning are available, none has been shown to be significantly superior. Some conditions may be more amenable to certain techniques of weaning, however.

POSITIVE-PRESSURE VENTILATION WITHOUT TRACHEAL INTUBATION

Noninvasive positive-pressure ventilation can be used during acute resuscitative efforts in the field and emergency department, in the operating room, and for sustained ventilatory support in the intensive care unit.

Bag-and-Valve System

With bag-and-valve systems, there is high risk for inadequate ventilation because of poor sealing between the mask and face as well as the need for two hands to secure a tight fit.

Esophageal Obturator Airway

The esophageal obturator airway can be described as a facemask with an esophageal obturator to divert flow into the trachea and to prevent gastric insufflation. The esophageal obturator airway was designed to establish a patent airway by personnel with a wide variety of skill and experience. Studies have shown a greater success rate in securing an airway with esophageal obturator airway (98.3%) than with endotracheal intubation (76.9%) in the prehospital setting. The superiority of esophageal obturator airway to endotracheal intubation in the prehospital environment, however, remains to be demonstrated. When using the esophageal obturator airway, efforts should be made to overventilate the patient pending arterial blood gas measurements, since the adequacy of ventilation with this device is not predictable. Potential adverse consequences include tracheal intubation, reduced V_{T}s, supraglottic obstruction, esophageal trauma or rupture, and gastric rupture. Contraindication for esophageal obturator airway insertion because of poor mask seal include edentulous patients and individuals with unusual facial morphology.

Pharyngeal Tracheal Lumen Airway

The pharyngeal tracheal lumen airway has a long tube (with stylet) and a short tube, both with inflatable cuffs. It does not require a facemask. After insertion, both cuffs are inflated, and gas is delivered by positive-pressure through the shorter tube. If the chest wall rises with each breath, the long tube is in the esophagus. Ventilation should continue, and the occluding stylet should remain *in* the long tube to prevent aspiration. If the chest wall does *not* rise with each breath, the long tube is in the trachea, and ventilation must take place through the long tube (with the occluding stylet removed), keeping both cuffs inflated.

Laryngeal Mask Airway

Laryngeal mask airway is a modified endotracheal tube that is obliquely cut anteriorly and has an inflatable low-pressure cuff around the oblique lumen opening. The airway is blindly advanced over the tongue until resistance is met, and the cuff is inflated to isolate the glottic aperture from the pharynx. This device is associated with several problems, including the need for anesthesia on insertion and removal as well as coughing, laryngospasm, inability to protect the airway, and down-folding of the epiglottis.

Positive-Pressure Ventilation Through a Mouthpiece

Previous studies have shown that a lip-seal mouthpiece, held in place by a harness, can be used for nocturnal positive-pressure support in patients with neuromuscular disease. Another application is for postoperative patients who experience short-term difficulty after extubation. Problems with this technique include aspiration pneumonia, dental malocclusion, temporomandibular joint problems, and leakage of delivered V_T through the nose or mouth.

Nasal Mask or Facemask Interfaces for Positive-Pressure Ventilation

Positive-pressure ventilation can be delivered through a full facemask or a nasal mask. The nasal mask offers the advantage of reduced likelihood of aspiration of gastric contents. There can be significant leakage of gas through the mouth, however. When a full oronasal facemask is used, there should be a safety valve to allow for entrainment of room air in the event of mechanical failure.

Noninvasive Positive-Pressure Ventilation to Prevent Tracheal Intubation in Acutely Ill Patients

Continuous Positive Airway Pressure for Patients with Acute Respiratory Failure

With CPAP, a constant positive airway pressure is maintained throughout the inspiratory and expiratory phases of the respiratory cycle. Mask CPAP has been used to treat patients with cardiogenic pulmonary edema and ARDS. Because of conflicting reports on its utility and safety, further research is necessary before definitive recommendations can be made for this form of noninvasive respiratory support.

Continuous Positive Airway Pressure by Mask for Patients with Lower Airway Obstruction

In patients with obstructive airway disease, CPAP can reduce inspiratory effort and improve alveolar ventilation by reducing expiratory bronchiolar collapse. The reduced inspiratory work can come at the expense of increased expiratory work to prevent hyperinflation, however. Further studies are necessary to define the patient population most likely to derive benefit from CPAP delivered by mask.

Continuous Positive Airway Pressure by Mask for Patients with Atelectases

Delivery of CPAP by mask can facilitate resolution of atelectases, although it does not prevent the development of postoperative pulmonary complications.

Continuous Positive Airway Pressure by Mask for Patients with Tracheobronchomalacia

Sputum clearance can be improved in patients with tracheobronchomalacia by CPAP through pneumatic stenting of the airway. CPAP can also relieve dyspnea and facilitate reexpansion of collapsed lung parenchyma.

Noninvasive Positive Pressure Ventilation

Modes of noninvasive ventilation include CPAP, pressure support ventilation, intermittent mandatory ventilation, assist control ventilation, and bilevel positive-pressure ventilation, which permits independent adjustment of inspiratory positive airway pressure and expiratory positive airway pressure. Typical initial settings are 10 cm H_2O for the former and 2 to 5 cm H_2O for the latter, which are then adjusted for patient comfort. If oxygenation is still poor, the pressures can be raised together, keeping the pressure gradient between them constant. For persistent hypercapnia, inspiratory positive airway pressure is increased to augment V_T. Potential complications of noninvasive ventilation include aspiration, patient intolerance, and leakage (loss of V_T).

More work is needed to identify patients most likely to benefit from noninvasive positive-pressure ventilation, to clarify the most efficacious manner in which it should be administered, and to define the associated risks.

EXTRACORPOREAL AND INTRAVASCULAR GAS EXCHANGE DEVICES

Technique of Extracorporeal Life Support

Extracorporeal life support (ECLS) refers to extracorporeal passage of blood through a gas exchange device, or oxygenator, and then return of the blood to a major artery or vein to assist respiration or support blood flow in settings of reversible heart or lung dysfunction (Table 5–30). In the ECLS circuit, blood is drained from the vena cava, pumped through the oxygenator, warmed by a water-jacketed heat exchanger, and returned to a major artery or vein. *Venoarterial bypass* provides cardiac (i.e., blood flow) and respiratory

Table 5–30. COMMON ACRONYMS FOR TYPES OF ARTIFICIAL CARDIAC OR PULMONARY SUPPORT

ECLS	Extracorporeal life support
ECMO	Extracorporeal membrane oxygenation
ECCOR or $ECCO_2R$	Extracorporeal CO_2 removal
$PECCO_2R$	Partial extracorporeal CO_2 removal
ECLA	Extracorporeal lung assist
CPS	Cardiopulmonary support
CPB	Cardiopulmonary bypass
LVAD	Left ventricular assist device
RVAD	Right ventricular assist device
IVOX	Intravascular oxygenator

support (i.e., oxygenation and ventilation), whereas *venovenous bypass* provides respiratory support only.

Venous drainage is accomplished through large-bore, high-flow catheters placed percutaneously or by cutdown into the internal jugular vein, femoral vein, iliac vein, or right atrium (decreasing order of preference). Blood is returned through the common carotid artery, femoral artery, aortic arch, or axillary artery in venoarterial circuits, or through the internal jugular vein, femoral vein, or iliac vein in venovenous circuits. Patients are systemically given heparin before cannulation and during bypass to maintain activated coagulation time at 160 to 200 seconds. Blood products can be given through the circuit to maintain the hematocrit at 30% to 40% and platelets over 100,000/μL, and to replace consumed clotting factors. Other fluids (parenteral nutrition, medications) should be maximally concentrated and can also run through the circuit.

Ultrafiltration can be added to the pressurized portion of the circuit between the pump and the oxygenator through a dialysis membrane. Other modalities, such as slow continuous ultrafiltration and continuous arteriovenous hemofiltration, with or without dialysis, can also be used.

When used for ventilatory support, ECLS allows "lung rest" from high FIO_2 and ventilatory pressures. Once the patient is on ECLS, the ventilator is turned down to more moderate FIO_2 and airway pressures. Once pulmonary function improves sufficiently, the bypass flow is gradually reduced according to the PaO_2 and $PaCO_2$ until the ECLS is less than 10% of the patient's metabolic needs. The mechanical ventilation is then increased as needed for oxygenation and ventilation.

During weaning from ECLS, the patient is "tried off" the oxygenator by clamping its inflow and outflow, but opening the bridge allows continuous circulation through the bypass cannulas. If hemodynamics and gas exchange are stable for 2 to 4 hours, one can consider withdrawing ECLS. If the patient is unable to tolerate the weaning trial, he or she should be returned to ECLS and another attempt made in 24 to 48 hours.

When the patient no longer requires ECLS, percutaneous

venous catheters are removed and the puncture sites are closed. Surgically placed catheters are removed after operative exposure of the vessels. The veins that were used are repaired or ligated as indicated.

Patient Selection

Selection of Neonates

Extracorporeal life support is standard therapy for respiratory failure due to meconium aspiration, infant respiratory distress syndrome, persistent pulmonary hypertension, persistent fetal circulation, pneumonia or sepsis, or congenital diaphragmatic hernia. Various predictors of mortality can be used to select appropriate patients. Early cranial ultrasound and cardiac echocardiography are done to exclude any intracranial bleed or major cardiac anomaly, respectively. Contraindications include estimated gestational age less than 32 weeks, major chromosomal aberration, major cardiac anomaly, and bleeding.

The overall survival rate for neonates requiring ECLS is 83%. The survival rate is highest with the meconium aspiration syndrome (93%) and lowest with congenital diaphragmatic hernia (58%).

Selection of Pediatric and Adult Patients

Respiratory Failure

Indications and exclusion criteria for older and adult patients are listed in Table 5–31.

Cardic Failure

Venoarterial ECLS is typically used as preoperative support of a failing heart ("bridge to transplant") after cardiac surgery or heart transplantion when the cardiac index is low.

Table 5–31. INDICATIONS AND CONTRAINDICATIONS FOR THE INSTITUTION OF EXTRACORPOREAL LIFE SUPPORT FOR PEDIATRIC AND ADULT PATIENTS

Indications
Total static lung compliance < 0.5 mL · cm $H_2O^{-1} \cdot kg^{-1}$
Transpulmonary shunt $> 30\%$ on $F_{IO_2} \geq 0.6$
Reversible respiratory failure
Time on mechanical ventilation ≤ 5 days (10 days absolute maximum)

Exclusions
Potential for severe bleeding
Time on mechanical ventilation 11 days or greater
Necrotizing pneumonia
Poor quality of life (those patients with metastatic malignancy, major central nervous system injury, or quadriplegia)
Age > 65 years

Results

The most common complication during ECLS is bleeding. Other complications include mechanical problems with the circuit, poor limb perfusion distal to the catheters, and trauma to cannulated vessels with resultant thrombosis or stenosis. Neonatal respiratory failure is associated with a high survival rate after the use of ECLS. The prognosis is poorer for older patients. This technology is both exhausting and costly and cannot be considered standard therapy at this time.

The Intravascular Oxygenator

The intravascular oxygenator is used to augment gas exchange, thereby allowing a decrease in VE and ventilatory pressures, thus reducing barotrauma. This is an implantable intracorporeal respiratory support device that is inserted into the femoral or internal jugular vein and that resides in the vena cava, where it is unfurled. The fibers expand to occupy the lumen of the vena cava.

The small-diameter, hollow fibers are made of siloxane-coated microporous polypropylene and carry O_2 from distal to proximal end, where a negative pressure is applied. Gas exchange occurs by means of diffusion across the fiber wall. Effluent gas can be measured for CO_2 concentration. The maximum CO_2 removal capability is approximately one third of the metabolically produced CO_2. The device is less efficient at O_2 transfer to venous blood.

HYPERBARIC OXYGEN IN CRITICAL CARE

Increasing the ambient pressure increases dissolved O_2 in plasma, making more O_2 available to the tissues. Hyperoxia results in peripheral vasoconstriction and reduction in tissue blood flow. It can be useful for cerebral edema, crush injury, burns, and so forth.

Pharmacology of Hyperoxia

Antibacterial Effects

Hypoxia in ischemic tissue can support the growth of anaerobic bacteria. Therefore, during hyperbaric O_2 therapy, there is an increased production of O_2 free radicals, which are directly toxic to the anaerobic bacteria. In addition, the killing of anaerobic bacteria by leukocytes depends on the generation of O_2 free radicals in lysozomes.

Cellular Effects

Hyperbaric O_2 therapy minimizes the leukocyte adherence to endothelium of the microcirculation, improving blood flow and decreasing detriment to O_2 transport through the microcirculation.

Oxygen Toxicity

Pharmacology

Exposure to increased O_2 results in higher production of reactive O_2 species (superoxide anion, hydroxyl radical, hydrogen peroxide, and singlet O_2). Toxicity of these O_2 species depends on both dose and duration of O_2 exposure.

Organ Effects

BRAIN. O_2 toxicity can produce a wide variety of symptoms, ranging from mild paresthesias to generalized convulsions. Factors that increase the risk of central nervous system toxicity include hypercapnia, exertion, and water immersion (in divers). Prophylactic anticonvulsant therapy probably reduces the risk of convulsions when using treatment schedules with significant risk of central nervous system toxicity.

LUNGS. Tracheobronchitis is the first manifestation of O_2 toxicity. Functional abnormalities include decreased forced vital capacity and CO transfer factor. Continued exposure to O_2 results in hyaline membrane formation and proliferation of type II pneumocytes; fibrosis occurs later. The *maximum* safe inspired PO_2 is based on central nervous system toxicity limits, and the *duration* is limited by pulmonary effects.

EYES. Repetitive hyperbaric O_2 therapy sessions can result in myopia, which occasionally is partially reversible. They may also predispose to cataract formation.

PERIPHERAL NERVES. Some patients experience paresthesias, usually fingers or toes, that normally resolve within a day or two.

Uses of Hyperbaric Oxygen for Specific Diseases

Gas Bubble Disease

SPECTRUM OF GAS BUBBLE DISEASE

ACCIDENTAL BUBBLE INJECTION. Intra-arterial injection of gas can result in acute stroke, myocardial infarction, or cardiac arrest. Iatrogenic arterial gas emboli are usually seen during diagnostic procedures, cardiopulmonary bypass, pulmonary barotrauma, and penetrating lung trauma. Venous injection of air can enter the arterial circulation by crossing the pulmonary circulation directly or by means of a patent foramen ovale.

GAS EMBOLISM IN DIVERS. Pulmonary overpressurization is the mechanism by which arterial gas embolism occurs in scuba divers. Once bubbles have entered the arterial tree, the signs and symptoms are due to infarction of end organs. The most common syndromes involve the brain.

IN SITU BUBBLE FORMATION. When a gas is dissolved in a liquid, an acute reduction in ambient pressure can allow the gas to come out of solution. Bubbles can form in any tissue but appear to have a predilection for joints, spinal cord, brain.

TREATMENT

PREHOSPITAL TREATMENT. In addition to the standard principles of resuscitation, the patient should be well hydrated with either oral or intravenous fluids. The highest FIO_2 should be administered as supplemental O_2 washes out blood and tissue nitrogen stores, hastens bubble shrinkage, and ameliorates hypoxia. Conscious victims should be placed in the supine position, and unconscious victims at risk for vomiting should be placed in the lateral decubitus position.

PHYSICAL REMOVAL OF GAS. Aspiration from the superior vena cava or right atrium from an appropriately placed catheter can be life-saving with massive venous gas embolism. In most instances, however, physical removal of gas bubbles from the vascular system is not feasible.

COMPRESSION. Increasing ambient pressure reduces the volume of tissue gas bubbles. Recompression therapy remains the mainstay of treatment for tissue gas. Early treatment is more likely to have complete relief of symptoms than late therapy.

Specific Treatment Protocols

The most commonly used treatment schedules were developed by the U.S. Navy. If a single hyperbaric O_2 treatment does not resolve all symptoms, repetitive treatments are required until a patient has no symptoms or improvement stops.

ADJUNCTIVE MEASURES

CORTICOSTEROIDS. The potential value of corticosteroid administration in patients with decompression illness is unknown.

ANTICOAGULATION. The potential benefits of anticoagulation are weighed against the tissue hemorrhage that can accompany spinal cord and inner ear decompression illness. Therefore, there is no clear agreement on the use of anticoagulation at this time. Nonsteroidal anti-inflammatory drugs with antiplatelet activity are commonly administered to patients without neurologic decompression illness. No benefits other than analgesia have been documented, however.

LIDOCAINE. The mechanism of effect of lidocaine is speculated to be reduction of intracranial pressure and increased cerebral blood flow. No controlled human data are yet available.

FLUOROCARBONS. Because fluorocarbons have a high solubility, intravenous administration can result in faster bubble resolution. Further human studies are pending.

Poisonings

CARBON MONOXIDE

Acute CO toxicity results in multiple organ dysfunction, particularly of the central nervous system. Common reported symptoms and signs include headache, nausea, vomiting, confusion, and loss of consciousness. Reasonable indications for the use of hyperbaric O_2 therapy in CO poisoning include a COHb level of 25% or higher, neurologic impairment, cardiac abnormalities (ischemia, arrhythmia, ventricular failure), and significant exposure during pregnancy. Hyperbaric O_2 treatment is best given within the first few hours. A single treatment is usually sufficient to reduce the COHb to acceptable levels.

OTHER POISONS

Hyperbaric O_2 therapy can also be useful for cyanide poisoning (plastic combustion), hydrogen disulfide, and carbon tetrachloride poisoning.

Necrotizing Infection

CLOSTRIDIAL INFECTIONS

Anaerobic bacteria lack antioxidant defenses and the growth of these organisms is inversely related to tissue P_{O_2}. Hyperbaric O_2 therapy can increase O_2 delivery to infected and uninfected tissues. Hyperbaric O_2 treatments are provided daily until the infection is under control. The literature supports a lower mortality rate in patients with clostridial infections treated with hyperbaric O_2 therapy.

NONCLOSTRIDIAL BACTERIAL INFECTIONS

Nonclostridial necrotizing infections are often mixed aerobic and anaerobic infections. Although the same principles of clostridial infections apply, many of these infections are more indolent and the clinical benefit of hyperbaric O_2 is more difficult to discern.

MUCORMYCOSIS

Rhinocerebral mucormycosis is due to an infection with fungi and usually occurs in patients with diabetes. Hyperbaric O_2 therapy can increase the tissue P_{O_2} and enhance killing of the organism.

Head Injury

Because hyperbaric O_2 decreases cerebral blood flow, it can reduce intracranial pressure. This decrease in intracranial pressure is transient, however, and does not occur when cerebral autoregulation is absent. No data support routine use of hyperbaric O_2 in this situation.

Thermal Injury

Patients treated with hyperbaric O_2 therapy for CO poisoning who also have burns show more rapid healing and less infection than burned patients not treated with hyperbaric O_2. Accumulating evidence shows a benefit of hyperbaric O_2 for the treatment of burns.

Other Indications

Hyperbaric O_2 therapy has been used to support tissue oxygenation transiently in patients with severe anemia who cannot be readily crossmatched or in patients who refuse transfusions.

CHAPTER 6
Visceral Dysfunction and Renal Failure

PART A
Visceral Dysfunction

Juan B. Ochoa, MD

THE ACUTE ABDOMEN

The collection of a *history and physical examination* is the first essential step in the diagnosis of acute abdominal pathology. During this initial assessment, the clinician addresses the following questions:

1. What is the degree of physiologic compromise? Does the patient require immediate resuscitation or cardiovascular monitoring?
2. Are additional tests necessary?
3. Does the patient require urgent surgery?

The threat to cardiorespiratory *homeostasis* is a frequent reason for consulting the intensive care specialist about patients with acute abdominal pathology. The clinician has to assess the degree of compromise to each system and decide the need for invasive cardiorespiratory monitoring and intervention. Intervention can be minimal, such as electrocardiographic monitoring and pulse oximetry, or can be elaborate, such as pulmonary artery catheterization, endotracheal intubation, and mechanical ventilation. The degree of chronic organ dysfunction present before the initiation of the current abdominal problem is a significant determinant of the need for aggressive cardiopulmonary management.

Acute abdominal pathology may be associated with significant intravascular volume and electrolyte alterations. Such patients frequently are dehydrated to the point of becoming hemodynamically unstable. Immediate fluid resuscitation becomes a priority. Renal perfusion and function is evaluated by monitoring urinary output.

CONCEPT: Acute abdominal pathology can alter the function of distant organs and systems to the point of threatening the patient's immediate survival. The intensivist must evaluate the situation and intervene when homeostasis is threatened.

Diagnostic tests should not endanger resuscitation and the restoration of homeostasis. They complement the assessment done by the clinician, however, and often are helpful in determining the need for surgery. The value of clinical assessment decreases when patients are under sedation or are receiving narcotic agents or have altered states of consciousness. Under these conditions, clinicians have to rely more heavily on the information obtained through imaging technologies and laboratory values. Diagnostic testing should not delay surgical intervention if it is clinically indicated, however. Laboratory testing helps to determine the presence of intra-abdominal infection or inflammation and chemical alterations seen in specific conditions such as pancreatitis.

Imaging technology has altered the diagnosis and management of the acute surgical abdomen. Because it can detect pathologic conditions with a great degree of specificity, computed tomography (CT) has become the gold standard for the diagnosis of many intra-abdominal disease processes. It is not as sensitive as other technologies in detecting hollow visceral pathology. Another significant drawback of CT is that the patient has to be transported out of the intensive care unit to a special procedure room. Transport of the patient, especially if he or she requires invasive monitoring or mechanical ventilation, is difficult and can be dangerous if supervision is not appropriate.

Peritoneal lavage is an accepted diagnostic tool for the evaluation of trauma victims. The role of peritoneal lavage in the work-up of other patients is less well established. Laparoscopy is also useful in the evaluation of patients with acute abdominal pain. Performed at bedside, laparoscopy may play a significant role in the future evaluation of intensive care patients.

CONCEPT: *Diagnostic tests give additional information about the patient's condition. They should not interfere with adequate patient management or delay any necessary surgical intervention.*

A critical decision to be made in the treatment of patients with acute abdominal pain is whether they require *surgical intervention.* A wrong decision can subject already critically ill patients to added stress. Timing is of the essence. Obviously, patients with uncontrolled intra-abdominal bleeding (i.e., ruptured abdominal aneurysm) benefit from emergent intervention. Conversely, patients with intra-abdominal sepsis may benefit from a short period of aggressive fluid resuscitation and antibiotics. In some patients, surgery may not be necessary or desirable. Examples of this are feeble patients with ruptured but contained duodenal ulcers or patients with uncomplicated pancreatitis.

Intraoperative management of a patient with an acute surgical abdomen requires close collaboration between the surgeon and anesthesiologist. Inherent anesthetic risks in this patient population include aspiration, hemodynamic instability, and pulmonary dysfunction. The anesthetic plan has to be modified accordingly by performing rapid sequence induction and by using anesthetic agents that minimally compromise the cardiovascular system. Aggressive intraoperative monitoring and fluid management may be necessary.

Surgical management must be tailored to a patient's special needs and characteristics. Decision making is guided by the objective of correcting the underlying pathology, taking into account the patient's physiologic condition. Decisions about the extent of surgery, exteriorization of the bowel, the techniques of wound closure, and the use of drains require sound judgment by the surgeon.

Postoperative survival is determined by the patient's physiologic ability to respond to the disease process and the surgical trauma. Physiologic response to supernormal values with an increase in cardiac output, oxygen delivery, and consumption is necessary for survival. Aggressive fluid management and hemodynamic monitoring help obtain these goals.

CONCEPT: *A close understanding of the patient's physiologic condition is necessary when the patient is taken to surgery. Intervention by both surgeons and anesthesiologists has to be tailored to patient needs.*

Prevention of complications has to be a priority for the health care team that cares for patients with acute abdominal pathology. Compulsive pulmonary care helps prevent atelectasis, pneumonia, and, ultimately, respiratory failure. Meticulous care of wounds, drains, and invasive lines is necessary to prevent secondary infections. Finally, a low threshold for detection and management of intraoperative complications, such as the formation of intra-abdominal abscesses, is essential. Intra-abdominal abscesses can be unidentified sources of sepsis in critically ill patients. Drainage is a mainstay of management.

On occasions, patients who are already in the intensive care unit for other reasons have *acute abdominal manifestations* suggestive of intra-abdominal processes. These patients, whose senses are often compromised and who may be unable to communicate with the clinician, constitute a significant challenge for the intensivist and the surgeon. Certain pathologic processes are especially frequent in the intensive care unit, including ileus, upper gastrointestinal bleeding, acalculous cholecystitis, intestinal ischemia, and pancreatitis.

Abdominal distention and ileus occur frequently in critically ill patients. They are seen in patients with sepsis, shock, or respiratory pathology, or in the presence of significant fluid and electrolyte abnormalities such as hypokalemia and hypomagnesemia. Management of ileus includes the use of nasogastric suction and decompression, and the correction of its underlying cause.

Upper gastrointestinal bleeding secondary to stress ulceration can occur in critically ill patients. The widespread use of ulcer prophylaxis has helped to decrease the incidence of this complication. When upper gastrointestinal bleeding occurs, however, endoscopic diagnosis, as well as the replacement of abnormal losses and the correction of bleeding abnormalities, is the standard treatment. Surgical correction is occasionally needed.

Acalculous cholecystitis occurs in patients with prolonged illnesses, especially those receiving total parenteral nutrition for long periods. Signs of acalculous cholecystitis can be insidious and requires a significant degree of suspicion. Ultrasonography and nuclear medicine studies have to be used judiciously for a correct diagnosis. Management includes percutaneous or surgical drainage or cholecystectomy.

A disastrous consequence of low-flow states is the presence of intestinal ischemia and necrosis. Severe systemic toxicity, acidosis, and hematologic changes such as leukocytosis and thrombocytopenia, along with abdominal distention and ileus, should point to the diagnosis. Bowel resection is necessary when necrosis is present.

Pancreatitis can occur as a consequence of surgical manipulation or metabolic disturbances in the intensive care unit. Serious pancreatitis is rare under these circumstances.

CONCEPT: *Intensive care patients who have acute gastrointestinal symptoms constitute a special group with unique clinical presentations and often require a different diagnostic approach and management.*

FAILURE OF THE GASTROINTESTINAL TRACT BARRIER

The gastrointestinal tract serves two important functions—to absorb water and nutrients, and to act as a barrier to the transfer of microbes and their products (i.e., toxins) into the systemic circulation. When this barrier fails, microbes and toxins can enter into the systemic circulation. As a result, the immune system can be activated sufficiently to produce a *systemic inflammatory response.* Thus, in contrast to previous thinking, it has been hypothesized that a dysfunctional gastrointestinal tract is a continuing source of bacteria and bacterial products during multiple organ systems failure. The idea that the gut is actually the motor that fuels the systemic inflammatory response syndrome and, ultimately, multiple organ systems failure has been called the gut hypothesis.

Translocation is the passage of microbes or their products through an otherwise anatomically intact mucosal barrier. Microbes and their products can traverse the mucosal barrier through microscopic discontinuities in the epithelium, or they can be transported across through a transcellular pathway. Absorption of macromolecules across the mucosal barrier is a known normal event. It appears, however, that translocation can be accelerated during pathologic states.

Permeability refers to the passage of hydrophilic compounds and ions across the epithelial barrier. Permeability is essential for absorption of water and electrolytes that traverse through paracellular channels adjacent to the enterocytes. Permeability is dynamically regulated during physiologic conditions. A marked increase in mucosal permeability can be seen during pathologic conditions.

CONCEPT: *A dysfunctional gastrointestinal tract can become abnormally permeable, permitting the passage of bacteria and their products into the systemic circulation.*

Evidence that bacterial translocation contributes to morbidity and mortality in critically ill patients has been slowly accumulating from both experimental and human observations. In the laboratory, bacterial translocation or hyperpermeability has been re-created when the host is subjected to a number of insults, such as thermal trauma, hemorrhage, immunosuppression, total parenteral nutrition, postischemic reperfusion, and endotoxemia. Some of these insults share common pathophysiologic mechanisms, such as intestinal ischemia. Mucosal intestinal ischemia can be measured in vivo through gastric tonometry. Mucosal acidosis, also measured by tonometry, suggests tissue hypoperfusion and has been associated with a lethal outcome in critically ill patients.

Nutritional, hormonal, and immunologic factors can promote translocation. For example, total parenteral nutrition is associated with increased bacterial translocation, which is abrogated when glutamine is added. Derangements in IgA-mediated mucosal immunity can also promote translocation, whereas hormones that have trophic effects on the gastrointestinal mucosa, such as bombesin, appear to decrease it.

Microorganisms appear to have different abilities to penetrate the mucosal epithelial barrier. For example, gram-negative aerobes appear to translocate easily, but anaerobes rarely do so. Alterations in the composition of the normal gut flora, such as with the use of antibiotics, may be associated with overgrowth of more pathogenic organisms and enhanced translocation.

An increased incidence of bacterial translocation has been documented in patients with nonstrangulated intestinal obstruction and with hemorrhagic shock. The precise role of gut barrier dysfunction as a mechanism of disease is unclear, however, and the contribution of translocation and hyperpermeability to morbidity and mortality in critically ill patients has not been established. Despite this, the accumulating evidence is too compelling to be dismissed as unimportant. A healthy and functional gastrointestinal tract is an essential goal in the care of critically ill patients. Simple recommendations to obtain this goal include the following:

Prevent gastrointestinal disuse and atrophy. Enteral nutrition should be used whenever possible. An aggressive approach to feeding the patient is warranted. Supplementation of dietary formulas with glutamine should be considered.

Use antibiotics judiciously. Overgrowth of microorganisms, such as gram-negative aerobes, should be prevented.

Maintain adequate perfusion to the gastrointestinal tract. Gastric tonometry can be helpful in assessing adequate mucosal perfusion.

CONCEPT: *Evidence of bacterial translocation and its contribution to multiple organ failure is slowly accumulating. Simple recommendations, such as early enteral feeding, provide the basis for its prevention.*

PANCREATITIS

Pancreatitis is a fascinating disease with a spectrum of clinical presentations that ranges from mild and self-limited to severe and potentially fatal. Its diagnosis and management require the skills and training of several specialties. *Acute pancreatitis* refers to a sudden onset of symptoms in the absence of morphologic and functional changes before and after the appearance of symptoms. *Chronic pancreatitis* presents with waxing and waning symptoms and morphologic changes to the pancreas. In many cases, differentiating acute from chronic pancreatitis is difficult. Fat necrosis, edema, and infiltration of the pancreas with inflammatory cells are seen with acute pancreatitis. Fibrosis and atrophy are seen with chronic pancreatitis.

Biliary stone disease and *alcoholism* are the known causes of about 80% of the cases of pancreatitis in a given population. Other causes of pancreatitis are drugs, metabolic diseases such as hyperlipidemia, traumatic causes (including surgery), and infectious diseases. In a small percentage of cases, a clear cause is not identified.

The classic symptom of acute pancreatitis is a constant epigastric pain that may radiate to the midback and that is accompanied by significant nausea and vomiting. Nausea and retching typically continue even after the stomach has been emptied of its contents. Physical examination may show signs of systemic compromise, including dehydration, vascular collapse, poor ventilatory effort, and mental alterations. Abdominal examination reveals guarding and tenderness in, but not necessarily limited to, the epigastrium.

CONCEPT: *The diverse presentation of pancreatitis provides a challenge to the clinicians who care for these patients. Identification of the cause permits adequate treatment and, in some cases, prevention of recurrence.*

Laboratory and imaging studies are useful in establishing a correct diagnosis and in determining the severity of the attack and the overall prognosis. Measurement of *serum amylase* levels is useful in suggesting the diagnosis but lacks the specificity necessary to rule out other causes of intra-abdominal pathology, such as intestinal ischemia or perforated bowel. Serum lipase levels, amylase clearance, and serum amylase isoenzymes are all used to make an accurate diagnosis. *CT* has become the gold standard of imaging techniques for establishing the diagnosis of pancreatitis, since it has a high degree of specificity and sensitivity. Dynamic contrast-enhanced CT has been used in predicting the severity of the attack. The use of CT by interventional radiologists may be beneficial in the management of some of the complications of pancreatitis.

Most patients have a relatively uneventful course of acute pancreatitis. About 10% of patients, however, have more severe attacks and are at high risk for complications and death. Ideally, high-risk patients should be identified early and the need for closer monitoring and intensive care management determined. A number of tools involving the measurement of clinical and laboratory parameters have been developed for this purpose. In 1974, Ranson and colleagues showed that certain alterations of clinical and laboratory parameters were predictive of mortality. Ranson's criteria

Table 6–1. RANSON'S CRITERIA

On admission
Age >55 years
White blood cell count >16,000/mm^3
Blood glucose >200 mg/dL
Lactate dehydrogenase >350 IU/L
Glutamic-oxaloacetic transaminase >250 SFU/dL
During initial 48 hours
Hematocrit decrease >10%
Blood urea nitrogen rise >5 mg/dL
Serum calcium <8 mg/dL
PaO_2 <60 mm Hg
Base deficit >4 mEq/L
Fluid sequestration >6 L

remain the most widely used for evaluation of the severity of a pancreatitis attack (Table 6–1).

CONCEPT: The judicious use of laboratory and imaging techniques helps in establishing the diagnosis and determining the severity of the disease process.

The diagnosis of pancreatitis usually is clear after adequate laboratory and imaging information has been collected and interpreted. Surgical exploration is sometimes the only way of establishing the diagnosis, however. The goals of therapy include the following:

1. Resuscitation and stabilization. Intravascular volume contraction secondary to gastrointestinal losses and retroperitoneal fluid exudation may be particularly significant and has to be dealt with aggressively. Urinary output should be closely monitored. Hemodynamic monitoring may be necessary for meticulous resuscitation. Electrolyte imbalances such as hypocalcemia and hypomagnesemia should be identified and corrected. In some patients, respiratory compromise due to local and systemic inflammatory effects is significant. An indwelling arterial catheter permits frequent analysis of blood gases and helps identify patients in need of mechanical ventilatory support.
2. Management of pain. For the most part, narcotics are used. Demerol is preferred over morphine to prevent spasm of the sphincter of Oddi when gallstone pancreatitis is suspected. A nasogastric tube is used in patients with significant nausea and vomiting. Nasogastric tube suction has not been shown to alter the natural course of the disease, however, but may be of benefit in relieving symptoms. Antacids and histamine$_2$ blockers can prevent stress ulcer bleeding.
3. Control of pancreatic inflammation and enzymatic secretion. All therapies discussed earlier are aimed at maintaining physiologic homeostasis while the inflammation and enzymatic autodigestion of the pancreas subsides. Ideally, clinicians should be able to control the pancreatitic process itself. With this as a goal, many therapies have been suggested but none has gained wide acceptance. Attempts at reducing pancreatic secretion include the use of glucagon, somatostatin, atropine, or calcitonin. Aprotinin, procainam-

ide, and gabexate, among others, have been used as protein inhibitors to prevent enzymatic autodigestion. Reducing inflammation through the use of prostaglandin inhibitors has been tried. Peritoneal lavage has been used in severe attacks, but randomized trials have failed to prove its benefit.

The treatment of biliary stone disease causing pancreatitis has changed dramatically with the use of new technologies of endoscopy and laparoscopy. In general, treatment of biliary tract stones is instituted when the pancreatitis has resolved in order to prevent recurrence. Endoscopic sphincterotomy and stone removal have replaced open surgical procedures, and laparoscopy is now the standard procedure for cholecystectomy.

CONCEPT: *Independent of the cause, the treatment of pancreatitis is aimed at adequate resuscitation, control of pain, and management of inflammation.*

There are numerous *systemic* and *local complications* of acute pancreatitis. Systemic complications tend to occur early during the attack and include cardiovascular collapse, respiratory insufficiency, renal failure, and disseminated intravascular coagulation. An aggressive approach is the key for the prevention of these complications. Local complications, including pancreatic necrosis, pseudocysts, and pancreatic ascites, are secondary to the effects of inflammation or to the accumulation of pancreatic secretions. These can become infected by bacterial translocation or after surgical or interventional procedures.

Sterile pancreatic necrosis has traditionally been managed expectantly, although some advocate surgical intervention. Pseudocysts are initially monitored expectantly, but many physicians advocate drainage if they cause symptoms, grow, or fail to disappear within a reasonable time. Pancreatic ascites and pleuropancreatic fistulas result from major duct disruption and are especially difficult to manage.

In contrast to the tendency of expectant management in sterile complications, the presence of infection demands aggressive intervention. Infected pancreatic pseudocysts can be managed by percutaneous drainage. Infected pancreatic necrosis is treated with open surgical débridement. Adequate antibiotic coverage for gram-negative enteric organisms should be used as an adjunct to surgical treatment.

SEVERE LIVER DISEASE

Few patients provide as great a challenge to the intensivist as those with liver disease. Severe liver disease has the potential of affecting virtually any organ or system in the body, with the possibility of serious complications. The availability of *liver transplantation* has dramatically changed an otherwise bleak outcome. Transplantation has given many patients the chance of recovering health and of leading normal and productive lives. The intensivist is faced with the task of managing the patient through the different stages before and after transplantation. The most frequent causes for admission to the intensive care unit include cirrhosis,

Table 6–2. MOST COMMON CAUSES OF END-STAGE LIVER DISEASE (CIRRHOSIS)

Alcoholism
Viral hepatitis
Autoimmune liver disease
Metabolic disorders
  Wilson disease
  Alpha$_1$-antitrypsin deficiency
  Hemochromatosis
Toxicity from drugs
  Isoniazid
  Methyldopa
  Acetaminophen
Biliary disease
  Primary biliary cirrhosis
  Sclerosing cholangitis
Vascular disorders
  Congestive heart failure
  Budd-Chiari syndrome (hepatic vein thrombosis)

fulminant hepatic failure, and the perioperative care of transplant recipients.

CONCEPT: *Liver transplantation has dramatically changed the care of the patient with severe liver disease.*

Cirrhosis

There are many causes of liver cirrhosis (Table 6–2). Regardless of the cause, *end-stage liver disease* is characterized by a series of physiologic alterations in different organ functions. Knowledge of these alterations is paramount for the patient's adequate treatment and ultimate survival.

Hemodynamic alterations are characterized by a high cardiac output with a low systemic vascular resistance. Blood volume is increased, but pulmonary artery occlusion pressure is normal. Pulmonary artery pressure is normal in most patients but is elevated in a small percentage.

Respiratory alkalosis, with Pa_{CO_2} levels in the range of 30 to 35 mm Hg, is characteristic of cirrhosis (Table 6–3). The cause of this finding is unclear. Mild hypoxemia with an increased alveolo-arterial oxygen tension difference is also

Table 6–3. TYPICAL CARDIOPULMONARY PROFILE IN PATIENTS WITH CIRRHOSIS

Cardiac index: 4.5–5.25 L/min/m^2
Systemic vascular resistance: 400–900 dynes · s · cm^{-5}
Pulmonary artery occlusion pressures: 4–6 mm Hg
Mean pulmonary arterial pressure: 12 mm Hg
Arterial blood gases
  P_{CO_2}: 30–35 mm Hg
  P_{O_2}: 65–85 mm Hg
  Alveoloarterial oxygen tension difference: 20–30 mm Hg

common. Hypoxemia is probably a result of several respiratory abnormalities, including an abnormal distribution of ventilation and intrapulmonary shunting. Elevation of the diaphragms due to ascites may also be a contributing factor. In some patients, hypoxemia is present or increases in the upright position (orthodeoxia).

Avid sodium retention by the kidney is characteristic of cirrhosis. This results in a total body water and sodium excess. Other common electrolyte abnormalities include hypokalemia and a reduced excretion of bicarbonate, which results in metabolic alkalosis.

Drug metabolism is altered in cirrhotic patients. Drugs whose metabolism is affected include bronchodilators, antibiotics, corticosteroids, and histamine blockers. Careful dosing and frequent determinations of serum levels, when available, are necessary. If narcotics are used, morphine is preferred over meperidine, since metabolism of the latter is decreased.

CONCEPT: *Characteristic alterations in organ physiology are seen in patients with end-stage liver disease.*

Life-threatening complications frequently cause patients to be admitted to the intensive care unit. The most common complications include gastrointestinal bleeding, hepatic encephalopathy, ascites, and renal failure.

Gastrointestinal hemorrhage is a serious complication in cirrhotic patients and should be managed promptly and aggressively. Hemodynamic stability has to be evaluated and corrected promptly. Adequate resuscitation includes the use of large-bore intravenous lines and blood products to correct the anemia and coagulation abnormalities frequently present. Endotracheal intubation should be performed if there is any question of the patient's ability to maintain and protect his or her airway. This may be difficult to perform because of hematemesis, and adequately trained and experienced personnel should undertake the procedure.

The causes of gastrointestinal bleeding include variceal bleeding (esophageal or gastric), duodenal ulcers, and esophageal (Mallory-Weiss) tear. Early use of endoscopy helps in determining the correct diagnosis and establishing an adequate treatment plan.

Ulcer disease causes 40% to 50% of all gastrointestinal bleeding in cirrhotic patients. Initial management includes use of histamine blockers, sucralfate, or proton pump inhibitors (omeprazole). Endoscopic hemostatic therapy is used when an active bleeding site is determined. Surgery is occasionally necessary to control ulcer bleeding.

Bleeding from esophageal varices carries a grave prognosis, with an average mortality rate of 50%. Several forms of therapy are used to control bleeding:

1. Reduction of portal blood flow. Vasopressin and somatostatin reduce splanchnic blood flow by different mechanisms. Propanolol has also been used, but its only proven role is as a prophylactic agent to prevent bleeding.
2. Balloon tamponade achieves temporary control of bleeding in 42% to 90% of the patients. It is associated with

many complications, however, including aspiration, gastric and esophageal mucosal necrosis, and esophageal rupture. Rebleeding is frequent after the balloon has been deflated.

3. Endoscopic sclerotherapy is more effective than pharmacologic agents alone and is as effective as balloon tamponade in controlling variceal bleeding. Complications include ulcerations of the esophagus with rebleeding, esophageal tears, mediastinitis, bronchoesophageal fistulas, and pleural effusions. Patients subjected to endoscopic band ligation of bleeding esophageal varices have fewer complications and a better survival rate than those who undergo sclerotherapy.

4. Transvenous intrahepatic portosystemic shunts can be created through a percutaneous transjugular approach. Their use provides a nonoperative approach to portal decompression. The procedure itself requires significant expertise and advanced technology, however.

5. The creation of surgical portosystemic shunts has been effective in controlling variceal hemorrhage. Surgical decompression of the portal system is associated with high morbidity and mortality, however, and is now used less frequently.

Hepatic encephalopathy is another major complication of cirrhosis and is believed to be secondary to inadequate hepatic degradation of toxins. Toxins implicated in the pathogenesis of encephalopathy include ammonia and abnormal concentrations of aromatic amino acids, fatty acids, and bacterial toxins. Encephalopathy has a wide extent of clinical presentations, ranging from subclinical changes to hepatic coma and brain death. It is customary to grade the degree of encephalopathy into four clinical stages (Table 6–4). A

Table 6–4. STAGING OF HEPATIC ENCEPHALOPATHY

Stage	Personality	Thought Process	Electroencephalographic Findings	Asterixis and Clonus
I	Sloppy personal habits	Difficulty with calculations	Normal or subtle changes	Absent
II	Loss of attention; inapropriate behavior	Confusion; abnormal sleep pattern	Slowing	Present
III	Short attention span; noncooperation with examination	Accentuated disturbance in thought process; extended sleep cycle (most of the time)	Triphasic waves	Present
IV	Coma	Little or no response to noxious stimuli	Delta waves	Absent

complete neurologic evaluation is necessary to rule out cerebral trauma and intracranial bleeding.

Careful attention to cardiopulmonary homeostasis is essential in patients with encephalopathy. Patients who are unable to protect their airways should be intubated. Maintaining an adequate circulating blood volume is essential. Treatment of encephalopathy is done by decreasing the accumulation of ammonia and other toxins. Most of the ammonia in the body comes from bacterial degradation of nitrogenous products (e.g., blood) in the gastrointestinal tract. Lactulose is metabolized by bacteria in the gut into small organic acids. Acidification of the colon produces diarrhea and inhibits ammonia production and absorption. Neomycin reduces the bacterial count and thus decreases ammonia production. Use of sedatives and narcotics should be minimized in patients with encephalopathy.

The formation of *ascites* is a result of the outpouring of fluid into the abdominal cavity and is due to increased hydrostatic pressure in the hepatic sinusoids and the splanchnic capillary bed. In addition, there is avid retention of sodium by the kidney. The mechanism of sodium retention is not clearly understood, but several hypotheses have been proposed. The most recent hypothesis suggests that sodium and water retention is the result of arterial dilatation and underfilling.

Treatment of ascites is geared toward restricting the sodium intake and promoting diuresis. Diets should reduce the sodium intake to 10 to 40 mEq/d. Diuretic therapy generally involves the use of furosemide and spironolactone. Spironolactone therapy is started alone, and furosemide is added if no response is observed in 3 to 5 days. Doses of both drugs should be increased in a stepwise manner until a response is observed. Complications secondary to diuretic therapy include azotemia, electrolyte abnormalities, and hepatic encephalopathy.

Paracentesis is performed in patients who cannot achieve control of ascites by sodium restriction and diuresis alone. Large-volume paracentesis is more effective than diuretic therapy in decreasing the ascites and has fewer complications. Another tool for reducing ascitic accumulation is peritoneovenous shunts. Such shunts are associated with their own risks and complications, however.

Oliguria occurs frequently in cirrhotic patients as a result of disease or as a secondary effect of treatment. The major causes of oliguria are prerenal azotemia, acute tubular necrosis, and hepatorenal syndrome. The differentiation between these causes is established by an adequate assessment of the circulating blood volume and evaluation of both plasma and urine creatinine and electrolytes. Circulating blood volume should be restored if volume depletion is encountered, and excessive diuretic use should be stopped. Nephrotoxic drugs should be avoided. Patients with hepatorenal syndrome are extremely difficult to treat, unfortunately, and usually die of complications of their disease if liver transplantation is not available.

Spontaneous bacterial peritonitis accounts for 60% of all serious infections in patients with cirrhosis. Gram-negative organisms are generally identified. The associated mortality rate is as high as 30%. Seventy per cent of survivors experience recurrence within 1 year. Clinical symptoms such as abdominal tenderness and fever may not be present. When spontaneous bacterial peritonitis is suspected, a peritoneal tap should be performed. A polymorphonuclear leukocyte count in the ascitic fluid greater than 500/μL is a positive indicator. A cephalosporin or ampicillin plus a β-lactamase inhibitor is used for treatment.

CONCEPT: *Complications of cirrhosis include gastrointestinal bleeding, encephalopathy, ascites, renal failure, and spontaneous bacterial peritonitis. Each of these complications is associated with a high mortality rate.*

Fulminant Hepatic Failure

Fulminant hepatic failure is a sudden onset of liver failure in a patient without preexisting liver disease. It is characterized by a prolonged prothrombin time and hepatic encephalopathy within 8 weeks of onset of symptoms. Causes include hepatitis A or B, the use of hepatotoxic drugs or substances, and metabolic causes such as Wilson's disease. Independent factors that affect prognosis in fulminant hepatic failure are listed in Table 6–5.

No specific treatment is available for fulminant hepatic failure. The goal is to support the patient until hepatic regeneration occurs. It is crucial to prevent or to promptly identify complications such as encephalopathy, respiratory failure, infection, coagulopathy, gastrointestinal bleeding, renal failure, and cerebral edema.

The primary cause of death for 60% to 70% of the patients is cerebral edema. Intracranial pressure monitoring devices are used to guide therapy. The use of CT scans of the head is important for the surveillance of intracranial bleeding.

The mortality rate associated with fulminant hepatic failure is high, ranging from 40% to 85%. Orthotopic liver transplantation is quickly becoming the treatment of choice, with a reported survival rate of 50% to 90%.

CONCEPT: *Supportive treatment while liver regeneration oc-*

Table 6–5. FACTORS THAT AFFECT PROGNOSIS IN FULMINANT HEPATIC FAILURE

Factors
Age
Cause
Degree of liver function affected
Severity of encephalopathy
Prolongation of prothrombin time
Factor V level
Serum bilirubin
Systemic physiologic abnormalities
Arterial pH
Serum creatinine
Other
Alpha-fetoprotein level

curs is the traditional way of managing fulminant hepatic failure. Liver transplantation has become the best option for survival, however.

SEVERE GASTROINTESTINAL HEMORRHAGE

Documented gastrointestinal bleeding is defined as severe when it produces hemodynamic instability or a significant blood loss as determined by a decrease in the hematocrit by 6% to 8% or the need for blood replacement. Initial assessment includes a brief history and physical examination. *Resuscitation* should begin simultaneously by starting two large-bore intravenous lines (14–16 gauge). Crystalloid replacement and blood products are used to maintain hemodynamic stability, an adequate hemoglobin concentration and platelet count, and a satisfactory prothrombin time (Table 6–6). Placement of central venous lines, Swan-Ganz catheters, and invasive arterial monitors depends on severity of the bleeding, age of the patient, and preexisting cardiopulmonary status.

CONCEPT: *Gastrointestinal bleeding is a true emergency with life-threatening consequences. Resuscitation must be started while the cause and site of bleeding are sought and a definitive treatment is designed.*

Upper gastrointestinal bleeding occurs proximal to the ligament of Treitz; the source of *lower gastrointestinal bleeding* is found distal to this. Determining the site of bleeding requires clinical insight and a rational use of available technology. The presence of hematemesis or blood in the nasogastric tube aspirate points to upper gastrointestinal bleeding, whereas the rectal passage of bright red blood suggests lower gastrointestinal bleeding. These signs are not totally reliable, however, and false-positive or false-negative assumptions may be made. Endoscopy, noninvasive and invasive radiologic techniques, and surgery are used in localizing the source, determining the cause, and treating the bleeding.

Esophagogastroscopy reveals the source of upper gastrointestinal bleeding in 90% of cases. The patient should be hemodynamically stable for the procedure. Airway protection by endotracheal intubation is essential if the patient is at risk of aspiration. *Colonoscopy* is equally valuable in cases of lower gastrointestinal bleeding and should be used as the first-line procedure.

Table 6–6. GOALS OF CRYSTALLOID AND BLOOD PRODUCT REPLACEMENT

Achieve hemodynamic stability
Heart rate <100 bpm
Systolic blood pressure >100 mm Hg
Blood product relacement if:
Hematocrit <24%
Platelet count <50,000/mL
Prothrombin time >15 seconds

CONCEPT: Endoscopy has become the standard tool for localizing the site of bleeding and identifying its cause.

Upper gastrointestinal bleeding is a common medical emergency and accounts for some 300,000 hospital admissions each year. Determination of the cause is central for both short- and long-term management and prevention of recurrence. The most common causes reflect the population served by a given hospital (Table 6–7). Most patients present with self-limited hemorrhaging. Fifteen to 20% of patients have active bleeding, however, with a mortality rate of 30% to 40%. These patients can benefit from the various acute therapies available.

Peptic ulcers are the most frequent cause of upper gastrointestinal bleeding in the United States and are responsible for some 100,000 hospitalizations per year. Prognosis is adversely affected by many factors, including age greater than 60 years, comorbid medical illnesses, shock, coagulopathy, onset of bleeding in a hospitalized patient, the requirement for multiple transfusions, and the presence of an ulcer crater at or near specific vessels (i.e., left gastric or gastroduodenal artery).

Medical treatment includes the use of histamine$_2$ blockers, sucralfate, and omeprazole. Medical treatment has been found to significantly decrease frequency of transfusions, rebleeding rates, need for surgery, and mortality rates. Endoscopic therapy has become essential in the modern management of ulcer bleeding. The goal of endoscopy is to coagulate or thrombose the underlying artery at the bleeding site. This can be done by contact thermal coagulation, laser devices, and injection of epinephrine, polidocanol, or alcohol into the bleeding site. The different methods of coagulation appear to have similar efficacy and safety. Surgery is indicated in patients with exsanguinating bleeding or in whom bleeding recurs after two sessions of endoscopic therapy. Surgery remains an alternative when there are large, visibly pulsating vessels that are not amenable to endoscopic therapy.

Esophageal variceal bleeding secondary to portal hypertension is the second most common cause of severe upper

Table 6–7. CAUSES OF SEVERE UPPER GASTROINTESTINAL BLEEDING*

Diagnosis	Occurrence (%)
Peptic ulcer	55
Gastric or esophageal varices	14
Angioma	6
Mallory-Weiss tear	5
Tumor	4
Erosions	4
Esophagitis	4
Other	8

*From Los Angeles Medical Center and West Los Angeles Veterans Administration Medical Center (n = 948).

gastrointestinal bleeding. It is associated with high short- and long-term mortality rates. Liver transplantation can improve the prognosis in selected patients. Medical management includes the use of vasopressin or somatostatin. Balloon tamponade, endoscopic sclerotherapy, and endoscopic variceal band ligation are used in conjunction with medical treatment.

Other causes of upper gastrointestinal bleeding include esophagitis, Mallory-Weiss tear, angiodysplasia, upper gastrointestinal tumors, and aortoenteric fistulas. The principles of initial assessment and resuscitation are similar for all causes, but there is a great variation in treatment modalities.

Severe lower gastrointestinal bleeding generally manifests itself as hematochezia. However, hematochezia can also be a manifestation of upper gastrointestinal bleeding. The most frequent causes of lower gastrointestinal bleeding are colonic angiomas and diverticulosis. Other causes are polyps, cancer, colitis, and hemorrhoids. Diagnosis is generally made by colonoscopy. In some cases, angiography and technetium-99m red blood cell scanning are needed for diagnosis. In a small percentage of cases, laparotomy is a last and desperate effort to coerce otherwise uncontrollable bleeding.

Spontaneous cessation of bleeding is the rule in 70% to 90% of patients. In the remaining 10% to 30%, urgent therapy is usually required. Treatment involves colonoscopic hemostasis, angiographic embolization, or surgery.

Colonic angiomas, most frequently localized to the right colon, are successfully treated by endoscopic coagulation 80% of the time. Diverticular bleeding may be severe, although such bleeding stops spontaneously 70% of the time. Twenty per cent of patients with diverticular bleeding require surgical intervention. Colon cancer can occasionally present with severe lower gastrointestinal bleeding. Colonoscopy is used for diagnosis and initial hemostasis. Definitive management involves surgical resection. Ulcerative colitis on occasions manifests as severe lower gastrointestinal bleeding. Medical therapy is generally attempted, but a subtotal colectomy may be needed if medical therapy fails.

CONCEPT: *The cause of gastrointestinal bleed determines its treatment.*

ACUTE GASTROINTESTINAL DISORDERS

Acute life-threatening emergencies can arise throughout the length of the gastrointestinal tract. The intensivist gets involved in the care of these patients when the disease process produces severe physiologic compromise, when the preexisting medical conditions place the patient at risk for acute decompensation, or when the emergency occurs in a patient already admitted to the intensive care unit for other reasons.

Gastrointestinal emergencies can be broadly classified into several categories—obstruction, perforation, inflammation and infection, and bleeding. Gastrointestinal bleeding has already been discussed. A brief summary of the clinical presentation, diagnosis, and principles of management of other emergencies follows.

Obstruction can occur in any part of the gastrointestinal tract from the pharynx to the anus. It can be acute or chronic and can arise from external compression or internal obturation. The physiologic consequences are secondary to the abnormalities produced in the gastrointestinal tract and include a loss of absorption and the potential for fluid loss, electrolyte abnormalities, bacterial translocation, vascular compromise with ischemia, and necrosis of the bowel.

The cause, presentation, evaluation, and treatment vary with the site of obstruction. Esophageal obstruction generally is secondary to ingested food or a foreign body that has become impacted at a site of previous esophageal disease. Esophageal disease is an emergency when there is imminent risk of perforation or aspiration. Gastric outlet obstruction presents as a chronic process associated with nonbilious vomiting, weight loss, and hypochloremic metabolic alkalosis. Small bowel obstruction, on the other hand, is more commonly seen as an emergency, with manifestations of bilious vomiting, crampy abdominal pain, distention, and dehydration. Colon obstruction manifests itself with constipation and abdominal distention.

Emergency management of life-threatening complications may be necessary with gastrointestinal tract obstruction. For example, small bowel obstruction can progress to strangulation and bowel necrosis. In this case, adequate fluid resuscitation, correction of the electrolyte abnormalities, decompression of the bowel with the use of a nasogastric tube, and early surgery may be necessary. In complicated cases or in patients with associated preexisting conditions, the intensive care unit is the best place for adequate treatment.

Perforation can occur anywhere along the length of the tract and is generally accompanied by the spillage of intraluminal contents, which usually are contaminated or which cause a severe inflammatory reaction. Free perforations are an emergency and should be managed as such. An aggressive approach consisting of prompt diagnosis, fluid management, antibiotics, and surgery gives the patient the best chances for survival and minimizes complications.

Ischemia most often presents in the territory of the superior mesenteric artery and compromises the entire small bowel and the right colon. Ischemia results from arterial emboli or arterial or venous thrombosis. In a small number of critically ill patients, mesenteric ischemia is secondary to low-flow states, hemodynamic instability, and the use of vasopressors. Patients typically complain of severe abdominal pain with an initial equivocal physical examination. If patients go untreated, their clinical picture rapidly progresses to one of severe acidosis, hypotension, and systemic compromise. Diagnosis may be difficult, and precious time can be lost with unnecessary testing. Surgery, with revascularization if possible, can be lifesaving. If necrosis is present, resection of the bowel offers the only chance of survival. Resection of large portions of the small bowel results in the short-gut syndrome and makes the patient dependent on parenteral nutrition for long-term survival.

A broad range of *inflammatory* and *infectious processes* can affect the gastrointestinal tract. Clinical presentations vary and can be difficult to diagnose in an intensive care setting. Often, gastrointestinal tract infection is seen in debilitated or immunocompromised patients or is the result of treatment itself. For example, candidal esophagitis is frequently seen in patients with transplants who are receiving antirejection treatment.

The management of infectious processes of the gastrointestinal tract involves an adequate microbiologic diagnosis, targeted antimicrobial management, and treatment of the disease process itself. *Clostridium difficile* colitis is frequently seen as a consequence of antibiotic use. The clinical presentation ranges from an asymptomatic carrier state to acute fulminant colitis. In a small number of patients, *C. difficile* colitis is a life-threatening infection causing septic shock and organ failure. Colectomy is indicated in these cases.

CONCEPT: *Acute gastrointestinal emergencies can be life-threatening. Aggressive resuscitation, judicious use of antibiotics, and prompt surgical intervention can be lifesaving. The intensive care unit is instrumental in the adequate management of these patients.*

PART B

Renal Failure

Rinaldo Bellomo, MD, FRACP

ASSESSMENT OF RENAL FUNCTION

Critically ill patients frequently experience a clinically significant deterioration in renal function. In fact, 5% to 15% of patients experience either a doubling of their serum creatinine levels from before admission to the intensive care unit (ICU) or an increase in serum creatinine levels above 200 µmol/L (about 2 mg/dL). Such degrees of renal dysfunction complicate pharmacologic management and necessitate great caution with the administration of intravenous fluids at a time when aggressive resuscitation is often needed. When renal dysfunction is severe and renal replacement therapy (hemodialysis or hemofiltration) is necessary, its presence becomes a major therapeutic and financial burden with serious implications for overall patient prognosis. It is likely that almost all critically ill patients develop some kind of renal dysfunction during the course of their illness, but our ability to detect it is limited. Generally, only a small number of scientifically inaccurate but clinically useful tests are routinely available in the ICU to assess kidney function.

Serum creatinine is a clinically reasonable gauge of glomerular filtration rate (GFR) when great precision is not necessary. It rarely is in clinical practice. The serum creatinine concentration depends on muscle mass, volume of distribution, rate of production, intestinal degradation, tubular secretion, and GFR. Serum creatinine has a well-described steady-state relation to creatinine clearance (Fig. 6–1), which is not easily predicted in critically ill persons. Such patients have a varying degree of muscle mass as a result of their illness and a rapidly changing and expanded volume of distribution for creatinine because of fluid resuscitation. Furthermore, serum creatinine is an insensitive marker of change in renal excretory function early in the course of kidney disease. A 30% decrease in GFR, for example, may increase the serum creatinine concentration only from the low-normal to the high-normal value range. If the baseline value is unknown, as in most cases, this major decrease in GFR may go unrecognized. Finally, once a renal insult has occurred, the serum creatinine level continues to increase until a new steady state is reached at which excretion and filtration are matched. This increase is seen even though no further renal injury is taking place.

CONCEPT: *Serum creatinine is an inaccurate but clinically*

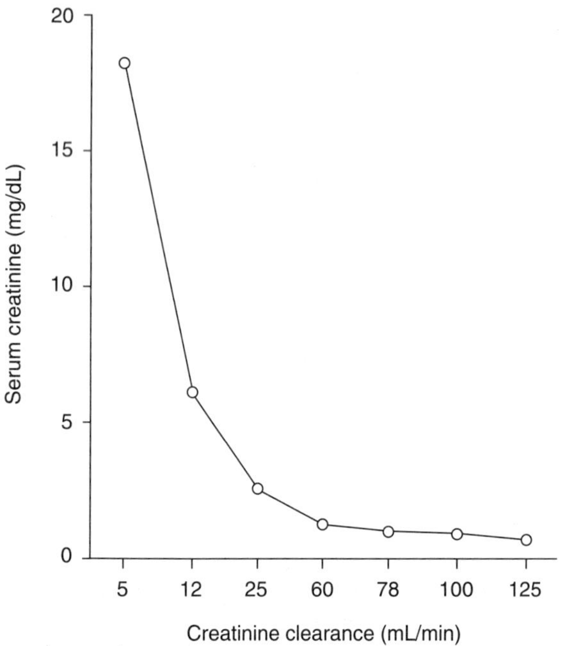

Figure 6–1. Diagram illustrating the relation between the serum creatinine concentration and the creatinine clearance, a good measure of true glomerular filtration rate (GFR). As can be seen, the serum creatinine is an insensitive marker of loss of GFR, because it starts to increase only when nearly 70% of GFR has been lost.

useful marker of renal dysfunction. It is particularly inaccurate at times when accuracy is most needed—in early renal injury and during rapidly changing renal function.

A more accurate way of assessing renal function is to measure the patient's *creatinine clearance*. This measurement is not commonly done in the ICU, since its findings rarely offer any major diagnostic insights, prognostic advantages, or therapeutic implications. At times, short collection periods (4 hours) can be used in the ICU to gauge renal function more accurately. Such short collection periods are close in accuracy to the standard 24-hour urine collection but lose their accuracy in the presence of severe oliguria. The GFR is obtained as follows:

$$GFR = U_{creat} \times V/P_{creat}$$

where U_{creat} is the concentration of creatinine in the urine; V is the volume of urine produced over a given period; and P_{creat} is the concentration of creatinine in plasma. This calculated GFR is still subject to inaccuracies that may be due to either rapid changes in function or the effect of drugs (trimethoprim or cimetidine) that interfere with the correct measurement of creatinine. Nonetheless, the measurement of creatinine clearance collected over a short period represents a step toward better assessment of renal function. Because creatinine clearance is approximately equal to the GFR and because of the cumbersome nature of collecting urine over time, equations have been developed to estimate creatinine clearance from the serum creatinine measurement. The most commonly used equation is that developed by Cockroft and Gault:

$$\text{creatinine clearance} = (140 - \text{age in years}) \times \text{lean weight (in kg)}/72 \times \text{serum creatinine}$$

The expression is multiplied by 0.85 for females. This equation, although widely used in stable patients, has not been validated in the critically ill, in whom the relation between the rapidly changing GFR and the serum creatinine concentration is less predictable, as previously discussed.

Serum urea nitrogen is another widely used serologic marker for the clinical assessment of renal function. It is less accurate than the serum creatinine but continues to be used clinically as a marker of uremic intoxication and a guide to the need for dialytic therapy. Although widely used for this purpose in patients with chronic renal failure, this measure has not been validated in those with acute renal failure. Urea nitrogen production fluctuates markedly depending on the patient's diet and catabolic state, as well as the presence of gastrointestinal blood. Because of the widespread use of total parenteral nutrition, impairment of renal function in ICU patients is often associated with a disproportionate increase in serum urea nitrogen compared with serum creatinine. This is particularly true in transplant patients who receive corticosteroids for immunosuppression. In these patients, the serum urea concentration may not provide even a semiaccurate guideline to the state of GFR or the need for dialytic therapy.

CONCEPT: *Serum urea nitrogen concentration in critically ill patients is a complex and composite signal that cannot be used alone to indicate the presence of intravascular fluid depletion, severe renal impairment, marked catabolism, or the need for dialytic therapy.*

Other tests of excretory renal function are clinically less useful and rarely performed. These tests include the measurement of renal blood flow with *P*-aminohippurate and of GFR with technetium-99m DTPA. The latter is sometimes useful in the evaluation of early renal allograft dysfunction, and both are used in the ICU only for research purposes.

The fractional excretion of sodium (FE_{Na}) is calculated according to the following equation:

$$FE_{Na} = U_{Na} \times V/GFR \times S_{Na}$$

where U_{Na} is the urinary sodium concentration; V is the volume of urine excreted during the period studied; GFR is the glomerular filtration rate (typically calculated simultaneously by means of the creatinine clearance); and S_{Na} is the serum sodium concentration. This equation can be used clinically with the formula being simplified to:

$$FE_{Na} = U_{Na}/S_{Na} \times S_{cr}/U_{cr} \times 100 \text{ (expressed as percentage)}$$

where S_{cr} is the concentration of creatinine in serum, and U_{cr} is the concentration of creatinine in urine. This simplified formula can help distinguish prerenal from renal parenchymal failure in the setting of acute renal dysfunction. Its accuracy, however, is severely limited in the presence of previous renal dysfunction, and the therapeutic implications of the test are unclear in critically ill patients. Such patients, in fact, already receive optimal fluid resuscitation.

Other derangements of electrolyte excretion and acid-base control accompany the development of acute renal failure (hyperkalemia, hyperphosphatemia, and metabolic acidosis) and may require specific treatment (especially hyperkalemia), but both types of derangement are insensitive and nonspecific markers of renal dysfunction.

RENAL IMAGING IN THE INTENSIVE CARE UNIT

Imaging of the kidney, although not a way of directly assessing renal function, provides useful information about the cause of renal failure and degree of previous renal damage if renal function before ICU admission is unknown. A plain radiograph of the abdomen, by allowing assessment of kidney size and presence of parenchymal calcification, may be of some clinical use, but the most commonly used modality in the acute situation is ultrasonography. A renal ultrasound is mandatory for any case of acute renal dysfunction, as renal outflow obstruction cannot be reliably diagnosed clinically. The technique is easily performed at the bedside and has no morbidity. It also permits the assessment of kidney size and provides useful information on the state of the renal parenchyma. In rare cases, renal ultrasonography will not detect clinically significant obstruction. In this situation, if obstruction is strongly suspected clinically, retrograde pyelogram and cystoscopy must be performed.

RECOMMENDATION: *In all patients admitted to the ICU with acute renal failure or who develop acute renal failure within the ICU, a renal ultrasound must be performed to exclude obstruction.*

Other imaging techniques (computed tomographic scanning scanning of the abdomen, angiography) are only rarely indicated (e.g., suspected perinephric abscess not detected on ultrasound, suspected acute renal arterial or venous thrombosis).

USEFUL INVESTIGATIONS IN ACUTE RENAL FAILURE

The most common renal syndrome seen in the ICU is acute renal failure. A number of investigations beyond those previously described are typically necessary to assess the patient. Full urine analysis, with microscopy and culture, should be performed in all patients admitted with acute renal dysfunction. Urinary tract sepsis must be excluded, the urine assessed for any evidence of proteinuria and hematuria, and the sediment inspected for the presence of white cells, fragmented red cells, or casts. The presence of white cells, fragmented red cells, or casts suggests ongoing parenchymal inflammation (active sediment). In cases of interstitial nephropathy, the presence of urinary eosinophils is a useful, although insensitive, diagnostic clue. In cases of acute tubular necrosis, large numbers of free tubular epithelial cells or tubular cell casts may be found together with coarse granular casts.

If rhabdomyolysis is suspected as a cause of renal failure, testing of the urine and of blood for free myoglobin and measurement of serum muscle enzyme activity are useful diagnostic methods. If a pulmonary–renal syndrome is suspected, chest radiography, serologic testing for inflammatory markers, and testing for specific autoantibodies (antineutrophil cytoplasmic antibodies, anti–glomerular basement membrane antibodies, or collagen disease–related autoantibodies) are necessary. If the hemolytic-uremic syndrome or thrombotic thrombocytopenic purpura is suspected, microscopic examination of blood films and testing for evidence of hemolysis are of great diagnostic utility. In some situations, the diagnosis of parenchymal kidney disease is made, but its cause and nature remain obscure. A kidney biopsy then becomes necessary and can be performed in ventilated patients with the assistance of ultrasonographic guidance.

ACUTE RENAL FAILURE

Typically, the major renal disorder of interest to physicians treating critically ill patients is the syndrome of acute or rapidly progressive renal failure. Although clinicians are familiar with the syndrome of rapidly (over hours to days) increasing serum urea nitrogen and creatinine concentrations and decreasing urine output, the definition of acute renal failure is not generally agreed on. It remains undetermined when acute renal dysfunction should be called failure, what the duration of severe oliguria (<400 mL/d [measurements are not adjusted for sex, age, and lean body mass]) should be, and what constitutes acute tubular necrosis as opposed to prerenal kidney injury with slow recovery. Furthermore, histologic evidence is lacking that acute renal dysfunction, as seen in critically ill patients with multiple organ dysfunction and sepsis, is indeed the so-called acute tubular necrosis of ischemic experimental models of acute renal failure. Although our understanding of human acute renal failure is incomplete, current opinion holds that acute changes in the adequacy of oxygen supply to the medulla, especially to the thick ascending loop of Henle (which lives in an ischemic penumbra at the best of times) are most likely responsible for initiating the cascade of events leading to the loss of excretory function and decreased urine output. A summary of this pathogenetic view of acute renal failure is presented in Figure 6–2.

Much time is often spent trying to establish clinically whether one is dealing with prerenal (functional) or full parenchymal (acute tubular necrosis) renal failure. Several tests have been proposed to assist in this diagnostic process. Typically, patients with prerenal kidney dysfunction have a low urine sodium concentration, urine-to-plasma creatinine ratio far higher than 20:1, high urine osmolality, benign urine sediment, and fractional excretion of sodium below 1%. A typical situation is rarely seen in the ICU, however, and these tests have serious limitations of diagnostic accuracy in elderly patients, those with previous renal dysfunction, those who have recently received diuretics, and those who have had recent aggressive fluid resuscitation. Only the clinical course of the patient eventually provides a substantial clue to the correct diagnosis. In addition, in critically ill patients, renal injury is a continuum and neat pathophysiologic subdivisions may be misleading. Finally, the clinical implications of this diagnostic process and its utility in the ICU remain unclear. In this setting, aggressive, invasively monitored resuscitation always occurs with any clinically significant hemodynamic, hemorrhagic, or septic insult. Such resuscitation is always aimed at maintaining optimal intravascular and extravascular volume states under all circumstances.

RECOMMENDATION: *In the presence of acute renal dysfunction, always determine whether the patient is adequately volume resuscitated, and, if the answer is unclear, consider which physiologic data (e.g., central venous pressure, cardiac output,*

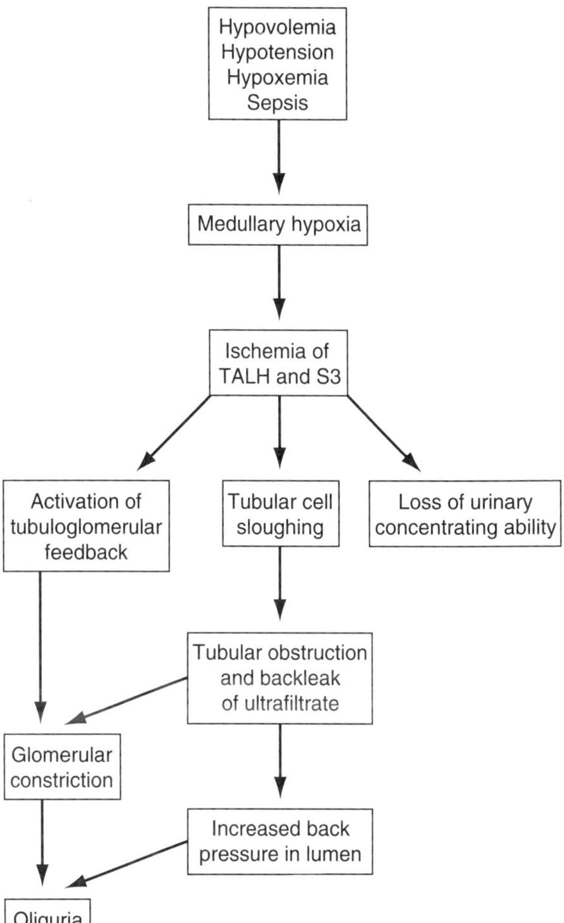

Figure 6–2. A simplified diagram of the most accepted model of the pathogenesis of acute renal failure in the setting of prerenal injury. The central mechanism revolves around inadequate oxygen delivery to the thick ascending loop of Henle (TALH) and the distal part of the proximal tubule (S3). Once this component of the nephron is damaged, a series of mechanisms are activated that lead to oliguria and, if severe, anuria.

pulmonary occlusion pressure, mean arterial pressure) is needed to obtain such information and guide further therapy.

Given these warnings, it still remains somewhat conceptually and clinically useful to subdivide patients with acute renal failure into those with prerenal, renal, and postrenal causes. Of these, the prerenal causes are by far the most common in patients in the ICU. Practically any insult that diminishes the blood and oxygen supply to the kidney (e.g., hemorrhage, hypotension, cardiogenic or septic shock) is capable, depending on its severity, of inducing renal failure. Kidney (parenchymal) disease is also an important cause of renal failure. Acute glomerulonephritis and various forms of vasculitis, as well as numerous exogenous or endogenous toxins, can induce acute renal failure. Of these, iatrogenic toxins cannot be overemphasized. Drugs (especially aminoglycosides, nonsteroidal anti-inflammatory agents, and radiocontrast dyes) are a common cause of iatrogenic renal failure, which can be avoided or rapidly treated if recognized.

RECOMMENDATION: *In all patients with acute renal failure, a detailed review of past and current medications is perhaps the single most important diagnostic step.*

Postrenal failure is common in the community but less common in the ICU. Nonetheless, because it can be treated effectively, it must always be considered and initially excluded by ultrasonography. Table 6–8 is an abbreviated list of the most common causes of acute renal failure.

It is sometimes important to distinguish acute renal failure or chronic renal failure presenting with an acute illness from a sudden deterioration in renal function. In the absence of previous information on the patient's renal function, the distinction can be difficult. A number of clinical clues can assist in this process, including the presence of shrunken kidneys; widespread cystic changes or calcifications on ultrasonography; normochromic, normocytic anemia at the onset of the acute illness; a history of symptoms that suggest chronic renal failure; and the presence of bony radiologic changes suggestive of renal osteodystrophy. These findings suggest preexisting and clinically important chronic renal failure.

Complications

The typical complications of acute renal failure include the development of the uremic state, which is characterized clinically by the retention of metabolic toxins and development of a bleeding diathesis, pericardial inflammation, and progressive encephalopathy. Biochemical derangements involve all major electrolytes. Solute retention leads to hyperkalemia, hyperphosphatemia, hypocalcemia, and hypermagnesemia. Water retention leads to hyponatremia. Sodium retention leads to peripheral edema and, later, pulmonary edema. Inadequate acid excretion invariably results in progressive metabolic acidosis.

Intermediate metabolism is affected and protein catabolism is accelerated. The homeostatic derangements seen in acute renal failure translate into serious morbidity and a tendency to develop gastrointestinal bleeding, arrhythmia, pulmonary edema, and infection. In critically ill patients, several additional problems are associated with acute renal failure. They include difficulties in accurately and safely

Table 6–8. MAJOR CAUSES OF ACUTE RENAL FAILURE

DIMINISHED KIDNEY PERFUSION
Any cause of hypotension or hypovolemia
Septic, cardiogenic, and hemorrhagic shock
Major trauma
Severe vomiting or diarrhea
Extensive burns
Adrenal insufficiency
Diabetic ketoacidosis
Pancreatitis
Hepatorenal syndrome
Crush injury
RENAL PARENCHYMAL DISEASE
Disorders affecting the glomerulus
Goodpasture's syndrome
Thrombotic thrombocytopenic purpura
Hemolytic uremic syndrome
Wegener's granulomatosis
Polyarteritis nodosa
Microscopic polyarteritis
Disorders affecting the interstitium
Exogenous nephrotoxins
Antibiotics
Anesthetic agents
Contrast media
Chemotherapeutic drugs
Heavy metals and organic solvents
Calcium
Urate
Paraproteins
Tumoral infiltration
Hypersensitivity reactions
Bacterial, viral, or fungal infections
OBSTRUCTION TO RENAL OUTFLOW
Mechanical causes of urinary tract blockage
Benign prostatic hypertrophy
Cancer of the prostate and bladder
Retroperitoneal fibrosis
Bilateral renal calculi
Bilateral papillary necrosis

adjusting the dosage and dosing interval of the multiple drugs usually necessary for patient treatment, in safely delivering adequate nutritional supplementation, and in avoiding fluid overload. In these patients, the development of acute renal failure signals a likely increase in morbidity and markedly increases the difficulty of clinical management.

CONCEPT: *Acute renal failure is not just a disease of the kidneys but a state of physiologic derangement involving the entire body.*

Management

The most important step in the management of acute renal failure is its prevention. Unfortunately, no single drug or procedure can secure the preservation of renal function. Renal protection, therefore, particularly in the critically ill, requires attention to several clinical details. Renal perfusion and adequate intravascular volume must be maintained. Experimental and human data indicate that renal autoregulation of perfusion fails at about 65 to 80 mm Hg of mean arterial pressure. Such failure may occur at higher pressures in elderly patients and those with a history of hypertension or renovascular disease. A decrease in renal blood flow of about 30% results from a pressure drop from 80 to 60 mm Hg in a healthy individual; in a septic patient with high oxygen organ consumption and humorally mediated renal vasoconstriction, a similar decrease in blood pressure can be disastrous.

CONCEPT: *The maintenance of adequate renal perfusion pressure is an important therapeutic goal of resuscitation and kidney protection.*

In patients with increased intra-abdominal pressure (e.g., from ileus, ascites, peritonitis, pneumoperitoneum, intra-abdominal bleeding) in whom renal perfusion pressure equals mean arterial pressure minus intra-abdominal pressure, the maintenance of a mean blood pressure of at least 80 mm Hg is particularly important. In some patients, decompression of the abdominal cavity becomes the only way that renal perfusion pressure and function can be maintained. The maintenance of renal perfusion pressure in critically ill patients can be achieved initially by the administration of intravenous fluids, which should be invasively monitored. Despite the administration of fluids and the achievement of a state of both high cardiac output and high pulmonary occlusion pressures, some patients remain oliguric and hypotensive. Further administration of fluids in these patients is of unproven benefit, and restoration of renal perfusion pressure in this setting is best achieved by the introduction of vasopressors such as norepinephrine.

CONCEPT: *After effective fluid resuscitation has been safely accomplished, additional intravenous fluids are likely to induce pulmonary edema without any further beneficial effect on the kidneys.*

CONCEPT: *Vasopressor drugs, which can induce renal failure in animal models at mean blood pressures of 150 mm Hg, can prevent acute renal failure when used, after adequate fluid resuscitation, to increase the patient's mean blood pressure from 50 or 60 to 80 mm Hg.*

A number of drugs have been proposed as protective to the kidneys, but there is no scientific evidence of their effectiveness. For each one, including mannitol, furosemide, and prostaglandins, various rationales have been offered but not proved. The administration of so-called low-dose dopamine (1–2 μg/kg/min) has been proposed as a way of protecting the kidney from prerenal injury. Evidence of increased renal blood flow during the intravenous infusion of low-dose dopamine in healthy subjects has been used to support its use in the critically ill. No scientific evidence indicates any protective effect in the critically ill, however, or in any patient or animal at risk of developing acute renal failure. In fact, there is some evidence to the contrary. Until further data are available, the routine administration of dopamine cannot be recommended. As previously stated, existing obstruction must be removed and nephrotoxic drugs discontinued if at all possible.

If renal failure becomes established, the intensivist encounters a number of important issues. First is the need to preserve homeostasis, which includes the prevention or correction of fluid and electrolyte imbalances. Second is the need to prevent the complications of uremia, which may require the introduction of renal replacement therapy. Third is the need to prevent further injury to the recovering kidney, which requires attention to hemodynamic support throughout the period of established renal failure and the provision of adequate nutritional support. In most of these areas, no scientific evidence supports any particular approach. A number of principles, however, should guide management at this stage:

1. The so-called conservative approach (trying to treat the patient without dialysis) is untenable in critically ill patients on mechanical ventilation.
2. Waiting for the development of uremic complications (e.g., fluid overload, pericarditis, encephalopathy, severe acidosis, severe hyperkalemia) before initiating artificial renal support (hemodialysis or hemofiltration) makes no sense in any patient, particularly the critically ill. In some way, it is akin to waiting for near cardiopulmonary arrest before intubating and mechanically ventilating a patient with obvious pulmonary edema, tachypnea, and hypoxemia.
3. Restricting protein intake in acutely ill patients in an attempt to diminish the frequency of dialytic therapy results in a severe negative nitrogen balance with associated protein wasting. Protein and calorie administration in critically ill patients with acute and renal failure should be no different from that of other critically ill patients. Uremia should then be controlled as necessary by means of hemofiltration or dialysis.

CONCEPT: *Early artificial support of the kidneys, maintenance of fluid and electrolyte homeostasis, and provision of appropriate nutritional supplementation are sensible and important therapeutic goals in critically ill patients with acute renal failure.*

CHOICE OF RENAL REPLACEMENT THERAPY

Three major modalities of renal replacement therapy are currently in use—intermittent hemodialysis, peritoneal dialysis (intermittent or continuous), and continuous hemofiltration with all of its technical variations.

Because of a high risk (15–20%) of peritonitis, limited solute clearances, and metabolic and respiratory side effects, peritoneal dialysis is rarely used in critically ill patients.

Intermittent hemodialysis has been the standard form of renal replacement therapy for decades, both in chronic and acute renal failure. Unfortunately, this technique has a number of serious limitations in the critically ill. It is associated with the induction of hypotension, particularly when rapid fluid removal is undertaken in hemodynamically unstable and pressor-supported patients. It triggers hypoventilation and hypoxemia, often results in inadequate fluid removal, and corrects electrolyte imbalances so rapidly that major shifts can induce arrhythmia, the development of cerebral edema, and, in some patients, the disequilibrium syndrome. Standard hemodialysis also exposes the patient to bioincompatible membranes, which activate a number of humoral proinflammatory molecules (complement and cytokines) that may aggravate organ injury. These adverse side effects

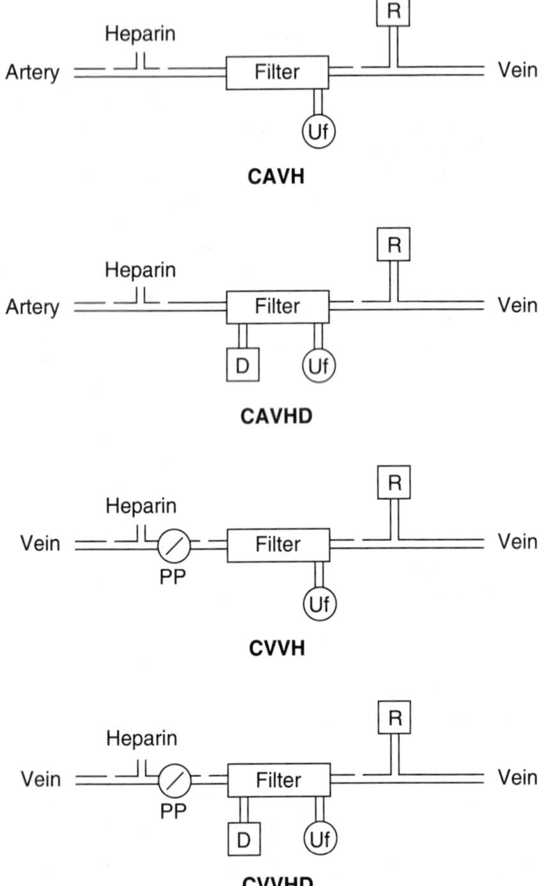

Figure 6–3 *See legend on opposite page*

of standard hemodialysis often have significant morbid repercussions in ICU patients.

Continuous hemofiltration has been developed during the past decade and is based on the use of a biocompatible, highly porous membrane that functions as an artificial glomerulus. By removing large volumes of fluid (which are separately replaced to avoid hypovolemia), this method achieves blood purification and controls uremia. It has the advantage of maintaining hemodynamic stability; achieving adequate solute removal and steady control of uremia, fluids, and electrolytes; using biocompatible membranes; and allowing the easy administration of nutritional support fluids and blood. The initial technique, continuous arteriovenous hemofiltration, used the patient's own blood pressure to drive blood through the hemofilter. Subsequent developments have used a slow countercurrent dialysate flow through the hemofilter to achieve higher urea clearances, such as in continuous arteriovenous hemodiafiltration. The use of peristaltic pumps maintains blood flow through the filter as in continuous venovenous hemofiltration or continuous venovenous hemodiafiltration and avoids the need for arterial puncture. Finally, if controlled (100–200 mL/h) slow fluid removal with no fluid replacement and countercurrent slow (1–2 L/h) dialysate flow is undertaken the technique of slow continuous ultrafiltration with dialysis can be implemented. The versatility of hemofiltration-based renal replacement therapy is obvious. The circuits for these techniques are summarized in Figure 6–3.

Figure 6–3. The four major techniques of hemofiltration. In continuous arteriovenous hemofiltration (CAVH), blood is driven by the patient's blood pressure from an artery to a vein. As it crosses the hemofilter, ultrafiltrate (Uf) is produced, and a degree of urea clearance is achieved. The lost fluid is replaced as needed with saline-based replacement fluid (R). The extracorporeal circuit is usually anticoagulated with heparin and contains multiple sampling ports (breaks in top lines of circuit).

During continuous arteriovenous hemodiafiltration (CAVHD), the same circuit is used, but urea clearance is enhanced by the administration of dialysate (D) to the nonblood compartment of the filter. This results in diffusive molecular clearance in addition to the convective clearance associated with hemofiltration alone.

Continuous venovenous hemofiltration (CVVH) uses single venous access with a double-lumen hemodialysis catheter. Blood, therefore, must be driven through the circuit by means of a peristaltic pump (PP) to generate ultrafiltrate.

The addition of a diffusive component to CVVH results in the technique of continuous venovenous hemodiafiltration (CVVHD). Once again, blood must be pumped through the circuit by a peristaltic pump, and dialysate is delivered to the nonblood compartment of the filter to enhance urea clearance. The circuit often requires anticoagulation with prefilter heparin.

The most effective mode of renal replacement in the critically ill remains undetermined, since no randomized controlled study directly comparing these approaches has ever been undertaken. In the United States, intermittent hemodialysis is the dominant mode, whereas hemofiltration is most frequently used in Europe. The current recommendation is that renal replacement therapy be individualized. It would be unwise, for instance, to use intermittent hemodialysis to treat a patient with the adult respiratory distress syndrome, acute renal failure, severe peripheral edema, and a vasopressor-dependent unstable circulation. However, hemofiltration may be phased out in this type of patient once there is physiologic stability, resolution of edema, and improvement of cardiovascular and respiratory function. Likewise, a head-injured patient with increased intracranial pressure, cerebral edema, and acute renal failure can experience life-threatening intracranial hypertension if hemodialyzed. After a few days of hemofiltration and resolution of the cerebral edema, however, conventional hemodialysis is an acceptable alternative. Decisions about the choice of renal replacement therapy in the critically ill are best made after consultation involving both the critical care physician and the nephrologist and with a clear understanding of the local medical and nursing expertise in the available techniques.

CONCEPT: *Numerous approaches to renal replacement therapy exist in the acute setting. Tailoring renal replacement therapy to each patient's needs is both possible and advisable.*

Despite the advances in renal support, acute renal failure continues to be associated with a high mortality rate in the ICU. This is not only because loss of renal function makes management more difficult and induces a morbidity of its own but also and principally because, in the setting of multiple organ failure, renal function is a marker of illness severity (as recognized in many illness severity scoring systems). Thus, these patients die with, not of, acute renal failure.

Because the prognosis of multiorgan failure will be altered only when effective therapies that address its causes have been developed, the prognosis of acute renal failure in the ICU will not be noticeably improved until that time. On the other hand, preventing the specific morbidity related to renal failure may save numerous patients, and, in this regard, the use of hemofiltration offers some promise.

HEPATORENAL SYNDROME AND RHABDOMYOLYSIS

The hepatorenal syndrome and rhabdomyolysis are two causes of acute renal failure that have some peculiar features requiring a brief separate discussion. The hepatorenal syndrome is the development of acute renal failure in the setting of severe liver dysfunction and without other recognized causes. This syndrome appears to be characterized by a state of renal vasoconstriction and by urine sodium concentrations (<10 mmol/L) consistent with severe prerenal kidney failure. The functional nature of this syndrome has been supported by the successful return to normal function of kidneys from patients with the hepatorenal syndrome following their transplantation into a healthy recipient. The diagnosis of the hepatorenal syndrome, however, is extremely difficult in the ICU. In this setting, the distinction between the hepatorenal syndrome and other causes of prerenal failure is blurred by the simultaneous presence of multiple sources of renal injury. Many of these patients with severe hepatic failure, for instance, have diuretic-induced intravascular volume depletion because of attempts to control their ascites. Some of them experience further fluid losses because of lactulose-induced diarrhea (to control encephalopathy) and abdominal paracentesis; in many cases, gastrointestinal bleeding further complicates the clinical picture. In addition, systemic vasodilation and the multiple arteriovenous shunts found in end-stage liver disease induce a hypotensive state, and, in the presence of tense ascites, the renal perfusion pressure of a patient with a failing liver is marginal at best.

Whatever the pathogenesis of acute renal failure in patients with progressive and severe hepatic dysfunction, attention must be paid to their intravascular and extravascular fluid status. Invasive monitoring is often necessary. If diuretic therapy is being undertaken, close monitoring of renal function and intravascular pressures is advisable. If paracentesis is planned, adequate simultaneous colloid administration may be beneficial and hypotension should be avoided. If gastrointestinal bleeding occurs, resuscitation should be prompt and invasively monitored.

Severe rhabdomyolysis can be induced by many physical and chemical insults and may result in the development of acute renal failure. The pathogenesis includes fluid sequestration, hypovolemia, diminished renal perfusion, toxicity of the heme moiety in an acidic environment, and obstruction by myoglobin casts in the tubules. Because of these particular features, it has been recommended that vigorous fluid replacement be undertaken as soon as possible from the time of injury and that alkalinization of urine be achieved by the administration of sodium bicarbonate. Although scientific evidence is lacking that alkalinization of urine is of additional benefit to aggressive and early fluid resuscitation, much anecdotal clinical evidence supports this therapy and its safety justifies its use in most instances.

CHRONIC RENAL FAILURE: SPECIAL CONSIDERATIONS

A number of patients with chronic renal failure are admitted to the ICU. In these patients, the development of an acute illness may trigger complete renal dysfunction, which can require renal replacement therapy and which occasionally can fail to resolve. One must be aware of the presence of chronic renal impairment to minimize renal injuries.

The preservation of an adequate intravascular and extravascular volume state is particularly important. Mild to moderate edema should not be aggressively treated with diuretics. Fluid losses should be promptly replaced under invasive monitoring. Vasopressors should be used only after adequate fluid resuscitation has taken place. Many of these patients have hypertension. Because poor control of their blood pressure significantly worsens renal function, tight control is mandatory and can require the use of intravenous antihypertensive agents.

Finally, these patients are particularly susceptible to the injurious effects of nephrotoxic drugs. Caution is advised before aminoglycoside antibiotics, nonsteroidal anti-inflammatory agents, or intravenous radiologic contrast dyes are used. If their use cannot be avoided, steps should be taken to monitor renal function regularly and to maintain a degree of intravascular and extravascular volume expansion.

DRUG–KIDNEY INTERACTIONS

Most drugs and their metabolites are excreted by the kidney. Renal dysfunction, therefore, has clinically important effects on their pharmacokinetics. These effects in turn require dose and dose interval adjustments, increasing the likelihood of drug-induced side effects. Several basic principles of pharmacokinetics must be understood when prescribing drugs in critically ill patients with renal failure. Renal failure may affect the bioavailability of nonparenterally administered drugs. If the drug is administered parenterally, renal failure, as well as the effects of volume resuscitation and extracellular space expansion, may affect its volume of distribution. This alteration is clinically important, since knowledge of the volume of distribution for a given drug allows the physician to predict the peak concentration. Gentamicin, for instance, has a volume of distribution of 20 L in the average noncritically ill patient. The administration of a loading dose of 120 mg will, therefore, result in a peak concentration of 120 divided by 20, or 6 mg/L (in the low therapeutic range). If the same dose is given to a volume-expanded, recently resuscitated, septic, critically ill patient with acute renal failure (expected volume of distribution, 40 L), it will result in a peak concentration of only 3 mg/L, a subtherapeutic level. The clinical consequences are obvious. The gentamicin loading dose for such a patient should be in the range of 320 to 350 mg.

RECOMMENDATION: *For many antibiotics, achieving adequate peak levels is of major therapeutic significance. Knowing the predicted volume of distribution in a given patient is mandatory before administration is begun.*

Renal failure results in diminished drug clearance. Drug clearance is defined as the rate of elimination of a solute relative to its plasma concentration. Clinically, clearance is used to indicate the volume of plasma from which a drug has been completely eliminated per time unit. Most drugs are cleared by the kidney by first-order kinetics: the plasma concentration of the drug diminishes exponentially from its initial level at time zero to zero at time infinity. This rate of disappearance is typically expressed in terms of biologic half-life ($t_{1/2}$) defined as the time needed for a drug's concentration to decrease one half the equilibration value. The $t_{1/2}$ of a given drug can be calculated with a reasonable degree of accuracy if its volume of distribution is known. The volume of distribution can be easily calculated from the dose administered, and its equilibration value can usually be measured 30 minutes after parenteral administration of the drug. The rate of clearance must also be known. This is typically close to the patient's creatinine clearance, which either can be directly measured over a 4- to 6-hour period or can be estimated using standard formulas as previously described. Such predictability of $t_{1/2}$ derives from the fact that its decrease in serum concentration follows an inverse natural logarithmic course:

$$t_{1/2} = 0.693 \times \text{volume of distribution/clearance}$$

The way in which renal dysfunction affects the excretion of several drugs used in the ICU and their metabolites is summarized in Table 6–9.

RECOMMENDATION: *For potentially toxic drugs or for drugs that require target peak and trough levels, dosing should be based on calculations of expected pharmacokinetics. Such calculations should be constantly adjusted to the patient's change in renal function and volume state.*

Table 6–9. INTENSIVE CARE DRUGS MOST COMMONLY AFFECTED BY ACUTE RENAL FAILURE AND GUIDELINES FOR DOSAGE

	Dose According to Creatinine Clearance		
	>60 mL/M	10–60 mL/M	<10 mL/M
Acyclovir	5 mg/kg q8h	5 mg/kg q12–24h	5 mg/kg q48h
Gancyclovir	5 mg/kg q8h	2 mg/kg q24h	1.2 mg/kg q24h
Amikacin	7 mg/kg q12h	5 mg/kg q24h	4 mg/kg q48h
Gentamicin	2 mg/kg q12h	1.5 mg/kg q16h	1.5 mg/kg q72h
Tobramycin	2 mg/kg q12h	1.5 mg/kg q16h	1.5 mg/kg q72h
Cefamandole	2 g q6h	1 g q8h	1 g q12h
Cefotaxime	2 g q8h	2 g q12h	1 g q12h
Cefotetan	2 g q12h	2 g q24h	1 g q24h
Ceftazidime	1 g q8h	1 g q12h	0.5 g q24h
Ceftriaxone	2 g q24h	1 g q24h	1 g q24h
Penicillin G	2 MU q4h	1 MU q4h	1 MU q6h
Ampicillin	1 g q6h	1 g q8h	1 g q12h
Imipenem	1 g q8h	1 g q12h	0.5 g q12h
Piperacillin	4 g q6h	3 g q6h	2 g q8h
Cloxacillin	0.5 g q6h	0.25 g q6h	0.25 g q6h
Vancomycin	0.75 g q12h	0.75 g q24h	1 g q5–7d
Ciprofloxacin	0.5 g q12h	0.25 g q12h	0.5 g q24h
Fluconazole	0.2 g q24h	0.1 g q24h	0.1 g q24h
Famotidine	40 mg q24h	20 mg q24h	20 mg q48h
Cimetidine	0.3 g q8h	0.3 g q12h	0.3 g q24h

If renal dysfunction is complete, the accumulation of renally excreted drugs is inevitable unless appropriate dosage adjustments are made. Many drugs, in fact, have other routes of excretion that will eventually lower their serum concentration. Vancomycin, which can be given once a week in patients with renal failure, is a typical example. The implementation of renal replacement therapy (hemodialysis or hemofiltration) also has a clinically important impact on drug clearance, requiring appropriate dose adjustments. Typically, hemodialysis removes drugs with a molecular size smaller than 500 daltons that do not have a major degree of protein binding. Thus, it removes gentamicin but not vancomycin (molecular weight, 1140 daltons). Hemofiltration and derived techniques, on the other hand, slowly but effectively removes drugs with low protein binding, even if their molecular weight is higher than 1000 daltons.

Tables 6–10 and 6–11 offer dosing guidelines for several drugs during artificial renal support.

RECOMMENDATION: *If a patient is receiving renal replacement therapy, tables should be consulted before drug administration so that appropriate therapeutic levels are achieved and toxic levels avoided. Tailoring of drug therapy is mandatory.*

DRUG-INDUCED NEPHROTOXICITY

Because the kidney is the route of excretion of many drugs and their concentrations are particularly high in the renal parenchyma, the organ is particularly vulnerable to drugs and toxins. In critically ill patients, other mechanisms of

Table 6–10. DIALYTIC CLEARANCE OF DRUGS COMMONLY USED IN THE INTENSIVE CARE UNIT

NEGLIGIBLE CLEARANCE DURING INTERMITTENT HEMODIALYSIS

Antibiotics
- Cefotetan, clindamycin, cloxacillin, nafcillin, doxycycline, vancomycin, amphotericin B, itraconazole, ketoconazole, azidothymidine, erythromycin, ciprofloxacin

Cardiovascular drugs
- Amiodarone, disopyramide, propafenone, esmolol, labetalol, metoprolol, digoxin, diltiazem

Miscellaneous drugs
- Morphine, propoxyphene, benzodiazepines, phenytoin, cimetidine, famotidine, omeprazole, cyclosporin A, prednisone

SIGNIFICANT CLEARANCE DURING INTERMITTENT HEMODIALYSIS (postdialysis redosing recommended)

Antibiotics
- Aminoglycosides, most cephalosporins, imipenem, aztreonam, ampicillin, piperacillin, sulfamethoxazole–trimethoprim, flucytosine, metronidazole, isoniazid, acyclovir, ganciclovir

Other drugs
- Ranitidine, cyclophosphamide, sotalol, captopril, allopurinol, atenolol, N-acetylprocainamide

Table 6–11. DOSAGE OF SOME INTENSIVE CARE DRUGS REMOVED DURING CONTINUOUS HEMOFILTRATION TECHNIQUES*

Cefuroxime	750 mg q12h
Tobramycin	120 mg q24h
Amikacin	250–500 mg q24h
Imipenem	500 mg q12h
Metronidazole	500 mg q8h
Ceftazidime	500 mg q12h
Gentamicin	80–100 mg q24h
Vancomycin	500–1000 mg q24h
Ciprofloxacin	500 mg q24h
Piperacillin	4 g q8h

*These values are approximate and depend on the type of hemofiltration technique in use.

renal injury (e.g., hypovolemia, hypotension, sepsis) can increase the injurious effect of nephrotoxic drugs. For these reasons, drug-induced renal failure is common in hospitals. Several drugs make up the bulk of those responsible for clinically significant renal injury. Aminoglycosides, for instance, are a common cause of iatrogenic renal failure, with an overall incidence of 5% to 15% of patient treatment courses. In critically ill septic patients, their contribution to the development of renal failure may be subtle and difficult to recognize in the presence of multiple factors capable of affecting renal function. The clinical pattern of aminoglycoside nephrotoxicity is characterized by the initial appearance of lysosomal enzymes in the urine, followed by polyuria and by a decrease in GFR. Typically, the urine sodium concentration is greater than 40 mEq/L and renal failure is nonoliguric, occurring 7 to 10 days after the initiation of treatment. Oliguria, however, may be seen with concomitant sepsis and hypotension, and the typical presentation is rarely seen in critically ill patients. Several risk factors predispose the patient to the development of aminoglycoside-induced renal failure (Table 6–12).

RECOMMENDATION: *If a critically ill patient with renal dysfunction requires antibiotics, aminoglycosides should be used only when mandated by bacterial antibiotic sensitivity studies and in the absence of equally efficacious antimicrobial drugs.*

Radiologic contrast media are also an important cause of drug-induced acute renal failure, particularly in patients with previous chronic renal impairment. They are now the most common cause of drug-induced acute renal failure. Several risk factors (Table 6–13) predispose the patient to contrast media–induced renal failure, with diabetes and a serum creatinine measurement over 2 mg/dL being of particular importance. Typically, this kind of acute renal failure is of the oliguric type, with the increase in serum creatinine beginning 24 hours after the insult and peaking at 72 to 96 hours. Prevention is the best therapeutic strategy. In patients at risk, modalities that avoid contrast media are preferable,

Table 6–12. RISK FACTORS FOR THE DEVELOPMENT OF AMINOGLYCOSIDE TOXICITY

High dosage and prolonged administration
High trough levels
Use of concurrent nephrotoxins
Vancomycin
Amphotericin B
Cisplatin
Cyclosporin A
FK-506
Radiographic contrast media
Nonsteroidal antiinflammatory drugs
Concurrent renal injury
Intravascular volume depletion
Hepatic disease
Sepsis
Hypotension
Disorders of acid-base status and of electrolytes
Hypercalcemia
Hypomagnesemia
Hypokalemia
Metabolic acidosis
Factors related to patient status
Old age
Chronic renal impairment
Previous treatment with aminoglycosides

but, if contrast must be used, the quantity administered should be minimized and appropriate fluid administration and maintenance of diuresis should be pursued at the same time (Table 6–14).

RECOMMENDATION: Do not administer contrast media to patients with chronic renal failure and diabetes unless absolutely necessary and unless appropriate steps have been taken to maintain diuresis and to provide appropriate volume expansion before, during, and after administration.

Table 6–13. RISK FACTORS FOR CONTRAST MEDIA–INDUCED ACUTE RENAL FAILURE

Chronic renal failure (serum creatinine >1.5 mg/dL)
Diabetes
Age >60 years
Hypertension
Exposure to other nephrotoxins
Radiocontrast injection >2 mL/kg
Multiple studies with contrast media
Dehydration
Hyperuricemia
Liver disease
Cardiac failure
Solitary kidney
Multiple myeloma
Proteinuria

Table 6–14. GUIDELINES FOR THE PREVENTION OF CONTRAST MEDIA–INDUCED ACUTE RENAL FAILURE

GENERAL MEASURES

Remove other nephrotoxins.
Minimize amount of contrast administered.
Avoid intravascular volume depletion.

SPECIFIC STEPS

Infuse 500 mL of 5% mannitol at 100 mL/h beginning 1 hour before the procedure.

or

Infuse 1500 mL of 0.45% saline beginning 4 hours before the procedure and 250 mL of 20% mannitol within 1 hour of exposure to the contrast agent.

or

Infuse 500 mL of 20% mannitol with 100 mg of furosemide for each mg/dL of serum creatinine at an infusion rate of 20 mL/h beginning 1 hour before the procedure and continuing for at least 6 hours. Simultaneously replace urine output 1:1 with intravenous fluids.

or

Infuse 1500 mL of 5% dextrose in 0.45% saline over 4 hours before the procedure and 125 mL/h of the same solution for 4 hours thereafter.

Other drugs used in critically ill patients can induce acute renal failure. Acyclovir-induced renal dysfunction is dose dependent and usually can be prevented by the administration of sufficient amounts of fluids. Amphotericin B can induce potassium wasting and a form of distal tubular acidosis. Over time, a dose-related nonoliguric renal failure develops that is often associated with hypomagnesemia. Mannitol, if given in large doses (as in cases of refractory intracranial hypertension), can induce renal ischemia and failure. Many other agents—such as nonsteroidal anti-inflammatory drugs, angiotensin-converting enzyme inhibitors, methotrexate, and cisplatin—can also induce acute renal failure, but they are rarely used in critically ill patient. Cyclosporin A and FK-506, which are used for recipient immunosuppression during solid organ and bone marrow transplantation, are more commonly seen in the modern ICU. Both can induce vasoconstriction, interstitial nephropathy, and renal dysfunction either acutely or chronically. Therefore, their dosage and their blood levels require constant monitoring.

CHAPTER 7

Endocrinology and Metabolism and Pharmacologic Principles

PART A

Endocrinology and Metabolism

J. Harlan Meyer, MD, PhD

The endocrine system is vital to the normal physiologic processes of homeostasis, growth, reproduction, and the utilization and storage of energy. As such, endocrine disorders can have profound influences throughout the body, and recognition of these disorders is vitally important so that treatment can be instituted in a timely fashion. Delay in treatment can result in increased morbidity and mortality. In the critical care setting, endocrine dysfunction occasionally occurs as the primary illness resulting in hospitalization. More commonly, however, endocrine disorders exist either as a chronic condition that is concurrent with an acute serious illness or as a secondary development of an acute illness. This chapter summarizes some of the more common endocrine and nutrition problems encountered in the critical care setting.

THYROID GLAND

Physiology

Thyroid hormone synthesis depends on active transport of iodide into thyroid follicular cells, a process stimulated by thyroid-stimulating hormone (TSH) produced in the pituitary gland. Subsequently, oxidization of iodide, organification of iodine into thyroglobulin molecules, and coupling reactions result in the formation of iodothyronines, which are then cleaved to produce the two thyroid hormones, thyroxine (T_4) and triiodothyronine (T_3). Once released, T_3 and T_4 exist both free and bound to proteins, including T_4-binding globulin (TBG), T_4-binding prealbumin (TBPA), and albumin. In contrast to T_4, T_3 is not appreciably bound to TBPA. Whereas T_4 is the predominant hormone released from the thyroid gland, T_3 is actually the physiologically active form of thyroid hormone and either is released directly from the thyroid or is produced in the periphery from intracellular deiodination of T_4 at its outer ring. Deiodination of the inner ring leads to formation of the hormonally inactive reverse T_3 (rT_3), which provides another level at which thyroid hormone activity can be regulated.

TSH release is subject to positive stimulation by hypothalamic thyrotropin-releasing hormone (TRH), the stimulatory input of which is counterbalanced by feedback inhibition of thyroid hormones on the TSH-secreting cells of the pituitary gland. This produces a system that tightly regulates the plasma levels of thyroid hormones, but any number of factors that affect the pituitary gland or thyroid gland can cause disruption in the normal regulation of thyroid hormone levels (Table 7–1), leading to either hyperthyroidism or hypothyroidism.

Laboratory Assessment

To assess a patient's thyroid status, plasma TSH, T_4, and T_3 levels are measured. TSH values are usually suppressed in the setting of hyperthyroidism, except in the case of a TSH-producing adenoma. In hypothyroidism, TSH values are typically elevated, although pharmacologic influences of medications on TSH secretion can confound the typical picture (Table 7–1). T_4 measurements are complicated by the fact that T_4 exists predominantly bound to proteins, the levels of which vary as the result of a number of different conditions, as outlined in Table 7–2. Thus, measurement of total T_4 needs to be corrected to assess the amount of physiologically active free hormone accurately. This can be done by using a T_3 resin uptake test, which can be used to derive a calculated free T_4 index, or by directly measuring the free T_4 levels by radioimmunoassay or equilibrium dialysis. When uncertainty exists as to the validity of free T_4 index measurements, it is frequently helpful to obtain one of these two latter studies. T_3 levels are typically elevated in hyperthyroid states and low in hypothyroidism. In certain cases, hyperthyroidism may be due to isolated increases in T_3 levels, so-called T_3 toxicosis. Thus, evaluation of a

Table 7–1. FACTORS AFFECTING HYPOTHALAMIC-PITUITARY-THYROID AXIS

	Stimulation	Inhibition
Hypothalamic TRH production	Norepinephrine Dopamine	T_3, T_4 Glucocorticoids
Pituitary TSH production	TRH	Estrogens Glucocorticoids Dopamine T_3, T_4 Somatostatin

Thyroid gland hormone production	TSH
	Iodine
	Catecholamines
	HCG
	Cold exposure
		Iodine
		Medications
		  Lithium
		  Antithyroid medications
		  Para-aminosalicylic acid
		  Ethionamide
		Dietary goitrogens
		Malnutrition

Abbreviations: HCG = human chorionic gonadotropin; TRH = thyrotropin-releasing hormone; TSH = thyroid-stimulating hormone.

Table 7–2. CAUSES OF THYROID-BINDING PROTEIN ABNORMALITIES AND EFFECTS ON THYROXINE LEVELS

	Hyperthyroxinemia	Hypothyroxinemia
T_4-binding globulin	Increased levels	Decreased levels
	Estrogens	Androgens
	Pregnancy	Acromegaly
	Acute hepatitis	Nephrosis
	Acute intermittent porphyria	Asparaginase
	Chronic active hepatitis	Glucocorticoids
	Primary biliary cirrhosis	Cirrhosis
	Inherited elevations in TBG levels	Inherited reductions in TBG levels
T_4-binding prealbumin	Increased T_4 binding	
Albumin	Familial dysalbuminemic hyperthyroxinemia	

suppressed TSH level should include determination of not only the T_4 level but also the total T_3 level. It is rarely necessary to determine a free T_3 level.

Hyperthyroidism

Pathophysiology and Manifestations

The differential diagnosis for elevated thyroid hormone levels is shown in Table 7–3. Euthyroid hyperthyroxinemia represents a laboratory finding only; patients appear normal clinically. In true hyperthyroidism, numerous clinical manifestations are seen, although elderly patients may display few overt signs. Symptoms include nervousness, sweating, palpitations, weight loss, fatigue, weakness, oligomenorrhea, increased appetite, eye complaints, hyperdefecation, diarrhea, and anorexia. Signs of hyperthyroidism include tachycardia or arrhythmia, goiter, tremor, exophthalmos, lid retraction, hyperreflexia, fine hair, and skin changes. A bruit may also be noted over the thyroid bed. TSH levels are typically suppressed, although an exception occurs in the setting of a TSH-secreting pituitary adenoma, in which pituitary hypersecretion of TSH causes hyperthyroidism.

Diagnosis

Once it has been determined that a patient has true hyperthyroidism as opposed to euthyroid hyperthyroxinemia, the cause needs to be determined, since the treatment provided depends on the underlying cause. In cases in which the patient exhibits proptosis, the diagnosis of Graves' disease

Table 7–3. CAUSES OF HYPERTHYROXINEMIA

Euthyroid Hyperthyroxinemia

- Protein-binding abnormalities
  - Familial dysalbuminemic hyperthyroidism
  - Increased T_4-binding globulin
  - T_4-binding prealbumin binding abnormalities
- Anti-T_4 antibodies
- Thyroid hormone resistance
- Acute psychiatric illness
- Medications
  - Heparin (abnormal laboratory finding)
  - Propranolol
  - Amphetamines
  - Oral contrast
  - Amiodarone

Hyperthyroidism

- Graves' disease
- Thyroiditis
- Toxic multinodular goiter
- Autonomous solitary nodule
- Struma ovarii
- Trophoblastic tumors
- Metastatic thyroid cancer
- Factitious
- Pituitary adenoma

can be readily established. In other cases, however, it can be difficult to determine the underlying cause, and a radioactive iodine uptake and scan are useful in determining the cause of the hyperthyroidism. Uptake is diminished in thyroiditis and increased in Graves' disease. A toxic nodule is seen on a scan as a focal area of increased uptake.

Therapy

Mild cases of hyperthyroidism can be treated on an outpatient basis. Thyroiditis-associated hyperthyroidism is typically a self-limited state that lasts several months and then resolves spontaneously. In this process, thyroid tissue destruction results in the release of preformed thyroid hormone. Thyroid hormone synthesis inhibitors are not effective, therefore, and therapy relies on the use of β-blocking medications to reduce the peripheral manifestations of hyperthyroidism. Among the β-blockers, propranolol has the additional theoretic advantage of inhibiting the conversion of T_4 to T_3. With the exception of TSH-producing adenomas, all other causes of hyperthyroidism are best treated by agents that lower the rate of thyroid hormone synthesis, using either the antithyroid medications, propylthiouracil and methimazole, or iodine-131 thyroid ablation. Concomitant use of β-blockers can help ameliorate the systemic manifestations of hyperthyroidism until thyroid hormone levels can be lowered through the use of I^{131} or antithyroid medications. Amiodarone-associated hyperthyroidism may be extremely difficult to treat with propylthiouracil or methimazole; perchlorate has been used in such difficult cases.

Severe cases of hyperthyroidism may necessitate hospitalization of the patient, and thyroid storm, the most severe form of hypothyroidism, should initially be treated in an intensive care environment. General measures include repletion of fluids lost due to sweating, vomiting or diarrhea, and antipyresis with acetaminophen. Salicylates should be avoided, since these compounds displace thyroid hormone from plasma-binding proteins, resulting in further elevations in the amounts of free thyroid hormones. The following specific treatment steps should occur simultaneously:

1. Inhibition of thyroid hormone release from the thyroid gland through the use of SSKI (saturated solution of potassium iodide) 5 drops every 6 hours, sodium iodide, 250 mg intravenously every 6 hours, or ipodate sodium (Oragrafin), 1 g/d. Ipodate sodium also inhibits conversion of T_4 to T_3 and thus is particularly effective.
2. Blockade of the hyperadrenergic state by means of β-blockers. A typical dosage of propranolol is 40 to 80 mg orally or 2 mg intravenously every 6 hours, but this agent should be used with caution in patients with heart failure. Esmolol has also been used and, because of its short half-life, can be advantagous in the setting of heart failure.
3. Administration of glucocorticoids (e.g., 2 mg dexamethasone every 6 hours), which inhibits release of thyroid hormone from the thyroid gland and also inhibits conversion of T_4 to T_3.

4. Administration of antithyroid medications; PTU is preferred over methimazole because of its ability to inhibit T_4 to T_3 conversion. A typical dosage of PTU is 300 to 400 mg every 4 hours. If necessary, PTU and methimazole can be crushed and administered through a nasogastric tube, or methimazole can be delivered rectally.

When these medical therapies are used in combination, almost all patients can be treated satisfactorily. Surgical treatment is almost never required but occasionally is necessary in the rare case of hyperthyroidism refractory to medical therapy or in the case of a large hyperfunctioning goiter that is compromising the airway or other nearby structures.

Hypothyroidism

Pathophysiology and Manifestations

Hypothyroidism is a relatively common diagnosis and rarely requires hospitalization. Signs and symptoms of hypothyroidism include weakness, dry and coarse skin, lethargy, slow speech, periorbital or facial edema, cold intolerance, coarse hair, tongue thickening, weight gain, constipation, peripheral edema, hoarseness, menorrhagia, and dyspnea. Hypothyroidism can result from either impaired thyroid gland function (primary hypothyroidism) or from hypothalamic-pituitary disease (secondary hypothyroidism). The differential diagnosis for hypothyroxinemia is outlined in Table 7–4.

Diagnosis

In primary hypothyroidism, T_3 and T_4 levels are low and TSH levels are elevated. Other diagnostic studies used in primary hypothyroidism include measurement of antithyroglobulin or antithyroid microsomal antibodies, but such studies rarely contribute to appropriate patient management. In secondary hypothyroidism, TSH levels may be low or atypically normal in the setting of low thyroid hormone levels. It is imperative to discriminate euthyroid hypothyroxinemia from secondary hypothyroidism, since TSH levels may be normal in both situations. Typical symptoms and signs of hypothyroidism can be helpful in discriminating true hypothyroidism from euthyroid hypothyroxinemia, since such findings usually are absent in euthyroid persons. Further discrimination can be done by measuring free T_4 levels, which are normal in euthyroid hypothyroxinemia but low in true hypothyroidism.

Therapy

Treatment is provided in the form of synthetic levothyroxine, which is hepatically metabolized to yield T_4. In all but the most profound cases of hypothyroidism, treatment can be initiated as an outpatient. Levothyroxine is typically administered orally, but it can be given intravenously for hospitalized patients unable to take oral medications. If given intravenously, the dose should be reduced to half the oral dose to correct for bowel absorption. For a young, otherwise

Table 7–4. DIFFERENTIAL DIAGNOSIS OF HYPOTHYROXINEMIA

Euthyroid Hypothyroxinemia

- Reduced TBG levels
  - Acromegaly
  - Androgens
  - Nephrotic syndrome
  - High-dose glucocorticoids or ACTH
  - Asparaginase
  - Protein-losing enteropathy
  - Hepatic cirrhosis
  - Inherited TBG deficiencies
- Altered T_4 protein binding
  - Phenytoin
  - Carbamazepine
  - Rifampin
  - Salicylates

Primary Hypothyroidism

- Autoimmune thyroiditis
- Iodine deficiency
- Hormone biosynthetic defects
- Iatrogenic
  - Postsurgical
  - Post–I^{131} treatment
  - Post-irradiation
- Antithyroid agents
  - Dietary goitrogens
  - Medications
    - Methimazole, propylthiouracil
    - Lithium
    - Ethionamide
    - Phenylbutazone
    - Topical resorcinol

Secondary Hypothyroidism

- Pituitary disease
  - Sheehan's syndrome
  - Hypophysitis
  - Pituitary tumor
  - Craniopharyngioma
  - Meningioma
  - Trauma
  - Medications (e.g., dopamine)
- Hypothalamic disease
  - Tumor (e.g., germinoma)
  - Histiocytosis X
  - Sarcoidosis
  - Trauma

Abbreviations: ACTH = adrenocorticotropic hormone; TBG = T_4-binding globulin.

healthy adult, the typical oral starting dosage can approximate full replacement dosages, often in the range of 75 to 125 μg/d. Elderly patients, particularly those with underlying cardiac disease, may need to be started at considerably lower dosages, around 25 μg, to avoid exacerbating cardiac disease. Dosages can then be increased gradually to reach full maintenance dosages. In primary hypothyroidism, a TSH level drawn approximately 6 to 8 weeks after the patient has been on maintenance therapy is used to confirm normalization of the thyroid status. Unfortunately, the TSH test cannot be used in cases of secondary hypothyroidism, and a T_4 level, in conjunction with the patient's clinical response, must be used to judge adequacy of therapy.

In patients diagnosed with hypothyroidism during a preoperative evaluation, mild to moderate hypothyroidism frequently has little adverse effect on surgical complications. Both increased rates of intraoperative hypotension and heart failure and increased rates of postoperative gastrointestinal and neuropsychiatric problems have been reported, but such findings were not accompanied by any significant impairment of wound healing or blood loss, or by any significant change in days of hospitalization or change in mortality. Thus, if surgery is needed, it should not be postponed. Thyroid hormone therapy can usually be initiated as soon as hypothyroidism is diagnosed, irrespective of timing with reference to the surgery. The one exception to this is patients with angina who are undergoing cardiac bypass. In such patients, thyroid hormone replacement is best deferred until after surgery, since thyroid hormone replacement presumably increases myocardial oxygen demands.

Myxedema coma, representing the most severe form of hypothyroidism, is associated with a high mortality rate and should therefore be managed in an intensive care setting. Precipitating factors for this condition include infection, trauma, and use of central nervous system depressants. Other than coma, manifestations include severe edema, pronounced hypothermia, bradycardia, hypotension, and areflexia. Hypercapnia and hyponatremia may be present, and seizures may occur. The mortality rate associated with this condition is high, but prompt institution of therapy can lead to clinical improvement within several hours of starting therapy. Thyroid function tests obtained to confirm the diagnosis should not delay initiation of therapy, since delay of appropriate treatment worsens prognosis. Initially, intravenous levothyroxine is administered as a single 200- to 300-μg bolus, followed by daily doses of 100 μg. Correction of the severe hypothyroid state accelerates the metabolism of steroids, so even a mild state of adrenal insufficiency existing before levothyroxine therapy may be converted to a full adrenal insufficiency crisis if supplemental steroids are not provided. To prevent this potential complication, 100 mg hydrocortisone should be administered every 8 hours for the first day and then tapered. Additional steps often necessary in myxedema coma include ventilatory assistance and correction of dilutional hyponatremia by administration of intravenous saline solutions and avoidance of hypotonic solutions. External warming should be avoided, because it can precipitate vascular collapse.

Sick Euthyroid State

The sick euthyroid condition is a common diagnostic dilemma in critically ill patients. In this state, both total T_4

and T_3 levels are diminished, and rT_3 levels may be increased. Free T_4 levels, as measured by equilibrium dialysis or radioimmunoassay, are often normal but may be slightly elevated or depressed. The discrepancy between total T_4 levels and free T_4 levels is a result of a higher fraction of T_4 being in the free state. TSH levels are frequently normal or only slightly elevated. Studies have failed to show any beneficial effect of thyroid hormone supplementation on clinical outcome in critically ill patients with a euthyroid sick state. Furthermore, there is no consistent evidence that thyroid hormone supplementation improves outcome in transplantation procedures, coronary revascularization procedures, or renal failure. Thus, hormone therapy cannot be advocated in any of these circumstances.

ADRENAL GLAND

Physiology

The adrenal gland, located superior to the upper pole of the kidney, is composed of an external cortex and an internal medulla. Within the cortex, three different layers exist both structurally and functionally. The outer zona glomerulosa produces aldosterone, the middle zona fasciculata produces cortisol, and the inner zona reticularis secretes androgens as well as lesser amounts of glucocorticoids. In the adrenal medulla, chromaffin cells produce catecholamines, which are released in response to activation of cholinergic preganglionic neurons. Corticosteroids and catecholamines produced in the adrenal medulla are vitally important to normal physiologic processes and stress responses, and deficiencies in any of these systems can adversely affect a patient's ability to cope with illness.

Typically, the hypothalamic-pituitary-adrenal (HPA) axis closely regulates the production of glucocorticoids. Hypothalamic corticotropin releasing hormone (CRH), transported in the portal circulatory system to the adenohypophysis, stimulates adrenocorticotropic hormone (ACTH) secretion from pituicytes. In turn, ACTH stimulates adrenal steroidogenesis by accelerating the rate-limiting step of cholesterol side-chain cleavage. Stress increases CRH levels, with consequent increases in both ACTH and cortisol levels. Adrenal steroids, on the other hand, exert negative feedback effects on both hypothalamic secretion of CRH and pituitary secretion of ACTH. Another short feedback loop occurs through ACTH's inhibitory actions on hypothalamic CRH neurons.

Glucocorticoids secreted by the zona fasciculata have a wide range of effects throughout the body, which occur predominantly through alteration of cell protein synthesis. One effect of these steroids is alteration of immune cell function whereby immune responses are lessened by glucocorticoids. Not only do steroids significantly affect immune cell function, but immune cells themselves can stimulate the HPA axis at both the pituitary and adrenal gland levels.

Other effects of glucocorticoids include mood changes, enhanced muscle catabolism, sodium retention, reductions in gastrointestinal calcium absorption, impairment of renal calcium excretion, and impairment of linear bone growth in children.

Aldosterone synthesis in the zona glomerulosa is regulated predominantly by renin, which is secreted by the juxtaglomerular cells of the kidney. Renin stimulates the conversion of angiotensinogen to angiotensin I, which then undergoes conversion to angiotensin II by angiotensin-converting enzyme within the lungs. Angiotensin II in turn stimulates the synthesis of aldosterone. Other stimulatory factors include potassium, ACTH, and vasopressin; inhibitory influences are exerted by dopamine, atrial natriuretic factor, and somatostatin. Aldosterone acts to stimulate sodium reabsorption in the renal distal tubule and collecting ducts, thereby causing water retention and increases in intravascular volume. Potassium excretion is enhanced as a consequence of sodium–potassium exchange across renal tubular epithelial cell surfaces.

Adrenal Insufficiency

Pathophysiology

Activation of the HPA axis by the stress of severe illness, trauma, or surgery results in elevations in glucocorticoids that are correlated with severity of illness. In patients with septic shock, baseline levels of cortisol are typically higher than 300 nmol/L. If the HPA axis is not fully responsive at each of the hypothalamic, pituitary, and adrenal gland levels, however, adrenal insufficiency can ensue. Primary adrenal insufficiency, indicating inadequate response at the level of the adrenal glands, is most commonly the result of autoimmune destruction of the adrenal glands. Secondary adrenal insufficiency is associated with pituitary or hypothalamic dysfunction and can be due to a number of causes. Table 7–5 lists potential causes of both primary and secondary adrenal insufficiency. Exogenous steroid administration is a frequent cause of adrenal insufficiency, and chronic use results in impairment of hypothalamic, pituitary, and adrenal gland function. These actions occur relatively quickly; suppression can occur with as little as 20 to 30 mg/d prednisone administered for 1 week. Rifampin, barbiturates, and phenytoin can enhance cortisol metabolism and precipitate adrenal insufficiency in patients with limited adrenal reserves. Levothyroxine treatment in a patient with concurrent hypothyroidism and hypoadrenalism can also precipitate severe adrenal insufficiency by enhancing cortisol metabolism.

Manifestations and Diagnosis

Clinical manifestations of adrenal insufficiency are detailed in Table 7–6. If such a condition is suspected, a random serum cortisol level should be obtained. A random cortisol

Table 7–5. CAUSES OF ADRENAL INSUFFICIENCY

Primary Adrenal Insufficiency

- Tuberculosis
- Fungal infections
- Adrenal hemorrhage
- Adrenal gland metastatic infiltration
- Amyloidosis
- Acquired immunodeficiency syndrome
- Adrenoleukodystrophy
- Congenital steroid enzyme blockages
- Medications that block cortisol synthesis
  - Ketoconazole
  - Etomidate
  - Aminoglutethimide
  - Metyrapone

Secondary Adrenal Insufficiency

- Tumors
  - Pituitary adenomas
  - Craniopharyngiomas
  - Metastatic disease
- Granulomatous disease
  - Sarcoidosis
  - Histiocytosis X
  - Tuberculosis
- Autoimmune hypophysitis
- Trauma
- Pituitary surgery
- Pituitary irradiation
- Pituitary infarction
- Exogenous steroid administration

level above 500 nmol/L (18 μg/dL) argues against adrenal insufficiency, but many normal patients do not manifest such high levels and an ACTH test must therefore be performed. In this test, 250 μg synthetic ACTH (Cortrosyn) is administered intravenously and blood samples are obtained before and 45 minutes afterward. Postadministration cortisol levels greater than 500 nmol/L indicate adequate adrenal gland function and rule out primary adrenal insufficiency. Unfortunately, secondary adrenal insufficiency cannot be eliminated by such a result, particularly if the patient has suffered from recent head trauma or undergone recent cranial surgery. In cases of postadministration levels less than 500 mmol/L, a 3-day ACTH stimulation test can be useful, producing progressive increases in serum cortisol levels and urinary 17-hydroxycorticosteroid (17-OHCS) concentrations in cases of secondary adrenal insufficiency but causing no such increases in primary adrenal insufficiency. Insulin-induced hypoglycemia, metyrapone administration, or CRH stimulation can also be used to test the hypothalamic and pituitary components of the HPA axis and thereby to evaluate the possibility of secondary adrenal insufficiency. Helpful imaging studies include computed tomographic (CT) scans of the adrenal glands to evaluate adrenal gland hemorrhage, atrophy, or infiltration, as well as head or sella CT or magnetic resonance imaging (MRI) scans to evaluate pituitary or

Table 7–6. MANIFESTATIONS OF ADRENAL INSUFFICIENCY

Symptoms
Weakness
Fatigue
Anorexia
Nausea
Vomiting
Abdominal pain
Diarrhea
Salt craving
Myalgias
Arthralgias
Light-headedness
Confusion
Signs
Abdominal tenderness
Fever
Hypotension
Weight loss
Vitiligo
Auricular calcification
Laboratory Findings
Hyponatremia
Hyperkalemia
Hypercalcemia
Eosinophilia
Hypoglycemia
Azotemia
Anemia

hypothalamic lesions. High cortisol levels have been found to be typical in patients with sepsis; low-normal random or stimulated cortisol values in critically ill patients can thus reflect subtle inadequacies within the HPA axis. These possibilities need to be taken into account when evaluating such patients.

Therapy

Prompt treatment of adrenal insufficiency is necessary to avoid significant morbidity or mortality. Patients suspected to have adrenal insufficiency should have blood drawn for cortisol and ACTH determination, and should then immediately be given 1 mg dexamethasone or 100 mg hydrocortisone every 6 to 8 hours until the patient has stabilized. Dexamethasone does not cross react to any great extent with cortisol in assays and thus is the preferred agent, since it does not interfere with any diagnostic studies. Patients may need aggressive intravenous fluid therapy using normal saline with 5% dextrose. In adrenal crisis, 2 to 3 L should be administered as quickly as possible, watching for signs of fluid overload. Hemodynamic monitoring may be necessary. Mineralocorticoids are not acutely useful since sodium-retaining effects may not be manifested for several days, although patients with primary adrenal insufficiency eventually require mineralocorticoid replacement as part of their chronic maintenance regimen. Once the patient has been stabilized, a Cortrosyn stimulation test can be performed to confirm the diagnosis of adrenal insufficiency.

After stabilization, precipitating factors for the acute adrenal insufficient state should be sought and treated if possible. As permitted by concurrent illness, steroid doses can be tapered to maintenance levels, typically 20 mg hydrocortisone each morning and 10 mg each evening. Alternatively, 5 mg prednisone each morning and 2.5 mg each evening can be used. When chronic mineralocorticoid therapy is necessary, fludrocortisone acetate can be used at an initial dosage of 0.1 mg/d with final dosages based on potassium levels, blood pressure, and body fluid status. Under-repletion is associated with hyperkalemia and hypotension, whereas over-replacement causes hypertension, hypokalemia, metabolic alkalosis, and heart failure.

Isolated Hypoaldosteronism

Occurring in the setting of normal glucocorticoid secretion, isolated hypoaldosteronism manifests primarily as hyperkalemia, potentially associated with weakness, arrhythmias, and sudden death. A mild hyperchloremic metabolic acidosis may also be observed. Causes of such isolated hypoaldosteronism are given in Table 7–7. Also, critically ill patients may have impaired aldosterone synthesis relative to renin-angiotensin levels. The diagnosis should be suspected in hyperkalemic individuals who have normal renal function or only mild renal insufficiency. To confirm the diagnosis, plasma aldosterone and renin levels can be measured after an upright posture has been maintained for 3 to 4 hours,

Table 7–7. CAUSES OF HYPOALDOSTERONISM

- Reduced angiotensin levels
- Reduced renal renin production
  - Diabetes mellitus
  - Acquired immunodeficiency syndrome
  - Systemic lupus
  - Chronic renal disease
  - Congenital defects
  - Medications
    - Heparin
    - β-blockers
    - Antibiotics
    - Nonsteroidal anti-inflammatory agents
- Reduction in angiotensin II receptors
- Aldosterone synthetic defects
  - Autoimmune disease
  - Heparin administration
  - Hemochromatosis
  - Hypoparathyroidism
  - Congenital enzyme deficiencies
- Reduced angiotensin-converting enzyme levels

and a Cortrosyn stimulation test should be performed to rule out the possibility of primary adrenal insufficiency. Typically, no therapy is required for mild cases of isolated hypoaldosteronism, although medications that suppress renin secretion should be avoided if possible. Oral potassium intake may need to be reduced. In severe cases, fludrocortisone acetate can be administered in a dosage of 0.1 to 0.3 mg/d. Other therapeutic options include diuretics, oral sodium bicarbonate treatment, and potassium-binding resins.

Cushing's Syndrome

Pathophysiology, Manifestations, and Diagnosis

Cushing's syndrome, a state of elevated glucocorticoid levels, may be due to a pituitary adenoma (Cushing's disease), an adrenal adenoma, adrenal carcinoma, ectopic ACTH, or ectopic CRH. Bilateral adrenal macronodular hyperplasia and micronodular dysplasia are other rare causes of Cushing's syndrome. If manifestations of Cushing's syndrome are present (Table 7–8), initial screening studies should be performed using either an overnight 1-mg dexamethasone suppression test or a 24-hour urine collection for free cortisol. Failure of the post-dexamethasone 8 AM serum cortisol level to suppress to less than 140 nmol/L suggests Cushing's syndrome. Likewise, an elevated 24-hour urinary free cortisol level also suggests Cushing's syndrome. False-positive tests can occur in obese, depressed, or alcoholic patients. Confirmation of Cushing's syndrome relies on a low-dose dexamethasone suppression test in which 24-hour urine free cortisol and 17-OHCS levels are measured before and during administration of 0.5 mg dexamethasone every 6 hours for 48 hours. Suppression of the second-day 17-

Table 7–8. MANIFESTATIONS OF CUSHING'S SYNDROME

Weight gain, obesity
Hirsutism
Facial plethora
Moon facies
Bruising
Acne
Polyuria
Hypertension
Osteoporosis, compression fractures
Weakness
Oligomenorrhea or amenorrhea
Impotence
Enlarged fat pads
Hyperpigmentation
Abdominal striae
Edema
Renal calculi
Glucose intolerance
Hyperlipidemia

OHCS levels to below 2.5 mg/d and free cortisol levels to below 20 mg/d indicates a normal response.

Once the diagnosis of Cushing's syndrome has been confirmed, Cushing's disease must be discriminated from nonpituitary causes of hypercortisolism. This differentiation can often be made on the basis of the response to a high-dose dexamethasone test, using either a standard 2-day urine study (2 mg dexamethasone administered every 6 hours for 48 hours; normal response: post-dexamethasone suppression of 24-hour urinary 17-OHCS and free cortisol levels to below 50% of baseline) or an overnight high-dose study (8 mg dexamethasone administered at 11 PM; normal response: suppression of post-dexamethasone 8 AM plasma cortisol levels to below 140 nmol/L). Other helpful studies include plasma ACTH levels, which are suppressed by adrenal tumors but elevated in cases of Cushing's disease or ectopic ACTH syndrome; inferior petrosal sinus venous sampling, which can localize an ACTH-secreting pituitary adenoma; and metyrapone administration. In the last study, metyrapone increases urinary 17-OHCS levels in Cushing's disease but suppresses 17-OHCS levels in cases of adrenal sources of hypercortisolism. Ectopic ACTH syndrome is associated with subnormal increases in 17-OHCS values following metyrapone administration. Imaging studies that may be helpful include sella MRI or CT scans to evaluate potential pituitary lesions, chest radiographs and CT scans to evaluate ectopic ACTH or ectopic CRH sources, and abdominal CT scans to reveal adrenal lesions. Nuclear imaging scans occasionally used include iodocholesterol scans for steroid-secreting tumors and labeled somatostatin scans for ectopic ACTH or CRH sources.

Therapy

Trans-sphenoidal resection of a pituitary adenoma is the appropriate treatment for Cushing's disease, and adrenal adenomas or carcinomas are treated by adrenalectomy. Localization and resection of ectopic ACTH sources should be attempted where possible. Successfully treated patients may manifest hypocortisolemia for up to 12 months after cure, and maintenance steroid therapy is needed during these periods. Additionally, supplemental stress doses are necessary in times of illness or injury.

Cushing's disease not adequately treated by initial surgery may need reoperation or pituitary irradiation, although these treatments leave a number of patients with persistent hypercortisolism. In such patients, or in patients with an unresectable ectopic source of ACTH or CRH, medical or surgical adrenalectomy may be necessary. Medical adrenalectomy of varying degrees can be achieved with mitotane, aminoglutethamide, metyrapone, ketoconazole, or trilostane. It has been suggested that patients undergoing surgical adrenalectomy have preoperative pituitary irradiation to reduce the chance of postoperative pituitary hyperplasia (Nelson's syndrome). Bilateral surgical adrenalectomy is the treatment of choice in patients with bilateral micronodular or macronodular disease.

Hyperaldosteronism

Pathophysiology and Manifestations

Hypersecretion of aldosterone, which occurs most frequently in women and which has a peak incidence between the ages of 30 and 50 years, accounts for less than 1% of cases of hypertension. Hyperaldosteronism can be classified as being either primary, indicating inappropriate hypersecretion of aldosterone by the adrenal gland in the absence of any stimulation, or secondary, resulting from processes such as congestive heart failure, cirrhosis, or nephrotic syndrome. This discussion is confined to primary hyperaldosteronism, which manifests as hypertension and hypokalemia and which can result from a unilateral adenoma, adrenal carcinoma, bilateral adrenocortical hyperplasia, or glucocorticoid-responsive hyperaldosteronism. The differential diagnosis for hypokalemia includes 11-β-hydroxylase deficiency, inherited or glycyrrhizic acid–associated 11-β-hydroxysteroid dehydrogenase deficiency, 17-hydroxylase deficiency, Liddle's syndrome, Bartter's syndrome, vomiting, diuretic use, and laxative abuse.

Diagnosis

Confirmation of hyperaldosteronism can be done by collecting a 24-hour urine sample for aldosterone and determining a plasma renin activity level. Plasma aldosterone and renin levels obtained after 3 hours of upright posture can be used in lieu of a 24-hour urine collection; a plasma aldosterone/plasma renin ratio of greater than 25 suggests hyperaldosteronism and the need for further evaluation. Confirmation of hyperaldosteronism can be achieved by intravenous infusion of 2 L of normal saline over 4 hours, which should normally suppress aldosterone levels to less than 10 ng/dL at the completion of the saline infusion. Alternatively, 25 mg captopril can be given to confirm a state of hyperaldosteronism (normal response: 2-hour post-captopril plasma aldosterone/plasma renin activity ratio below 50).

Discrimination of adenoma versus bilateral hyperplasia can rely on (1) abdominal CT scan studies or (2) changes in 8 AM supine and noon erect aldosterone and renin levels. Aldosterone and renin levels typically rise slightly from 8 AM to noon in cases of adrenal hyperplasia, but in adrenal adenomas, renin levels remain suppressed and aldosterone levels paradoxically fall because of declines in ACTH values. Glucocorticoid-remediable hyperaldosteronism can be diagnosed empirically through a trial of dexamethasone treatment or through genetic testing for the underlying genetic defect.

Therapy

Unilateral adrenalectomy is the treatment of choice for adenoma- or carcinoma-associated primary hyperaldosteronism. In contrast, medical treatment is indicated for patients with bilateral adrenal hyperplasia. Spironolactone and amiloride are helpful in treating hypokalemia, although additional antihypertensive medications may be necessary for adequate blood pressure control. Glucocorticoid-remediable hyperaldosteronism is treated with low-dose glucocorticoids.

Pheochromocytoma

Pathophysiology

Excessive catecholamine production due to pheochromocytomas is a rare problem. These tumors are typically benign and solitary, but about 10% are malignant and 10% are bilateral. Most pheochromocytomas are located within the adrenal gland, but tumors also can be located at extrarenal sites, including sympathetic ganglia within the abdomen or thorax, the organ of Zuckerkandl, and locations such as the bladder, brain, or neck. Pheochromocytomas occur sporadically, as part of the multiple endocrine neoplasia type II syndromes or associated with von Recklinghausen's disease or von Hippel–Lindau disease.

Manifestations

Pheochromocytomas cause less than 1% of cases of hypertension. The most common clinical manifestations are diaphoresis, headache, and palpitations; other manifestations include dyspnea, postural hypotension, flushing, tremor, angina, nausea, diarrhea, and a sense of impending doom. Physical findings include tachycardia, hypertension, orthostatic hypotension, tremor, and weight loss. An abdominal mass may be palpable. Laboratory findings can include hyperglycemia, glycosuria, hypertriglyceridemia, hypercalcemia, and an elevation in hematocrit.

Diagnosis

Diagnosis can be achieved with 24-hour urine assays to determine the presence of increased levels of free catecholamines, vanillylmandelic acid, and metanephrines. Alternatively, a clonidine suppression test can be performed in which plasma catecholamine levels are determined before and after clonidine administration. Catecholamine levels fall after clonidine administration in normal patients but do not fall in patients with pheochromocytomas. Patients must remain supine at least 30 minutes before initiation of such testing and should have an intravenous catheter inserted for blood drawing well in advance of the testing to minimize stress associated with venipuncture and consequent artifactual disturbance of plasma catecholamine levels. CT or MRI scans can help to localize pheochromocytomas, which markedly enhance on T2-weighted MRI images. Iodine 131 meta-iodobenzylgaunidine scintigrams can be used in cases in which standard imaging studies are unable to locate the tumor.

Therapy

Pheochromocytomas are managed with surgical excision. Patients should be provided with adequate α-blockade before surgery by administration of phenoxybenzamine, prazosin, or doxazosin. Because patients often have reduced vascular volumes, preoperative hydration is necessary to prevent vascular collapse once the tumor has been removed. If patients manifest tachycardia or arrhythmia, β-blockers are administered once the patient has been adequately α-blocked. Beta-blockers should never be administered before α-blockade in patients with suspected pheochromocytoma, since they can cause a hypertensive crisis.

Intraoperative monitoring is necessary and should include both an arterial catheter and a pulmonary arterial catheter. Hypertension occurring during surgical resection of a pheochromocytoma should be managed with phentolamine or sodium nitroprusside. Atropine-like agents and halogenated anesthetics should be avoided. Although catecholamine levels may remain elevated for about a week postoperatively, hypertension can be cured by surgery in about 75% of patients. Of the remaining 25%, most cases of hypertension can be managed with antihypertensive medications. Malignant pheochromocytomas that cannot be surgically resected should be treated with α- and β-blockers.

GLUCOSE HOMEOSTASIS

Diabetes

Diabetes affects 5% of the United States population and represents a major healthcare problem not only because of its common nature but also because of the potential for severe consequences such as diabetic ketoacidosis, hyperosmolar hyperglycemic nonketotic coma (HHNC), and long-term complications, such as retinopathy, nephropathy, coronary artery disease, stroke, and peripheral vascular disease.

Pathophysiology

Effects of insulin include stimulation of glucose transport into cells, triglyceride synthesis, and glycogenesis as well as inhibition of lipolysis, gluconeogenesis, glycogenolysis, and ketogenesis. In type I diabetes mellitus, hyperglycemia can occur as a consequence of an absolute insulin deficiency secondary to destruction of beta cell mass, often as a consequence of autoimmune processes. Alternatively, a relative insufficiency in the amount of insulin required to maintain euglycemia may be present (type II pattern). In this pattern, insulin resistance is present, and though there is a relative deficiency of insulin, on an absolute basis, plasma insulin levels may be elevated. This hyperinsulinemia can lead to hypertension, hyperlipidemia, and atherosclerosis (syndrome X). Medication-associated diabetes (e.g., due to thiazides or glucocorticoids) or other disease-associated diabetes (e.g., secondary to pancreatitis, pancreatic cancer, hemochromatosis, Cushing's syndrome, or acromegaly) can result in either a type I or type II pattern, depending on the degree of insulin secretion impairment as well as the degree of insulin resistance.

Patients with previously undetected glucose intolerance or frank diabetes frequently display worsened glucose control when subjected to the stress of illness and hospitalization. Such effects are mediated by stress-related increases in catecholamine, cortisol, and glucagon levels, in combination with the effects of growth hormone. Each of these so-called counter-regulatory hormones impairs one or more specific actions of insulin, leading to accelerated glycogenolysis, gluconeogenesis, lipolysis, and ketogenesis. Hyperglycemia itself can exert direct effects on the pancreas and impair insulin secretion, further worsening glucose control.

Treatment

Inadequate treatment of a diabetic patient can lead to hyperglycemia, ketoacidosis, dehydration, and electrolyte abnormalities. Wound healing may be impaired, and neutrophil phagocytic function may be impaired as a consequence of hyperglycemia, leading to increased risk for gram-positive and gram-negative infections. To prevent such problems, it is imperative that adequate glucose control be maintained throughout the course of a patient's hospitalization, with optimal plasma glucose levels ranging from 90 to 180 mg/dL. Because of the significant stress responses associated with severe illness or injury, oral hypoglycemic agents are typically inadequate in the critical care setting to achieve such control. Thus, insulin therapy is usually required and is best provided as a continuous intravenous infusion, since the 5-minute plasma half-life of insulin and a 20-minute biologic effect provides a maximal degree in flexibility for titrating insulin dosages.

In critically ill adults, therapy can be initiated using a protocol similar to that outlined in Table 7–9, but these broad guidelines need to be tailored to the individual patient. Hourly glucose monitoring in the initial stages of therapy allows appropriate titration of the insulin infusion rate. In patients with significantly elevated blood sugar levels, glucose-containing intravenous fluids should be minimized as much as possible until plasma glucose levels reach approximately 250 mg/dL. Similar insulin infusion protocols can also be used in patients receiving total parenteral nutrition or continuous tube feedings. Pediatric patients should receive initial insulin doses of 0.05 U/kg/d along with adequate glucose- and potassium-containing parenteral fluids, and subsequent adjustments in insulin dosage should be based on regular blood glucose monitoring.

Diabetic Ketoacidosis

Pathophysiology

Diabetic ketoacidosis is associated with significant morbidity and mortality: up to 10% of diabetic deaths may be associated with this condition. Ketoacidosis can exist in isolation or can occur with concurrent hyperosmolarity. In fact, diabetic ketoacidosis–associated mortality has been found to correlate more with the degree of hyperosmolarity than with acidosis. Development of diabetic ketoacidosis results from insulin levels insufficient to adequately counteract the effects

Table 7–9. THERAPY OF DIABETES: ADULT PATIENTS

Blood Glucose Level Above 250 mg/dL

1. Prepare insulin at concentration of 0.1 U/mL of isotonic saline.
2. Initiate insulin therapy at 3 U/h.
3. Administer intravenous fluids: half normal saline or normal saline with 10 to 20 mEq/L KCl. Discontinue potassium infusion if the serum potassium level exceeds 5.5 mEq/L. Give supplemental potassium infusions if serum potassium level is below 3.5 mEq/L.
4. Monitor capillary blood glucose level hourly. When the blood glucose level is below 250 mg/dL, see protocol outlined below.
5. Add 0.5 U/h if the blood glucose level remains over 250 mg/dL. When the blood glucose level is below 250 mg/dL, see protocol outlined below.

Initial Blood Glucose Level Below 250 mg/dL

1. Administer intravenous fluids: half normal saline or normal saline with 5% to 10% dextrose and 10 to 20 mEq/L KCl infused at a rate to deliver 10 g glucose and 2 mEq potassium per hour. Potassium administration is based on serum potassium, as noted above.
2. Initiate insulin therapy at a rate of 0.25 to 0.35 U insulin per gram of administered glucose. Prepare initial insulin solution at concentration of 0.1 U/mL of isotonic saline.
3. Monitor capillary blood glucose level every hour initially. Once blood glucose is controlled and has stabilized, reduce monitoring frequency to every 2 to 4 hours. If blood glucose is:
   - 90–180 mg/dL: Continue current insulin infusion rate.
   - >180 mg/dL: increase insulin infusion rate by 0.5 U/h.
   - <90 mg/dL: decrease insulin infusion rate by 0.5 U/h.
   - <70 mg/dL: hold insulin infusion for 1 hour, then lower prior rate by 0.5 U/h and resume if blood glucose level exceeds 70 mg/dL.

*Ratio of insulin infused per gram of glucose depends on the level of stress and the degree of insulin resistance. Ratios can approach 0.7 to 1.0 U/g in patients after coronary bypass surgery. Initial ratios can be 0.1 to 0.2 U/g in patients with minimal stress and initial blood sugar levels in the 90- to 140-mg/dL range.

of glucagon, catecholamines, cortisol, and growth hormone, all of which can increase in the setting of illness or trauma. Precipitating factors for ketoacidosis include inadequate insulin therapy, infection, abdominal disorders (e.g., ischemic bowel or perforated viscus), myocardial infarction, hyperthyroidism, and trauma. Medications (e.g., glucocorticoids, thiazides, phenytoin, pentamidine, dobutamine, and terbutaline) have also been implicated in the development of diabetic ketoacidosis. As a consequence of increased counter-regulatory hormone levels and reduced insulin levels, enhanced lipolysis occurs, releasing free fatty acids, which are then metabolized to form the ketoacids, acetoacetate, and β-hydroxybutyrate. Glycogenolysis and gluconeogenesis are increased, and an osmotic diuresis ensues from the hyperglycemic and ketoacidotic state, leading to dehydration and hypovolemia. Electrolytes, including sodium, potassium, phosphorus, magnesium, and calcium, are lost through the urine in significant quantities.

Manifestations

Signs, symptoms, and common laboratory values in diabetic ketoacidosis are given in Table 7–10. The anion gap acidosis is due mostly to elevated levels of acetoacetate, β-hydroxybutyrate, and acetone. Lactate may play a minor role in the acidosis. Bedside test strips primarily measures acetoacetate. Because β-hydroxybutyrate and acetoacetate can exist in 20:1 ratios, particularly in patients with tissue hypoxemia, false-negative results can occur if bedside test strips are relied on. It may therefore be more useful to observe serum acetone levels or the magnitude of the anion gap acidosis when treating patients. This method can be complicated by the occasional condition in which the anion gap acidosis occurs simultaneously with a metabolic alkalosis that results from vomiting, diuretic use, or alkali ingestion. In such cases, the serum pH is higher than expected based on PCO_2 measurements. Measurements of serum sodium often indicate hyponatremia, but this needs to be corrected for hyperglycemia by adding 1.6 mEq/L to the measured serum sodium for each 100 mg/dL of glucose that exceeds 100 mg/dL. A corrected sodium level that is elevated indicates severe intracellular dehydration. Serum potassium is typically elevated because of acidosis-associated shifts of this cation from the intracellular to extracellular fluid space. Nonetheless, total body potassium levels are significantly depleted. Other laboratory findings include elevated blood urea nitrogen (BUN)

Table 7–10. DIABETIC KETOACIDOSIS

Symptoms
Polyuria
Polydipsia
Oliguria
Fatigue
Anorexia
Nausea and vomiting
Abdominal pain
Muscle cramps
Dyspnea
Signs
Dehydration
Tachycardia
Hypothermia
Coma
Hypotension
Hyperventilation
Acetone breath
Laboratory Findings
Hyperglycemia
Serum ketones
Anion gap acidosis
HCO_3^- <15 mEq/L
pH <7.3
Leukocytosis
Serum Na^+ variable
Serum K^+ variable

and creatinine levels, reflecting dehydration and hypovolemia. Magnesium deficiencies may be 0.5 to 1.0 mEq/kg of body weight. Body phosphorus levels are frequently depleted, although initial serum levels may be normal or elevated secondary to acidosis-associated extracellular shifts in phosphorus.

Therapy

Appropriate treatment of diabetic ketoacidosis relies on the key components of hydration, insulin therapy, and correction of electrolyte abnormalities. Initially, blood sugar levels should be monitored hourly and electrolytes checked every 2 hours until the serum bicarbonate value reaches 15 mEq/L or greater. Thereafter, blood work can be obtained at 4- to 6-hour intervals until the acidosis is resolved and the patient can tolerate oral intake. BUN, creatinine, calcium, and phosphate levels can be checked initially at 4- to 8-hour intervals, depending on baseline values. Urine output should be monitored closely, and bladder catheterization may be necessary. Other steps that may be necessary include insertion of a nasogastric tube in comatose patients and oxygen administration if the PO_2 is less than 80 mm Hg. Finally, evaluation and treatment of any underlying illness precipitating the ketotic state should be undertaken.

Hydration corrects hypovolemia, improves serum glucose levels, and represents the primary treatment of diabetic ketoacidosis. In adults, initial fluid repletion should be accomplished by administering normal saline at a rate of 1 to 2 L during the first hour, followed by 500 to 1000 mL/h during the next 4 hours and then 250 mL/h for 4 hours. Initial infusion rates can be halved if the patient has only modest volume depletion and half normal saline should be used in lieu of normal saline if the initial serum sodium level is greater than 150 mEq/dL. When serum glucose levels reach 250 to 300 mg/dL, intravenous fluids should be altered to include 5% to 10% dextrose in addition to saline. Such glucose allows maintenance of euglycemia while permitting delivery of adequate amounts of insulin necessary to rectify persistent acidosis.

In children, fluid correction must be done cautiously to prevent the complication of cerebral edema. Normal saline should be administered in 10- to 20-mL/kg boluses as rapidly as necessary to correct hypotension and restore tissue perfusion. Subsequently, an estimated fluid deficit of 10% should be corrected during the first 24 to 26 hours, in combination with normal maintenance fluids (approximately 1500 $mL/m^2/d$) and replacement of fluid losses due to vomiting or diarrhea. To reduce the risk of cerebral edema, total fluids should not exceed 4 $L/m^2/d$.

Insulin therapy in adults can be initiated with a 10-U intravenous bolus, followed by a continuous intravenous infusion at a rate of 0.1 U/kg/h. This infusion rate can be doubled every 2 hours if the glucose level does not fall by 50 to 100 mg/dL or if there is no improvement in acidosis in that period. Therapy in children can be initiated with a 0.1-U/kg intravenous bolus, followed by a continuous infusion at a rate of 0.1 U/kg/h. If no improvement in acidosis occurs after 2 hours of therapy, the rate can be increased to 0.15 to 0.2 U/kg/h. For both adults and children, if blood glucose levels fall too low despite administration of glucose-containing fluids, insulin infusion rates can be halved. Once plasma ketones and acidosis have resolved and the patient is able to tolerate oral intake, he or she can be switched from intravenous insulin therapy to subcutaneous insulin therapy. In previously known diabetic patients, usual doses of short- and intermediate-acting insulin can be reinstituted. In newly diagnosed patients, total insulin dosage of 0.2 to 0.3 U/kg/d should be initiated. This can be given as a mixture of one third short-acting and two thirds intermediate-acting insulin, with two thirds of the total amount given in the morning and one third in the evening. To prevent recurrence of hyperglycemia insulin infusions should not be turned off until 1 to 2 hours after the first subcutaneous insulin injection has been given.

Electrolyte therapy is also critical to the successful treatment of diabetic ketoacidosis. As mentioned, total body potassium stores may be severely depleted, despite normal or elevated initial blood potassium levels. Potassium can be administered at 20 mEq/h if the initial serum potassium is between 4 and 5 mEq/L, but it can be given at rates of 30 to 40 mEq/h if initial potassium levels are less than 3 mEq/L. Bicarbonate therapy should be restricted to cases in which plasma pH is less than 7.0 or in which serum bicarbonate is less than 5.0 mEq/L, since bicarbonate therapy can cause hypokalemia, Na^+ overload, delayed metabolic alkalosis, and paradoxical worsening of cerebral acidosis. If bicarbonate is used, 44 mEq sodium bicarbonate (one ampule) should be mixed in half normal saline and infused over 2 hours until the pH has returned to 7.2 and serum bicarbonate level has exceeded the critical value of 5 mEq/L. With reference to serum phosphate, although serum levels may be diminished, there is no proven benefit to aggressive phosphate repletion. If desired, however, phosphate can be given as a potassium salt for significantly low serum phosphate levels. Magnesium may also need repletion.

Complications

Cerebral edema occurs most frequently in pediatric patients less than 5 years of age and in newly diagnosed type I diabetics. Manifestations include a severe headache, labile blood pressures and body temperatures, reduced awareness, and seizures. The risk for cerebral edema can be reduced by ensuring a gradual reduction in blood glucose, averaging 75 mg/dL/h, and by using normal saline rather than half normal saline if serum osmolality is falling precipitously. Cerebral edema should be treated with intubation, hyperventilation, fluid restriction, dexamethasone, and 0.25 to 1.0 g/kg mannitol administered intravenously over 20 minutes. Another potential complication is pulmonary edema, which typically afflicts young patients with severe acidosis. Manifestations include the symptom of dyspnea, the physical findings of hypoxia and rales, and infiltrates observed on chest radiographs. Such manifestations dictate appropriate monitoring of volume status using a central venous catheter and extremely cautious fluid replacement. Multiple thromboses may be observed during treatment of diabetic ketoacidosis, and prophylactic low-dose heparin, 5000 U subcutaneously every 12 hours should be considered.

Hyperosmolar Hyperglycemic Nonketotic Coma

Occurring most frequently in elderly patients with type II diabetes mellitus and rarely affecting children, hyperosmolar hyperglycemic nonketotic coma (HHNC) is associated with significant hyperglycemia (glucose > 600 mg/dL) and profound hyperosmolality (> 320 mOsm). Serum pH and serum bicarbonate level are typically normal, although acidosis with a serum pH below 7.3 is present in 33% of cases. In such cases, acidosis may be due to lactate, uremia, or, to a small extent, accumulation of ketoacids.

Pathogenesis

Potential precipitating factors of HHNC include infection, myocardial infarction, strokes, intravenous hyperalimentation, burns, and medications (glucocorticoids, diuretics, phenytoin, β-blockers, and calcium channel blockers). Although insulin levels in patients with HHNC are typically sufficient to prevent lipolysis and ketogenesis, they are insufficient to stimulate peripheral glucose utilization and to prevent hepatic glycogenolysis, gluconeogenesis, and significant hyperglycemia. An osmotic diuresis and volume depletion result, which in turn lead to further rises in serum glucose levels and worsening of the patient's condition.

Manifestations and Therapy

For any elderly patient who presents with altered mental status, HHNC should be considered in the differential diagnosis. Other symptoms are similar to those for diabetic ketoacidosis (see Table 7–10). Patients may be profoundly dehydrated and hypotensive and may present with focal neurologic findings and seizures. As is true for diabetic ketoacidosis, the mainstay of treatment for patients with HHNC is fluid repletion. Patients should be administered 1 L normal saline over the first half hour and then provided another 1 L if they remain hypotensive. Subsequently, half normal saline can be used. In elderly patients, half of the fluid deficit should be corrected during the first 12 to 24 hours, and the remainder should be corrected in the next 24 to 48 hours. A central venous catheter is helpful in patients with prior congestive heart failure and in those with significant renal insufficiency. In conjunction with fluid rehydration, an insulin infusion should be used, administered in a manner similar to that outlined in Table 7–9. To prevent too rapid a reduction in blood glucose, however, it may be necessary to use a lower initial infusion rate, in the range of 0.05 U/kg/h. When the blood glucose approaches 250 mg/

dL, dextrose must be added to the intravenous fluids. Potassium repletion is almost certainly required.

Hypoglycemia

Pathophysiology

Clinical hypoglycemia may be diagnosed if the blood glucose level is below 50 mg/dL (45 mg/dL in children) in the setting of neuroglycopenic symptoms that resolve after the low blood glucose has been corrected. Physiologic defense mechanisms to protect against hypoglycemia include reduction in insulin levels and increases in glucagon and catecholamine levels, which enhance glycogenolysis, gluconeogenesis, and lipolysis. Cortisol and growth hormone play a permissive role in glycogenolysis and gluconeogenesis. In the outpatient setting, hypoglycemic symptoms are most often attributed to an idiopathic postprandial syndrome, in which the patient has typical hypoglycemic symptoms but a normal blood sugar level. In the critical care setting, however, documented hypoglycemia can arise from a number of causes (Table 7–11).

Manifestations and Diagnosis

Hypoglycemia results in symptoms and signs of neuroglycopenia and hyperadrenergism. The adrenergic manifestations of sweating, weakness, anxiety, tremor, tachycardia, and pallor typically occur first. Further decreases in blood glucose may elicit neurologic manifestations such as headache, confusion, focal neurologic deficits, seizures, coma, and even death. Evaluation of hypoglycemia depends on documentation of hypoglycemia and determination of concurrent insulin and C-peptide levels. Hyperinsulinemia is present when the plasma insulin level is greater than 5 μU/mL at the time the blood glucose level is less than 40 mg/dL. Endogenous hyperinsulinemia should have a concurrently elevated C-peptide level and should prompt further diagnostic studies to look for an insulinoma. On the other hand, suppression of the C-peptide level suggests exogenous insulin as the cause of hypoglycemia. Sulfonylurea ingestion should be associated with elevations in both insulin levels and C-peptide levels. Toxicology screens should be able to detect the presence of sulfonylureas, thus allowing discrimination between an insulinoma and ingestion of these medications. Additionally, insulin antibodies should be measured and adrenal insufficiency should be considered. Empirical treatment with hydrocortisone should be considered in cases in which adrenal insufficiency is a possibility, pending appropriate diagnostic evaluation with a measurement of the cortisol level and performance Cortrosyn stimulation test. With reference to the many other potential causes of hypoglycemia (see Table 7–11), further diagnostic studies may be necessary if the cause of hypoglycemia is uncertain after these tests.

Therapy

Appropriate treatment dictates that euglycemia be restored as rapidly as possible. Adults should be given 50 mL of

Table 7–11. CAUSES OF HYPOGLYCEMIA

Fasting Hypoglycemia
Medications
Insulin
Sulfonylureas
Sulfa-based medications
Pentamidine
β-Blockers
Disopyramide
Salicylates
Ethanol
Quinine
Malnutrition
Abrupt cessation of total parenteral nutrition
Seizures
Organ failure
Liver disease
Cardiac disease
Renal disease
Sepsis
Insulinoma
Non–beta cell tumors
Autoimmune hypoglycemia
Insulin antibodies
Insulin receptor antibodies
Endocrine dysfunction
Adrenal insufficiency
Hypothyroidism
Growth hormone deficiency
Postprandial Hypoglycemia
Rapid gastric emptying
Idiopathic
Artifactual Hypoglycemia
Polycythemia
Leukocytosis
Pediatric Hypoglycemia
Congenital defects in carbohydrate, fat, and protein metabolism
Ketotic hypoglycemia
Neonatal hypoglycemia
Reye's syndrome
Nesidioblastosis

50% dextrose intravenously, but if severe neuroglycopenic symptoms are present (e.g., seizure or coma) and intravenous access cannot be achieved, glucagon can be administered intramuscularly. Thiamine should be administered before glucose if there is concern about possible malnutrition, so as to prevent Wernicke-Korsakoff syndrome and neurologic damage. After the acute D_{50} infusion, patients should receive 10% dextrose intravenously at a rate that can maintain blood glucose levels over 100 mg/dL. If such levels cannot be achieved despite intravenous administration of 10% dextrose at rates of 200 mL/h, 100 mg hydrocortisone and 1 mg glucagon should be added to each liter of 10% dextrose fluid. Diazoxide also can be used in refractory cases (3–8 mg/kg/d in 5% dextrose). When euglycemia has been restored and the patient is able to eat, a high-carbohydrate diet (>300 g/d) should be started.

Children should be treated initially with a bolus of 25% dextrose (0.5 g/kg) followed by a continuous infusion of 10% dextrose. Glucagon can be administered either intravenously or intramuscularly (0.1 to 0.3 mg/kg up to maximum of 1 mg), as may hydrocortisone (5 mg/kg/d). Diazoxide can again be used in refractory cases, with the enteral route preferred to prevent the hypotension associated with this medication (enteral dosage, 10 mg/kg/d; intravenous dosage, 1 mg/kg by slow infusion while monitoring blood pressure).

NUTRITIONAL THERAPY

Starvation, chronic wasting diseases, and hypercatabolic states induced by severe infections or trauma can significantly disturb normal organ and tissue functions as a consequence of those physiologic mechanisms that are activated to respond to states of negative energy balance. Clinical outcome in critically ill patients can thus be significantly worsened if patients do not receive appropriate nutrient replacement during their illness. Such treatment is guided by a thorough understanding of nutrient requirements, various treatments, and physiologic responses that occur in the setting of nutritional deficiency.

Starvation

Body carbohydrate stores, chiefly in the form of glycogen, constitute about 200 to 300 g in a 75-kg adult man, whereas protein and fat stores constitute 10 to 15 kg and 11 to 22 kg, respectively. Pure protein and glycogen contain 4 kcal/g, and pure triglycerides contain 9 kcal/g. In the body, however, energy density is somewhat lower: fat tissue stores are approximately 8 kcal/g, and carbohydrates and proteins are stored at an energy density of about 1 kcal/g. A negative energy balance necessitates utilization of body energy stores to maintain key physiologic processes, most notably the maintenance of glucose and ketone delivery to the brain as well as maintenance of energy supplies to the liver, kidney, and intestine. Nutrients and energy are also required for the preservation of body structural integrity. In response to starvation, compensatory mechanisms can be grouped into early and late stages.

Early stages: When faced with inadequate energy intake, carbohydrate stores are the first to be mobilized, although such stores can provide energy for a maximum of approximately 24 hours. This mobilization results from decreased insulin levels and increased glucagon levels that enhance glycogenolysis, thus releasing glucose from glycogen stores. Additionally, adipose tissue hormone–sensitive lipase is activated, thereby releasing free fatty acids that provide energy to muscle and liver and glycerol, which can be metabolized to yield glucose. Falling insulin levels also result in protein hydrolysis and transamination of pyruvate and α-ketoglutarate to form alanine and glutamine. Alanine can then be utilized as a substrate for gluconeogenesis to provide glucose to the brain, whereas glutamine serves as an energy substrate for the gut and lymphocytes and as a substrate for ammonia synthesis by the kidney.

Late stages: With sustained starvation, fats are used increasingly as a source of energy in an effort to preserve proteins. A significant elevation in serum free fatty acid concentrations occurs as a consequence of enhanced lipolysis as well as impaired fatty acid re-esterification into triglycerides. These free fatty acids can then be metabolized to form ketones, and in later stages of starvation, such ketones assume an increasingly important role in meeting the energy needs of the brain.

Aside from metabolic compensations, prolonged starvation can have various other manifestations. Cortisol and growth hormone levels increase, whereas IGF-1 levels decrease. Thyroid hormone and gonadotropin levels also may decrease, leading to amenorrhea and reduced metabolic rates. Renal function may be impaired, anemia can occur, and both cardiac output and blood pressure are frequently decreased. Other effects include reduced T-lymphocyte function, complement levels, and secretory immunoglobulin levels, allowing for an increased incidence of infections, particularly gram-negative bacterial sepsis.

Severe malnutrition in children can manifest as kwashiorkor or marasmus. In both syndromes, weight loss, failure to grow, and reductions in organ size, body protein content, and plasma proteins can occur. Kwashiorkor, however, is distinguishable from marasmus on the basis of increased extracellular water with associated edema, ascites, and anasarca. Kwashiorkor can develop from marasmus, particularly under the influence of carbohydrate feeding. In such cases, carbohydrate-induced insulin increases and a secondary reduction in muscle protein breakdown decreases the levels of free amino acids available to the liver for production of albumin, thereby causing edema. Variations of these syndromes also may be seen in adults who have profound wasting and major fluid shifts between intracellular water and extracellular water in the setting of protein-calorie deficiency or trauma. It is important that such changes in distribution be considered, because inappropriate fluid administration can exacerbate fluid imbalances in critically ill patients.

Effects of Injury and Sepsis

Protein catabolism and metabolic rates are significantly increased under conditions of severe injury or illness. Energy reserves can be depleted at a rate up to 10,000 kcal/d, and nitrogen losses up to 40 g/d can occur. To help cope with such significant deficits, gluconeogenesis is increased. This occurs through insulin-resistant mechanisms, since the addition of exogenous insulin does not alter gluconeogenesis rates, in contrast to the state in normal individuals wherein insulin suppresses gluconeogenesis. Insulin resistance, arising from elevations in cortisol, growth hormone, catecholamine, and glucagon levels, can contribute to enhanced fatty acid oxidation, mild acidosis, and elevated blood glucose levels. Accelerated protein catabolism in combination with the low energy density of body protein (1 kcal/g) can lead to weight loss that seems exceedingly high in comparison with a patient's overall metabolic rate. Further weight loss can arise from cytokines that cause anorexia and weight loss, such as tumor necrosis factor, interleukin-1, and interleukin-6. These catabolic responses may be adaptive for the first 5 to 7 days after illness or injury, but subsequent prolongation of these processes may be associated with wasting and multisystem organ failure.

Evaluation of Nutritional Failure

Patients should be questioned about appetite, anorexia, diarrhea, weight loss, and swallowing difficulties. Other factors that can affect nutritional state include alcohol intake, drug use, socioeconomic status, and cultural influences. A food diary or calorie count can allow assessment of dietary intake. Examination of the patient for factors that increase energy requirements (e.g., fever, burns, labored breathing, trauma) is important, as is inspection for physical signs or symptoms of nutritional deficiency (e.g., muscle wasting, dermatitis, keratosis, mucosal ulcerations, glossitis, tetany, paresthesias, growth retardation, osteomalacia, delayed wound healing, goiter, depression). Ecchymoses, epistaxis, and other bleeding tendencies can also reflect nutritional deficiency.

Height and weight should be determined. Ideal body weight in males is calculated by estimating 106 lb for the first 5 feet and 6 lb for every further inch; normal body weight in females should be estimated on the basis of 100 lb for the first 5 feet and 5 lb for every inch thereafter. The ratio of actual weight to ideal weight can provide a rough measure as to the severity of malnutrition: ratios of 90% to 100% correspond to mild states of malnutrition, ratios of 50% to 90% and ratios of less than 50% correspond to moderate and severe malnutrition, respectively.

Laboratory tests should include a blood count (including total lymphocyte count), blood smear, reticulocyte count, and plasma osmolality. Blood glucose, sodium, potassium, chloride, bicarbonate, calcium, phosphate, magnesium, and iron should be measured in addition to the BUN, creatinine, albumin, total protein, cholesterol, and triglycerides. Serum transferrin, fibronectin, ferritin, retinol-binding protein, vitamins, essential fatty acids, and trace elements can also be determined. Serum albumin levels decrease in states of protein deprivation but may not accurately measure nutritional status, since the lower synthesis rates of albumin may be partly countered by reduced rates of protein catabolism.

A variety of derived values have been developed to quantify a patient's nutritional status. One such value, the prognostic nutritional index (PNI), has been found to correlate with the risk of complications in the postoperative period.

This value is calculated from a patient's albumin level, delayed cutaneous hypersensitivity (DCH) measurement, transferrin level, and triceps skinfold (TSF) thickness:

$$\text{PNI} = 158 - 16.6 \cdot \text{albumin (g/dL)} - 0.78 \cdot \text{TSF (mm)} - 0.2 \cdot \text{transferrin (mg/dL)} - 5.8 \cdot \text{DCH (graded 0, 1, or 2)}$$

The creatinine-height index, which relates the 24-hour urine creatinine output to the height, has been used, but this measure is not valid in patients with trauma or rhabdomyolysis. Values less than 60% of the expected value indicate a significant loss in lean body mass.

Nutritional Requirements

Energy Requirements

Energy requirements—dictated by basal metabolic rate, age, sex, and body surface area—are also affected by physical activity, eating, growth, pregnancy, lactation, and processes such as trauma or sepsis. Resting energy requirements can be calculated by the Harris-Benedict equation:

$$\text{Men: kcal/24 h} = 66.473 + 13.7516 \times \text{weight (kg)} + 5.0033 \times \text{height (cm)} - 6.7550 \times \text{age (years)}$$

$$\text{Women: kcal/24 h} = 655.0955 + 9.5634 \times \text{weight (kg)} + 1.8496 \times \text{height (cm)} - 4.6756 \times \text{age (years)}$$

Alternatively, a metabolic cart and indirect calorimetry can be used to provide a more accurate assessment of energy expenditures, using the modified Wier formula, which relates oxygen and carbon dioxide gas exchange to energy utilization.

Protein Requirements

Nitrogen balance, reflecting the summed rate of nitrogen retention and nitrogen loss, can be calculated using 24-hour urine collections:

$$\text{Nitrogen balance} = \text{nitrogen intake} - (\text{urine urea nitrogen level} + 4)$$

where: nitrogen intake is protein intake in grams $\div$ 6.25 and 4 represents the magnitude of stool and skin nitrogen losses and nonurea nitrogen losses. A normal nitrogen intake of 10 to 30 g/d typically suffices to replace normal nitrogen losses. A number of factors can influence nitrogen losses and expenditures, however, and thus can affect the amount of nitrogen intake necessary to maintain equilibrium. For example, nitrogen excretion rates increase proportionally to the metabolic rate. Fasting elicits a gradual adaptation in nitrogen excretion such that nitrogen excretion decreases from 6 to 8 g/d in the initial stages of fasting to 3 to 4 g/d as the fasting state is prolonged. Similarly, inadequate protein intake causes gradual reductions in nitrogen excretion rates.

Despite such compensatory changes, nitrogen deficits occur even in healthy individuals faced with short-term dietary reductions. After uncomplicated moderate surgery, deficits may persist for a week but can then easily be repleted with oral feeding. If nitrogen requirements are increased because of extensive wound healing, sepsis, or hyperthermia, however, deficits can be exacerbated. Losses associated with transudates, exudates, gastrointestinal losses, burns, and hemorrhage can worsen nitrogen deficits, leading to impaired liver and gut function. Inadequate protein intake decreases the gut's ability to digest food, possibly because protein is needed to produce gastrointestinal secretions. In the liver, the rate of albumin synthesis rapidly decreases in response to reduced protein intake. The muscle also may be significantly affected, since catabolism of muscle tissue is required to help compensate for reduced protein intake. The net result of such derangements can be increased vulnerability to infection, failure of wound healing, and organ failure.

Refeeding after a period of reduced intake produces a net increase in body nitrogen, which is manifested chiefly as increased liver, kidney, and muscle proteins. Peak nitrogen retention rates last only 4 to 7 days, after which nitrogen retention slows. Positive nitrogen balance can be achieved by providing a high protein intake, even if the total calories are less than metabolic requirements. Such an effect of proteins to modulate nitrogen balance independent of other factors is termed *anabolic drive.* On the other hand, increasing carbohydrate and fat dietary content can also increase nitrogen retention, thereby revealing the complex interaction of proteins and nonproteins to regulate nitrogen balance.

Fats

Dietary fat is composed primarily of long-chain fatty acids, including the saturated palmitic and stearic acids, and the unsaturated oleic and linoleic acids, and linolenic acid. Medium-chain fatty acids also contribute to the total fat dietary content. Linoleic and linolenic acids are unable to be synthesized from nondietary sources and are thus considered essential fatty acids. Lack of these essential fatty acids can manifest as a rash and may appear within 10 days after starting fat-free total parenteral nutrition (TPN). Provision of intravenous lipid solutions prevents this problem.

Enteral Nutritional Therapy

Enteral nutrition, by virtue of preventing gut atrophy and possibly reducing translocation of bacteria across the gut wall, is the preferred route of nutritional delivery. Whenever possible, natural foods should be administered orally. If this is not possible, supplemental enteral diets can be administered either orally or through nasogastric, nasoduodenal, gastrostomy, gastrostoduodenal, or jejunostomy tubes. Enteral liquid feeding can be prepared from fresh foods that contain all essential nutrients or from commercial liquid diets. Depending on the preparation, these fluids contain 53 to 211 nonprotein calories per gram of nitrogen in non–renal failure formulations; 1500 to 3000 mL administered daily meets the United States recommended daily allowances for necessary nutrients.

Patients with normal renal function should receive approximately 1.5 to 2 g/kg/d of protein. Protein intake needs to be decreased for patients in whom BUN increases to approximately 80 mg/dL or creatinine increases to 3 mg/dL. In patients with preexisting renal insufficiency or renal failure, dialysis may be necessary if BUN or creatinine increases are not prevented by reducing protein intake to the minimum 25 to 50 g of protein that is necessary to prevent a significant catabolic state. Carbohydrates should be administered at rates of 100 to 500 g/d. Levels in excess of 500 g can cause hyperglycemia, hepatomegaly, and elevations in serum hepatic transaminase levels. Fats should be provided at a rate of 1 to 3 g/kg/d. To guard against vitamin deficiencies, a multivitamin preparation can be administered daily.

Although bolus feeding into the stomach represents a more physiologic mode of nutrient administration, it can increase the risk of aspiration in elderly patients or patients with impaired levels of consciousness. Bolus feeding also is associated with more frequent episodes of feeding intolerance in patients with malabsorption and short bowels. On the other hand, continuous enteral feeding reduces the risk for aspiration and increases tolerance to feeding, but it also increases the risk for bacterial contamination. To reduce this risk, formulas should not be maintained at room temperature for longer than 12 hours. Jejunal feeding can be done on a continuous basis or through small but frequent meals.

Parenteral Nutritional Therapy

Total parenteral nutrition delivered through a central venous catheter may be necessary for critically ill patients unable to tolerate adequate enteral feeding. In addition, preoperative TPN for at least 1 week reduces morbidity and mortality in severely malnourished individuals. The potential fluid retention associated with parenteral administration of saline and utilization of carbohydrate as the sole caloric source can be reduced by use of TPN solutions that contain a mixture of carbohydrates, amino acids, fats, minerals, and vitamins. TPN can also be used to provide constant daily infusions of drugs, such as insulin, histamine$_2$ blockers, metoclopramide, aminophylline, and steroids. By so doing, materials and personnel time can be reduced, and extraneous fluids can be minimized.

Fluid and nutrient administration should meet but not exceed nutritional requirements, since administration of glucose in excess of utilization can cause elevations in alkaline phosphatase, hepatic enzymes, and bilirubin, and cause metabolic acidosis in patients with renal insufficiency. Overfeeding can also result in hyperglycemia, which leads to impaired white blood cell function, liver steatosis, and respiratory decompensation because of the increased minute ventilation needed to cope with increased carbon dioxide production.

Energy

Glucose, containing 3.4 kcal/g, provides most of the calories in TPN. In nondiabetic patients, glucose should be given at a rate of approximately 2 mg/kg/min, or about 200 g glucose per day in a 70-kg individual, to mimic endogenous glucose liver production. In contrast, hyperglycemic diabetic patients should be provided glucose at a rate of about 1 mg/kg/min in conjunction with appropriate insulin therapy until euglycemia is reached, after which glucose infusion rates can be increased by about 50 g/d. In critically ill patients, excessive energy requirements dictate an infusion rate of about 4 mg/kg/min. This rate should be considered maximal, and increasing glucose infusion rates beyond this can cause some of the problems outlined earlier, including hyperglycemia, liver abnormalities, and increased respiratory demands. Blood glucose values should be monitored regularly, and exogenous insulin should be used to maintain euglycemia in patients receiving nutritionally appropriate glucose infusions.

Nitrogen

A positive nitrogen balance is frequently not possible in the intensive care setting and should not be the goal of TPN. Rather, TPN should limit excessive catabolism of proteins and thereby reduce the total nitrogen deficit. A negative nitrogen balance of 0 to 5 g/d can be considered moderate, whereas deficits greater than 5 g/d should be considered severe. TPN solutions, providing protein in the form of crystalline amino acids, should deliver about 1.5 to 2.0 g/kg/d of protein. However, appropriate rates for amino acid administration are guided by the BUN value. The amount of amino acid given should not raise the BUN level above 30 mg/dL in normal patients. In patients with baseline BUN levels above 30 mg/dL, the infusion should not raise the level to greater than 40 mg/dL. In patients with BUN levels above 40 or 60 mg/dL, increases should not exceed 60 or 80 mg/dL, respectively. Patients with BUN values greater than 80 mg/dL should receive infusions only at rates that do not further elevate their BUN levels.

Fats

Addition of fats to parenteral fluids spares proteins and reduces problems associated with excessive carbohydrate refeeding. Fat calories should not exceed 30% of the total calories provided and should be administered continuously over a 24-hour period, since bolus administration can induce fat uptake in reticuloendothelial cells, thereby impairing immune defense mechanisms. Intravenous lipid emulsions available in the United States consist solely of long-chain triglycerides derived from safflower or soybean oils. Medium-chain triglycerides may be used routinely in the future, since these lipids have been shown in animal models to cause less impairment of the reticuloendothelial cell function. Also, medium-chain triglycerides are directly transported into mitochondria, in contrast to long-chain triglycerides, which depend on carnitine-based transport into the mitochondria. Because carnitine levels are decreased in stress, medium-chain triglycerides may be a more efficient energy source during stressful conditions.

Electrolytes

SODIUM. Malnourishment can increase total body sodium concentrations, and particular care must be taken when administering TPN to avoid causing fluid overload in malnourished patients who are elderly or who have cardiopulmonary disease. If possible, sodium intake should be restricted to 50 to 60 mmol/d in these patients, although volume status frequently assumes priority over sodium infusion in critically ill patients. Adequate repletion of sodium in patients with gastrointestinal disease may require 100 to 200 mmol/d. Whenever possible, replacement rates for sodium and potassium should be guided by monitoring all fluid and electrolyte losses.

POTASSIUM. Malnutrition can cause significant depletion of total body potassium stores: 50- to 70-kg adult patients may have total body potassium deficits of 800 to 900 mmol at the time TPN is initiated. To maintain body stores, 40 to 50 mmol of potassium is needed each day, and repletion of deficient stores may require 80 to 120 mmol/d of potassium. Children can undergo repletion at a rate of 2 mmol per 100 kcal of energy intake, since growth deposits 60 to 80 mmol of potassium per kilogram of weight gain. Glucose infusions increase the need for potassium, and about 3 mmol of potassium is retained per gram of retained nitrogen.

MINERALS. The minerals magnesium, phosphorus, and calcium are critical components of TPN. To maintain magnesium equilibrium, estimated replacement rates range from 0.125 to 0.187 mmol/kg/d; in children and pregnant or lactating women, however, replacement rates of 0.25 mmol/kg/d have been recommended. Patients with short bowels may need 0.5 to 0.6 mmol/kg/d of magnesium. Malnourished patients may have significant magnesium depletion, and intakes of 15 mmol/d can help replete deficiencies and can improve nitrogen balance. Calcium should be provided at a minimum rate of 12 to 15 mmol/d. Serum phosphorus levels can be significantly reduced by glucose-only parenteral regimens, but a combination of glucose and lipids does not pose such a risk. The recommended repletion rate from all sources, including both phosphate compounds and phospholipids infused in the lipid fraction, is to provide phosphorus in a 1:1 molar ratio with calcium.

Complications

The requirement of a central venous line to deliver TPN can cause complications because of line infection and central line–associated thrombosis. Signs of infection, including fever, elevations in white blood cell counts, and hyperglycemia, should be evaluated with blood cultures drawn by peripheral venipuncture as well as from the central venous line. The incidence of line infections can be reduced through strict aseptic insertion techniques and proper dressing and line care. The second major complication associated with central venous lines is thrombosis of either the catheter or the vein in which the catheter is inserted. Addition of 6000 U/d heparin to the TPN solution to raise the partial thromboplastin time (PTT) values to 28 to 30 seconds reduces the incidence of such thrombosis. Patients with platelet counts below 100,000/mm^3 may require lower doses of heparin. Patients who smoke, who are obese, or who have inflammatory bowel disease, pancreatitis, or certain cancers are at increased risk for thrombosis because of accelerated PTT values (<25 seconds). Such patients should receive heparin in an amount to raise PTT levels to greater than 25 seconds.

Special Circumstances

DIABETES. When TPN is administered to diabetic patients, insulin can be added to the TPN admixture in an initial amount estimated on the basis of the patient's routine insulin requirements. If the preadmission insulin requirements are unknown, initial insulin dosages in the TPN admixture should approximate 0.1 U insulin per 1 g dextrose delivered, although supplemental insulin delivered through a separate intravenous line may be necessary to maintain adequate control of blood sugars. For reasons of economy, as well as because of the variability in insulin delivery rates associated with insulin adherence to intravenous tubing, it is safest to underestimate the amount of insulin added to the TPN admixture. Glucose should be monitored at a minimum of every 4 to 6 hours to ensure adequate glucose control; additional insulin can be administered subcutaneously or intravenously as necessary. About two thirds of the day's supplemental insulin requirement can be added to the TPN solution the following day to help maintain glucose control.

PULMONARY DYSFUNCTION. TPN administration limits the loss of pulmonary musculature as well as the impairment of host defense mechanisms that can occur in states of malnutrition. Accurate delivery of energy requirements is imperative in ventilator-dependent patients, since inadequate energy delivery results in catabolism of diaphragmatic and accessory musculature, whereas excessive calories can increase carbon dioxide production and minute ventilation. A metabolic cart can be helpful in guiding therapy. Respiratory dysfunction can be minimized by delivering no more glucose than 4 mg/kg/min and by using intravenous lipids. Lipids must be used with caution, however, in patients who have adult respiratory distress syndrome, since lipid-containing TPN can worsen pulmonary function. Unless contraindicated by liver or renal disease, proteins should be administered at a rate of 1.5 g/kg/d.

RENAL DISEASE. In patients unable to tolerate enteral feeding, TPN can be used to prevent excessive catabolism associated with acute renal failure. Protein is administered at a rate of 1.5 g/kg/d, but this may need to be decreased if BUN values rise. Dialysis can be used to control nitrogen retention and to prevent uremia. Essential amino acids and nonessential amino acids are infused in a 1:1 ratio. Branched-chain amino acids (e.g., leucine, isoleucine, valine), which are required for protein synthesis and as an energy source for peripheral skeletal muscle, are not metabolized by the liver and therefore decrease the formation of BUN. Thus, in patients with uremia, a branched-chain amino acid–enriched formulation is recommended. Protein delivery is usually decreased to 1 g/kg/d, but this may need further reduction if BUN values rise.

LIVER DISEASE. Most patients with significant liver disease are overloaded with total body water and sodium. Thus, volume associated with TPN delivery needs restriction, and diuretic therapy may be necessary to allow adequate delivery of proteins and calories. Lipid infusion can reduce glucose intolerance and hepatic lipogenesis. Protein can usually be provided at a rate of 1.5 g/kg/d, but in cases of severe hepatic encephalopathy, its administration may need to be restricted to 1 g/kg/d. Although controversial with respect to efficacy, use of branched-chain amino acids can be of benefit by reducing BUN production and subsequent hepatic encephalopathy.

In patients with liver transplants, TPN can be used in both the preoperative and postoperative periods. TPN infused over 5 to 7 days preoperatively can provide calories (30 kcal/kg/d) and protein (1 g/kg/d) that will help in the injury response after surgery. In patients with BUN values greater than 100 mg/dL, hepatic encephalopathy, or hepatic coma, branched-chain amino acids should be given in a ratio of 1:1 with standard amino acid formulations. The postoperative period may be complicated by total body water overload, which may then limit the amount of fluid that can be administered as TPN. Despite this, TPN decreases morbidity and shortens intensive care stays after liver transplantation.

OBESITY. Obese patients who require TPN should receive protein in the normal amount (1.5 g/kg/d) but should receive about 500 kcal less than expected resting energy expenditures. This is 8 to 10 kcal/lb and 10 to 12 kcal/lb in females and males, respectively. This regimen promotes lipolysis and reduces glucose intolerance. Lipids should not be administered unless hyperglycemia is a problem.

ACQUIRED IMMUNODEFICIENCY SYNDROME. Marasmic protein-calorie malnutrition is a common occurrence in acquired immunodeficiency syndrome (AIDS), and patients with AIDS have minimal energy reserves when faced with the stress of injury or illness. TPN can be provided to patients unable to tolerate enteral feeding, with total calories provided at a rate based on lean body mass and proteins provided at a rate of 1.5 g/kg/d, based on the patient's usual weight. As a consequence of elevated levels of tumor necrosis factor, interleukin-1, and α-interferon, hypertriglyceridemia is frequently observed in patients with AIDS. Lipid infusion should be withheld in patients with triglyceride levels greater than 400 mg/dL to prevent complications associated with hypertriglyceridemia.

PART B

Pharmacologic Principles

Michael L. Hess, MD

Clinical pharmacokinetics is the study and characterization of the time course of drug absorption, distribution, metabolism, and excretion and the relationship of these processes to the intensity and time course of therapeutic and adverse effects of drugs in humans. Multiple system organ dysfunction in critically ill patients predisposes to large interindividual variability in each phase of drug disposition.

Absorption

The pharmacokinetic description of the extent of drug absorption is termed *bioavailability.* When a drug is administered intravenously, it is completely available systemically, or 100% bioavailable, as opposed to orally administered drugs, which pass through the gastrointestinal tract or liver before entering the general circulation. Impaired oral bioavailability may result from incomplete disintegration or dissolution, resulting in poor absorption or significant biotransformation and extraction of the drug by the liver. Gut wall edema, stasis, and alterations in gastric or intestinal blood flow, as well as concurrent therapy with anticholinergics and narcotic analgesics, account for delayed or incomplete drug absorption and altered gastrointestinal transit time in the critically ill. Gut wall absorptive capacity is diminished after hemorrhagic shock. Bioavailability may be decreased by 70% to 80% for drugs such as phenytoin coadministered with antacids or enteral feeding routes. Coadministration of enteral feedings may speed or delay the rate or extent of absorption of various drugs. Individual absorption characteristics of each drug must be examined before relying on the adequacy of this route of administration.

Bioavailability considerations also exist with intravenous, intramuscular, subcutaneous, rectal, and aerosol drug delivery routes. A decrease in bioavailability of as much as 50% can occur when intravenously administered nitroglycerin and diazepam bind to the polyvinylchloride constituent of intravenous tubing. Subcutaneous, intramuscular, and rectal routes of administration are not recommended, except for subcutaneous heparin, in the ICU. Aerosolization of drugs such as epinephrine, β_2-receptor agonists, lidocaine, anticholinergics, and corticosteroids has been shown to be reliable in the critically ill because of the extensive alveolocapillary membrane surface area. Bronchodilation associated with aerosolized β_2-receptor agonists exceeds that achieved orally and is similar to that attained after intravenous administration. The intravenous route is the primary medication delivery mode in the ICU. In spite of accurate, high-technology infusion control devices, delays in drug response may occur when drug concentrations are changed without priming the intravenous tubing.

Distribution

The relationship between the amount of drug in the body and the plasma concentration after absorption and distribution is expressed by a proportionality constant called the apparent volume of distribution (V). It reflects a nonphysiologic compartment into which the drug disperses and may be affected by body size, physiochemical characteristics of the drug, tissue binding, plasma protein binding, and regional blood flow. The early part of the serum concentration-time curve is the distributive phase and primarily represents drug diffusion from the intravascular space into extravascular fluids and tissue. Knowledge of drug volumes of distribution is helpful in choosing adequate loading doses to achieve rapid therapeutic effects, particularly for drugs such as theophylline, anticonvulsants, antiarrhythmics, and many antibiotics.

The concentration of plasma proteins, which changes dramatically in response to critical illness, may also affect drug distribution. Albumin, prealbumin, and transferring concentrations decrease in patients with burns, cancer, chronic bronchitis, diabetes mellitus, heart failure, liver disease, malnutrition or sepsis, and uremia. Albumin concentration decreases significantly after trauma. Acidic drugs, which bind to albumin, exhibit a larger, unbound fraction in hypoalbuminemic patients, potentially producing a greater pharmacologic effect. The concentration of acute phase-reactant proteins, including α_1-acid glycoprotein, increases in patients with burns, cancer, epilepsy, infection, myocardial infarction, surgery, and trauma. Alpha$_1$-acid glycoprotein increases three- to fourfold after severe multiple trauma, reaching peak concentrations by the sixth day after injury, and remains elevated for 15 to 21 days. In this situation, increased binding of basic drugs (e.g., lidocaine) may lead to decreased effect, necessitating greater than usual doses. This effect reverses with recovery from the acute injury phase.

Clearance

Clearance is a term based on the concept of the whole body acting as a drug-eliminating system. Clearance is the sum of the individual clearance rates of the various drug-eliminating organs. Many drugs are metabolized by the liver or excreted unchanged in the urine. Decreased glomerular filtration (GFR), as may be seen in low cardiac output states, decreases renal elimination and drug clearance.

Generally, a linear relationship exists between renal drug clearance and creatinine clearance (Cl_{cr}), which is often used as a marker for GFR. Patients may demonstrate low-normal serum creatinine values because of immobility, age, or malnutrition and yet have significantly impaired GFR and drug clearance.

Because aminoglycoside antibiotics are filtered but minimally secreted and reabsorbed, aminoglycoside clearance has been shown to be a more accurate predictor of GFR than Cl_{cr} in critically ill medical patients. Doses of other filtered drugs can be altered on the basis of aminoglycoside clearance. Linear regression equations and empirical recommendations are available to modify dosage regimens before characterization by serum concentration monitoring. The effects of dialysis, ultrafiltration, hemodiafiltration, and peritoneal removal techniques on drug elimination have been well documented. Water-soluble drugs with small distribution volumes, low protein binding, and a substantial renal component to total body clearance demonstrate greater dialytic removal, requiring dosage replacement after dialysis.

Decreases in liver functional capacity consistent with hypoalbuminemia, hyperbilirubinemia, and prolongation of partial thromboplastin time are seen in alcoholic cirrhosis and biliary stasis. Antipyrine, a marker of oxidative capacity, and lorazepam, a marker of glucuronidation, have been used to demonstrate decreased enzymatic function in head trauma patients. On the other hand, glucuronidation is preserved in burn trauma patients. Drugs depending primarily on enzymatic function rather than liver blood flow for clearance are considered low-extraction drugs and may require dosage adjustment in patients with liver dysfunction. An exception to this is phenytoin, a low-extraction drug whose dosage requirements may continue to increase in neurotrauma patients, with either induction of metabolism as a result of influences of stress on hepatic metabolic activity or decreases in protein binding. Specific recommendations for dosage adjustment of hepatically cleared drugs are available. Further study is needed to elaborate on the interrelationships of organ dysfunction and drug clearance. Preliminary information suggests a decrease in hepatic clearance of drugs metabolized through oxidation by the P450 isoenzyme in patients with renal failure.

Microsomal enzyme function is decreased by interleukin-1, interleukin-6, tumor necrosis factor, interferon, and endotoxin, whereas no effect of these cytokines has been demonstrated on glucuronidation. The cytokines appear to bind to receptors on the surface of the hepatocytes during the acute phase response. Cytokine suppression of hepatocyte fixed-function oxidation and subsequent reduction in drug clearance may have significant clinical importance warranting further investigation.

The influence of mechanical ventilation and positive end-expiratory pressure (PEEP) on drug clearance is a consideration in critically ill patients. Mechanical ventilation and PEEP additively decrease cardiac output, hepatic and renal blood flow, GFR, and urine flow. A 22% decrease in lidocaine clearance, consistent with a reduction in hepatic blood flow, has been demonstrated after initiation of mechanical ventilation. The role of invasive mechanical assist devices, such as balloon counterpulsation, in altering drug disposition needs elaboration.

Recommendations for Optimizing Pharmacotherapy

Specific pharmacologic endpoints should be set to provide optimal therapeutic effect with minimum toxicity. Knowledge of the alterations in both pharmacokinetic and pharmacodynamic behavior of drugs in critically ill patients is fundamental to setting appropriate endpoints and individualizing pharmacotherapy regimens. Physiologic modifications resulting from acute illness change not only the drug effects but also the monitoring endpoints. Patient assessment and pharmacotherapeutic individualization become very dynamic processes.

Common problems encountered in optimizing drug therapy regimens include (1) underestimating the time required for a regimen to reach steady state, (2) misinterpreting the physiologic parameters chosen as therapy endpoints, and (3) failing to anticipate the altered response resulting from either pharmacokinetic or pharmacodynamic changes. Assessment of the time required to reach steady state is a function of the estimated change in drug half-life. Clinicians must have knowledge of customary drug half-lives and then estimate the likely prolongation in half-life resulting from concurrent organ dysfunction. For most drugs, blood for serum concentration monitoring can be drawn after four half-lives have elapsed. Drugs with a narrow therapeutic range given intermittently may warrant assessment of both peak and trough concentrations for dosage individualization. If doses have been appropriately spaced (i.e., one to two half-lives apart), steady state can be assumed after the third dose in most cases. Administration of a loading dose, large enough to account for the potentially enlarged volume of distribution for water-soluble drugs, is recommended when immediate drug effects are desired. Steady state may not be attained in patients with rapidly changing organ function, necessitating clinical reassessment with each administered dose.

Misinterpretation of physiologic parameters can lead to grossly inaccurate assessment of organ function. Low or normal serum creatinine values should not imply unaffected GFR or drug clearance. Hyperbilirubinemia, hypoprothrombinemia, and hypoalbuminemia correlate better with decreased hepatic function than elevated transaminase values for most drugs.

Failure to recognize that critical illness may be responsible for exaggerated drug effects can lead to significant overdosing of drugs. Centrally acting agents, neuromuscular blockers, opioids, theophylline, and histamine$_2$ receptor antagonists are examples of medications with the potential to alter response and disposition in critically ill patients. Dosage titration to minimally effective concentrations or pharmacologic response is recommended to avoid prolonged, unwanted effects or toxicity. The prolonged half-life portends delayed elimination and continued effect beyond that expected in non-ICU patients.

PROVIDING PHARMACEUTICAL SERVICES IN CRITICAL CARE AREAS

Critical Care Pharmaceutical Services

The unique and complex drug-related issues surrounding the critically ill patient have stimulated the growth of this area of practice. Approximately 6% to 20% of ICU admissions are drug related, and more than 50% of iatrogenic cardiac arrests are caused by medications. The ICU patient receives, on average, 6 to 9 drugs per day and 8 to 12 different drugs during an ICU stay. Examples of commonly prescribed drugs include antibiotics, analgesics/sedatives, agents for stress ulcer prophylaxis, antiarrhythmics, and antianginal drugs.

It is well recognized that ICU patients have altered pharmacokinetics and pharmacodynamics. Changes in organ blood flow, changes in fluid status, dysfunction of drug-eliminating organs, and altered plasma proteins account for many of these changes. Examples of drugs with known pharmacokinetic alterations in critically ill patients include aminoglycosides, β-lactam antibiotics, lidocaine, vancomycin, phenytoin, theophylline, and midazolam. The critical care pharmacist applies principles of pharmacology and physiology to design regimens to achieve and maintain therapeutic serum concentrations of many drugs rapidly and to optimize monitoring. A pharmacist-coordinated theophylline dosing system in a medical ICU (MICU), for example, resulted in fewer serum theophylline concentrations and less inappropriately obtained serum levels (15% versus 40%). Much attention has been focused on the increased distribution volume of the aminoglycosides in critically ill patients and the subsequent need for large loading doses to achieve therapeutic concentrations. Furthermore, pharmacist-managed aminoglycoside therapy achieved a significantly lower mortality rate. Thus, an important function of the critical care pharmacist involves dosing and monitoring of drugs using pharmacokinetic principles. However, more studies are needed to continue to document the impact of therapeutic drug monitoring on outcome and associated costs.

Implementing Critical Care Pharmacy Services

With automated dispensing technology (Pyxis, Meditrol, Sur-Med, ATC 212, Medispence), the physical size of the satellite may decrease. However, a pharmacy facility is still needed, preferably within close proximity to the critical care patient area. Standard procedures for preparation and dilution will produce a more consistent product that has the flexibility to be relabeled for another patient, thereby minimizing waste. However, individualized formulation will still be needed for many patients to minimize fluid overload. Pharmacists have demonstrated successful improvements in the fluid status of ICU patients by individualizing preparation techniques.

Additionally, the pharmacist must have a strong knowledge base in critical care to anticipate and initiate therapy recommendations when the order is written. This will require good communication skills and an effective working relationship with the critical care team. The drug dose should be evaluated on the basis of renal-hepatic function estimates and the appropriate therapeutic drug monitoring initiated. Other important roles of the critical care pharmacist are in nutritional support, pharmacokinetic dosing, profile review for elimination of unnecessary drug therapy, and report of adverse drug reactions. The pharmacist must provide education to other health professionals on the team and may be called on to obtain a medication history. These patient-focused services have been projected to require 13 hours per day in one 20-bed surgical ICU.

Critical care pharmacists must document their contributions to patient care. The record of pharmacist drug therapy evaluations should be a part of the medical record just as is standard for other personnel. Optimally, pharmaceutical care plans will be developed around the problem-oriented analysis of drug therapy selection, dosing, monitoring, and follow-up for desired outcome. To facilitate efficient service, the members of the critical care team should develop practice guidelines and algorithms for selection and use of drugs in their ICU population. These guidelines (or critical paths) must consider optimal drug therapy outcome and the potential costs of the therapy. An important challenge for critical care pharmacists is to assess the impact of the pharmaceutical care services on patient outcome. Reports of outcome assessment should be used by committees such as critical care, pharmacy and therapeutics, and infection control as evidence of continuous drug use improvement or continuous quality improvement. The objective evaluation of outcome also will be needed to determine the role of new and more expensive therapies.

DRUG MONITORING

Studies show that therapeutic drug monitoring (TDM) improves the therapeutic response and decreases the length of hospital stay, number of adverse reactions, and number of inappropriate serum drug concentrations in the general hospital patient population.

Pharmacokinetic Analysis

To use pharmacokinetic forecasting methods and maximize the benefit of serum drug concentration monitoring, the timing of obtaining drug samples is essential. Serum drug concentrations are obtained once steady-state conditions have been achieved. The time required to achieve greater than 90% of the pharmacokinetic steady state, when the rate of drug input is equal to the rate of drug elimination, is at least three and a half elimination half-lives. Drug concentration samples should be obtained 2 to 4 hours after the administration (peak) of rapid-release medications, immediately before the next dose (trough) for slow-release or anticonvulsant and antiarrhythmic medications, and at any time after steady state has been attained during a constant-rate intravenous infusion. Distributional characteristics of drugs also need to be considered. Serum samples for drugs should be obtained after distribution between plasma and tissues has taken place to avoid misinterpretation of increased predistributional serum concentrations. Alternatively, plasma concentrations of many drugs a few hours after hemodialysis are low because of slow redistribution from tissues and therefore should not be used for dosage predictions.

Dosing nomograms are generally useful to estimate initial drug dosing, but usually they perform poorly in comparison with individualized pharmacokinetic monitoring.

Antimicrobials

High peak-dose concentrations of gentamicin and tobramycin in the range of 5 to 10 μg/mL produce an optimum response. This translates into a desirable peak-dose concentration of 20 to 40 μg/mL for amikacin. Early achievement of gentamicin therapeutic concentrations increases the cure rate in patients with sepsis, pneumonia, and wound and urinary tract infections. However, renal toxicity may occur in up to 25% of patients and is more common with gentamicin and amikacin peak levels of greater than 10 and 38.5 μg/mL, respectively, as well as with increased trough levels (more than 2 or 8 μg/mL, respectively). Other predisposing factors for renal toxicity are prolonged therapy (greater than 11 days), use of diuretics and nephrotoxic agents, increased initial serum creatinine, female gender, liver disease, old age, shock, and congestive heart failure (CHF). Risk factors for ototoxicity are the same as for renal toxicity. Aminoglycoside-induced ototoxicity is not reversible, is usually difficult to detect, and occurs in 2% to 10% of patients receiving aminoglycosides.

Published nomograms of aminoglycoside dosing are generally of little use in critically ill patients. Individualized dosing with peak and trough serum drug concentrations should be used to maximize efficacy and minimize toxicity. Aminoglycoside concentrations can be obtained in all patients; however, aminoglycosides are inactivated in vitro by semisynthetic penicillins, and samples that contain high concentrations of these drugs should be placed on ice and analyzed immediately or frozen before analysis. Serum vancomycin concentration monitoring is most useful in patients who exhibit decreased renal function, receive concurrent nephrotoxic drugs, or suffer from life-threatening methicillin-resistant staphylococcal or enterococcal sepsis. Peak concentrations of 20 to 40 μg/mL and trough concentrations of 5 to 10 μg/mL are generally sufficient, and serum drug concentrations should not be obtained more frequently than once weekly.

Amphotericin B is often used in patients who receive concurrent aminoglycoside or vancomycin therapy. The risk for amphotericin B–induced nephrotoxicity with potassium and magnesium wasting is decreased by administering sodium supplements, avoiding dehydration, and limiting the cumulative dose to less than 4 to 5 g. Although some clinicians advocate the use of alternate-day amphotericin B dosing to decrease nephrotoxicity, little evidence supports this practice. Monitoring for amphotericin-induced nephrotoxicity includes serum concentrations of creatinine, magnesium, and potassium.

Anticoagulants

The prothrombin time (PT) is sensitive to decreases in factors II, VII, and X and is used to measure warfarin anticoagulation. The test is performed by adding calcium and thromboplastin to citrated plasma. Because commercial thromboplastins have different sensitivities to the reduction of vitamin K–dependent factors, variable PT ratios (patient-laboratory control value) may be reported for the same level of anticoagulation. The international normalized ratios (INRs) standardize the PT ratios according to the World Health Organization's reference thromboplastin and should be used to monitor warfarin anticoagulant response.

The activated partial thromboplastin time (APTT) is sensitive to inhibition of factors IIa, IXa, and Xa and is the standard parameter of heparin anticoagulation monitoring. Prolongation of the APTT versus laboratory control of 1.5 to 2.5 times provides adequate anticoagulation and minimizes the risk for bleeding. The APTT should be measured before and 6 hours after the initiation of the heparin infusion, with subsequent measurements taken once daily.

The primary adverse effect of warfarin and heparin is bleeding, which can be reversed with fresh-frozen plasma, factor concentrates, vitamin K (warfarin), and protamine (heparin). Elderly patients, those with comorbid conditions, and those who receive more intensive anticoagulation are at greater risk for major bleeding episodes. Heparin may cause a bimodal incidence of thrombocytopenia, requiring monitoring of the platelet count every 2 to 3 days. The early thrombocytopenia occurs within 2 to 4 days and reverses with continued heparin treatment. The delayed thrombocytopenia, an autoimmune reaction, occurs after 7 to 10 days in less than 5% of patients but requires discontinuation of the drug.

Anticonvulsants

Phenytoin, valproic acid, and phenobarbital are used in the prevention and treatment of generalized and focal seizures in the ICU. Phenytoin undergoes zero-order (saturable) hepatic elimination. The drug is 90% bound to albumin. Decreases in protein binding in hypoalbuminemia, renal failure, and jaundice, and following displacement reactions with other drugs, can significantly increase drug clearance with resultant decreases in total but not free drug concentrations. The total phenytoin concentration is usually a good indicator of clinical response, but free serum phenytoin concentrations show a better correlation with clinical response in patients with altered serum protein binding. Therefore, free serum drug concentrations should be measured when the potential for altered protein binding exists. Phenytoin absorption is significantly decreased by enteral feedings, and the intravenous route is preferred in these patients. When one is using the oral suspension or parenteral phenytoin sodium, the daily dose should be split into two or three doses to avoid peak concentration toxicity. Phenytoin trough serum concentrations should be measured approximately 24 hours after a loading dose and once every 5 to 10 days thereafter until the patient has been stabilized.

Valproic acid has a relatively short half-life (9 to 18 hours) and is administered several times daily. Longer dosing intervals with higher doses may be equally effective but increase the risk for gastrointestinal side effects. Unlike the other anticonvulsants, valproic acid decreases hepatic enzyme drug-metabolizing capacity, and the dose of other anticonvulsants may need to be reduced during polytherapy. Valproic acid is a low-extraction-ratio drug that also exhibits dose-dependent protein binding, with resultant wide fluctuations in both total and free drug concentrations. Serum drug concentrations may also vary significantly in different oral preparations. Peak plasma concentrations are usually reached after 3 to 8 hours with the enteric-coated preparation and within 2 hours with other oral dosage forms. Valproic acid trough concentrations should be obtained every 2 to 3 days after the initial loading dose until the patient is stable.

Phenobarbital undergoes rapid and complete absorption from oral and intramuscular sites. The drug is 50% bound to albumin, and an increased therapeutic effect or risk for toxicity is expected in patients with severe hypoalbuminemia. Phenobarbital is metabolized by the liver and induces hepatic enzyme metabolism of other drugs. The renal clearance accounts for 40% of total clearance and is increased five- to tenfold with urinary alkalinization. Phenobarbital exhibits a linear dosage-concentration relationship, making dosage adjustments easy. The drug has a very long half-life (96 hours), and frequent sampling for serum concentrations is useful only in patients in whom toxicity or inadequate therapy is suspected.

Antiarrhythmic Agents

Quinidine and Procainamide

Quinidine and procainamide are class Ia antiarrhythmics and are used extensively for both ventricular and supraventricular arrhythmias. Quinidine is strongly bound to both albumin and α_1-acid glycoprotein; protein binding is decreased in liver disease and increased after trauma and surgery and during myocardial infarction owing to increases in α_1-acid glycoprotein levels. Because quinidine is a high-extraction-ratio drug, changes in plasma protein binding directly alter free drug concentrations, and drug toxicity would most likely occur in patients with poor hepatic blood flow and decreased protein binding. Increased oral bioavailability resulting from decreased first-pass metabolism would also be expected in heart failure patients. Quinidine is metabolized to several active metabolites, of which 3-OH quinidine is the most important.

Procainamide is 50% renally eliminated; the remainder is metabolized to active *N*-acetyl procainamide (NAPA), which is 85% renally eliminated. Procainamide is only 15% bound to albumin, and clearance and plasma concentrations are not altered by protein-binding changes. Liver, renal, and cardiac insufficiency decrease procainamide clearance. Procainamide concentrations should be obtained in patients with these conditions, and dosing should be adjusted accordingly. The significance of NAPA as a contributor to antiarrhythmic activity and drug-induced torsades de pointes is controversial, and NAPA concentrations should be obtained only in patients with renal insufficiency or in patients who show signs of drug toxicity.

Lidocaine

Lidocaine (class Ib) is frequently chosen in the treatment of ventricular arrhythmias because of its low incidence of hemodynamic complications. However, the drug has a narrow therapeutic concentration range and clinically important central nervous system toxicity. Lidocaine is a high-extraction-ratio drug, and its clearance is dependent on cardiac function and hepatic blood flow. Approximately 70% of lidocaine is bound to albumin and α_1-acid glycoprotein, and drug toxicity is correlated with increasing amounts of total and free drug. Lidocaine protein binding is decreased in patients with hypoalbuminemia and is increased after myocardial infarction. The renally eliminated metabolites monoethylglycinexylidide and glycinexylidide possess 80% to 90% and 10% to 26%, respectively, of the antiarrhythmic potency of lidocaine but have not been correlated to adverse events during lidocaine therapy. Lidocaine clearance is decreased by congestive heart failure and other low-flow states and liver disease. Monitoring of lidocaine toxicity is difficult because of the initial subtle signs of toxicity and the significant number of patients who may require lidocaine concentrations greater than 6 μg/mL for arrhythmia control.

Digoxin

Therapy with digoxin should be monitored carefully because the agent is known to cause practically any type of arrhythmia but primarily atrioventricular (AV) junction tachycardia. The absorption of digoxin is dependent on the preparation used, with tablets being the least bioavailable (70% to 80%) and the liquid-filled capsules the most (90% to 100%). The currently accepted therapeutic range of digoxin is 0.8 to 2.0 ng/mL, but treatment of atrial fibrillation may require concentrations of 1.6 ng/mL or greater. The risk for digoxin toxicity is increased by hypokalemia, hypercalcemia, hypothyroidism, and drug interactions (quinidine, verapamil, and spironolactone). Nonspecific ECG changes (ST depression, T wave abnormalities, and QT shortening) do not correlate with drug effects. Serum digoxin concentration monitoring is further complicated by radioimmunoassay interference by a digoxin-like immunoreactive substance, an endogenous compound, which produces falsely elevated serum digoxin concentrations in neonates and patients with liver or renal impairment.

Antihypertensives

The metabolism of nitroprusside may lead to life-threatening cyanide or thiocyanate toxicity in patients with end-organ dysfunction. Most cyanide from nitroprusside reacts with thiosulfate to form renally eliminated thiocyanate. Normal hepatic clearance of cyanide by conversion to thiocyanate corresponds to a nitroprusside infusion of less than 2 $\mu g \cdot kg^{-1} \cdot min^{-1}$. Unmetabolized cyanide binds to cytochrome oxidase and blocks cellular respiration. Nitroprusside infusions in excess of 4 $\mu g \cdot kg^{-1} \cdot min^{-1}$ can produce toxic cyanide levels in 5 to 10 hours. The acute clinical manifestations of cyanide toxicity can range from headache, dizziness, tachypnea, and tachycardia to apnea, convulsions, and lactic acidosis. Patients with renal insufficiency are also at risk for the development of thiocyanate toxicity, which may manifest as confusion, hyperreflexia, hallucinations, convulsions, coma, and death. Nitroprusside should be dosed carefully in patients with hepatic dysfunction, and prolonged infusions exceeding 2 $\mu g \cdot kg^{-1} \cdot min^{-1}$ should be avoided. Serum thiocyanate concentrations should be measured in patients who receive nitroprusside infusions at rates exceeding 10 $\mu g \cdot kg^{-1} \cdot min^{-1}$ for more than 48 hours or who have renal insufficiency.

THEOPHYLLINE

Theophylline is commonly used for the treatment of respiratory disorders in the ICU and is one of the few drugs with a relatively well-defined dose-response relationship. Although the onset of activity with theophylline is delayed, pulmonary function (forced expiratory volume in 1 second or forced vital capacity) will improve 2% for each microgram per milliliter increase in serum theophylline concentrations of from 5 to 20 μg/mL. However, the risk for toxicity will increase from 0% to 7% over the same concentration range and may exceed 80% for concentrations greater than 25 μg/mL in some patients. Theophylline-induced seizures and arrhythmias (primarily sinus tachycardia, paroxysmal supraventricular tachycardia, or ectopic beats) may occur at 20 to 25 μg/mL, especially in older patients and in those with underlying neurologic and cardiovascular disorders.

DRUG ABUSE, OVERDOSE, AND WITHDRAWAL SYNDROMES

Recognition and Diagnosis

One of the best indicators of substance abuse problems is a history of drug abuse. It can be a chronic disorder; it is not uncommon for some people to return to drug use during stressful situations. A family history of drug use is significant. It is vital to go back at least two generations, because the problem will often skip a generation. Individuals who associate with known drug abusers also are at high risk. There is no stereotypic addict. Addiction involves patients from all racial, ethnic, and socioeconomic backgrounds.

The physical examination is also critical. We have all been taught the stigmas of cirrhosis, such as spider angiomas, rhinophyma, and palmar erythema, which can be helpful in recognizing the alcoholic patient. Intravenous drug users may have tracks over sites from intravenous injection. When injection drug use is suspected, it is important to look not only in the antecubital fossa but at other sites as well, because drug users will try to hide their use and may inject in the axilla, under the tongue, in breast veins, and in the dorsal vein of the penis. In individuals who have been unable to maintain good venous access, scars and ulcers may be present from subcutaneous injection. To disguise track marks, drug users will often draw elaborate tattoos that incorporate the tracks.

Other signs of heavy drug use include cigarette burns on the fingers and on the chest. Those who snort drugs will show inflammation of the nasal mucosa, and heavy chronic users may even shown perforation of the nasal septum. Hepatomegaly is common from alcohol use as well as from hepatitis and other problems associated with injection drug use. Murmurs also may be found from endocarditis.

Alterations in consciousness may also be present from drug use. Opioids and sedative-hypnotics can cause effects from sedation to coma. They will also decrease vital signs with decreased respirations, pulse, and blood pressure. Stimulants like cocaine or amphetamines cause hyperactivity and paranoia. Physically, they produce hyperthermia, agitation, tachycardia, and hypertension. Ocular manifestations of drug use include nystagmus with sedatives and alcohol. PCP (phencyclidine pepirdine) will cause both horizontal and vertical nystagmus. Opioids cause miosis and mydriasis in withdrawal except for meperidene, which produces mydriasis during intoxication. On funduscopic examination, microemboli have been seen occluding retinal vessels.

One of the best ways to confirm suspicions about drug use is through laboratory findings. Because of the high rates of trauma associated with drug use, urine toxicologic screens should be performed on all patients who present for critical care from trauma (Table 7–12). If there is concern about alcohol use, blood for alcohol levels can be drawn and sent to the laboratory or breath alcohol levels obtained. Elevations of liver enzymes, HIV infection, tuberculosis, and increased mean corpuscular volume could all be indicators of alcohol and other drug use. For toxicology, urine screens are superior to plasma levels because the drugs are concentrated in the urine. With urine toxicology, there is a window of opportunity, and a negative screen does not totally rule out that the person has not used those drugs in the recent past.

Table 7–12. DURATION OF DRUG DETECTION IN URINE AND LIMITS OF SENSITIVITY*

Drug	Approximate Duration of Detectability	Limits of Sensitivity
Amphetamine	48 h	100 ng/mL
Methamphetamine	48 h	100 ng/mL
Barbiturates		
Short-acting		
Hexobarbital		1.0 μg/mL
Pentobarbital	24 h	100 ng/mL
Secobarbital		100 ng/mL
Intermediate-acting		
Amobarbital		1.0 μg/mL
Butabarbital	48–72 h	0.5 μg/mL
Butalbital		1.5 μg/mL
Long-acting		
Phenobarbital	7+ d	1.0 μg/mL
Benzodiazepines	3+ d†	100 ng/mL
Cocaine		
Benzoylecgonine	2–3 d	50 ng/mL
Ecgonine methyl ester	2–3 d	50 ng/mL
Methadone	3+ d	0.5 μg/mL
Codeine	48 h	0.5 μg/mL
Morphine (heroin)	48 h	100 ng/mL
Propoxyphene	6–48 h	0.5 μg/mL
Cannabinoids	3–21 d‡	10 ng/mL
Phencyclidine	±8 d§	10 ng/mL

*Interpretation of detectability must take into account many factors: metabolism, physical condition, state of hydration, route and frequency of administration, and method of detection used.

†Therapeutic doses.

‡Dependent on frequency and chronicity of use.

§Poorly excreted in alkaline urine.

(Adapted from Schnoll SH, Lewis DE: Drug screening in the workplace: Pros and cons. Semin Occup Med 1986; 243–251, by permission of Thieme Medical Publishers.)

Treatment of Acute Intoxication

General Considerations

Recent years have seen the fortunate development of specific narcotic antagonists for some of the common drugs with abuse potential. The presence of these pure antagonists has provided not only rapid reversal of intoxication but also diagnosis of the intoxicating agent. In cases of coma of unknown origin, in addition to infusion of 50% glucose, naloxone (Narcan) and flumazenil (Mazicon) should be administered intravenously to determine whether the coma is secondary to hypoglycemia or opioid or benzodiazepine intoxication. Although intoxicated patients can become extremely agitated and at times violent, physical restraints should be avoided unless all other measures fail. When possible, chemical restraints should be used to control agitation and aggressive behavior.

Opioid Intoxication

Naloxone is an extremely safe drug that can be administered intramuscularly, subcutaneously, and intravenously in large quantities without any significant adverse effects. When administering naloxone, two important points must be kept in mind. First, naloxone is extremely short acting, its effects lasting 60 to 90 minutes. This duration of action is significantly shorter than almost all opioids except the ultrashort-acting drugs such as fentanyl and its analogs. Because of this, naloxone must be administered repeatedly or through continuous intravenous infusion to avoid relapse into coma. Second, naloxone can precipitate withdrawal in an individual who is dependent on opioids. However, this problem can be alleviated by titrating the amount of naloxone that relieves respiratory depression without precipitating withdrawal. All opioids are antagonized by naloxone, including the agonist/antagonists and the partial agonists.

Sedative-Hypnotic Intoxication

Sedative-hypnotic intoxication in conjunction with alcohol intoxication is one of the most frequent combinations seen in the emergency department. The recent release of flumazenil has been an important addition for the treatment of benzodiazepine intoxication and overdose. However, like naloxone, flumazenil is a short-acting preparation and, therefore, requires either repeated dosing every 30 minutes or intravenous infusion over time to cover the longer-acting effects of most benzodiazepines. Also, like naloxone, flumazenil can precipitate a withdrawal syndrome in an individual who is dependent on benzodiazepines. This effect can result in seizures and a major withdrawal syndrome.

Although flumazenil reverses most of the effects of a benzodiazepine overdose, it does not always reliably reverse respiratory depression. Flumazenil does not antagonize the effects of other sedative-hypnotics, including alcohol, barbiturates, and the nonbenzodiazepine, nonbarbiturate sleeping pills. Treatment of overdose with these drugs may require dialysis to clear the drug from the system because no antagonists of these drugs are currently available. When the drug has been taken orally, administration of activated charcoal can be important in reducing absorption of more drug into the body and preventing reabsorption of drug through the enterohepatic circulation. With both the opioids and the sedative-hypnotics, a withdrawal syndrome may develop as the intoxication clears. Therefore, it is important to monitor for withdrawal and treat it appropriately. Failure to do this will result in more severe problems and, with sedative-hypnotics, the potential for status epilepticus and delirium.

Psychostimulant Intoxication

The most common psychostimulant intoxication seen at this time occurs with cocaine. Cocaine overdoses are very common in the emergency department. Unlike the opioids and benzodiazepines, no specific antagonist is available for the effects of cocaine or other psychostimulants. Although cocaine itself is relatively short acting, there is evidence that some of its metabolites, particularly benzoylecgonine, may produce long-acting effects after cocaine has cleared. In addition, some of the cardiac effects of cocaine can occur a week to 10 days after the individual has stopped using the cocaine. Individuals who use alcohol with cocaine can synthesize coca ethylene, which may be more toxic than cocaine.

One of the most difficult problems associated with severe cocaine and other psychostimulant intoxication is the psychosis, which may be indistinguishable from a naturally occurring psychosis. This problem is best treated with high-potency antipsychotic medications, such as haloperidol. It is best to give haloperidol intravenously. Haloperidol may lower the seizure threshold. Therefore, care should be taken when it is administered. For excessive stimulation, an intravenously administered benzodiazepine can be very useful. Benzodiazepines should not be administered intramuscularly because of erratic absorption from the intramuscular injection site. Lorazepam intravenously has a duration of action of approximately 2 hours. Diazepam has a duration of action, when given intravenously, of about 30 to 40 minutes, and if an ultrashort-acting drug is necessary, midazolam could be used. Because respiratory depression can occur with the use of intravenous benzodiazepines, in particular midazolam, it is best to start with a low dose and titrate up on the basis of the clinical picture.

Arrhythmia is associated with cocaine use and can be treated with β-blockers and, if associated with myocardial ischemia, calcium channel blockers. All the psychostimulants can cause hypertension. Hypertensive effects usually ameliorate as the drug clears the system.

Cocaine is a short-acting drug with a duration of action of several hours. However, some of the amphetamines are long acting and, if taken in high doses, effects can persist for several days. To reduce the duration of these effects, acidification of the urine will enhance excretion of amphetamines. Acidification can be accomplished through the use of ascorbic acid, 500 mg three or four times a day, or ammonium chloride. However, the latter may produce hepatic toxicity. Once the urinary pH is less than 6.0, a diuretic should be administered to enhance drug excretion.

Phencyclidine Intoxication

Overdoses with PCP and other arycyclohexylamines, although not common in all parts of the country, can present very challenging clinical problems. The nonionized drug is frequently taken up by cells from which it cannot be excreted, resulting in a prolonged effect. One of the most severe problems with PCP is hypertensive crisis. Psychoses and catatonia can also occur with PCP intoxication. Individuals on PCP have also been known to become violent. The acute psychosis and agitation with PCP can be treated like treatment of amphetamines—use of intravenous haloperidol and benzodiazepines. The doses are similar to those used for psychostimulants.

PCP, like the amphetamines, is best excreted in an acid urine, which will significantly decrease the duration of effects from the drug. There is a 100-fold difference in the rate of excretion between pH 5.5 and pH 6. Once the pH is down to the 5.5 level, a diuretic should be administered. This will significantly decrease the duration over which PCP effects persist.

Hallucinogen Intoxication

With the recent increased use of hallucinogens, acute reactions are being seen in the emergency department. Of particular concern are seizures that can occur with high doses and the acute disorientation that results in confusion and severe anxiety. In severe cases, antipsychotics such as haloperidol have been shown to be effective in reducing some of these problems, and sedation can be effected with benzodiazepines. Problems with hallucinogens are rarely seen in the critical care setting unless the person is severely injured while intoxicated. The effects of these drugs can last up to 12 hours.

Solvent Intoxication

Acute problems with volatile inhalants are rare; however, they can be quite serious. The most significant is arrhythmias, which develop from the hydrofluorocarbons and other volatile substances that resemble some of the older general anesthetics. These arrhythmias occur from sensitization of the heart to catecholamines and have been fatal. Fortunately, the effects of these drugs are short lived. However, in patients in whom arrhythmias may persist, β-blockers may be effective in reducing the problems.

When withdrawing patients from dependency-producing drugs, it is important to reduce gradually the amount of drug the individual is taking. This can be safely done by reducing the dose of the drug at a rate of approximately 10% of the initial dose per day, resulting in a gradual withdrawal over approximately 10 days. In a stable individual for whom a long-acting drug is being used to effect the withdrawal, then a 20% per day taper can be used, completing the withdrawal in 5 days.

When selecting a drug to treat the withdrawal syndrome, the first choice should be one that shows cross-dependence and cross-tolerance with the drugs causing the withdrawal syndrome.

Opioid Withdrawal

Although street addicts are inordinately concerned about opioid withdrawal, rarely has anyone died from its effects. In most cases, opioid withdrawal is no more severe than a bad case of the flu, with lacrimation, rhinorrhea, nausea, vomiting, diarrhea, and piloerection. Traditionally, opioid withdrawal has been treated with methadone, a long-acting narcotic, or more recently in combination with the α_2-agonist clonidine. Methadone can cause problems because of its extremely long half-life and because it can accumulate over time in cases of hepatic or renal impairment.

The easiest way to deal with opioid withdrawal is to treat the signs and symptoms as they appear. An alternative approach is to use intravenous morphine. Morphine should be increased at a minimum of 1 mg per hour or as rapidly as 1 mg every 5 minutes until signs and symptoms of withdrawal are relieved. Once stabilized on morphine, the patient can either be maintained on that amount of morphine or withdrawn at a rate of 10% of the total daily dose each day. As the patient begins to recover and can be switched to oral medications, it is important to remember that the oral dose of morphine is six times the parenteral. If there is going to be a switch from parenteral to oral medication, it may be more satisfactory to switch the patient to methadone. The methadone can then be reduced to 5 mg per day in a fixed volume of liquid.

Sedative-Hypnotic and Alcohol Withdrawal

Withdrawal from alcohol and other sedative-hypnotics is the only life-threatening withdrawal. Patients in whom major withdrawal symptoms, such as delirium tremers, develop can have mortality rates as high as 5%. Therefore, it is important to treat major withdrawal vigorously. There is no correlation with the amount of drug or alcohol ingested or other medical conditions. Patients with a history of chronic alcohol dependence are often vitamin depleted; therefore, it is imperative to give thiamine and multivitamins with glucose to prevent the precipitation of Wernicke's and Korsakoff's syndromes.

In a patient with a history of alcohol or other sedative-hypnotic use, it is critical to begin prophylactic treatment to prevent the patient from going into sedative-hypnotic withdrawal. In most cases, a long-acting benzodiazepine or long-acting barbiturate such as phenobarbital can be used as treatment or prophylaxis for sedative-hypnotic and alcohol withdrawal. Phenobarbital is extremely long acting, with a half-life of more than 72 hours, and also is an enzyme inducer that could result in interference with the metabolism of other medications. However, if it can be used, phenobarbital is the treatment of choice. It is also available in many different dosage and delivery forms, allowing very precise dosage adjustments. Phenobarbital also has a long latency, which reduces its abuse potential. Long-acting benzodiazepines are converted to the long-acting form only on passage through the liver. Therefore, parenteral administration bypasses the liver, and the long-acting metabolites will not be generated.

Only three benzodiazepines can be given parenterally: midazolam, diazepam, and lorazepam. Midazolam is an ultrashort-acting benzodiazepine, and unless there is specific need for an ultrashort-acting medication, it should not be used. Diazepam intravenously has a half-life of about 30 minutes, and lorazepam intravenously has a half-life of about 2 hours. Therefore, the choice of medication will be based on specific need. Because the latency of intravenous benzodiazepines is very short (minutes), the drug can be titrated very rapidly to relieve withdrawal symptoms.

POISONING

Treatment Modalities

Decontamination

Decontamination of the eyes, skin, and gastrointestinal tract is the first and foremost task to perform in any poisoning emergency. Gastrointestinal decontamination involves the use of emetics, gastric lavage, oral sorbents, cathartics, and whole-bowel irrigation.

EMETICS

Ipecac is currently the emetic of choice. Contraindications to the use of ipecac include the potentially imminent onset or presence of a decreased level of consciousness or seizures, uncontrolled hypertension, and prior ingestion of acid or alkali. Ipecac is generally not indicated for low-viscosity petroleum distillate ingestions unless a toxic coingestant is implicated. The incidence of diarrhea and lethargy is 13% and 11.6%, respectively.

GASTRIC LAVAGE

Orogastric lavage is frequently used for gastric decontamination in the emergency department. Tracheal intubation should precede lavage in patients with seizures, depressed mental status, or an absent gag reflex. Lavage is contraindicated in patients with caustic ingestions. The complications include aspiration; airway obstruction; esophageal, gastric, or laryngeal damage; water intoxication in children when tap water is used; and gastrointestinal hemorrhage. Orogastric lavage is indicated in patients with life-threatening ingestions who reach medical attention within 1 to 2 hours postingestion and possibly longer with substances associated with delayed gastric emptying, such as anticholinergics.

ACTIVATED CHARCOAL

The maximum binding capacity of activated charcoal is dependent on its surface area, which ranges from 950 m^2/g to 200 m^2/g. Activated charcoal absorbs most drugs but is not very effective for alcohols, hydrocarbons, organophosphates, carbamates, cyanide, acids, alkali, lithium, and iron. The dosage should reflect an activated charcoal-to-drug ratio of 10:1. However, because the amount ingested is rarely accurately known, it is common practice to dose activated charcoal based on a patient's body weight (1 to 2 g/kg).

Enhanced Elimination

Alkalinization

Sodium bicarbonate therapy enhances the elimination of certain toxic drugs by altering drug ionization, and it also decreases toxicity by changing sodium gradients or receptor binding or by buffering acidemia. The drugs that respond to urine and serum alkalinization in this fashion include salicylic acid, phenobarbital, chlorpropamide, and the chlorophenoxyl herbicide 2,4-dichlorophenoxyacetic acid.

Sodium bicarbonate may also be useful in the treatment of overdose of other cardiotoxic drugs that produce a widened QT interval, including carbamazepine, procainamide, quinidine, and quinine. Sodium bicarbonate therapy for ethylene glycol, methanol, and isoniazid, as well as other drugs, is based on the buffering capability of bicarbonate and does not enhance elimination.

Multidose Activated Charcoal

The dosage of activated charcoal is approximately 50 to 100 g in adults for the first dose, given with a cathartic, and then about 20 to 50 g given at 2- to 4-hour intervals without a cathartic. Adverse reactions include vomiting, aspiration, and bowel obstruction. Diarrhea with dehydration may be seen when repeated doses of cathartic are mistakenly included with the multiple doses of activated charcoal. When activated charcoal is required in a patient with drug-induced vomiting, as in theophylline toxicity, ranitidine has been recommended as an antiemetic agent. Metoclopramide, ondansetron, or droperidol may also be used. Therapy should be discontinued if bowel sounds are absent, vomiting is persistent, or the level of the drug (and metabolites, when applicable) decreases to the therapeutic range.

Extracorporeal Modalities

Hemodialysis involves arterial to venous blood flow with diffusion of substances through a semipermeable membrane. Drugs and chemicals that are well dialyzed have low molecular weights, high water solubility, low lipid solubility, low plasma protein binding, low volume of distribution (low tissue binding), and a short distribution phase. Hemodialysis is routinely used in severe ethylene glycol, lithium, methanol, and salicylate poisonings. Although theophylline is cleared by hemodialysis, charcoal hemoperfusion is more effective than dialysis and is the procedure of choice. In some overdose patients, dialysis may also be indicated to manage refractory hyperkalemia, acidosis, renal failure, or vomiting overload.

Antidotes and Shelters: Controversies and New Issues

N-Acetylcysteine

N-Acetylcysteine (NAC) has been widely accepted as antidotal therapy for acetaminophen overdose. A remarkable hepatoprotective effect was demonstrated in patients who were treated with the oral NAC regimen.

FLUMAZENIL

Flumazenil is a 1,4-imidazobenzodiazepine that competitively inhibits benzodiazepines at the central receptors, effectively blocking their clinical effect. Contrary to popular belief, benzodiazepine overdose alone can cause death or serious morbidity. Coingestants often potentiate toxicity.

Flumazenil is an effective benzodiazepine antagonist that may decrease morbidity, complications, and therapeutic intervention required in patients with benzodiazepine overdose. The risk of precipitating convulsions in tricyclic antidepressant overdoses dictates that caution be taken when flumazenil is administered in patients with mixed drug overdoses with undetermined agents.

PHYSOSTIGMINE

Physostigmine is a reversible acetylcholinesterase inhibitor. As an uncharged, lipophilic, tertiary ammonium compound, physostigmine easily crosses the blood-brain barrier. The other reversible acetylcholinesterase inhibitors are quaternary ammonium compounds (edrophonium, neostigmine, pyridostigmine) and do not penetrate the blood-brain barrier. Although physostigmine is effective in reversing both central and peripheral manifestations of anticholinergic drug overdose, adverse reactions are common. Symptoms of a cholinergic crisis, including salivation, lacrimation, urination, defecation, and bronchorrhea, may occur if physostigmine is administered in the absence of true anticholinergic poisoning. Even when given in the setting of pure anticholinergic overdose, physostigmine may cause seizures. Physostigmine use in anticholinergic poisonings should be limited to patients with life-threatening manifestations who are unresponsive to other therapy. Physostigmine is not recommended in the treatment of cyclic antidepressant overdose because cardiac abnormalities unrelated to anticholinergic effects usually predominate as the cause of mortality.

A Review of Selected Toxic Agents

Acetaminophen

Acetaminophen (*N*-acetyl-*p*-aminophenol, APAP, paracetamol) is the most prevalent analgesic implicated in overdose today. The potential for a clinically significant overdose can be seen with acute acetaminophen ingestions of 150 mg/kg or of 7.5 to 10 g in an adult. The clinical presentation, primarily hepatotoxicity, is often delayed. Three general stages occur:

- *Stage I* can begin within hours, with symptoms of nausea, vomiting, and diaphoresis.
- *Stage II* occurs 24 to 48 hours after the ingestion, when gastrointestinal symptoms are minimal but hepatic injury

is progressing. Right upper quadrant abdominal pain and early liver function abnormalities are noted. The disproportionate rise in transaminase levels compared with the small increases in bilirubin concentration can help differentiate among acetaminophen-induced hepatic injury, viral hepatitis, and biliary obstruction.
- *Stage III* occurs 3 to 4 days after ingestion, when hepatic necrosis and liver function abnormalities peak. Hepatic encephalopathy, bleeding diatheses, and hypoglycemia may be present. By 7 to 9 days, most patients recover full hepatic function without evidence of cirrhosis. Other organ systems can manifest acetaminophen toxicity. Acute renal failure with or without hepatic involvement may occur. Treatment of acetaminophen overdose is based on identification of potential victims, decontamination, assessment of risk based on serum concentration and a nomogram, early therapy with NAC, intensive supportive care, and early consultation for liver transplantation in refractory patients.

Alcohols

Isopropanol, ethylene glycol, and methanol are the toxic alcohols that are commonly implicated in poisonings.

Ethylene glycol is found in antifreeze, deicers, and industrial solvents. Methanol is referred to as "wood alcohol," whereas ethanol is known as "grain alcohol." Methanol can be found in paint remover, duplicator fluid, gas line antifreeze, windshield washing fluid, solid canned fuel (4%), alternative fuels, denatured ethanol (added to ethanol to make it unfit to drink), and bootlegged whiskey (as a contaminant). Isopropanol is found in rubbing alcohol (although some rubbing alcohols contain ethanol), skin lotions, hair tonics, aftershave lotions, and glass cleaners.

- *Stage I* of ethylene glycol toxicity occurs over the first 30 minutes to 12 hours after ingestion and is predominantly characterized by central nervous system effects and acidosis. The poisoned patient has nystagmus and depressed reflexes and appears intoxicated, with Kussmaul's respirations owing to pronounced metabolic acidosis. Coma with focal seizures may develop, and tetany from hypocalcemia may ensue.
- *Stage II* occurs within the first 24 hours, when deposition of calcium oxalate crystals in the myocardium, lung, and vasculature causes multisystem complications, including hypertension, tachycardia, and pulmonary edema.
- *Stage III* (24 to 72 hours), oliguric renal failure develops.
- *Stage IV* is characterized by delayed neurologic sequelae that occur 6 to 15 days after the original insult. Patients present with hyperreflexia, ataxia, facial nerve paralysis, and other cranial nerve abnormalities.

Methanol, like ethylene glycol, is clear and odorless; however, in its crude form, it is bitter tasting, and this in part explains its use as an additive in denatured ethanol. Early central nervous system signs reflect inebriation, which may be followed by an asymptomatic period. The delayed effects begin after 6 to 36 hours, with vertigo, motor restlessness, delirium, blurred or whitened vision, hyperemia of the optic disk, dilated pupils, and occasionally blindness. The classic description of visual changes is "seeing as if through a blizzard." Pulmonary findings include Kussmaul's respirations owing to the severe acidosis caused by formate and lactate. Bradycardia is uncommon, and its presence confers a grave prognosis. Abdominal pain, vomiting, and diarrhea are common.

Isopropanol is clear, colorless, and bitter tasting and leaves the smell of acetone or "alcohol" on the breath. The neurologic symptoms of intoxication are similar to those of ethanol; however, isopropanol is twice as potent as ethanol, and this causes marked central nervous system depression, ataxia, headache, and depression of deep tendon reflexes. Gastrointestinal irritation, nausea, vomiting, abdominal pain, and hematamesis are common. Respiratory depression with progression to respiratory arrest and myocardial depression that causes hypotension can be seen in severe overdose.

A marked osmolar gap (0.2 mOsm/L for every 1 mg/dL of ethylene glycol) and an anion gap acidosis are present with ethylene glycol ingestions. Isopropanol produces an osmolar gap (0.17 mOsm/L for every 1 mg/dL of isopropanol) and ketonuria. The ketonuria is accompanied by only minimal acidosis and no glycosuria. Determination of serum acetone levels can be helpful.

The treatment of ethylene glycol and methanol poisoning is based on prevention of the formation of toxic metabolites. Gastric emptying may be effective early. Activated charcoal is ineffective. Ethanol administration should be started early to prevent the metabolism of ethylene glycol to glycoaldehyde and that of methanol to formaldehyde by competitively inhibiting the hepatic enzyme alcohol dehydrogenase. Ethanol can be administered orally or intravenously. The ethanol should be in solution of 20% or greater, and intravenous ethanol should be in solution of 5% to 10%. Begin treatment with an intravenous bolus of 7.9 to 10 mL/kg of 10% ethanol in 5% dextrose in water over 30 minutes. A maintenance infusion can be estimated at 1 to 2 $mL \cdot kg^{-1} \cdot h^{-1}$ of 10% ethanol in 5% dextrose in water; the higher end of the range should be chosen for the chronic drinker. A serum level of just over 100 mg/dL should be maintained. Acidosis should be aggressively treated with sodium bicarbonate.

Hemodialysis should be instituted early for ethylene glycol intoxication if the level is greater than 50 mg/dL or if a patient has metabolic or hemodynamic evidence of toxicity; for methanol intoxication, hemodialysis should be instituted if the methanol level is greater than 50 mg/dL or if a patient has clinical manifestations of toxicity, such as visual changes or acidosis. During hemodialysis, ethanol can be added to the dialysate bath to achieve a concentration of 100 mg/dL in the dialysate.

Specific additional therapies for an ethylene glycol overdose patient include administration of thiamine (100 mg intravenously per day) and pyridoxine (100 mg intravenously per day) to enhance the metabolism of glyoxylate. Specific therapies for methanol intoxication include administration of folic acid and its metabolite leucovorin (folic acid), which is a cofactor in the metabolism of formate. The dose is 1 to 2 mg/kg intravenously every 4 hours for six doses. Leucovorin, the active form, is preferred in patients who are already symptomatic. Isopropanol therapy is predominantly supportive; hemodialysis is reserved for patients with hypotension that is unresponsive to fluid administration. Isopropanol and acetone are effectively dialyzed, but the procedure is infrequently needed.

Alkalis, Acids, and Hydrofluoric Acid

Liquid, granular, and solid forms of alkali (usually sodium or potassium hydroxide) are present in many households. Liquid and granular forms can be found mostly in drain openers, oven cleaners, automatic dishwasher detergents, and other household cleaning products. Automotive airbags can also release a sodium hydroxide powder if they burst on impact. The tablets used to test urine for sugar (e.g., Clinitest) and tablets to clean dentures also contain alkali.

The mechanism of injury for acids and alkali differs. Alkali causes liquefaction necrosis during contact with and penetration of tissues. Destruction of protein and collagen, saponification of fat, and thrombosis of blood vessels occur within minutes after exposure. Acids, however, tend to cause coagulation necrosis and have more limited penetration. Hydrofluoric acid is a weak acid that dissociates poorly in solution. This property actually enhances the toxicity of the fluoride component. Although the free proton may contribute to tissue damage, as with other acids, it is the uncharged hydrogen fluoride complex that penetrates deeply into tissues. In the tissues, dissociation takes place, slowly releasing the strongly negative fluoride ions that bind avidly to calcium and magnesium.

Alkali symptoms may be deceptively mild compared with the mucosal damage and long-term sequelae following alkaline burns. For example, within minutes alkali can begin to penetrate the corneal stroma, interfering with sensory nerves and producing anesthesia. Penetration then continues, sometimes without pain, to involve the structures of the anterior chamber and retina, causing total blindness. In contrast, acid injuries are usually painful, are limited to the cornea, and only rarely cause blindness. Inhalation of either acids or alkali can produce coughing, stridor, and severe damage to the respiratory mucosa, leading to pulmonary edema and respiratory failure. Dermal exposure can produce first- to third-degree burns.

The treatment of all dermal and ocular exposures begins with copious irrigation and removal of contaminated clothing. Neutralization is not recommended. Ocular irrigation should continue until the ocular pH has returned to neutral range and all particulate material has been removed. Alkaline burns require irrigation for at least 1 hour and sometimes for up to 12 hours. Lid retractors and topical anesthetics are important adjuncts. The skin exposed to alkali should be washed until the soapy feeling has been removed. Ophthalmologic consultation is merited for all severe alkaline eye burns, and prolonged irrigation as well as use of topical mydriatrics, cycloplegics, antibiotics, steroids, and collagenase inhibitors may be required.

The airway and ventilatory status of patients with pulmonary inhalation is of the utmost importance. Rapid progression of pharyngeal and laryngeal edema may necessitate early intubation or cricothyroidotomy with subsequent tracheostomy.

Emesis and lavage are usually contraindicated for acid and alkali ingestions, and use of activated charcoal is ineffective. Hydrofluoric acid burns are treated with similar attention to decontamination and respiratory status, but calcium is used as an adjunct. Superficial skin burns can be treated with a topical gel of 2.5% calcium gluconate mixed as 3.5 g of USP calcium gluconate powder in 5 oz of surgical lubricant. This can be repeated as often as necessary to relieve pain. If pain is not relieved or if the burns are deep, subcutaneous calcium gluconate infiltration may be required. A 5% to 10% calcium gluconate solution is injected with a 30-gauge needle in a dose of 0.5 mL/cm^2 of affected tissue. Calcium chloride should never be infiltrated in place of calcium gluconate because it is very irritating. Intra-arterial infusions of calcium gluconate are less painful and may be more effective than subcutaneous injections for digital burns. Administration of large amounts of intravenous calcium chloride or gluconate may be required to prevent hypocalcemia in patients with systemic fluoride toxicity.

Beta-Blockers

The clinical manifestations following a β-blocker overdose vary in severity with the type and the amount of drug ingested. Some patients become symptomatic following ocular exposure to β-blocker–containing ophthalmic products. The cardiovascular manifestations are the major cause of morbidity and mortality. They include bradycardia, atrioventricular blocks, arrhythmias, and hypotension; with the partial agonists, especially pindolol, tachycardia and hypertension can occur. Other effects include bronchospasm, wheezing, dyspnea, delirium, lethargy, decreased level of consciousness, and seizures. Hypoglycemia may occur, especially in children, due to inadequate glycogen mobilization in response to epinephrine. Hyperglycemia has also been reported in chronic poisoning.

The treatment of β-blocker overdoses begins with immediate decontamination. Administration of activated charcoal and gastric lavage are the methods of choice for substantial ingestions, because the possibility for rapid cardiovascular collapse renders emesis unsafe. Multidose activated charcoal has been shown to enhance the elimination of several β-blockers. With sustained-release preparations, whole-bowel irrigation may be indicated. Cardiovascular effects predominate and should be treated aggressively with intravenous glucagon administration and a combination of fluid resuscitation, vasopressor agents, atropine therapy, and transvenous pacing. A Swan-Ganz catheter, transvenous pacer, intra-aortic balloon pump, and cardiopulmonary bypass are sometimes required to maintain adequate perfusion during an acute overdose. Bronchospasm can be treated with aminophylline and nebulized beta-agonists. When pharmacotherapy fails, hemodialysis or hemoperfusion may be considered for the more water-soluble agents with low volumes of distribution (specifically, atenolol and acebutolol); however, glucagon and other drug therapy should be used preferentially.

Calcium Channel Blockers

Death from overdose of calcium channel blockers has increased dramatically in frequency over the past decade. Cardiac toxicity usually predominates as the major cause of morbidity and mortality. Hypotension and cardiac arrhythmias, including sinus bradycardia, junctional rhythms, second- and third-degree heart block, and asystole, are commonly reported. Nifedipine acts primarily on the peripheral vasculature as a vasodilator and thus manifests fewer conduction delays and less myocardial depression when taken in overdose. Verapamil overdose more commonly causes arrhythmias, conduction blockade, and decreased myocardial contractility. Diltiazem overdose results in impairment of conduction and contractility to a greater extent than does nifedipine but to a lesser extent than does verapamil. Central nervous system effects include dizziness, lethargy, confusion, slurred speech, and rarely seizures. Hyperglycemia and lactic acidosis are not infrequent.

The treatment of calcium antagonist overdose patients involves decontamination, calcium and glucagon administration, and specific management of arrhythmias and hypotension that may involve multiple invasive techniques (e.g., Swan-Ganz catheterization, external or internal pacemaker placement, intra-aortic balloon pump, or cardiopulmonary bypass). Decontamination is primary and should begin with gastric emptying and administration of activated charcoal and a cathartic. Ipecac is contraindicated in patients who have ingested substantial quantities because rapid deterioration of mental and cardiovascular status can occur. In patients with large ingested amounts or who have taken sustained-release products, multidose activated charcoal and whole-bowel irrigation may be indicated.

Carbon Monoxide

Carbon monoxide is ubiquitous. It is the leading single agent implicated in suicide-related deaths. Firefighters and smokers are at increased risk for carbon monoxide poisoning. Methylene chloride (a paint stripper) and methylene iodide (used to analyze gem quality) are metabolized within hours to clinically significant amounts of carbon monoxide. Inhaled carbon monoxide rapidly diffuses across the alveolocapillary membrane and becomes bound to the four binding sites of hemoglobin. Those at high risk for carbon monoxide poisoning include fetuses, pregnant women, children younger than 15 to 16 years of age, and elderly people. Often, infants, children, and pets are the first to manifest symptoms of increased ambient carbon monoxide because they have increased metabolic demands. The symptoms of mild-to-moderate carbon monoxide poisoning are usually seen at carboxyhemoglobin levels of 10% to 30% and may include headache, dizziness, weakness, nausea, dyspnea, visual disturbances, irritability, and decreased concentration. The signs are mild tachycardia, tachypnea, mild systolic hypotension, vomiting, and confusion. In severe carbon monoxide poisoning, the carboxyhemoglobin level is usually over 30% to 50%, and findings include visual field defects, blindness, papilledema, retinal hemorrhages, adult respiratory distress syndrome, arrhythmias, hypotension, syncope, and angina. Neurologic features include intense headaches, subtle confusion that progresses to coma, seizures, agitation, cranial nerve deficits, increased deep tendon reflexes, hyperventilation, muscular rigidity, and ataxia.

The subacute and chronic manifestations can resolve over years or be permanent. The clinical findings in the delayed neurologic syndrome are widespread and include cortical blindness, psychosis, extrapyramidal rigidity, akinesia, aphasia, dementia, and choreoathetosis. More subtle findings include memory impairment, personality alterations, and parietal lobe dysfunction with visual agnosia, dyspraxia, dysnomia, and dysgraphia.

Common laboratory tests, including complete blood count, and chemistry determinations are not of value in the diagnosis of carbon monoxide poisoning. Arterial blood gas determinations are notoriously unreliable for assessing oxyhemoglobin level. Oxygen saturation determined by pulse oximetry is unreliable. Carboxyhemoglobin spectrophotometry has been the standard and is accurate for assessing current carboxyhemoglobin content; however, extrapolation back to the initial carboxyhemoglobin level (using the half-life) may be important in determining the need for hyperbaric oxygen therapy.

The therapy of mild-to-moderate carbon monoxide poisoning is controversial. Mild-to-moderate acidosis should not be aggressively treated, because hydrogen ions shift the hemoglobin dissociation curve to the right, thus enhancing oxygen delivery to tissues. The only currently accepted treatment of carbon monoxide poisoning is administration of oxygen. The indications for hyperbaric oxygen therapy are unknown, but guidelines have been proposed by various centers that offer hyperbaric oxygen therapy.

Cyanide

Cyanide can be inhaled as cyanide gas, injected, ingested, or absorbed through mucosal membranes and intact skin. Absorption is rapid (within seconds to minutes) by almost any route. Some compounds appear to have delayed absorption (30 minutes to 2 hours or longer) because cyanide is released as a product of metabolism.

Clinically, patients with cyanide poisoning present in extremis without signs that are specific for cyanide intoxication. The odor of bitter almonds is detectable for a genetically predetermined 65% of the population. Early symptoms include anxiety, agitation, flushing, tachycardia, tachypnea, and dizziness. These early symptoms are followed rapidly by the progressive onset of metabolic acidosis, seizures, coma, and cardiovascular collapse. The cellular extraction of oxygen from the blood decreases so profoundly that arterial and venous PO_2 and retinal artery and vein color are similar. Individual organ systems manifest the symptoms of hypoxemia.

Therapy is effective if instituted early in the course. Oxygen, decontamination, nitrites, and sodium thiosulfate are the mainstays of therapy. Initially, oxygen given by facemask or endotracheal tube should be employed to deliver as close to 100% inspired oxygen as possible. Administration of nitrites should not be delayed by decontamination procedures or by prolonged resuscitation in the field. Lavage is only helpful in patients with recent ingestions, and cyanide binds poorly to activated charcoal. Inhalation of amyl nitrite pearls produces a 5% methemoglobinemia, and one "ampule" of sodium nitrite (300 mg in 10 mL of a 3% solution) in an adult produces a methemoglobin level of approximately 20. As cyanide is slowly released from the cyanmethemoglobin compound, thiocyanate is formed and excreted in the urine. Intravenous administration of sodium nitrite should follow amyl nitrite therapy as soon as possible. Amyl nitrite therapy may be omitted if an intravenous route is already established. Following nitrite therapy, sodium thiosulfate should be given intravenously to provide additional substrate to allow formation of thiocyanate.

Cyclic Antidepressants

Antidepressant exposures were responsible for the largest absolute number of fatalities and largest fatality/exposure rate (0.66%) of all exposure categories in one study. Approximately 70% of individuals who have taken fatal overdoses of cyclic antidepressants are pronounced dead before medical assistance can be provided. The cyclic antidepressants include the tertiary amines (amitriptyline, imipramine, doxepin, trimipramine) and the secondary amines (nortriptyline, protriptyline, desipramine). Other cyclic antidepressants with significant toxicity include amoxapine, bupropion, and maprotiline. The oral absorption of the cyclic antidepressants is delayed in patients with overdose because of the delayed gastric emptying and ileus caused by these drugs' anticholinergic effects. These drugs are extensively protein bound ($> 90\%$) and highly lipophilic. The half-lives of the parent compounds and their active metabolites are very long (8 to 52 hours). Toxicity is likely if more than 20 mg/kg is ingested.

The clinical manifestations of cyclic antidepressant overdose are based on the four toxic mechanisms: direct muscarinic receptor blockade (anticholinergic), neurotransmitter reuptake blockade (adrenergic excess), α-adrenergic receptor blockade, and type I antiarrhythmic action. The direct anticholinergic effects include sinus tachycardia, ileus, urinary retention, pupillary dilation, mental status changes, coma, impaired sweating with hyperthermia, and possible seizures. Alpha-adrenergic receptor blockade contributes to hypotension by causing vasodilation and arteriolar dilation, and it can cause pupillary constriction. The type I antiarrhythmic action seen with cyclic antidepressants stems from sodium channel blockade. These agents cause direct myocardial depression, QRS prolongation, and ventricular arrhythmias.

Clinical manifestations stem directly from the drugs' mechanisms. The pupillary size is unreliable, but dry skin, ileus, urinary retention, and hyperthermia are common. The cardiovascular signs often include hypotension, which can be refractory, arrhythmias (sinus tachycardia, supraventricular tachycardia, ventricular tachycardia), and conduction disturbances. Neurologic findings commonly include central nervous system depression. Myoclonus, hallucinations, and choreoathetosis are less common. Seizures are especially frequent with amoxapine, bupropion, and maprotiline poisonings. The laboratory studies that may aid therapy and predict outcome include electrocardiography, serum drug level determinations, and arterial blood gas analysis. The treatment of cyclic antidepressant overdose patients can be very challenging. The mainstays of decontamination, multidose activated charcoal administration and lavage, are important in the early stages. The anticholinergic properties of cyclic antidepressants make lavage for up to 3 to 5 hours after ingestion worthwhile. Ipecac has no role in treatment of the cyclic antidepressant overdose. Repeated doses of activated charcoal over the first 24 hours shorten the elimination half-life of active metabolites.

Alkalinization of the serum is essential and can be accomplished by sodium bicarbonate infusion or bolus therapy, or by hyperventilation. Bicarbonate is effective in reversing QRS prolongation, ventricular arrhythmias, and hypotension but has no effect on cyclic antidepressant–induced seizures. However, the use of bicarbonate to correct any acidosis that develops with seizure activity is essential to prevent cardiotoxicity precipitated by acidosis. More clinical data support the use of sodium bicarbonate alkalinization than support hyperventilation therapy.

Multiple measures can be undertaken to control the variety of arrhythmias seen in these overdose patients, including serum alkalinization, antiarrhythmic therapy, administration of magnesium and rarely β-blockers, isoproterenol use, and overdrive pacing. Hypotension can be managed initially by fluid resuscitation; then α-adrenergic agonists such as norepinephrine should be used instead of dopamine. Although physostigmine is effective in reversing the anticholinergic effects in cyclic antidepressant overdose, it is not indicated because the cardiotoxic effects can worsen. Seizures should be treated sequentially with benzodiazepines (diazepam, lorazepam), phenytoin, and phenobarbital. If these modalities are ineffective, paralysis (vecuronium, pancuronium) and barbiturate coma should be considered early in the course.

Patients should be monitored for 24 hours after resolution of all signs and symptoms, assuming that they have been passing charcoal stools and have bowel sounds. Late complications usually are the result of aspiration, prolonged seizures, or anoxia during the acute illness. Delayed sudden death is rare, but cases of sudden death after apparent recovery from severe cyclic antidepressant overdose have been reported.

Hypoglycemic Agents

Oral hypoglycemic agents are more commonly implicated in poison exposures than in insulin use. The sulfonylureas are the only oral hypoglycemic agents available in the United States today. They can be divided into the first-generation compounds acetohexamide, chlorpropamide, tolazamide, and tolbutamide and into the more potent second-generation compounds flyburide and glipizide.

Prolonged absorption from massive subcutaneous administration of insulin is common in intentional overdose patients. The absorption of the oral agents varies tremendously, with peak levels ranging from 1 to 2 hours for glipizide to 6 hours for glyburide and tolbutamide. They are more than 90% protein bound and have low volumes of distribution. Chlorpropamide has the longest half-life, averaging 36 hours or even longer in the overdose state.

The clinical presentation can be delayed up to 24 hours (and possibly even 48 hours) after ingestion. Symptoms are the same as those seen in hypoglycemia, including diaphoresis, confusion, agitation, nausea, and tachycardia, which can progress to seizures, coma, bradycardia, and asystole if treatment is not instituted in a timely manner. Cutaneous examination of patients with large parenteral insulin exposures can reveal an erythematous, boggy injection site. Patients concurrently taking β-blockers may be at increased risk for accidental overdose and delayed diagnosis because the early signs of hypoglycemia in the presence of such therapy are masked. A disulfiram-like reaction has occurred in patients maintained on chlorpropamide following ingestion of ethanol. Sulfonylurea abuse can mimic an insulinoma.

Treatment is primarily supportive. Decontamination with emesis or lavage can be helpful when an acute ingestion of an oral agent is involved. Some workers advocate surgical debulking at the site of a massive insulin overdose. Activated charcoal has been shown to reduce absorption of chlorpropamide by 90%, although multidose activated charcoal was ineffective in reducing the plasma half-life. Urinary alkalinization to a pH of 8 can increase the urinary clearance of chlorpropamide fourfold. Intravenous glucose administration is the mainstay of therapy. Administration of 25 g of dextrose solution is appropriate initial therapy, but an infusion of 5% to 10% dextrose must follow. Oral glucose administration alone is insufficient, and recurrent hypoglycemia is common with oral therapy. Glucagon also has been used in the prehospital setting and in refractory cases but not as a substitute for glucose.

Iron

Iron poisoning is the leading cause of pediatric accidental ingestion fatalities in the United States. Iron has a direct irritant effect on the gastrointestinal mucosa. Additionally, when the iron-binding sites on the transferring, hemosiderin, and ferritin molecules become saturated, the serum free iron levels rise and systemic toxicity develops. Clinical toxicity is likely following ingestion of 40 to 60 mg/kg of elemental iron, although serious complications usually require ingestion of greater than 100 mg/kg. To estimate the severity of an ingestion, the amount of elemental iron must be calculated. For example, the sulfate salt of iron (ferrous sulfate) is 20% elemental iron; the gluconate salt, 12%; and the fumarate salt, 33%. Four stages of clinical toxicity occur:

- *Stage I* occurs within 30 minutes to 2 hours after ingestion. The findings include nausea, vomiting with hematemesis (and hypotension in massive overdoses), abdominal pain, and lethargy.
- *Stage II,* occurring 6 to 12 hours after ingestion, is also called the quiescent period because the patient may become asymptomatic.
- In *Stage III,* which takes place between 12 and 48 hours after ingestion, life-threatening complications occur, including metabolic acidosis, increased lethargy, coma, vasomotor collapse, gastrointestinal bleeding, and perforation.
- In *Stage IV,* which occurs 2 to 4 days after the ingestion, liver failure develops as a direct effect of iron on mitochondria in the liver.

Treatment for iron intoxication relies heavily on gastrointestinal decontamination and emptying. Activated charcoal is ineffective. Emesis may be induced when the estimated ingestion is 20 to 60 mg/kg and the patient is asymptomatic; however, following massive ingestion or in the symptomatic patient, lethargy may complicate emetic therapy. The safety and efficacy of oral lavage solutions (sodium bicarbonate, phosphate solutions) are questionable. Whole-bowel irrigation with polyethylene glycol electrolyte solutions has been used effectively in both adult and pediatric patients, with evidence of large amounts of undissolved iron remaining in the gastrointestinal tract.

The indications for deferoxamine chelation are not well defined. Intravenous or intramuscular therapy is generally recommended when the serum iron concentration exceeds 350 μg/dL or if a serum iron concentration cannot be obtained in a timely manner and the patient is symptomatic. In patients who present with hypotension or severe poisoning, the intravenous form of deferoxamine should be used. As chelated iron is excreted, the urine turns a pink to orange color. The resolution of this "vin rose" urine in patients has been used as a clinical endpoint for deferoxamine therapy. Not all patients exhibit a visible urinary color change; thus, this finding cannot be used as a reliable confirmation of suspected toxicity.

Isoniazid

Clinical intoxication can occur with INH overdoses of 10 to 30 mg/kg and death with doses greater than 50 mg/kg. Early signs and symptoms may include nausea, vomiting, abdominal pain, slurred speech, dizziness, and visual changes (mydriasis, blurring, nystagmus), although seizures may be the presenting symptom. Characteristically, severe intoxication produces seizures that may progress to status epilepticus, coma, and a refractory anion gap metabolic acidosis.

Treatment involves early gastric decontamination, activated charcoal administration, and aggressive management of the seizures and acidosis. Seizure activity, acidosis, and coma should be treated with pyridoxine. One gram of pyridoxine is administered for every gram of INH ingested, or 5 g are given initially if the amount of INH is unknown. Benzodiazepines, paralysis, and barbiturate coma may also be required to control refractory seizures. Peripheral neuropathy from pyridoxine is seen only with chronic administration of large doses. Acidosis results primarily from production of lactic acid during seizures. Hemodialysis, peritoneal dialysis, and exchange transfusion effectively clear INH but are not indicated in view of the efficacy of pyridoxine.

Lithium

Lithium has a very narrow therapeutic index, and serum levels above the therapeutic index range (0.8 to 1.2 mEq/L) result in toxicity. The main clinical effects are on the central nervous system, the kidneys, and the heart. Early nervous system findings are confusion, tremor, and hyperreflexia. Symptoms may progress to delirium, choreiform movements, spasticity, hallucinations, coma, and seizures. Long-term memory impairment and neurologic deficits have been documented following lithium toxicity. Renal damage with a gradual decline in glomerular filtration rate and a reversible vasopressin-resistant renal concentrating defect are seen in patients receiving chronic therapy. These changes result in dehydration and in the worsening of toxicity. Hypotension, arrhythmias, and electrocardiographic abnormalities that include diffuse T wave flattening, QT prolongation, and U waves are common. Symptoms of nausea, vomiting, and diarrhea may also be present. Other effects are blurred vision, nystagmus, dry mouth, hyperthermia or hypothermia, and profound weakness. Chronically, overmedicated patients have a greater risk of complications.

The treatment of the acute lithium overdose patient begins with gastric emptying. Activated charcoal does not absorb lithium well, and it is not indicated unless coingestants are present. Preliminary evidence does show that the exchange resin sodium polystyrene sulfonate binds lithium and prevents some absorption. The complications of sodium polystyrene sulfonate use include sodium overload, hypokalemia, hypocalcemia, nausea, vomiting, and constipation. Lithium carbonate is a poorly soluble lithium salt and can form bezoars. Whole-bowel irrigation with a polyethylene glycol electrolyte lavage solution has been shown to decrease the absorption of a sustained-release lithium preparation by 67% when compared with control therapy.

Once lithium has been absorbed, enhancing its elimination becomes important because the drug is not metabolized. In the past, treatment with saline diuresis and forced alkaline diuresis were used but have since been found to be dangerous and ineffective. Intravenous normal saline or 0.45% saline should be infused to maintain a normal urine output and to correct dehydration and sodium depletion. Hemodialysis is the treatment of choice, although the indications for its use are poorly defined. Peritoneal dialysis is less effective than hemodialysis. Serum lithium levels are an inaccurate reflection of tissue levels. Hemodialysis should be considered when the peak serum level (at least 6 hours after ingestion) is greater than 3.5 mEq/L, or when it is greater than 2.5 mEq/L with symptoms in a chronic overdose patient. However, patients often require dialysis at lower levels, especially symptomatic patients with chronic overmedication. Patients with renal insufficiency or renal failure cannot excrete lithium normally and should also undergo dialysis at lower serum levels. Following dialysis, a drug rebound occurs as the drug redistributes, and repeat hemodialysis may be required.

Monoamine Oxidase Inhibitors

Although the MAO inhibitors are rapidly absorbed from the gastrointestinal tract, reaching peak serum levels within 1 to 2 hours after an overdose, reaching the peak toxicity can take 6 to 24 hours. These compounds are highly protein bound and are rapidly metabolized by acetylation in the liver. The irreversible nature of MAO binding causes a delay in the resolution of clinical effects, pending the resynthesis of MAO. The clinical manifestations of overdose do not necessarily mimic the clinical effects of MAO inhibitor interactions. The onset of symptoms in overdose patients is often delayed for 6 to 24 hours. A wide range of symptoms has been described: excitement or agitation, sinus tachycardia, mydriasis, muscle rigidity, coma, or hyperthermia. Hypertension is present in only 17% of patients. Other symptoms include sweating, hyperreflexia, nystagmus, writhing or grimacing, tachypnea, seizures, hypotension, cardiac arrest, hallucinations, papilledema, and peaked T waves on electrocardiography. Recovery can be delayed for 3 to 7 days as MAO is synthesized.

Coingestants are of particular concern in patients taking MAO inhibitors. The food products known to cause toxicity (e.g., aged cheeses, wines (especially Chianti), fava beans, and pickled herring) often contain monoamines, such as tyramine, that are usually degraded in the gastrointestinal tract and liver by MAO. With MAO inhibition, undegraded monoamines enter the circulation and precipitate the release of large quantities of stored norepinephrine. This results in hypertension, tachycardia, headache, hyperthermia, and other hyperadrenergic symptoms. Similar symptoms occur with indirectly acting sympathomimetic amines (e.g., amphetamines, phenylpropanolamine, and pseudoephedrine), opioids (e.g., meperidine), and cocaine.

The treatment of MAO inhibitor overdose begins with aggressive decontamination. Use of activated charcoal with a cathartic is indicated, and gastric emptying may be valuable if the patient presents early. Urinary acidification is not recommended because excretion is only minimally enhanced and because the risk of renal failure secondary to rhabdomyolysis and myoglobinemia would increase. Supportive treatment is the mainstay of therapy. Hyperthermia must be treated immediately with external cooling and control of muscular activity. Administration of dantrolene sodium, a lipid-soluble hydantoin analog that directly relaxes skeletal muscle, has been shown to be effective. Seizures and agitation may be controlled with benzodiazepines or phenytoin. Potentiation of the sedative effects of barbiturates is possible; however, barbiturates may be used for the management of refractory seizures. Neuromuscular paralysis may be required if convulsions persist. Hypertension may be treated with nitroprusside or phentolamine. Beta-blocker use is contraindicated because the unopposed α-effects can lead to hypertension.

Salicylates

Clinical manifestations of acute salicylism may include mild confusion, tinnitus, and decreased auditory acuity. As the salicylate level in the serum and central nervous system increases, other symptoms begin to appear, including agitation or lethargy, vertigo, convulsion, hyperventilation, metabolic acidosis, coagulation abnormalities, nausea, and vomiting. Although fever is a hallmark of pediatric salicylism, its presence in adults is less frequent and a poor prognostic sign. If the serum salicylate levels increase, noncardiogenic pulmonary edema (rarely seen in pediatric salicylism), refractory seizures, and both are common. Chronic salicylism produces similar symptoms, although at much lower serum levels; however, chronic salicylism is often occult, and delays in diagnosis can result in increased mortality.

The combination of respiratory alkalosis and metabolic acidosis usually produces alkalemia in adults unless central nervous system depressants were also ingested or the overdose is severe. An overriding metabolic acidosis is more common in children. Fluid and electrolyte disorders are common and include dehydration, hypokalemia, hypocalcemia, and hyperglycemia or hypoglycemia. Therapy with intravenous bicarbonate can worsen hypokalemia. A paradoxical aciduria is also common. The central nervous system is the site of the lethal effects of salicylates.

Treatment of patients with suspected salicylate overdose includes recognition of the diagnosis, early gastric decontamination followed by multidose activated charcoal, urinary alkalinization, monitoring of serial serum salicylate levels (until a decline is confirmed), a close monitoring of fluid and electrolyte balance, and possibly hemodialysis. The effectiveness of urinary alkalinization without forced diuresis is based on the marked increase in urinary excretion of salicylate that occurs at a urinary pH of 7.5 to 8.0. Although rehydration is important, forced diuresis does not increase the efficacy of urinary alkalinization and is fraught with complications because salicylate-intoxicated patients are at risk for noncardiogenic pulmonary edema and cerebral edema. The indications for hemodialysis are primarily clinical. Dialysis should be considered and is often necessary in patients with a serum level of 100 to 120 mg/dL or with deteriorating clinical status (worsening acidosis, decline in mental status, seizures, noncardiogenic pulmonary edema). In chronic overdose, dialysis may be necessary for symptomatic patients with a salicylate level of greater than 60 mg/dL.

Strychnine

The clinical manifestations of strychnine poisoning occur rapidly. A prodromal phase of agitation, anxiety, and increased sensory awareness may precede the diffuse, painful muscle spasms that resemble seizures and characterize poisoning with this agent. These muscle spasms are tetanic and last 1 to 2 minutes; during this time, the patient often remains alert and without a postictal period, in contrast to that which occurs with true generalized seizures. All the muscles of the body are affected. Spasms of the strongest groups of muscles predominate and lead to opisthotonos, trismus, and the grin of risus sardonicus. The arms are flexed, the legs are in extension, and nystagmus can be seen. The increased sensory awareness continues, and loud noises, physical stimuli, or bright lights can precipitate diffuse spasms. The excessive muscular activity causes severe lactic acidosis, hyperthermia, rhabdomyolysis, and compartment syndromes. Diaphragmatic and chest wall spasms can lead to respiratory arrest. Long-term complications are usually a result of anoxia, hyperthermia, and renal failure, with resultant cerebral injury or multisystem organ failure. Primary renal, hepatic, pulmonary, or gastrointestinal effects do not seem to occur. The lethal dose of strychnine is estimated to be 1.5 to 2 mg/kg. Fatal serum levels range from 0.5 to 90 mg/L and do not accurately reflect toxicity.

The therapy starts with decontamination with administration of activated charcoal and gastric lavage. Emesis is contraindicated, and lavage should be limited to patients with recent ingestions because the stimulation may induce muscle spasms. Beyond the initial decontamination, care is largely supportive. The tetanic muscle spasms and convulsions can be treated initially with benzodiazepines, which may raise the threshold for convulsions and actually displace some of the strychnine bound to receptor sites. For refractory convulsions, intubation and neuromuscular blockade, general anesthesia, or barbiturate-induced coma are recommended. Phenobarbital has been recommended as the anticonvulsant of choice because of its longer duration of action and effect on the other inhibitory neurotransmitter, ψ-aminobutyric acid. Aggressive treatment of hyperthermia and rhabdomyolysis with cooling, hydration, urinary alkalinization, and neuromuscular blockade (to block persistent muscular hyperactivity) should be undertaken.

Superwarfarins

The superwarfarins are a number of agents within the two main groups of rodenticide anticoagulants. The hydroxycoumarin group, which contains warfarin, also contains the 4-hydroxycoumarins brodifacoum, defenacoum, bromadiolone, and coumatetralyl, which are considerably more potent and longer acting than warfarin. These products are often packaged as round, green-blue pellets, cakes, or powders and are sometimes left in areas accessible to toddlers. Hematologic effects in humans have been reported to last for 2 to 3 months and, in some cases, for 8 to 13 months.

The clinical effects of these rodenticides relate directly to their anticoagulant properties. Anticoagulation can present with epistaxis, cutaneous ecchymoses, bleeding gums, hemoptysis, melena, hematuria, or menorrhagia. Bleeding may begin within 24 to 48 hours of ingestion, and hematologic abnormalities can last for months or longer, especially in cases of chronic ingestion.

Laboratory evaluations can assist in uncovering the covert abuse of these substances. Elevations in prothrombin and partial thromboplastin times with normal mixing studies in the absence of malnutrition or liver disease should suggest the diagnosis. Therapy involves early decontamination with emesis or gastric lavage in addition to the administration of activated charcoal. If prolongation of the prothrombin time is already present, emesis and gastric lavage are contraindicated. The specific antidote for symptomatic patients is intravenous phytonadione (vitamin K_1). In adults, a minimum dose of 10 mg is given intravenously diluted in saline or in 5% dextrose in water and infused over 20 minutes. Initial doses of 25 to 400 mg have been required in patients with active bleeding. Neither vitamin K_4 (menadiol) nor vitamin K_3 (menadione) can reverse the effects of coumadin derivatives. The effects of intravenous vitamin K_1 may take 4 to 6 hours to manifest, so patients with hemodynamic compromise or active bleeding should receive fresh-frozen plasma.

SEDATIVES AND MUSCLE RELAXANTS IN THE INTENSIVE CARE UNIT

Clinically Useful Muscle Relaxants

Rocuronium Bromide

A new addition to the muscle relaxant armamentarium, rocuronium bromide (Zemuron), may prove useful in facilitating emergency ICU intubation. Rocuronium is a nondepolarizing neuromuscular blocking agent with a rapid-to-intermediate onset of action, dependent on the initial dose. The duration of action of rocuronium bromide, 0.6 mg/kg, is longer than that of succinylcholine and at this dose is approximately equivalent to the duration of other intermediate-acting neuromuscular blocking drugs. Clinical experience with this compound in the ICU is lacking, and usage patterns have yet to be determined.

Pancuronium Bromide

Pancuronium is a nondepolarizing muscle relaxant with a relatively long elimination half-life reported from 89 to 161 minutes, a volume of distribution of 241 to 280 mL/kg, and plasma clearance of 1.1 to 1.9 mL $\cdot$ kg^{-1} $\cdot$ min^{-1}. Pancuronium is excreted primarily by the kidneys, with 40% of the total dose administered recovered from the urine. In addition, 11% of the dose has been recovered from the bile. Dosage must be adjusted in patients with liver or renal disease. The major side effect of importance to the ICU clinician is tachycardia. Concomitantly, an expected increase in blood pressure and cardiac output has been noted. Because of its long half-life, pancuronium is usually administered in intermittent boluses, and dosage should be individualized with peripheral nerve stimulator titration. For endotracheal intubation, pancuronium should be administered in a bolus dose of 0.06 to 0.15 mg/kg.

After intravenous injection the patient will remain paralyzed for 45 to 90 minutes. Subsequent dosing of pancuronium should be from 0.01 to 0.05 mg/kg approximately each hour. If appropriate neuromuscular monitoring is used, the likelihood of inappropriate overdose will be minimized. The major disadvantages of overdose are prolongation of the neuromuscular block and prolonged ventilator dependence. Careful dosing is important in patients who have received or are receiving intravenously or intraperitoneally large doses of certain antibiotics that may themselves intensify an existing neuromuscular block or cause one independently. Antibiotics implicated are aminoglycosides (neomycin, streptomycin, kanamycin, gentamicin, and dihydrostreptomycin), tetracyclines, bacitracin, polymyxin B, colistin, and sodium colistimethate.

Atracurium Besylate

Atracurium is a nondepolarizing skeletal muscle relaxant with a duration of action of approximately one half to one third of that seen with pancuronium at initially equipotent doses. Time to onset decreases and duration increases with increasing doses. The dose required to produce 95% twitch height depression with a balanced anesthetic is 0.23 mg/kg, and initial doses of 0.4 to 0.5 mg/kg produce a maximum dose effect within 3 to 5 minutes of injection and good intubating conditions within 2 to 2.5 minutes in most patients. Under balanced anesthesia, recovery of twitch can be anticipated within 20 to 35 minutes after injection, and recovery to 25% of control is achieved at approximately 35 to 45 minutes after injection and is 95% complete at 60 to 70 minutes. Unlike with most other relaxants, repeat doses have no cumulative effect, and recovery from atracurium blockade is predictable in all clinical settings. Atracurium injection may cause histamine release, although in most instances reactions are mild and easily controlled. The possibility of a significant histamine reaction must be anticipated if an initial dose is 0.6 mg/kg or greater. Side effects may be minimized if the drug is given in divided doses over 1 to 2 minutes or if an infusion technique is used.

Appropriate dosing for intubation and initial muscle relaxation is 0.4 to 0.5 mg/kg. Dosage ranges of 0.005 to 0.01 $mg \cdot kg^{-1} \cdot min^{-1}$ have been successful in maintaining adequate operating conditions in most situations. The degradation characteristics of atracurium may make it most predictable in geriatric patients, who demonstrate variable organ perfusion and decreased capacity to metabolize compounds by conventional methods.

Vecuronium Bromide

Vecuronium is a nondepolarizing skeletal muscle relaxant of intermediate duration and is reportedly about one third more potent than pancuronium. The duration of effect is significantly less than that of pancuronium. When the drug is used in a continuous infusion for prolonged periods, the duration of effect is seldom increased beyond that expected from a single dose after cessation of the infusion. A dose of 0.08 to 0.15 mg/kg produces first depression of twitch within 1 minute and appropriate intubating conditions within 2.5 to 3 minutes. Subsequently, maintenance doses of 0.01 to 0.04 mg/kg may be administered every 20 to 30 minutes with minimal cumulative effect. Because of its elimination characteristics and lack of cumulative drug effects, vecuronium may be used successfully as a continuous infusion in the operating room and ICU. After an initial loading dose, an infusion of 0.075 to 0.10 $mg \cdot kg^{-1} \cdot h^{-1}$ has been used successfully for prolonged periods. In some series, recovery to 10% to 25% of control has occurred within 7 minutes of stopping the infusion, although longer times to recovery have been noted.

Doxacurium Chloride

Doxacurium is a recently released, long-acting, nondepolarizing muscle relaxant. Like all agents of this class, it binds competitively and reversibly to cholinergic receptors on the motor end-plate to antagonize the action of acetylcholine. Pharmacodynamically, it is two and one half to three times more potent than pancuronium and has a duration of action that is similar when administered in equipotent doses. The average effective dose (ED_{95}) is 0.025 mg/kg in adults receiving balanced anesthesia. When the drug is administered at this dose, the time to maximum block is approximately 9.3 minutes, with an average duration to 25% recovery of 55 minutes. At a dose three times ED_{95}, the time to onset of maximum block is reduced to 3.5 minutes, with a duration of 160 minutes. As with other agents of this class, the clinical response to the recommended dose exhibits considerable interpatient variability, and it is important to individualize doses carefully and follow recommendations for monitoring the depth of neuromuscular blockade.

The pharmacokinetics of doxacurium are similar in both young and elderly patients. Although there appears to be little or no accumulation with repeat administration, to avoid prolonged action careful determination of appropriate patient-specific dosing intervals must be performed. An anesthetic relaxant dose associated with appropriate intubating conditions in approximately 5 minutes is 0.05 mg/kg, with a duration of approximately 100 minutes. More rapid onset and longer duration are anticipated with 0.08 mg/kg doses. Maintenance doses of 0.005 mg/kg are advised.

Clinical Implications of Muscle Relaxant Use in the Intensive Care Unit

Central Nervous System Effects

Muscle relaxants have no known sedative or analgesic properties. They do not alter the perception of pain, and they act only at the neuromuscular junction of skeletal muscles. Normal pupil reactivity is preserved in patients receiving nondepolarizing muscle relaxants. Severe agitation is masked by these agents, and dosing of routinely prescribed sedatives and analgesics is difficult. Careful titration of muscle relaxant dose is important so that the patient will be able to respond visibly to noxious stimuli. Variations in pulse rate and blood pressure may be related to inadequate pharmacologic blunting of affect as much as to an acute hemodynamic insult.

Respiratory Effects

One of the most common uses of muscle relaxants in the ICU is to ensure adequate ventilation in the face of decreased pulmonary performance. A common use is to control the patient who is "fighting" the ventilator. Early patient assessment should recognize that, in many instances, the patient is reacting to inadequate ventilatory support to meet physiologic demands. Often, adjustment of PEEP, tidal volume, pressure support level, or ventilator rate will cause a dramatic improvement in the patient's sense of well-being, and agitation will decrease markedly. Dyspnea may have a physiologic basis because of inappropriate lung expansion secondary to the erosion of functional residual capacity common to the postoperative period and associated particularly with thoracic, upper abdominal, and some retroperitoneal procedures. In a number of patients, even the most careful adjustments have a minimal effect in controlling ventilator disharmony, which leads to an increased work of breathing, ventilation-perfusion mismatch, and possibly increases the risks of pulmonary baratrauma secondary to increased ventilator pressures. In these situations, muscle relaxants may be beneficial and increase the efficiency of ventilator support to the patient's benefit.

Sedation and the Use of Muscle Relaxants

Sedative-Hypnotic Drugs

Benzodiazepines are used frequently in the ICU, and midazolam has become the sedative of choice in some units because of its short elimination half-life, water solubility, and lack of adverse hemodynamic side effect. However, more recent reports indicate that dosage variability among patients may be high, and prolonged effects after continuous infusion have been noted. Patients acquire acute tolerance early during infusion, and if abrupt weaning is attempted, withdrawal is noted. This includes acute restlessness, tachycardia, marked blood pressure lability, hypermetabolism, and other symptoms that usually require reinstitution of the infusion. Midazolam remains a useful drug in ICU practice. Continuous infusion has become an increasingly accepted method of administration, and most patients tolerate the drug well.

Two other benzodiazepines, diazepam (Valium) and lorazepam (Ativan), are also popular. In contrast to diazepam, lorazepam and midazolam lack active metabolites and have more predictable elimination half-lives. This may be a disadvantage in situations in which weaning from a continuous infusion of any of the drugs is accompanied by agitation. Administration of a hypnotic with a longer duration of action may provide an opportunity to discontinue the short-acting agent without complications. It is important to provide adequate sedation in all situations in which a patient requires mechanical ventilation and associated administration of muscle relaxants. Monitoring adequacy of sedation in this patient population is extremely difficult because of vast changes in volumes of drug distribution, hemodynamic parameters, nutritional and protein concentration imbalances, and altered drug metabolic processes.

Narcotic Analgesics

The availability of new delivery systems and specific, short-acting narcotics such as fentanyl (Sublimaze), sufentanil (Sufenta), and alfentanil (Alfenta) may alter the more routine prescriptions for morphine sulfate and meperidine hydrochloride (Demerol). Indeed, complicated surgical dressing changes may be facilitated by appropriate use of these agents in combination with short-acting hypnotic agents.

Reversal Agents

Common practice dictates the use of either atropine or glycopyrrolate (Robinul) whenever acetylcholinesterase inhibitors are used. The three drugs in common use, and recommended dosing ranges, are as follows: (1) neostigmine bromide (Prostigmin), 2.5 to 5.0 mg/70 kg; (2) pyridostigmine bromide (Regonol), 0.1 to 0.20 mg/kg with a 25-mg maximum in a 70-kg patient; and (3) edrophonium chloride (Tensilon, Enlon, Reversol), 10 to 40 mg/70 kg. Use of atropine, 0.6 to 1.5 mg/70 kg, or glycopyrrolate, 0.5 to 1.0 mg/70 kg, provides an appropriate antimuscarinic dose and will promote the desired nicotinic effects. Of major importance in the ICU is that the effectiveness of these agents be documented before extubation, and restoration of neuromuscular transmission must be demonstrated with a peripheral nerve stimulator.

Analgesia

Perhaps for non-narcotic analgesics such as ketorolac, intermittent intravenous or intramuscular administration may be justified. Ketorolac can ordinarily be given in 30- to 60-mg doses either intravenously or intramuscularly. The agent can interfere with platelet aggregation. Therefore, the dosages may need to be adjusted or the drug entirely eliminated when thrombocytopenia develops or when an increased risk of bleeding exists.

The two different agents more commonly used for continuous infusion are morphine and fentanyl or derivatives such as alfentanil or sufentanil. Morphine remains a mainstay of intravenous therapy because of its reliable analgesic properties. In the average-size individual, dosages may range from 0.5 mg/hour to as high as 4 to 6 mg/hour, usually between 2 and 4 mg/hour. Because of its reliable respiratory depressant effects, mainly centering on reduction of rate, morphine can be used to aid in the mechanical ventilatory support of the patient in respiratory failure. The reduction in spontaneous rate during mechanical ventilation may promote better distribution of gases and overall enhancement of gas exchange. The fat solubility of fentanyl implies its rapid uptake and usage. Therefore, as opposed to the water-soluble morphine, it is less likely to accumulate, and fewer problems will potentially develop. In general, during continuous infusion, rates of up to 125 μg per hour of fentanyl can provide good-to-excellent analgesia and not result in any significant respiratory depression.

The narcotics used for epidural analgesia include morphine, fentanyl, and derivatives such as alfentanil and sufentanil. The fat solubility of fentanyl favors continuous infusion. The water solubility of morphine better lends itself to intermittent administration. However, in small dosages, the drug can be administered by continuous infusion. Ordinarily, fentanyl dosages of up to 1 μ/kg/hour will provide adequate analgesia without significant respiratory depression. When morphine is chosen, bolus administration of preservative-free drug of 4 to 6 mg every 8 to 24 hours usually proves to be adequate. For continuous infusion, most adults of average size will tolerate dosages of 0.1 to 0.5 mg/hour. Because of the large potential volume of the epidural space, the drugs must be mixed in sufficient volume to have effective action. Ordinarily, morphine is in 1 mg/mL and fentanyl in 5.0 μ/mL concentrations.

Supplements such as local anesthetics are often added to the epidural infusion, particularly with fentanyl. Such additives reduce the overall drug requirements while still providing excellent analgesia. The most often used local anesthetic is bupivacaine. It is usually delivered in concentrations of 1/8% to 1/16%. At such dosages, the local anesthetics are able to block the smaller sensory pain fibers and yet have little effect on the much larger motor fibers. Patients are still able to maintain ambulation and not experience the paralysis common when local anesthetics are used to provide operative analgesia.

Common complications of epidural analgesia include nausea, vomiting, pruritus, and urinary retention. The incidence varies between 20% and 50% in most series and relates to the actual drug dosage. Although most concerns are related to respiratory depression, the overall incidence is extremely low (approximately 1%). Other concerns include inadvertent penetration of the dura at the time of catheter placement. Drugs introduced into the epidural space at the same level can migrate through the hole and into the CSF. When inserted via the needle, the epidural catheter can penetrate the dura, resulting in drug administration into the subarachnoid space. Catheters can also be inadvertently placed in a vessel in the epidural space; consequently, unwanted intravenous infusion may occur. Both problems can be best detected by intermittent aspiration of the catheter to ensure that neither the clear CSF nor blood is present in the catheter. If so, usage of the catheter should be immediately discontinued.

Recently, interest has developed in non-narcotic agents for pain relief via epidural administration. Clonidine has been advocated most often. This α_2-adrenergic agonist can provide pain relief and can probably reduce overall narcotic requirements. Intrathecal drug administration has had limited use as a means of providing pain relief in the critically ill. The majority of experience has been obtained with the use of morphine in dosages of 0.25 to 1.25 mg in single-dose administration.

Patient-controlled analgesia (PCA) is another major mainstay of analgesic administration in critically ill patients. The technique appeals to most patients. It is obviously less invasive than epidural or intrathecal administration of agents. However, it does require that the patient be able at least to grasp the concept. Perhaps one of the greatest problems involves patients not attempting to push the button at the first sign of discomfort but rather waiting too long. This waiting results in uneven drug levels and can contribute to some of the problems such as hypertension and tachycardia that the analgesia is intended to prevent. In general, for most adults, morphine can be administered in 1.0- to 1.5-mg doses, with a 6-minute lockout time. This would result in a dosage schedule of 10 to 15 mg per hour.

Sedation

Today, benzodiazepines remain a mainstay of sedation therapy for critically ill patients. The most commonly used drugs are lorazepam and midazolam. These drugs can be administered by either continuous or intermittent infusion. Dosages range from 0.01 to 1.0 mg/kg/hour for midazolam to 0.1 to 2.0 mg/kg/hour for lorazepam. Most data suggest minimal impact on cardiovascular function with both lorazepam and midazolam. In higher concentrations, both drugs can suppress respiration, blood pressure, and cardiac output. Discontinuation of continuous infusions of midazolam generally allows return to baseline states within 30 to 40 minutes. Lorazepam has a half-life of 4 to 8 hours, and discontinuation may not result in rapid recovery.

Recently, a benzodiazepine-competitive antagonist (flumazenil) has become available. The agent may be administered as a single dose or by continuous infusion. Major benefits appear to be reversal of benzodiazepine overdose and a return to baseline state for other clinical reasons. Compared with the agents it is intended to reverse, flumazenil has a relatively short duration of action. Therefore, it may require either continuous infusion or frequent readministration of a single-bolus dose. It is recommended that flumazenil not be administered to patients on long-term benzodiazepine therapy for fear of untoward reactions.

Propofol is a nonbenzodiazepine sedative. The drug is also used in the operating room for induction technique as part of the administration of anesthesia. Because of its water insolubility, the drug is prepared in a lipid emulsion. Propofol elimination relies on liver blood flow and the ability to be rapidly conjugated by the liver. Only in severe liver disease would any accumulation be expected. The drug can have significant vasodilating properties of which the clinician should be aware. However, once a steady state is reached, this is no longer a problem. The usual dosage is between 0.2 and 0.4 mg/kg/hour.

Haloperidol decanoate (Haldol), a butyrophenone, has been used for sedation in elderly patients. After several days in the ICU, elderly patients may experience a disorientation syndrome, particularly in the evening. This effect often results in severe agitation. Intermittent dosages of haloperidol decanoate, 1 to 2 mg every 4 to 6 hours, seem to work quite well in this group to relieve the agitation.

CHAPTER 8

Infectious Diseases

Peter Linden, MD, DMD

INFECTIONS IN CRITICALLY ILL TRAUMA VICTIMS AND PATIENTS WITH HEMATOLOGIC MALIGNANCIES

The critically ill patient is at increased risk for nosocomial infection in comparison with other hospitalized patients, due to a diverse number of factors both extrinsic and intrinsic to the patient. Major extrinsic factors include increased exposure to antibiotic-resistant flora or to broad-spectrum antibiotic(s) that induce antibiotic resistance or select for resistant organisms, and the general "busy" ICU work environment, which may interfere with appropriate handwashing, glove wearing, and other cross-infection control policies. Intrinsic factors include local or systemic defects in the host defense that may predispose to a specific or broad category of infectious pathogens.

Common *local* breaches in the host defenses are intravascular access sites, bladder catheterization, the obstructed viscus, and tissue derangements from either a surgical wound or trauma. *Systemic* host defects are increasingly a major determinant of infection due to both opportunistic and nonopportunistic organisms. Such defects may be secondary either to the native disease or to therapeutic interventions such as chemotherapy, radiotherapy, or immunosuppression to suppress allograft rejection or graft-versus-host disease. The major categories of defective systemic host defenses are (1) granulocytopenia (absolute neutrophil count less than 1000/mm^3), usually due to myelosuppressive therapy or aplastic conditions; (2) cell-mediated (antigen recognition by the lymphocyte/macrophage cell lines, proliferation, and killing) immunodeficiency due to corticosteroids, antilymphocyte globulin or antibody, cytotoxic agents, and the acquired immunodeficiency syndrome (AIDS); and (3) humoral immunodeficiency (antigen-specific antibody production) due to immunosuppressive therapy, lymphoproliferative disease, bone marrow transplant, or prior splenectomy. Combinations of multiple local and systemic host defects are the rule rather than the exception when such patients require intensive care therapy.

In addition to these formal categories, a high prevalence of preexisting diseases (e.g., diabetes) or concomitant organ failure (e.g., renal or hepatic failure) may further predispose the host to infection.

Preventing Iatrogenic Infections

Infections arising in the ICU population may be secondary to either endogenous or exogenous pathogens. The majority of bacterial infections originate from endogenous flora that colonize a mucosal surface of the skin. This flora is often "modified" by the acquisition of bacteria or fungi indigenous to both the ICU patient reservoir and the inanimate environment. Such organisms are invariably more antibiotic-resistant and to a variable degree more virulent than the patient's own colonizing flora. The principal vectors of transmission are healthcare personnel with direct patient contact responsibilities. Frequent handwashing employed between contact with the inanimate environment and the patient and between different patient contacts is considered by many to be the single most efficacious procedure to interrupt the cycle of patient-to-patient cross-infection. Two per cent chlorhexidine is the optimal agent for handwashing; it is usually nonirritating at this concentration yet retains prolonged antimicrobial activity against most bacteria and yeasts and many viruses.

The Body Substance Isolation (BSI) policy was formulated on the assumption that all body substances are potentially infectious (Table 8–1). If properly employed, the measures of this policy should prevent both the transmission of infection to healthcare providers and cross-infection of nosocomial pathogens among patients. However, prospective evidence that nosocomial cross-infection rates are diminished by the existence and undertaking of BSI policy is lacking.

Preventing Bacterial Colonization of Infusion and Drainage Devices

Urinary Catheters

Approximately 40% of nosocomial infections originate from the urinary tract, and urinary catheters account for 80% of

Table 8–1. BODY SUBSTANCE ISOLATION

1. Gloves are worn for anticipated contact with blood, secretions, mucous membranes, nonintact skin, and moist body substances of all patients. (Handwashing is not necessary when gloves are worn unless the hands become visibly soiled.) Gloves are changed before another patient is treated.
2. After other types of patient contact, hands are washed.
3. Gowns, plastic aprons, masks, or goggles are worn when secretions, blood, or body fluids are likely to soil or splash on clothing, skin, or the face.
4. Soiled, reusable items, linen, and trash are contained to prevent leaking. Double-bagging is not necessary unless the outside of the bag is visibly soiled.
5. Needles (without recapping them) and sharp items are placed in puncture-resistant, rigid containers.
6. Private rooms are indicated for patients with some diseases transmitted exclusively or in part by the airborne route, such as pulmonary tuberculosis and other diseases listed in the Strict Isolation category of the CDC Guidelines for Isolation Precautions in Hospitals. Private rooms are also indicated for patients who soil articles in the environment with body substances.

(Data from Lynch P, Jackson MM, Cummings J, et al: Rethinking the role of isolation precautions in the prevention of nosocomial infections. Ann Intern Med 1987; 107:243.)

these. Bacteriuria occurs in 10% to 20% of patients catheterized for only one day, with a subsequent 5% to 10% risk of bacteriuria per day. Bacteriuria is a precursor to urinary tract infection (UTI); however, only 20% to 30% of bacteriuric patients will develop a UTI. The urinary catheter promotes bacteriuria by disturbing the protective mucopolysaccharide coating of the bladder thereby providing a direct conduit to the bladder, and it serves as a nidus for bacterial attachment and growth. The Centers for Disease Control and Prevention (CDCP) guidelines for urinary catheters recommend that catheters be reserved only for essential indications, be inserted under aseptic technique, and employ only a closed drainage system. Multiple investigative techniques, such as selective bowel decontamination, antibiotic or disinfectant bladder irrigation, urethral meatus cleansing, and antibacterial silver- or chlorhexidine-impregnated catheters, have not demonstrated consistent clinical or cost efficacy in reducing bacteriuria.

Preventing infections related to central and peripheral vascular catheters and respiratory assist devices is discussed subsequently in this chapter.

Infections in Critically Ill Trauma Victims

Altered Host Immunity

Blunt and penetrating injuries both cause an immunosuppressive state that correlates with the extent of the soft tissue injury and is multifactorial in nature. Total lymphocyte counts fall quickly following injury, and the proliferation of stimulated lymphocytes is suppressed. Anergy is a common manifestation; its presence correlates with length of hospital stay, incidence of infection, and overall mortality. B lymphocyte counts may also decrease after injury, with secondary declines in serum concentrations of immunoglobulin (Ig) G and IgM. Despite an early rise in the neutrophil counts, there is a reduction in their enzyme-mediated bactericidal activity and chemotaxis. Finally, activation of the inflammatory cytokine cascade has immune-altering effects and may be the most likely cause of multisystem organ failure in the absence of infection.

Approach to the Critically Ill Trauma Patient

Fever and leukocytosis are common in the early post-trauma period and often occur in the absence of true infection. Noninfectious causes include extensive soft tissue and bone injury, head injury, surgical manipulation of ischemic tissue, large soft tissue hematoma, transient atelectasis, or reactions to administered medications or blood products. Administration of therapeutic antibiotics, excluding prophylaxis, should be deferred until a focus of infection is established or is strongly suspected on clinical grounds. Progression to frank sepsis with or without hemodynamic compromise necessitates the use of empiric antibiotics directed at the most likely anatomic focus and inciting pathogens.

Surgical Wound Infections

Wound infection accounts for only 10% of all infections in postsurgical trauma patients. Clinical signs and symptoms characteristically occur more than 48 hours after surgery. *Staphylococcus aureus* causes the majority of infections; however, necrotizing infections or abdominal-perineal wounds are commonly polymicrobial, with gram-negative bacilli, enterococci, and anaerobes participating.

Intra-Abdominal Infection

Blunt trauma victims with negative abdominal CT scanning or diagnostic peritoneal lavage are unlikely to sustain intra-abdominal infection. Infrequent exceptions include acute acalculous cholecystitis or post-traumatic appendicitis. Blunt trauma may cause peritoneal soiling from a ruptured viscus. The higher risk of postoperative infection is seen with older victims, left-sided colon injury, multivisceral injury, high transfusion requirements, and a longer time period from peritoneal contamination to surgical debridement.

Penetrating abdominal injuries have a much greater risk of progressing to intra-abdominal infection. Intraoperative peritoneal lavage and postoperative antibiotic prophylaxis are the two most common interventions performed to minimize the frequency and severity of postoperative infection. Infection occurs only in the minority of such cases; however, these are often difficult to treat and may require serial CT scanning followed by percutaneous or repeat surgical drainage procedures of multiple fluid collections.

Sinusitis

This infection is not limited to the post-trauma population, but it does occur more frequently here owing to the use of nasotracheal tubes and concomitant facial trauma. Sinusitis is often unrecognized, as there may be few or no localizing symptoms or signs. Fewer than 50% of patients have purulent nasal discharge. Symptoms may appear as early as 48 hours after intubation but usually somewhat later. Complete opacification of the involved sinus noted on plain film radiographs or CT scan is suggestive but not diagnostic of sinusitis. Aspiration of the involved sinus or sinuses should be performed and the fluid sent to the laboratory for Gram's stain and culture. Therapy includes appropriate antibiotics, removal of the nasotracheal or nasogastric tubes, and temporary drainage of the sinus.

Post-Traumatic Central Nervous System Infections

Neurosurgical intervention or trauma that communicates with the central nervous system is a major predisposition for CNS infection. Patients with clinical or radiographic evidence of basilar skull fracture or patients with midface bone fractures may have an unrecognized cerebrospinal fluid (CSF) fistula. The majority of patients with CSF leaks have spontaneous closure without CNS infection. However, a patient with unexplained fever, leukocytosis, or altered mental status should be assessed for CNS infection. Lumbar puncture should be performed immediately unless there is a history of head trauma or focal signs suggestive of a focal lesion (hemorrhage, abscess) that would first necessitate a CT scan of the head.

Primary Bacteremia

Ten per cent of bacteremic trauma patients have no definite site of infection. Such instances are termed "primary bacteremia" and are due primarily to coagulase-negative staphylococci, *S. aureus*, enterococci, or a gram-negative bacillus. If concomitant signs of infection or sepsis are present, then antibiotic treatment is indicated. Persistence of the same organism during antibiotic therapy or relapse with the same organism after antibiotic therapy should prompt a search for an endovascular focus (e.g., endocarditis, suppurative thrombophlebitis, arteritis or mycotic aneurysm, infected prosthetic material).

Infections in Patients with Hematologic Malignancies

Granulocytopenia can be defined as an absolute neutrophil count (ANC) of less than 1000/μL. It is associated with hematologic malignancies, myelosuppressive therapy, bone marrow transplantation, and aplastic crises and thus frequently coexists with either deficiencies in cell-mediated immunity or humoral immunity. The ANC is inversely correlated with the incidence of infection, especially when counts fall below 100/μL, at which point the rates of bacteremia and overall infection increase dramatically. Though most granulocytopenic patients with infection manifest a fever, the classic signs of local inflammation are often muted or completely absent. Thus, fever is considered the early primary sign of infection, and its recognition has substantial therapeutic implications.

Pneumonitis is one of the most common and serious complications, with an associated mortality of 40% to 50% or higher. Major sites of infection are the upper alimentary canal (periodontium, oropharynx, and lower esophagus), lower colon and perianum, lungs, and integument. Major pathogens are the enteric gram-negative bacilli (e.g., *Escherichia coli, Klebsiella* sp.) and the aerobic gram-negative bacilli (*Pseudomonas* sp.). A significant trend during the past decade toward gram-positive infections (coagulase-negative staphylococci, *S. aureus*, enterococci, and alpha-hemolytic streptococci) has occurred. Fungal infection due to yeasts (*Candida albicans, Candida tropicalis*, and other non-albicans species) and mycelial forms (*Aspergillus* sp., *Mucor* sp.) rarely cause the first infectious episode, but these are prominent pathogens with prolonged granulocytopenia due to antibiotic selection factors and nosocomial exposure.

Diagnostic Process

Local clinical manifestations of infection may be subtle even in a severely infected patient. The clinician should attempt to elicit the presence of symptoms such as painful oral sores, skin lesions, cellulitis, sore throat, cough, dyspnea, painful or difficult swallowing, and perirectal pain or irritation. Meticulous evaluation of any peripheral or central intravascular device sites should be routine. Any episode of rigors, fever, unexplained hypotension or tachypnea, or other signs compatible with incipient sepsis warrant two separate cultures of blood obtained by peripheral venipuncture.

A chest radiograph is a mandatory part of the fever workup in the granulocytopenic patient. However, radiologic findings are often absent or minimal on the initial study due to the poor inflammatory response in the lung. New or progressive infiltrates should be interpreted with the bias that an infectious pneumonitis is present. A definitive diagnosis may require both semi-invasive and invasive procedures to determine the etiology of the pneumonitis. Several causes of noninfectious fever that warrant consideration in the granulocytopenic patient include pulmonary infiltrates, tumor, radiation pneumonitis, drug-induced pulmonary toxicity, and hemorrhage.

The upper and lower alimentary tract is another major source of infection and bacteremia in the granulocytopenic patient due to the high inoculum of indigenous bacteria and concomitant mucosal damage from recent cytotoxic chemotherapy. Esophagitis may present as difficult or painful swallowing and may be due to herpes simplex virus, cytomegalovirus, or *Candida* species. Upper endoscopy is the diagnostic procedure of choice. Colitis may present as diarrhea, abdominal pain, or distention. Confirmation of the diagnosis is best accomplished with colonoscopy.

Antibiotic Therapy in the Granulocytopenic Patient

The high probability that fever signals the presence of occult infection, coupled with the high potential for rapid clinical deterioration, necessitates immediate antimicrobial intervention. The selection of empiric antibiotic therapy can be guided with these general considerations:

1. The spectrum of coverage should include aerobic and facultative gram-negative bacilli and gram-positive cocci.
2. The antibiotic(s) should provide bactericidal activity.
3. Antibiotic combinations that expand the spectrum of coverage and provide synergistic activity are preferable.
4. If possible, potential toxicities should be minimized.

Classic proven regimens for empiric therapy include single-agent therapy ("monotherapy") with a third-generation cephalosporin (ceftazidime) or imipenem-cilastatin; combination therapy with a semisynthetic β-lactam with antipseudomonal activity and an aminoglycoside; or double β-lactam therapy. The latter may provide expanded coverage and synergism and avoid aminoglycoside-related nephrotoxicity; however, combinations of a β-lactamase inducer (ceftazidime) and a susceptible β-lactam (piperacillin) should be avoided. Monotherapy is not indicated for patients with documented gram-negative bacteremia or clinical sepsis.

Special considerations should also be given to granulocytopenic patients who reside in the ICU. Such patients may have had a more prolonged exposure to multiresistant nosocomial flora or indwelling vascular devices. Incorporation of vancomycin into the empiric regimen to cover methicillin-resistant *S. aureus* (MRSA), coagulase-negative staphylococci, and some strains of enterococci may be needed in such cases.

Amphotericin B is generally not employed for the initial febrile episode. Failure of patients to defervesce after 7 days of antibacterial therapy or microbiologic confirmation of fungal infection is a clear indication for amphotericin B. The drug is given intravenously in doses of 0.3 to 0.6 mg/kg/day and in higher doses (0.7 to 1.5 mg/kg/day) for more resistant fungal species (*Aspergillus* sp., *Mucor* sp., and some non-albicans species of *Candida*). Fluconazole has shown equal efficacy in catheter-related candidemia in nongranulocytopenic patients; however, evidence to suggest its efficacy over amphotericin B in the granulocytopenic host is insufficient. Superinfection with fluconazole-resistant fungal species such as *Candida krusei* and *Torulopsis glabrata* is also described.

The optimal duration of empiric antibiotic therapy depends on the clinical scenario. Patients with gram-negative or gram-positive bacteremia should receive 10 to 14 days of therapy, whereas serious nonbacteremic infections are treated for 7 to 10 days, provided the clinical response is adequate. It is not uncommon for fever and granulocytopenia to persist without a proven source of infection despite repetitive clinical and microbiologic examinations over several days. Antibiotics may be judiciously discontinued in such instances provided there is a continued reevaluation for persistent fever.

INFECTIONS IN THE SURGICAL CRITICAL CARE UNIT

Postoperative infections contribute significantly to morbidity and mortality in surgical ICU patients. The incidence of nosocomial infection is two- to fivefold higher in the surgical ICU patient population than in the general hospital population. Postoperative infections contribute significantly to this problem. Infections may arise due to a primary complication of the surgery (anastomotic leak, hemorrhage, dehiscence, devitalized tissue) or at distant locations (pneumonia, catheter sites) at which defenses are impaired in the perioperative period.

Wound Infection

The overall rate of postoperative wound infection approximates 7.5%, based on a landmark study 3 decades ago. The nature of surgery is a major independent variable that determines the risk for wound infection. Surgical wounds are classified by the following stratification: "clean" wounds involve no entry into the gastrointestinal, genitourinary, or respiratory tracts and have an overall wound infection rate of less than 2%; "clean-contaminated" wounds are those arising from elective surgery that enters the gastrointestinal, genitourinary, or respiratory tracts, and these wounds have a higher wound infection rate of 5% to 10%; in "contaminated" wounds there has been ongoing inflammation or gross spillage of gastrointestinal contents, and these have a 20% rate of wound infection; "dirty" wounds have gross purulence at the time of operation and have an extremely high rate of wound infection that may exceed 40%. Other major variables that have shown a direct association with increased wound infection rates include longer preoperative hospitalization period, razor shaving of the operative site the day before surgery, increased duration of operative time, prophylactic use of abdominal drains, and elective surgery in the presence of an active remote infection.

Clinical Presentation

Uncomplicated wound infection involves only the skin and subcutaneous tissues. Clinical signs usually occur between the fourth and eighth postoperative day and may consist of incisional pain or tenderness, warmth, or redness and swelling with fever. Appearance of these signs within 48 hours of surgery may suggest infection with a rapidly progressive and virulent pathogen such as Group A beta-hemolytic streptococcus or a *Clostridium* species. Management of these latter infections requires early and aggressive debridement of devitalized tissue, parenteral antibiotics usually with a penicillin G–containing regimen, and hyperbaric oxygen therapy, which shows benefit as an adjunctive measure. Routine wound infection management includes good operative drainage and meticulous wound care.

Prevention

Antibiotic prophylaxis has been convincingly shown to reduce the incidence of postoperative wound infection even for low-risk "clean" surgery. Several critical elements must be followed to achieve prophylactic efficacy: parenteral administration of the antibiotic(s) 30 minutes prior to the operative incision so as to obtain therapeutic serum and tissue levels, and selection of the antibiotic(s) that have activity against the microflora appropriate for the operative site (Table 8–2). The risk of infections in patients undergoing clean surgical procedures with prosthetic devices such as total hip replacement or implantation of cardiac valves or vascular grafts is low. However, infection in such settings may be catastrophic. Penicillinase-resistant antistaphylococcal agents (oxacillin, nafcillin) had been the mainstay of prophylaxis for such surgery. The increased incidence of *S. epidermidis* infection, which has some resistance to these agents, has led to a preference for either first-generation cephalosporins or vancomycin in prosthetic implantations and other clean surgical procedures.

Administration of prophylactic antibiotics beyond 24 hours into the postoperative period does not further reduce

Table 8–2. MICROORGANISMS MOST COMMONLY ISOLATED FROM SITES OF POSTOPERATIVE INFECTION

Infection Site	Aerobes	Anaerobes
Gastrointestinal		
Mouth	Streptococci	Bacteroides (other than *Bacteroides fragilis*), peptostreptococci, fusobacteria
Esophagus	Same as for mouth	Same as for mouth
Stomach	Enteric gram-negative bacilli, streptococci	Same as for mouth
Biliary	Enteric gram-negative bacilli, group D streptococci	Clostridia
Distal ileum	Enteric gram-negative bacilli	*B. fragilis*, peptostreptococci, clostridia
Colon	Same as for distal ileum	Same as for distal ileum
Gynecologic	Same as for distal ileum	Same as for distal ileum
Orthopedic	Staphylococci, streptococci	
Thoracic	Streptococci, pneumococci	Bacteroides (other than *B. fragilis*), peptostreptococci
Cardiovascular	Staphylococci, streptococci	
Urologic	Enteric gram-negative bacilli, group D streptococci	

the rate of infection and may increase the risk of drug toxicity or superinfection.

Peritonitis and Intra-Abdominal Abscess

Secondary bacterial peritonitis primarily occurs following the leakage of endogenous microflora from a diseased or traumatized intraperitoneal hollow viscus. The extent and severity of the peritoneal insult depend on the source and duration of contamination, the presence of devitalized tissue or fluid (hemoglobin, fibrin, bile), bacterial synergy, and the adequacy of the host response. Experimental models of intra-abdominal sepsis elucidated the role of bacterial synergy and the need to utilize antibiotic(s) with activity against both aerobes and anaerobes. Aerobes are responsible for the high early mortality in acute peritonitis. Culmination in a second-disease phase with the formation of intra-abdominal abscesses may occur because of the persistence of anaerobic bacteria.

Clinical Presentation

Abdominal pain is present in almost all patients with peritonitis or abscess. Patients with generalized peritonitis usually manifest diffuse involuntary guarding and tenderness; in contrast, these findings are localized in patients with a formed abscess. These symptoms are characteristically worsened by any movement.

Bowel sounds are usually diminished or absent, and distention may be present owing to paralytic ileus. Fever, leukocytosis with a left shift, and signs of hypovolemia are a common triad in peritonitis. A clinical diagnosis of acute peritonitis can be made accurately based upon a patient's history and physical findings. Helpful ancillary studies include plain or contrast radiography to demonstrate perforations, ileus, space-occupying lesions, or free fluid. Detection of discrete fluid collections requires ultrasound or CT scan of the abdomen. Peritoneal lavage (1 liter of normal saline instilled via a peritoneal catheter and examination of the drainage) may be diagnostic of peritonitis in the absence of detectable ascites. The presence of pus, bile, feces, or a fluid cell count greater than 500 neutrophils per cubic millimeter, or the presence of bacteria or food fibers on direct stains, is diagnostic of peritonitis.

Therapy

Early diagnosis and prompt therapy of secondary peritonitis are critical for a favorable outcome. A strong correlation between the interval from presentation to treatment determines the rates of perioperative morbidity and mortality. Abdominal exploration is indicated both to uncover the source of secondary peritonitis and for therapy. Therapy depends on whether the peritonitis is localized or diffuse.

Treatment Methods for Localized Infection

RESECTION. Certain conditions, such as gangrenous appendicitis, cholecystitis, bowel infarction, or perforated diverticulitis, are remedied by primary resection of the diseased tissue. Some conditions, such as peridiverticular abscess, may be approached with a combined modality: initial therapy with percutaneous drainage and antibiotics, followed by elective resection of the involved colon with primary reanastomosis.

DRAINAGE. Open incision and drainage is the optimal method for treating most abdominal abscesses, whereas percutaneous drainage for favorable abscesses is strongly advocated by some. However, percutaneous drainage is not advisable for the following: (1) complex abscesses (more than 2 septations, continuous with the gastrointestinal tract, thick debris, or with fungal elements); (2) more than two abscesses; (3) pancreatic abscesses; and (4) drainage pathways that traverse bowel or uncontaminated body cavities.

Treatment Modalities for Diffuse Intra-Abdominal Infection

A wide variety of approaches are employed for this condition.

SIMPLE DRAINAGE. Simple drainage of the peritoneal cavity after diffuse suppurative peritonitis is totally ineffective, probably because of walling off of the drain by fibrin deposition.

CONTINUOUS POSTOPERATIVE PERITONEAL LAVAGE. Irrigation catheters are placed at laparotomy for repeated peritoneal lavage until the effluent becomes totally clear or for an arbitrary duration of time. The technique usually involves instillation of 1 liter of saline over 5 to 10 minutes, 30 minutes of dwell time, and drainage over 25 minutes. It is notable that the majority of prospective studies show no survival advantage compared with conventional management.

INTRAOPERATIVE IRRIGATION. The use of intraoperative peritoneal irrigation with or without antibiotic-containing solutions is a widely practiced technique. The number of bacteria and adjuvant substances remaining in the peritoneal cavity is reduced; however, there is no reduction in mortality or in progression to abscess formation. Antibiotics include cephalothin (1 g/L), kanamycin (1 g/L), bacitracin (50,000 U/L), chloramphenicol, and other aminoglycosides. Rapid absorption of peritoneal antibiotics may cause high systemic concentrations and toxicity.

RADICAL PERITONEAL DEBRIDEMENT. This involves the complete exposure of the peritoneal cavity with removal of all free fluid, pus, and devitalized tissue. No favorable effect on outcome has been reported with this technique.

LEAVING THE PERITONEAL CAVITY OPEN. No closure is performed at the time of exploratory laparotomy, and the patient is returned to the operating room daily to break up loculations and debride dead tissue. Often a polypropylene mesh is used to prevent evisceration. The abdomen is closed when no further fluid collections or necrotic tissue is apparent. Possible advantages of this method include improved blood flow resulting from decreased intra-abdominal pressure, decreased bacterial burden, and prompt recognition of abdominal complications. Bowel perforation and fistula formation are the principal drawbacks.

Antibiotic Selection

Antibiotic therapy should be initiated as soon as the diagnosis is made and continued well into the postoperative period. The chosen antibiotics must have activity against both colonic aerobes and anaerobes, including *Bacteroides fragilis*. The antibiotics that are commonly used singly or in combination are listed in Table 8–3. The optimal duration of therapy is based in part on the clinical response; the persistence of leukocytosis without fever at the conclusion of the antibiotic course correlates with a 33% risk of ongoing or recurrent intra-abdominal infection. In one study, 79% of patients who were still febrile developed recurrent infection. Thus, antibiotics should be continued for a minimum of 5 to 7 days after laparotomy or until both fever and leukocytosis have resolved.

INFECTION AFTER SOLID ORGAN TRANSPLANTATION

Infectious complications remain the leading primary or associated cause of mortality for all categories of solid organ transplantation. Nevertheless, the proliferation of organ transplant centers has resulted in significant advances in the

Table 8–3. PARENTERAL ANTIBIOTIC AGENTS CURRENTLY USED FOR THERAPY OF INTRA-ABDOMINAL INFECTION

Combination Therapy	
*Aerobic Coverage**	
Amikacin	Ciprofloxacin
Aztreonam	Gentamicin
Cefotaxime	Tobramycin
Ceftriaxone	
Anaerobic Coverage†	
Chloramphenicol	
Clindamycin	
Metronidazole	
Single-Drug Therapy	
Aerobic-Anaerobic Coverage: Single Agents	
Ampicillin/sulbactam	Imipenem/cilastatin
Cefotetan	Piperacillin/tazobactam
Cefoxitin	Ticarcillin/clavulanic acid
Ceftizoxime	

*To be combined with a drug having anaerobic activity.
†To be combined with a drug having aerobic activity.

prevention, diagnosis, and treatment of post-transplant infection.

Epidemiology

The frequency and severity of infections are to a partial extent a function of the category of organ transplantation; both heart-lung and liver recipients experience higher overall rates of infection compared with kidney recipients. In addition, the frequency of certain infections may vary between organ transplant centers because of candidate selection policies and the intensity and quality of immunosuppression regimens.

Temporal Pattern

The time course of infections can be grouped into three consecutive but overlapping periods: (1) early infections within the first post-transplant month, (2) infections occurring in a middle period between the second and sixth month, and (3) late infections that may occur sporadically during the lifetime of the recipient. The sites and causes of the more common infections are shown in Table 8–4. Early infections are most commonly postoperative superficial or deep wound infections, often related to technical complications or graft dysfunction. Reactivated mucocutaneous herpes simplex virus (HSV) may also occur very early; however, its incidence is reduced by acyclovir prophylaxis.

Cytomegalovirus (CMV) is the dominant infectious threat during the intermediate period. Manifestations of CMV disease include a febrile syndrome (fever, malaise, and atypical lymphocytosis), focal invasive disease (pneumonia, hepatitis, enteritis), and disseminated disease. Invasive CMV disease appears to potentiate the risk of allograft rejection and the incidence of serious opportunistic infections caused by fungi and protozoa. Nosocomial exposure, antibiotic pressure, and the cumulative effects of immunosuppression also contribute to opportunistic infection between the second and sixth post-transplant months. Late infections are caused by endogenous latent pathogens that may become reactivated (*Mycobacterium tuberculosis*), relapsing forms of infection such as bronchitis in lung recipients, cholangitis in liver recipients with biliary duct disease, and urinary tract infections in kidney recipients. Infections with community-acquired pathogens (influenza, *Streptococcus pneumoniae, S. aureus*) may present with an atypical or fulminant course.

Sources of Pathogens Causing Clinical Disease in Organ Recipients

Pathogens that cause infection in the organ recipient are either endogenous (i.e., originating from within the host), exogenous (i.e., newly acquired from the environment, allograft, or transfused blood products), or possibly both. Endogenous organisms often exhibit the property of "latency" in which, after a variable period of iatrogenic immunosuppression, they reactivate to cause clinical disease. The proba-

Table 8–4. COMMON INFECTIONS AFTER SOLID ORGAN TRANSPLANTATION BASED ON THE TIME OF PRESENTATION

Early (Weeks 1–4)
All Solid Organ Recipients
Superficial wound infection
Bacterial pneumonia
Urinary tract infection
Catheter infection
Kidney Recipients
Pyelonephritis
Perinephric/parenchymal abscess
Liver Recipients
Cholangitis
Intra-abdominal abscess
Peritonitis
Hepatic abscess
Heart and Heart-Lung Recipients
Sternal wound infection
Mediastinitis
Empyema
Middle (Months 2–6)
Cytomegalovirus
Epstein-Barr virus (PTLD)
Legionellosis
Tuberculosis
Nocardia
Aspergillus
Pneumocystis
Late (After 6 Months)
Pneumocystis
Cryptococcosis
Herpes zoster virus
CMV retinitis
Community-acquired pathogens
Streptococcal pneumonia
Influenza

Abbreviations: PTLD = post-transplant lymphoproliferative disorder; CMV = cytomegalovirus.

bility of harboring these organisms at the time of transplantation depends upon prior subclinical or clinical infection (*M. tuberculosis*) or geographic origin (*Coccidioides immitis, Strongyloides stercoralis*). Seroprevalence studies show that certain organisms, such as Type I HSV, Epstein-Barr virus (EBV), and varicella-zoster virus (VZV) have predictably high rates of prior infection, with greater than 95% of adults demonstrating seropositivity. CMV is an important exception, with a variable range of 40% to 100% of seropositive adults.

Exogenous organisms may be transmitted from the inanimate or animate physical environment. Organ recipients are exquisitely sensitive to environmental contamination with microorganisms capable of causing infection. Outbreaks of nosocomial infections among cohorted transplant recipients may signal that a contaminated environmental source exists. Prominent examples include clusters of invasive aspergillosis caused by air contamination with *Aspergillus* spores, usually from hospital construction or defective air filtration units, and legionellosis from contamination of the hospital hot water supply with *Legionella* species.

The donor allograft is a proven source of potential pathogens unique to the organ recipient population. Serologic screening of donors has mostly eliminated potential pathogens like hepatitis B and C and human immunodeficiency virus 1 (HIV-1). Some transplant centers may electively use organs from hepatitis C–seropositive donors for recipients who are already hepatitis C–seropositive. The clinician's knowledge of the donor status for organisms such as cytomegalovirus, *Toxoplasma gondii,* and *Treponema pallidum* and the tracheal bacterial cultures of lung donors is important for guiding chemoprophylaxis in the recipient.

Role of Iatrogenic Immunosuppression

Solid organ recipients receive an induction and maintenance immunosuppressant regimen that usually combines a corticosteroid with either cyclosporine or FK-506 and perhaps azathioprine. Rejection episodes are usually managed with a corticosteroid bolus or recycle, or an antilymphocyte agent (OKT3, ALG [antilymphocyte globulin]). Though there are overlapping immunologic targets among some immunosuppressive drugs, the cause-effect association between certain categories of infection and the type of agent is well established. Corticosteroids cause a dose- and duration-dependent impairment of the neutrophil inflammatory response, macrophage antigen processing, antibody production, and cell-mediated immunity. These potentiate the risk of infection owing to a broad range of opportunistic and nonopportunistic bacteria and fungi. Notably, corticosteroids are not potent inducers of CMV or other invasive viral diseases.

Both cyclosporine and FK-506 appear to lower the risk-to-benefit ratio for infectious complications when compared with corticosteroid/azathioprine–based immunosuppression regimens used in the precyclosporine era. Much of this effect is mediated by the diminished need for prolonged high doses of corticosteroids. However, their select impairment of lymphocyte-derived interleukin-2 synthesis predisposes the recipient to de novo or reactivated infection with bacteria and especially the Herpesviridae family (CMV, HSV, EBV, VZV). The availability of serum or blood level monitoring is a unique refinement that allows the individualization of dosing.

Antilymphocyte therapy with either ALG or OKT3 is used in some transplant centers as an induction agent or for steroid-refractory rejection. Higher rates and greater severity of CMV disease are described in kidney, liver, and heart recipients receiving antilymphocyte therapy. These agents also are significant cofactors in the pathogenesis of EBV-mediated post-transplant lymphoproliferative disease (PTLD) in several reports.

Recent reports demonstrate that the elective withdrawal of corticosteroids after 3 months could be successfully accomplished in the majority of recipients without excess rejection or allograft loss. The recently discovered ability to detect host-donor chimerism in liver recipients is a landmark. It is hoped this will achieve host immunotolerance without incurring the infection-producing risks of iatrogenic immunosuppression.

Infections Related to the Transplant Operation

Both the allograft organ and the contiguous tissue structures are especially vulnerable to infection, particularly in the early post-transplant period. Kidney recipients are especially prone to urinary tract infections (UTIs), with either aerobic gram-negative bacilli or enterococci. UTIs occurring in the early post-transplant period may be refractory to conventional therapy and lead to severe sequelae (bacteremia, graft pyelonephritis). Rarely, graft nephrectomy is indicated for such cases. Prophylaxis with TMP-SMX (trimethoprim-sulfamethoxazole) or ciprofloxacin has shown a clear reduction in the rates of early UTI. Postoperative hematomas, lymphoceles, and urinomas resulting from technical errors potentiate the risk for deep perinephric wound infection. This may lead to mycotic aneurysm formation of the vascular pedicle, sepsis, and graft failure unless prompt and adequate drainage is performed.

The prolonged duration and extensive nature of liver transplant surgery results in the highest rate of early postoperative infection among all solid organ recipients. Such infections are principally intra-abdominal and closely related to the duration of surgery, type and viability of the biliary anastomosis, and adequacy of the graft vascular supply. Bile leakage from the reconstructed biliary anastomosis (choledochocholedochostomy or choledochojejunostomy) usually occurs within the first 2 post-transplant weeks and usually manifests as fever, bacteremia, or frank sepsis, with an elevated serum bilirubin level and localized peritonitis. Hepatic arterial insufficiency (thrombus, stenosis) is often the precipitating reason for the bile leak. Conventional management includes operative drainage and either immediate or delayed revision of the biliary anastomosis. Hepatic arterial thrombosis may present as relapsing enteric bacteremia, hepatic abscess, fulminant hepatic necrosis, or breakdown of the biliary anastomosis. Retransplantation or hepatic artery thrombectomy is the principal therapeutic option.

The most common sites of infection following heart, heart-lung, and lung transplantation involve the lung parenchyma, mediastinum, and pleural cavity. Mediastinitis occurs in only 2.8% of heart recipients but is a potentially devastating complication. Prior sternotomy, postoperative hemorrhage, staphylococcal pneumonitis, diabetes, and early rejection are associated risk factors. Contamination of the mediastinum may occur at the time of transplantation, from a sternal wound infection, or from leakage of secretions from the tracheal or bronchial anastomosis of lung recipients. *S. epidermidis* and *S. aureus* are the predominant organisms; however, gram-negative bacilli, fungi, *Mycoplasma hominis*, and *Nocardia* sp. are also reported. Incisional erythema and purulent drainage with an unstable sternum are common presenting signs. Treatment includes systemic antibiotics with open debridement and irrigation.

Pneumonia is quite prevalent in heart-lung and lung recipients and may occur as early as the second post-transplant day. Careful clinical and microbiologic evaluations are required since acute graft rejection may have a similar presentation. Therapy is guided by the results of donor tracheal cultures and diagnostic bronchoalveolar lavage or protected brushings.

Important Opportunistic Infections in the Solid Organ Recipient

Legionellosis

Legionella are low-frequency pathogens that may present as a community-acquired pneumonia in the late post-transplant period. Nosocomial epidemics of *Legionella* pneumonia due to a contaminated hospital water supply have been reported among transplant patients. Thus, any case of legionellosis in a transplant unit should prompt a search for nosocomial sources. The majority of patients will manifest a high-grade fever even in the presence of corticosteroid administration. Minimal or no sputum production is most common. Chest radiographic findings typically show uni- or multilobar alveolar infiltrates. Cavitary lesions are more common in transplant patients.

Since legionellosis has a nonspecific clinical presentation, early diagnosis necessitates strong clinical suspicion because special microbiologic methods are required. Rapidly available tests such as the *Legionella* gene probe or urine radioimmunoassay are especially valuable since they may prompt early therapeutic intervention. Culturing for *Legionella* still remains the diagnostic gold standard; however, cultures may not become positive for 3 to 5 days. Treatment delay is poorly tolerated in transplant recipients, so suspected cases should be treated empirically. Intravenous erythromycin (4 g/day) has the longest cumulative record of success, although its inhibition of oxidative hepatic enzymes may cause an undesired increase in serum cyclosporine and FK-506 levels. Other promising agents include ciprofloxacin and the newer macrolide, clarithromycin. Duration of therapy should be a minimum of 21 days, as relapses have been reported with shorter courses of treatment.

Tuberculosis

The incidence of tuberculosis among solid organ recipients is quite low considering the high number of predisposing factors in the pretransplant period (uremia, cirrhosis, alcoholism) and post-transplant period (immunosuppression). However, the rising incidence of tuberculosis in other immunosuppressed populations (HIV-infected) and the general population may result in higher rates of TB in the near future. Tuberculosis develops most commonly because of reactivation of dormant foci of mycobacteria as a result of the impairment of cell-mediated immunity from iatrogenic immunosuppression. However, solid organ recipients may develop pulmonary or disseminated primary disease following exposure to an active case of pulmonary tuberculosis in transplant units. The spectrum of clinical presentation may be both atypical and more diverse than in the nonimmunocompromised host. Included are (1) higher rates of extrapulmonary disease; (2) reactivated pulmonary disease presenting in the middle and lower lobes; (3) poorly visible or absent tissue granulomas; (4) higher rates of bone and joint disease; and (5) reactivated disease manifesting in the donor organ. Many transplant programs perform PPD (purified protein derivative) skin testing on prospective candidates to screen for prior TB infection; however, the sensitivity of this test is significantly diminished owing to cutaneous anergy.

Active or suspected tuberculous disease should be treated with a minimum of three first-line antituberculous agents. The efficacy of shortened 6-month regimens for transplant recipients is unknown and cannot be recommended at present. Risk factors for isoniazid (INH) or multidrug resistance (prior incomplete therapy, noncompliance or failed INH prophylaxis, exposure to resistant strain) will require a broader empiric regimen until definitive susceptibility results are available. Chemotherapy may be especially problematic due to hepatotoxicity (INH, rifampin, pyrazinamide) or the potentiation of cyclosporine and FK-506 metabolism by rifampin.

Nocardiosis

Nocardia sp. are gram-positive, rod-shaped bacteria with a characteristic branching and beaded morphology. These organisms are ubiquitous in nature and usually gain entry via inhalation of airborne organisms. Qualitative improvements in immunosuppression and perhaps the widespread use of trimethoprim/sulfamethoxazole for *Pneumocystis* prophylaxis may be responsible for a fall in the incidence of nocardiosis over the past decade. Clinical presentation is most often a subacute febrile illness with clinical and radiographic pulmonary disease. Hematogenous dissemination to the brain, skin, and other viscera is quite common. Sulfa drugs (TMP-SMX, sulfisoxazole, or sulfadiazine) have the longest cumulative record of efficacy when used for a duration of at least 3 to 6 months. Sulfa-intolerant individuals can be treated with minocycline and amoxicillin/clavulanic acid. Surgical drainage of abscesses is often required for refractory disease.

Candidiasis

Invasive disease caused by *Candida* species remains the most common fungal infection seen after solid organ transplantation. Serious *Candida* infection usually occurs within the first 2 to 3 post-transplant months. The spectrum of disease caused by *Candida* ranges from mucosal involvement only (stomatitis, esophagitis, cystitis) to bloodstream infection indicative of either a catheter-related source or multivisceral invasion. Candidemia itself is an insensitive marker of multivisceral invasion. Conversely, the presence of candidemia in any solid organ recipient should never be managed presumptively as a contaminant or catheter-related source until appropriate clinical and laboratory investigations are performed. The isolation of *Candida* sp. at multiple sites (e.g., urine, sputum, stool) has poor positive predictive value for the presence of visceral candidiasis. Diagnostic tests that are reliable indicators of serious *Candida* infection include the histopathologic demonstration of yeast or pseudohyphae in deep tissue specimens or positive cultures from a sterile body site (e.g., ascites, pericardial or joint fluid, CSF, blood).

Superficial *Candida* infections (stomatitis, esophagitis) are usually responsive to nystatin or fluconazole. Amphotericin B at a daily dose of 0.5 to 1.0 mg per kg is still the primary treatment for serious *Candida* infection. Fluconazole has shown equivalent efficacy to amphotericin B for catheter-related candidemia; however, its value in organ recipients with visceral disease is unproved. The efficacy of liposomal amphotericin preparations is currently being investigated.

Aspergillosis

Aspergillus sp. are filamentous fungi ubiquitous in the environment, but they may cause devastating invasive disease in solid organ recipients. The incidence of aspergillosis is highest within the first 3 post-transplant months due to the greater immunosuppression and nosocomial exposure in this period. Pathogenesis includes inhalation of airborne spores followed by invasion of the pulmonary parenchyma and hematogenous dissemination to multiple viscera, especially the central nervous system. The pulmonary manifestations are most often a febrile focal pneumonitis that may appear as solitary or multiple nodules with cavitation in some cases. Hemoptysis, although nonspecific, may be a clinical sign of angioinvasive disease. Less common sites of primary inoculation include the sinuses, surgical wounds, and skin.

A definitive diagnosis of invasive aspergillosis requires the demonstration of tissue-invasive hyphal forms, with dichotomous 45°-angle branching and growth of *Aspergillus* sp. from the specimen. Isolation of *Aspergillus* sp. from a respiratory specimen with a compatible clinical picture carries a fairly high predictive value that incipient or established invasive aspergillosis is present. Despite its propensity for hematogenous dissemination, *Aspergillus* species rarely grow in routine or fungal blood culture systems.

The attributable mortality of invasive aspergillosis exceeds 90% in some solid organ recipient populations even despite antifungal therapy. Factors that contribute to a poor outcome include difficulties in establishing an early diagnosis, poor in vivo response to amphotericin B, and fatal relapse after the completion of apparently adequate antifungal therapy. In addition to high-dose amphotericin B (1 mg/kg/day), surgical resection of isolated pulmonary, brain, or other visceral lesions should be considered. Itraconazole has been reported to achieve clinical cure or improvement in organ recipients with amphotericin-refractory invasive aspergillosis.

Cryptococcosis

Cryptococcus neoformans is a yeast pathogen with a strong tropism for the central nervous system that may cause meningitis or other visceral disease in the transplant recipient. Infection may occur many years after the transplant procedure. The lung is the portal of entry. Pulmonary manifestations are usually subclinical, although a febrile pneumonitis may occur in some patients. The meningeal syndrome is characterized by a subacute, progressive fever; headache; and visual disturbances with or without meningismus. Cerebrospinal fluid (CSF) shows a mononuclear pleocytosis, moderate elevation in protein level, and a normal or mildly depressed glucose level. Testing for CSF cryptococcal antigen has near 100% sensitivity and rapid turnover, whereas India ink stain is positive in only 50% of culture-positive specimens. Recommended therapy includes either amphotericin B (0.5 mg/kg/day) with 5-flucytosine (150 mg/kg/day) or fluconazole (400 mg loading dose and 200 mg/day maintenance dose). Intrathecal or intraventricular amphotericin B (0.1 to 0.5 mg/day) may improve outcome in refractory cases.

Viral Infections

Herpes Simplex Virus

Localized reactivated herpes simplex virus (HSV) infection may occur in the early post-transplant period. Orolabial lesions that appear as painful vesicles or ulcers are most common. Contiguous spread to the respiratory tract (tracheobronchitis) or alimentary tract (esophagitis) is well described. Disseminated cutaneous or visceral infection is rare but may cause life-threatening sequelae. Diagnosis rests on the demonstration of multinucleated giant cells or typical inclusions on cytologic or histologic specimens, positive culture, or immunofluorescent staining for HSV antigens. Intravenous acyclovir (15 mg/kg/day) remains the therapy of choice for HSV infection. Low-dose oral acyclovir (200 mg twice daily) provides effective HSV chemoprophylaxis.

Cytomegalovirus Infection

CMV remains the most common significant pathogen for all categories of solid organ transplantation. The virus is either transmitted to the host via the donor organ or blood products, or the recipient CMV strain undergoes reactivation. The CMV serologic status of the recipient is a major determinant for the risk and severity of CMV disease following transplantation. CMV-seronegative recipients who receive a CMV-seropositive allograft have a rate of CMV disease as high as 70%, with more serious morbidity, frequent clinical relapse, and occasional mortality. CMV-seropositive recipients experience a less severe spectrum of symptomatic disease regardless of the CMV status of the donor. The risks of CMV disease are also increased by prior use of antilymphocyte therapy.

Symptomatic CMV disease usually occurs between the second and sixth post-transplant month. Clinical manifestations are diverse, ranging from a febrile syndrome (fever, atypical lymphocytosis, CMV viremia) to serious focal or disseminated invasive disease. There is some predilection for CMV disease to occur in the allograft organ—i.e., pneumonitis in lung recipients, hepatitis in liver recipients. Diagnosis of invasive disease requires the demonstration of typical CMV inclusions in tissue or cytology or virologic evidence of CMV along with a compatible clinical picture. Rapid detection of early CMV antigens in fluid or tissue specimens has enhanced the clinician's ability to direct antiviral therapy sooner and in nonempiric fashion, compared with conventional cell culture methods.

Ganciclovir, a guanosine analog, is now the principal therapy for CMV disease. Recommended dosing is 5 mg/kg every 12 hours, with dose reduction required for renal insufficiency. The principal limiting toxicity is bone marrow suppression (leukopenia, thrombocytopenia). Foscavir is an alternative therapy, though cumulative experience with it is limited. CMV hyperimmune globulin has shown benefit in bone marrow recipients with CMV pneumonia. Its therapeutic benefit in CMV-seronegative solid organ recipients is currently under investigation.

Epstein-Barr Virus Infection

EBV is strongly linked to the development of PTLD, based on the isolation of EBV genomic DNA and viral protein in lymphatic and other affected tissues. EBV-related disease may be mild, with only a mononucleosis-like syndrome (fever, adenopathy, atypical lymphocytosis). The severe end of the spectrum includes nodal or visceral lymphoma disease with monoclonal surface markers. The median time from transplantation to PTLD is 3 to 5 months, though it may present years later. Favorable clinical response may be seen with only withdrawal or tapering of immunosuppression. Though acyclovir decreases the duration of EBV shedding, its actual clinical benefit remains unproved. Antineoplastic chemotherapy or surgical excision may be required for aggressive lymphomas.

Varicella-Zoster Infection

Primary varicella infection occurs in those rare recipients who lack protective immunity (no prior chickenpox) and are exposed to an incubating case of chickenpox. Such cases can be severe, with interstitial pneumonitis and multiorgan dissemination. Reactivated disease (shingles) occurs in 10% to 15% of VZV-seropositive recipients, often in the late post-transplant period. A single or multidermatomal cutaneous eruption of painful vesicles is the most common clinical presentation. High-dose intravenous acyclovir (30 mg/kg/day) shortens the clinical syndrome and viral shedding and may prevent progression to visceral dissemination. Varicella-zoster immune globulin (VZIG) should be administered to VZV-seronegative individuals with documented or suspected exposure to a case of chickenpox.

Chemoprophylaxis and Other Preventive Measures

The majority of solid organ transplant programs are now using oral TMP-SMX for *Pneumocystis* prophylaxis and some form of CMV prophylaxis. Selective decontamination of the gut with non-absorbed agents (colistin/gentamicin/nystatin) has shown benefit in liver recipients. Much disparity of opinion and practice exists for the use of INH prophylaxis in PPD-positive recipients, low-dose amphotericin B in recipients at high risk for candidiasis, and aerosolized amphotericin B or itraconazole for prevention of aspergillosis. Table 8–5 summarizes some of the common preventive and chemoprophylactic strategies.

BACTERIAL PNEUMONIA IN ADULT RESPIRATORY DISTRESS SYNDROME

Defense Mechanisms in the Respiratory Tract

The upper respiratory tract has several intrinsic defenses to prevent the gross contamination of the lower respiratory tree. These defenses may become compromised by both the underlying disease or iatrogenic intervention. The mucociliary apparatus and gag and cough reflexes prevent the gross contamination of the lower respiratory tract with inhaled or aspirated organisms. These mechanisms are complemented by specific immune components (e.g., secretory IgA and IgG) and nonspecific secreted components (e.g., lysozyme, surfactant, lactoferrin, and fibronectin) that enhance the entrapment and neutralization of bacteria. The final line of defense consists of bronchiole-associated lymphoid tissue and alveolar macrophages and their secreted soluble factors (lymphokines, tumor necrosis factor, interleukin-1), which propagate the inflammatory response to enhance microbicidal activity.

Colonization of the Respiratory Tract

The endogenous oropharyngeal flora of normal individuals is composed of nonpathogenic, gram-positive bacteria (viridans streptococci, lactobacilli) and anaerobes. Gram-negative bacilli are present in only 1% to 6% of normals. With the onset of critical illness and other common stresses in the ICU (general surgery, catabolism, renal failure), there is a shift in the composition of upper respiratory flora to gram-negative bacilli. This transition is mediated by the elaboration of proteases that alter the binding selectivity of epithelial cells via cleavage of surface-bound fibronectin. Subsequently, oropharyngeal colonization with potential gram-negative pathogens may lead to tracheobronchial colonization. Persistent tracheobronchial gram-negative colonization

Table 8–5. CHEMOPROPHYLAXIS AND OTHER PREVENTIVE MEASURES AFTER SOLID ORGAN TRANSPLANTATION

Pathogen(s)	Chemoprophylaxis	Other Measures
Herpes simplex	Acyclovir	
CMV	High-dose acyclovir	Vaccination*
	Ganciclovir*	CMV (−) products
	Hyperimmune CMV globulin*†	
Varicella	VZIG*	
Pneumocystis	Trimethoprim-sulfamethoxazole	
	Aerosolized pentamidine	
Toxoplasmosis	Pyrimethamine*	
Aspergillus	Itraconazole†	HEPA
	Aerosolized amphotericin B†	
Candida	Systemic amphotericin B	
	Nystatin	
Bacteria	Antibiotic (wound prophylaxis)	Gut decontamination
Mycobacterium tuberculosis	Isoniazid‡	
Streptococcus pneumoniae		Pneumovax

*In seronegative recipient.
†Investigational.
‡(+) purified protein derivative or high-risk exposure.
Abbreviations: CMV = cytomegalovirus; VZIG = varicella zoster immune globulin; HEPA = high-efficiency particulate air filtration.

is associated with a threefold risk increase for gram-negative pneumonia. These organisms may be acquired from the patient's intestinal reservoir or directly from the environment.

Pathogenesis of Pneumonia

Experimental evidence demonstrates that the probability of developing pneumonia is increased by a larger inoculum of bacteria or a larger aspirated volume. In normal animals, bolus delivery of 10^7 per ml or greater bacteria produces pneumonia. Moreover, preexisting lung injury, such as diffuse alveolar damage, reduces the critical inoculum threshold that will result in pneumonia. This is supported by a study of postmortem examinations of adult respiratory distress syndrome (ARDS) patients, which showed that more than 70% had bronchopneumonia. In humans, microaspiration of bacteria from a colonized oropharynx and tracheobronchial tree is the primary route of lung inoculation. Bacterial concentrations may be so very high (10^8 organisms per ml) that only small quantities of secretions will deliver a high inoculum. Cuffed artificial airways fail to provide protection against small-volume aspiration and may serve as a direct conduit to the lung both from healthcare givers and attached respiratory equipment.

The association of gastric acid neutralizing therapies (H-2 blockers, antacids) with increased gram-negative bacterial colonization of the stomach and higher rates of pneumonia indirectly supports the theory that retrograde migration occurs from the stomach to the oropharynx.

Pneumonia may commonly be superimposed on preexisting ARDS secondary to extrapulmonary processes and is extremely difficult to distinguish either clinically or radiographically. Antibacterial defenses, especially the alveolar macrophages and surfactant, are further impaired in ARDS due to the accumulation of interstitial and alveolar edema. Nosocomial pneumonias that occur consequential to ARDS are often polymicrobial due to the large inoculum of multiple organisms in the upper respiratory tract. Enteric gram-negative bacilli are the predominant pathogens, with *Pseudomonas aeruginosa* the most common species in most studies.

Clinical Aspects of Pneumonia

Nosocomial pneumonia is the third most common hospital-acquired infection. Generally, the risk of pneumonia increases with the duration of mechanical ventilation; in one analysis, the risk of pneumonia was 6.5% after 10 days, 19% after 20 days, and 28% after 30 days of ventilation. Few studies have analyzed the cause-effect relationship between nosocomial pneumonia and ARDS. Seidenfeld and associates demonstrated that 21% of patients had pneumonia that precipitated ARDS and 53% had pneumonia after established ARDS. Pneumonia developing within 4 days of ventilation has been designated early onset; pneumonia occurring after 4 days is termed late onset. This distinction has a biologic basis, as early onset pneumonias appear secondary to aspiration whereas late onset pneumonias have a different pathogenesis.

Frequency estimates of pneumonia, especially in ARDS, are hampered by the inadequacy of current diagnostic methods. The clinical triad of fever, leukocytosis, and purulent tracheobronchial secretions has a high prevalence in ARDS uncomplicated by pneumonia. Moreover, the mere presence of pathogenic organisms in respiratory secretions is an unreliable discriminator. Anderson and associates examined autopsies of patients dying with respiratory failure; 58% had histologic pneumonia; however, one third of this group lacked clinical signs of pneumonia. The remaining 42% without histologic evidence of pneumonia had clinical evidence of pneumonia in 20% of the cases. The poor correlation between clinical criteria and histopathology has been duplicated by others. Many investigators have proposed other radiologic or microbiologic criteria to enhance diagnostic accuracy. These include positive blood or pleural fluid cultures and progressive or cavitating radiographic infiltrates; however, the overall sensitivity of such criteria is low.

Sampling of respiratory secretions from the lower respiratory tract with quantitative microbiologic methods has shown a variable correlation with gold-standard definitions of pneumonia. Growth of 10^3 colony-forming units (CFU)/mL from a protected specimen brush (PSB) has correlated with pneumonia in animal and human studies. Quantitative bronchoalveolar lavage (BAL) has a diagnostic threshold of 10^4 CFU/mL; however, it is more prone to contamination with upper airway bacteria than is a PSB. Protected BAL that employs a proximal bronchus-occluding balloon has shown better results (sensitivity 97%, specificity 92%) by reducing contamination. Antibiotic therapy reduces the predictive value of both quantitative PSB and BAL. Thus, when possible, bronchoscopic specimens should be obtained prior to starting antibiotic therapy. Finally, Gram's staining of cytocentrifuged BAL specimens that demonstrate greater than 7% alveolar cells with intracellular organisms is another accurate discriminator of pneumonia (80% predictive value).

The mortality rate of nosocomial pneumonia is reported as between 55% and 75%. When pneumonia and ARDS coexist, mortality is reported as high as 80%. Mortality is also related to the microbial etiology of pneumonia; Fagon has shown significantly greater mortality for pneumonia due to *Pseudomonas* sp., *Acinetobacter* sp., and *S. aureus* than other gram-negative bacilli.

Prevention of pneumonia has centered on the use of selective-digestive decontamination to diminish pathogenic colonization. Although such intervention reduces the frequency of pneumonia, overall mortality remains unchanged. Application of topical antibiotics to the oropharyngeal mucosa is advocated based on animal studies; however, concern exists that such intervention promotes antibiotic resistance. Current investigation is focused upon the reduction of bacterial adherence to the respiratory epithelium and promoting the integrity of the intestinal mucosal barrier to prevent translocation.

CATHETER-RELATED INFECTIONS AND ASSOCIATED BACTEREMIA

Catheter-related bacteremia develops in approximately 50,000 patients annually in the United States. More than 90% of these infections are associated with central venous or arterial catheters. Notably, 45% of these occur in the intensive care unit population, in whom use of such indwelling devices is highest.

Definitions

The terms commonly used in this area are often imprecise and prone to subjective interpretation. The following definitions are generally accepted:

- *Catheter colonization*: ≥ 15 colonies of bacteria (positive semiquantitative culture) in the absence of associated bacteremia or obvious local clinical signs of infection.
- *Catheter-related infection*: a positive semiquantitative culture result with local or systemic signs of infection attributable to the catheter site.
- *Catheter-related bacteremia*: simultaneous isolation of the same organism from a catheter segment (quantitative or semiquantitative methods) and a peripheral blood culture.

Pathogenesis

The prevailing hypothesis for catheter-related bacteremia is that bacteria immediately recolonize the antiseptic-prepared skin at the catheter entrance site. Bacteria may then propagate distally along the external catheter surface within the subcutaneous tract and eventually into the vascular system. The overwhelming majority of catheter-related bacteremias are caused by coagulase-negative staphylococci and *S. aureus*, both of which commonly reside on the skin. These species have also been identified with electron microscopy adhering to the catheter surface. A second mechanism is colonization of the catheter hubs, with distal intraluminal propagation into the circulation. Third, hematogenous seeding of the intravascular portion of the catheter from a distant focus of infection may occur uncommonly. A fourth mechanism is contamination of the infusate, though this risk is considered very low.

Risk Factors

Some common risk factors for infectious catheter complications can potentially be altered or controlled.

ANATOMIC SITE. Recent studies suggest a higher infection rate for central venous and pulmonary arterial catheters inserted via the internal jugular vein when compared with the subclavian vein. This may be due to excessive catheter motion; contamination of the site from respiratory flora, particularly in the presence of a tracheostomy stoma; and difficulty in maintaining a sterile occlusive dressing. When placed and maintained in appropriate fashion, it is notable that femoral venous catheters show no higher infection rate than other sites.

DURATION OF CATHETER SITE USE. The incidence of catheter-related infection is directly proportional to the duration of catheter site use. The rate of infection occurring before 3 days is very low. Global recommendations for the duration of catheter placement at a given site are not applicable to all patients since the likelihood of infection is multifactorial. Catheters should be removed when they are no longer needed or if a catheter-related infection is suspected.

SEVERITY OF ILLNESS. Multiple studies have demonstrated significantly higher rates of catheter-related infection in patients with superimposed sepsis or longer durations of prior hospitalization.

Diagnostic Techniques

The semiquantitative technique developed by Maki and colleagues is the most widely used, based on its proved reliability and simplicity of method. This culture is performed by rolling a 5-cm catheter segment (preferably the intracutaneous segment) across a blood-agar plate and subsequently counting the number of colonies per plate. A positive culture is defined as 15 or more colonies per plate, although a positive culture may represent catheter-related bacteremia, local catheter infection, or catheter colonization.

Cultures of the intracutaneous segment and the tip have the highest diagnostic sensitivity overall. Quantitative blood cultures obtained through the catheter may offer an acceptable diagnostic alternative in those patients with difficult venous access or permanent indwelling devices in whom empiric catheter removal is preferably avoided. Catheters in place for a short time period (less than 5 days) with no clinical suspicion of infection may not require routine culture.

Catheter and Site Maintenance

Two per cent chlorhexidine appears to be the most efficacious cutaneous antiseptic, with a 2.3% incidence of catheter-related infection versus 7.1% and 9.3% for alcohol and povidone-iodine, respectively. Chlorhexidine possesses activity against nearly all nosocomial bacteria and yeasts and provides residual cutaneous antibacterial activity hours after application. Topical antimicrobial combination ointments (e.g., polymyxin-neomycin-bacitracin) confer only modest protection and are used primarily for peripheral catheter sites.

The majority of published investigations strongly suggest that transparent polyurethane dressings actually augment the risk of catheter-related infection for central venous catheters when compared with simple dry gauze dressings. One meta-analysis reported a 53% increased risk for peripheral catheters and a 63% to 78% increased risk for central venous catheters. Transparent dressings trap skin moisture, which creates a favorable condition for bacterial colonization.

Replacement Schedules and Guide Wire Exchange

Recent studies support the general guideline of not routinely changing central venous catheters at a specific time interval since no significant lowering of the infection risk could be demonstrated. Moreover, performing new central venous sticks on a fixed schedule incurs both a higher risk of complications and greater expense. Alternatively, leaving the catheter in place for an indefinite period is problematic since the cumulative risk of infection increases with time. Studies that examined the outcome of catheter sites maintained with the use of a guide wire exchange have shown variable results, ranging from protection against catheter infection to an increased rate of catheter-related bacteremia.

Guide wire exchange is generally an appropriate strategy when a new catheter is needed or when catheter-associated bacteremia is suspected and there is no evidence of established infection at the catheter site. If the semiquantitative culture of the removed catheter is positive, then the new catheter should be removed and replaced with another catheter at a different site. Guide wire exchanges should be performed with a meticulous chlorhexidine scrub of the external catheter surface and a 10-cm circumferential area of skin around the insertion site, followed by an exchange of sterile gloves and application of sterile towels. A sterile guide wire should be inserted into the distal lumen hub, ensuring that the wire does not contact the external surface of the hub. A chest x-ray film generally is not required after guide wire exchange.

Novel Technologies

Several new innovations have shown promising, though not consistent, results in achieving a reduction in catheter-related infection. (1) An attachable subcutaneous cuff of bovine collagen impregnated with silver ions (Vitacuff, Vitaphore Corporation, Plainsboro, NJ) significantly reduced catheter-related infection; however, overall rates of bacteremia were not reduced and the cuff has questionable efficacy against *Candida* species. (2) Antiseptic-coated catheters (silver sulfadiazine and chlorhexidine) achieve a twofold reduction in catheter colonization and a fourfold reduction of bacteremia. (3) Antibiotic-coated catheters have also successfully reduced the rates of catheter-related infection and associated bacteremias.

CENTRAL NERVOUS SYSTEM INFECTION

Infections occurring within the CNS are especially challenging, from both a diagnostic and a therapeutic perspective. A diverse range of pathogens may produce CNS infection; characteristically, however, CNS infection presents as only two stereotypical syndromes: acute meningitis syndrome with rapid onset of symptoms of less than 48 hours, and subacute CNS infection syndrome in which the onset of symptoms is more gradual. Table 8–6 summarizes the etiolo-

Table 8–6. ETIOLOGY OF ACUTE AND SUBACUTE SYNDROMES OF CENTRAL NERVOUS SYSTEM INFECTION

Acute meningitis syndrome (rapid onset [<24–48 h] of fever, headache, and/or meningismus, with early impairment of higher integrative functions)	
Common:	Pyogenic meningitis (pneumococcal, meningococcal, *Haemophilus*, other)
Uncommon:	Viral encephalitis (especially herpes simplex), subarachnoid bleed, and brain tumor (with rupture)
Rare:	Viral meningitis, granulomatous meningitis (cryptococcal, mycobacterial), carcinomatous meningitis, and brain tumor
Subacute CNS infection syndrome (subacute onset [>24–48 h] of fever, headache, and/or meningismus, with no or gradual impairment of higher integrative functions)	
Common:	Viral meningitis, viral encephalitis, pyogenic meningitis
Uncommon:	Brain abscess, brain tumor, granulomatous meningitis
Rare:	Cerebrovascular accident, carcinomatous meningitis

gies of acute and subacute syndromes of CNS infection. Noninfectious pathology, especially neoplasms and hemorrhage, may closely mimic the signs and symptoms of CNS infection.

Bacterial Meningitis

Bacterial meningitis is a pyogenic infection of the cerebral ventricles and subarachnoid space that is usually confined to the CSF. The brain parenchyma is usually not invaded in uncomplicated bacterial meningitis except for neonatal cases of *Citrobacter freundii* and *Haemophilus influenzae* meningitis and *Listeria* meningitis in adults in whom abscess or cerebritis may occur. However, even without parenchymal invasion, significant adverse CNS sequelae may occur because of bacterial toxins, cortical blood vessel occlusion, nerve root damage, hydrocephalus due to impaired CSF flow, and cytokine-induced capillary leakage with edema formation. Infectious agents gain access to the CNS by three principal routes: (1) bacteremia with seeding of the CSF via the vessels supplying the choroid plexus and pia; (2) direct invasion across the meninges (e.g., surgery, trauma, or via emissary veins from contiguous foci); or (3) extension of a parenchymal brain abscess into the CSF.

The limited host defenses of the CNS allow for unimpeded bacterial multiplication. The neutrophil response is normally delayed and qualitatively impaired because of the lack of phagocytic surfaces in the large CSF-filled spaces. CSF contains little immunoglobulin or complement to assist in bacterial killing. This normal deficiency of CNS host defenses explains the necessity for bactericidal antibiotic activity to minimize morbidity and mortality from bacterial meningitis.

Clinical Course

Acute Meningitis Syndrome

Patients presenting with an acute meningitis syndrome exhibit dramatic deterioration once meningeal symptoms (vomiting, stiff neck, headache) appear. Patients appear "toxic," and higher integrative functions may rapidly worsen over hours and culminate in obtundation in severe cases. Focal neurologic signs (excluding Todd's paralysis) or papilledema may be present in meningitis; however, these signs should prompt a diagnostic workup for a focal lesion (abscess).

A "rapid therapy" approach should be implemented for patients with the acute meningitis syndrome. Antibiotics must be administered in the first 30 minutes. Therapeutic delays to perform a difficult lumbar puncture or await the results of CSF studies or radiologic tests are poorly tolerated. A diagnostic and therapeutic algorithm for acute meningitis is shown in Figure 8–1.

Subacute Central Nervous System Infection Syndrome

Bacterial meningitis should be included in the differential diagnosis of patients presenting with a more gradual onset of headache, stiff neck, and fever. Other etiologies may include non-pyogenic organisms (viruses, fungi, *Mycobacterium* sp.), brain abscess, HSV encephalitis, and noninfectious pathology. A "rapid diagnosis" approach is required to pinpoint the cause and begin directed therapy. Laboratory findings that suggest bacterial meningitis include a peripheral leukocyte count of over 10,000/mm^3, CSF pleocytosis greater than 1000/mm^3, CSF protein greater than 100 mg/dL, or CSF glucose less than 40 mg/dL. An antibiotic should be administered empirically within several hours when there is positive or suggestive evidence for a bacterial etiology. A diagnostic and therapeutic algorithm for subacute meningitis syndrome is shown in Figure 8–2.

Therapy of Bacterial Meningitis

Most cases of community-acquired bacterial meningitis in previously healthy adults are caused by *S. pneumoniae*, *Neisseria meningitidis*, and rarely *H. influenzae*. High-dose parenteral penicillin (18 to 24 million U/day) traditionally has been the antibiotic of choice. However, the increasing prevalence of penicillin resistance among pneumococci—intermediate resistance (minimum inhibitory concentration over 0.1 μg/mL) or highly resistant (minimum inhibitory concentration greater than 1.0 μg/mL)—has necessitated changes in the therapeutic approach. Thus, initial therapy for adults with community-acquired bacterial meningitis should include a third-generation cephalosporin (cefotaxime, ceftriaxone) that has activity against penicillin-resistant pneumococci. Suspected or documented cephalosporin-resistant pneumococci require parenteral vancomycin. Despite

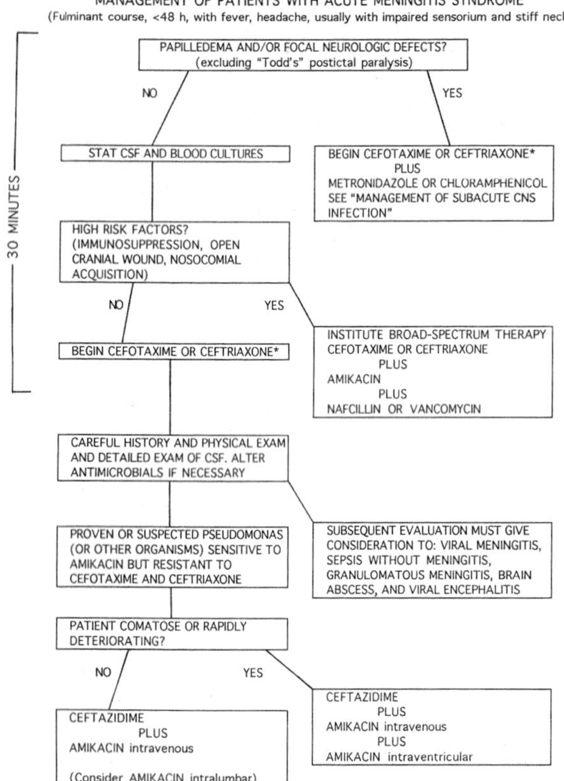

Figure 8–1. Algorithm for the management of patients with the acute meningitis syndrome. (*Consider adding vancomycin as empiric coverage against high-level penicillin-resistant pneumococci that may also be resistant to cephalosporins. See Table 139–3 in the *Textbook of Critical Care* for specific antimicrobial doses.)

its excellent CNS penetration and in vitro activity, chloramphenicol has been associated with clinical failures in high-level, penicillin-resistant pneumococcal meningitis. Elderly or immunosuppressed patients may develop meningitis caused by gram-negative bacilli or *Listeria monocytogenes*. Ceftazidime (8 g/day) is the preferred third-generation cephalosporin for enteric gram-negative meningitis, whereas high-dose ampicillin (12 g/day) is indicated for *Listeria*. Intraventricular aminoglycoside administration may be required for poor responders to cephalosporin or for multiresistant gram-negative bacilli.

Meningitis due to *S. aureus* should be clinically suspected in neurosurgical patients, trauma patients with CSF communicating injuries, or patients with concomitant or recent seri-

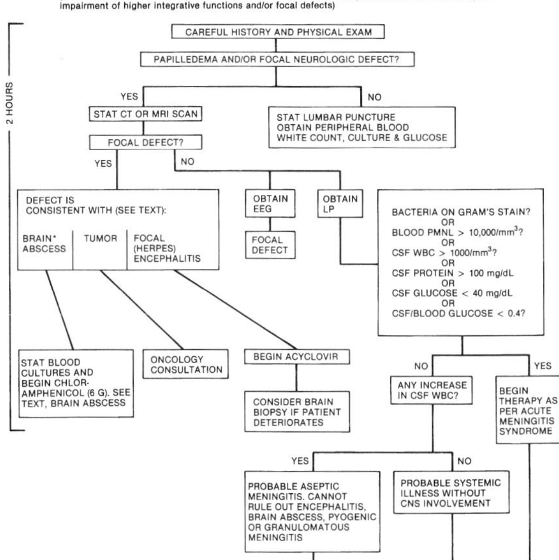

Figure 8–2. Algorithm for the management of patients with subacute CNS infection syndrome. (*If CT not diagnostic, multiple antimicrobial therapy may be indicated pending further evaluation.)

ous staphylococcal infection (endocarditis, pneumonia). Nafcillin (12 g/day) is adequate for methicillin-susceptible strains; however, vancomycin is required for methicillin-resistant strains.

The duration of antibiotic therapy depends on the inciting pathogen and the clinical response. Pneumococcal and meningococcal meningitides usually fail to relapse after 7 days of appropriate parenteral antibiotics. The response to meningitis due to gram-negative bacilli is more variable. In poor responders, repeat CSF cultures and Gram's stain should be monitored on a daily basis. Antibiotic therapy is recommended to extend an additional 7 days after CSF cultures become sterilized. Unexplained persistence of fever or neurologic relapse requires appropriate tests for a brain abscess, a parameningeal collection, or endocarditis.

Adjunctive treatment of bacterial meningitis with corticosteroids has been shown only to benefit children with *H. influenzae* meningitis (intravenous dexamethasone, 0.6 mg/kg/day for 4 days). Although anecdotal reports show a benefit of corticosteroids in adult meningitis for intracranial hypertension, routine corticosteroid use for adults is not advised.

Meningitis may occur in the setting of concomitant sepsis from an extra-CNS source, or, less commonly, meningitis may seed the bloodstream and cause a secondary sepsis. Meningococcemia with sepsis is an especially fulminant syndrome with a high case-fatality rate. Hypotension in that setting may reflect adrenal insufficiency that does require steroid replacement.

Other local complications include the impairment of cranial and spinal nerve roots, cerebral infarction, hydrocephalus, and subdural effusion. Fifteen per cent of patients experience impaired ocular movement, and eleven per cent develop hemiparesis or quadriparesis. Focal defects may resolve during recovery.

Brain Abscess

A brain abscess develops from a localized area of parenchymal cellulitis and culminates in frank necrosis and suppuration. Characteristically, a hyperemic peripheral capsule and some degree of edema surround the inflammatory area. The underlying presumed cause of brain abscess has changed from an untreated contiguous focus (middle ear, mastoids, sinuses) in the preantibiotic era to hematogenous spread from distant foci of infection or unknown primary sites. Aerobic and anaerobic streptococci are the most common isolated species. Other causes include enteric gram-negative bacilli, staphylococci, pneumococci, *Nocardia* sp., *Aspergillus* sp., and amebae.

Clinical Course

The symptoms and signs from brain abscess usually evolve in a subacute fashion (7 to 14 days) and include headache, low-grade fever, and focal neurologic signs. Asymptomatic lesions that suddenly rupture into the ventricles or subarachnoid space will cause dramatic acute deterioration. Other specific CNS signs relate to the size and location of the abscess and are difficult to distinguish clinically from other space-occupying lesions. Examination of CSF may demonstrate a pleocytosis, elevated protein, and normal or decreased glucose. Lumbar puncture should be avoided in the presence of focal lesions with mass effect, edema, or midline shift because of the risk of cerebral herniation.

Computed Tomography and Magnetic Resonance Imaging

Both these imaging techniques are valuable in assessing the response to therapy and the need for surgical or radiographically guided drainage or just continued surveillance. CT scanning has limited sensitivity in detecting cerebritis, microabscesses, and brain stem and cerebellar lesions. Gadolinium-enhanced MRI is superior for the detection of such lesions.

Therapy

The selection of antibiotics is based on the results of aspirate cultures and ability to cross the blood-brain barrier. If available, positive cultures from extra-CNS suppurative foci or the blood may guide the initial therapeutic regimen. Therapeutic neurosurgical intervention is required for deterioration caused by space-occupying effect, aspiration to obtain specimens for culture, and abscesses that fail to respond to antibiotics. Corticosteroids should be reserved for clinically significant edema.

Viral Infections of the Central Nervous System

All components of the CNS are vulnerable to viral infection. The dominant clinical syndrome may be a meningitis, encephalitis, or myelitis or a combination of these. CNS invasion is usually secondary to viremic seeding from a primary extraneural site of viral invasion and replication. A second major route of CNS access is neuronal spread (e.g., rabies virus, HSV). Viruses exhibit a selective affinity for regions of the CNS; enteroviruses and mumps viruses usually involve the ependyma and subarachnoid space; arthropod-borne and rabies viruses involve the parenchyma and cause encephalitis; and HSV-I causes temporal lobe encephalitis whereas HSV-II usually causes meningitis. Such affinities are not absolute.

Acute Viral Meningitis

This entity is commonly termed *aseptic meningitis,* since no CSF pathogen is isolated. Viral meningitis is rarely seen after age 40 years. Peak incidence is during the summer or fall. Patients are usually otherwise healthy young adults with a several-day prodrome of constitutional symptoms (chills, myalgias, malaise) culminating in headache, photophobia, stiff neck, nausea, and vomiting. CSF findings consist of a lymphocytic pleocytosis (neutrophils may predominate very early in the syndrome), a normal glucose level, and mild protein elevation. Symptoms are self-limiting, with resolution of meningeal signs in 7 to 10 days, though constitutional symptoms may persist for up to 6 weeks.

Viral Encephalitis

An impaired level of consciousness disproportionate to the degree of systemic illness is the hallmark symptom of encephalitis. Actual parenchymal invasion by the virus occurs. The presentation is typically an acute febrile illness with headache. Other neurologic signs may include behavioral or speech disturbances, seizures, or hemiparesis.

Herpes Simplex Encephalitis

HSV encephalitis is distinguished from the great majority of viral encephalitides because it is treatable with early administration of intravenous acyclovir. The mortality of untreated cases may exceed 70%. The temporal lobes are the predominant site, which results in aphasia, anosmia, temporal lobe seizures, and focal neurologic defects. The level of consciousness may range from mild confusion to lethargy or frank coma. Temporal localization is demonstrable by electroencephalogram, CT, and MRI. Suggestive clinical and radiologic findings should prompt empiric intravenous acyclovir (15 mg/kg/day for 10 or more days) therapy since a definitive early diagnosis may be difficult to achieve. CSF polymerase chain reaction is often diagnostic. A rising titer of HSV antibodies in the CSF is also confirmatory; however, this may not occur until 1 week or more into the illness.

CNS Infection and Patients with AIDS

Owing to the high incidence of CNS pathology in AIDS, the presence of headache or altered mental status requires an anatomic study (CT, MRI) to rule out a mass lesion(s). The three most common lesions are toxoplasmosis, lymphoma, and progressive multifocal leukoencephalopathy. Contrast enhancement is usually present in toxoplasmosis and lymphoma; however, radiologic distinction between the two may be difficult. The absence of serum *Toxoplasma* antibodies (at 1:2 dilution or greater) makes the diagnosis of toxoplasmosis very improbable. Toxoplasmosis is quite responsive to antimicrobial therapy (pyrimethamine/sulfadiazine), but lifelong therapy is required to prevent relapse.

Cryptococcal meningitis is another common CNS infection in the AIDS population that rarely presents with a mass lesion. Several features that distinguish cryptococcal meningitis in AIDS from transplant recipients are the higher serum and CSF titers, and higher rates of relapse in AIDS patients (see Infection After Solid Organ Transplantation).

Paradural Abscess

Anatomic differences favor the occurrence of abscess formation in the subdural space in the skull and the epidural space in the vertebral column. Precipitating causes for both are usually contiguous infection, surgery, trauma, or hematogenous spread.

CRANIAL SUBDURAL ABSCESS (EMPYEMA). This has a symptom complex similar to brain abscess. The paranasal sinuses, ears, and mastoids are the most common primary sites of infection. Nonhemolytic streptococci, pneumococci, *Haemophilus* sp., anaerobes, and staphylococci cause most infections. Gram-negative enteric bacilli may be associated with middle ear and mastoid sources.

SPINAL EPIDURAL ABSCESS. This classically evolves through four clinical phases: (1) spinal ache, or "backpain"; (2) nerve root pain; (3) radicular weakness; and (4) paralysis. Any patient with back pain associated with fever, localized vertebral tenderness, and sensory or motor deficits should be considered to have a spinal epidural abscess until proved otherwise. MRI is the most sensitive screening study and may confirm the presence of cord compression, drainable paraspinal foci, and concomitant vertebral osteomyelitis. The differential diagnosis should include degenerative disk disease and metastatic tumor. Clinical differentiation may be achievable by MRI or may require neurosurgical exploration.

Emergency neurosurgical decompression is indicated to relieve incipient or actual cord compression, for debridement, and to obtain specimens for Gram's stain and culture. Conservative management with parenteral antibiotics only has been successful in patients who have no initial neurologic signs and show early resolution of their back pain and leukocytosis. However, appropriate caution is advised since dramatic neurologic deterioration may occur weeks into conservative therapy. *S. aureus* causes the majority of community-acquired spinal epidural abscesses and can be treated with nafcillin. Vancomycin is indicated when the prevalence of methicillin-resistant *S. aureus* is high. Risk factors for a gram-negative bacilli include recent urinary tract infection, decubitus ulcers, and vertebral surgery. In such instances, a third-generation cephalosporin with or without an aminoglycoside should be administered until definitive culture results are available.

A diagnostic and treatment algorithm is shown in Figure 8–3.

LABORATORY DIAGNOSIS OF INFECTION

Specimen Collection

Clinical interpretation of microbiologic tests depends upon the proper collection, transportation, and processing of the specimen. Specimens obtained from normally sterile body sites (e.g., blood, CSF, joint fluid) should not be contaminated by indigenous flora of the skin or mucous membranes. If possible, tissue specimens are preferable to swab specimens. Transportation to the laboratory should be prompt and in a vehicle that prevents contamination and preserves fastidious organisms. Antibiotic therapy should be deferred prior to specimen collection if the clinical situation permits.

Respiratory Specimens

Bronchoscopic methods that obtain lower respiratory specimens while avoiding oropharyngeal contamination are discussed in the section on Bacterial Pneumonia in Adult Respiratory Distress Syndrome. Local anesthetic agents (e.g., lidocaine) that are usually applied during bronchoscopy should be avoided as they possess antibacterial activity. In nonintubated patients who are unable to expectorate sputum, transtracheal aspiration is an option; however, it is less commonly used now due to the ease of bronchoscopic sampling and has associated complications (hemoptysis, subcutaneous emphysema, aspiration, and cellulitis).

Blood Specimens

Demonstration of pathogens in the bloodstream is often the first confirmation of underlying infection and allows directed antimicrobial therapy. Blood is ideally collected by direct venipuncture with sterile needle and syringe or vacuum tube sets. Blood collection performed exclusively from

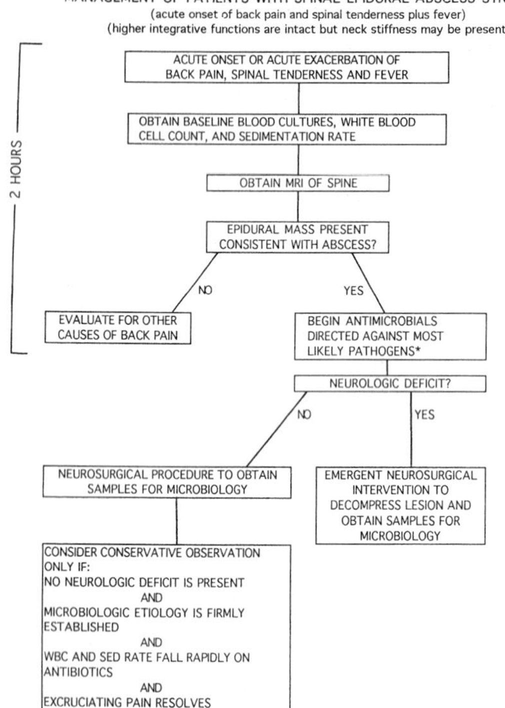

Figure 8–3. Algorithm for the management of patients with spinal epidural abscess syndrome. If MRI cannot be performed, myelography (the lateral cervical approach may be required), high-contrast CT, or CT-myelography may be an acceptable alternative to localize an epidural abscess. (*If abscess drainage can be performed promptly, antimicrobial drugs may be withheld until specimens for microbiologic analysis are obtained; they can then be immediately administered in the operating room or radiology suite.)

indwelling catheters should be avoided since positive results may indicate hub or lumen colonization only rather than true bacteremia. Skin should be sequentially disinfected with 70% alcohol, followed by 2% iodine or iodophor for 1 minute. The volume of collected blood depends upon the volume of broth in the commercial blood culture system; the optimal ratio of blood to broth is 1:10 per bottle. Bacteremia is best detected by drawing two or three blood culture sets over several hours from different venipuncture sites. Practically, it may be possible to obtain only two sets just minutes apart due to the need for antibiotics in rapidly deteriorating patients. Special bottles with antibiotic-neutralizing resins are an alternative in the antibiotic-treated patient.

Urine Specimens

Critically ill patients usually have urine specimens collected from an indwelling bladder catheter. The proper collection method is with a needle and syringe through the clamped catheter tubing. Urine catheter tips should not be submitted for culture as they may reflect only catheter colonization. Urine specimens should be transported to the laboratory as soon as possible and set up for culture within an hour of collection.

Direct Examination of Specimens

Direct microscopic examinations are categorized as either wet mounts or stained smears. In critically ill patients, their rapid availability enhances their diagnostic value in early management of infections.

Wet Mounts

The selection of techniques for direct examination of a fluid specimen depends on the clinical suspicion for a particular organism: (1) phase contrast (bacteria, spirochetes), (2) India ink (*Cryptococcus*), or (3) potassium hydroxide (fungi).

Stained Smears

Gram's Stain

Gram-stained smears of body fluids may demonstrate both inflammatory cells and the morphology and staining characteristics of bacteria. Overinterpretation of the stain should be avoided, particularly in abscesses or from antibiotic-treated patients, since such conditions may alter the predicted appearance of bacteria. Gram's stain of certain specimens may also provide information about the quality of the specimen (e.g., squamous epithelial cells in sputum demonstrate oropharyngeal contamination) or may predict a significant culture threshold (e.g., two or more bacteria per oil-immersion field of unspun urine predict significant bacteriuria).

Acid-Fast and Fluorescent Stains

Mycobacteria resist acid decolorization, which allows their identification by either the Ziehl-Neelsen method (hot carbolfuchsin) or the Kinyoun method (cold concentrated carbolfuchsin). Both methods will stain mycobacteria red in sputum and other specimens. Auramine will stain mycobacteria a bright yellow under fluorescent illumination.

Fluorescein-tagged fluorescent antibody stains may demonstrate a wide range of respiratory pathogens (*Legionella* sp., *P. carinii, Francisella tularensis*, and certain viruses). Silver staining is the method of choice for fungi in tissue or for *P. carinii*, and Giemsa stains of blood smears are the common method to detect malarial parasites.

Detection of Microbial Products

Counterimmunoelectrophoresis (CIE) is the established method for the detection of capsular polysaccharide antigens of *H. influenzae, S. pneumoniae*, and *N. meningitidis* in CSF. Some laboratories will perform CIE on serum, sputum, and urine, although careful clinical discrimination is required since the specificity and sensitivity in these specimens is less than that for CSF. Latex agglutination for cryptococcal antigen is highly sensitive in CSF and to a somewhat lesser extent in serum. Enzyme-linked immunosorbent assay (ELISA) has shown high sensitivity for detection of antigens from rotavirus, gonorrhea, and *L. pneumophila*.

Culture Methods

Physicians need to be aware of which culture methods are routine and which require special collection methods or specific communication with their microbiology laboratory or referral laboratory. Specimens are usually processed for groups of organisms, such as rapidly growing bacteria (aerobic and anaerobic), mycobacteria, fungi, chlamydiae, and viruses. Rapidly growing bacteria are usually isolated by inoculating a variety of agar media that are incubated aerobically or anaerobically. Common bacteria can usually be isolated on blood agar, whereas fastidious organisms (*Haemophilus* and *Neisseria* sp.) require an enrichment media such as chocolate agar. MacConkey agar is a selective agar for the growth of enteric gram-negative bacilli.

Mycobacteria can be isolated on specialized media (Löwenstein-Jensen) between 2 and 6 weeks, depending on the species. Detection within a week is possible using liquid media containing ^{14}C-labeled substrates.

Fungi may grow on routine bacterial media made selective with the addition of antibacterial agents. Some species may be slow growing and require incubation at 30°C and 37°C. The lysis-centrifugation method (isolator tubes) may enhance the isolation of molds from the bloodstream.

Viruses and chlamydiae can be isolated by animal inoculation, or by inoculation of egg embryos or mammalian cell cultures. Cell culture methods (e.g., human foreskin fibroblast) may support the isolation of some viruses.

Respiratory Specimens

Sputum, transtracheal aspirates, and bronchoscopic specimens are usually cultured on blood agar with CO_2 (pneumococci, staphylococci), chocolate agar with CO_2 (*Haemophilus* sp.), and MacConkey agar (gram-negative bacilli). Mycobacteria and fungi require prolonged aerobic incubation. *Legionella* species require selective media (charcoal-yeast extract) but usually grow within 5 days.

Blood Specimens

After the inoculation of blood into liquid medium and incubation at 35°C, examinations are performed several times daily for turbidity and measurement of CO_2 release from ^{14}C-labeled substrate. Blind subcultures of negative broths can also be performed. Special methods are required for slow-growing organisms (*Brucella* sp., yeasts), and those from antibiotic-treated patients (resin-removal bottles or lysis centrifugation).

Urine Specimens

Quantification of organisms is used to differentiate bladder or upper urinary tract infection (over 100,000 organisms/mL) from urethral and perineal contaminated specimens (less than 10,000 mixed organisms/mL). However, any growth of a potential pathogen may be significant in catheter or suprapubic specimens or in urine specimens from antibiotic-treated patients.

Antimicrobial Susceptibility Tests

Rapid and accurate susceptibility testing of bacteria is critical for guiding antibiotic selection in critically ill patients. In vitro susceptibility is only one of many factors (native host defenses, inherent severity of the infecting agent(s), and surgical drainage) that determine outcome. Organisms are regarded as susceptible if they are inhibited in vitro by a concentration of the antibiotic that is lower than achievable serum concentration with the usual dosage. Susceptibility and resistance are expressed as the minimal inhibitory concentration (MIC) of the antibiotic required to inhibit growth of a defined population of organisms.

MIC determinations are performed by the inoculation of 10^5 organisms/mL into serial twofold dilutions of antimicrobial agents in tubes (macrobroth method) or microtiter wells (microdilution method). The macrodilution method is reliable but time consuming and expensive. The microdilution method produces comparable results to the macrobroth method for gram-positive organisms; however, it produces onefold lower dilution results for enteric gram-negative bacilli. Agar dilution is a third method, in which 10^4 organisms/mL are inoculated onto antimicrobe-containing plates.

MICs should generally be at least twofold to fourfold lower than the mean achievable antibiotic level. Most laboratories deliver a qualitative report expressed by predetermined resistance categories based on achievable serum antibiotic concentrations. Many laboratories perform the disk diffusion method for the majority of nonblood bacterial isolates. Disk diffusion measures the zone of growth inhibition around an antimicrobe-containing disk. Results are reported as susceptible, intermediate, or resistant. Anaerobes cannot be tested by disk diffusion.

Both MIC and disk diffusion methods require overnight incubation in addition to the 24 hours required to isolate the organism. Automated systems that determine susceptibility based on photometric methods have a much shorter turnaround time (3 to 7 hours) and are comparable to MIC results provided there is strict adherence to the manufacturers' guidelines. Such systems are especially valuable to the critically ill patient in whom prompt and appropriate antibiotic selection may greatly influence outcome.

For all methods, the choice of antimicrobial agents to be tested depends on the organism, site of isolation, and local patterns of susceptibility and antimicrobial usage. Some laboratories will test only certain antimicrobial agents if in vitro resistance has already been shown to a panel of conventional agents. Special testing for beta-lactamase production is important for *H. influenzae* and *S. aureus*. Testing for synergy between combinations of antibiotics is usually not required, since in vivo synergy is usually predictable for common combinations of agents, such as beta-lactams and aminoglycosides.

Monitoring Antimicrobial Levels

Measurement of concentrations of antimicrobial agents in serum and other body fluids can confirm that therapeutic drug levels are present while potentially toxic levels are avoided. Gentamicin and tobramycin trough levels of greater than 2 μg/mL and amikacin levels of greater than 10 μg/mL are associated with nephrotoxicity. Reversible hematopoietic toxicity due to chloramphenicol occurs with serum concentrations of greater than 25 μg/mL. To ensure interpretability of the result, all specimens must indicate the sampling time; time, dose, and route of administration; and concomitant drugs being administered.

ANTIMICROBIAL THERAPY IN THE CRITICAL CARE SETTING

Selection of Antibiotics

Several historic and clinical factors must be considered when deciding on the empiric antibiotic regimen in a critically ill patient: (1) Is the infection community-acquired or hospital-acquired? The susceptibility of the inciting pathogen(s) in a community-acquired infection is invariably broader than hospital-acquired flora in which complex antimicrobial resistance patterns are commonly established. (2) What is the patient's underlying disease(s)? Certain conditions predispose to infection with a stereotypic range of organisms owing to specific defects in the host defense (e.g., diabetics experience polymicrobial infections with *S. aureus* and anaerobes). (3) What is the suspected primary focus of infection? There is a predictable association of the anatomic focus and the endogenous colonizing microflora, even with anatomic or functional abnormalities. (4) Has the patient received antibiotics in the recent past? Infections occurring during or shortly after antibiotic therapy are likely to be caused by a more resistant pathogen. Additionally, patients who develop infection while on antibiotics may have growth suppression in the actual culture specimen, resulting in false-negative results.

The appropriate selection of antimicrobials for empiric therapy also has an important pharmacologic foundation. (1) Bactericidal antibiotics kill bacteria without the assistance of native host defenses whereas bacteriostatic agents provide adequate therapy when host defenses are intact. Antibiotics with cell wall activity (natural and semisynthetic penicillins, cephalosporins, vancomycin) are generally bactericidal; however, they possess only bacteriostatic activity against enterococci (cephalosporins have no enterococcal activity). Classic examples of bacteriostatic antibiotics include the tetracyclines, macrolides, and clindamycin. Though bactericidal activity offers theoretical advantages, the only three proved clinical situations in which a beneficial outcome is evident are meningitis, infective endocarditis, and serious infection in the neutropenic host.

(2) The antibiotic susceptibility pattern of the pathogen(s) within the institution should be a major determinant of the choice of antibiotic(s). It is not uncommon that the microflora prevalent in the ICU population have the highest rates of multidrug resistance, particularly among certain species (e.g., *S. aureus, Enterococcus faecium, Pseudomonas* sp., *Enterobacter* sp.).

(3) The distribution and elimination characteristics of the antibiotic. Infections confined to specific fluid compartments such as bile, urine, or CSF may be refractory to antibiotic therapy despite in vitro activity if the agent does not reach adequate levels at that site. Toxicities may also be potentiated by preexisting impairment of the major elimination route of the antibiotic.

(4) Dose and dosing intervals should be chosen based on the pathogen's MIC, severity of infection, patient size, and ease of drug elimination.

(5) The toxicity profile of the antibiotic is important for the overall clinical outcome. Factors that contribute to toxicity may be avoided or monitored.

When culture and sensitivity results are available, the antibiotic regimen should be reassessed and tailored to the narrowest effective spectrum, with the least toxic and least expensive agents. Such practice will reduce the risks of superinfection and antibiotic-related complications (*C. difficile* colitis, antibiotic-associated diarrhea). The long-term benefit of selective antibiotic use is to minimize the "antibiotic pressure," which promotes antimicrobial resistance in the overall hospital and ICU patient population.

The details of the pharmacokinetics and pharmacodynamics of the major antibiotic classes are beyond the scope of this text. This material was extensively covered in Chapter 133 of *Textbook of Critical Care.*

CHAPTER 9
Hematology/Oncology

Herbert E. Jacob, MD, FACP, FCCP

HEMATOLOGY

Diagnosis and Management of Bleeding Disorders

Approximately 80,000 patients die each year in the United States of uncontrolled bleeding, and 50% of all deaths in this country can be attributed to thrombotic disorders like myocardial infarction, cerebrovascular accident, or pulmonary embolism. Thus, disorders of hemostasis transcend all medical specialties. The ability to establish an accurate diagnosis rapidly and institute appropriate therapy represents a major challenge to the critical care physician.

Normal Hemostasis

Three ingredients are required for normal clotting to occur. After a vessel is severed, it must retract and constrict, functioning platelets must be available in adequate numbers (the formation of the white thrombus), and adequate and functional coagulation proteins must be available to generate the fibrin mesh (red thrombus).

The injury of the vessel exposes subendothelial connective tissue, of which microfibrils and collagen are the most important constituent. Platelets adhere to the exposed collagen and release a number of substances stored in the alpha granules and dense bodies, including thromboxane A_2, which cause more platelets to aggregate and thus form the platelet plug (white thrombus) that temporarily seals the vessel. The activated platelet also undergoes membrane changes, making it possible to assemble clotting factors on its surface that ultimately generate thrombin, the enzyme responsible for fibrinogen activation.

Bleeding could occur if platelets are not present in sufficient numbers or are functionally deficient to form the white thrombus or if there is some problem with the coagulation system such that functional fibrin is not deposited in and around the white thrombus. In this case, after an initial period of hemostasis, the white thrombus will break up and rebleeding will occur.

The history and physical examination can give clues as to whether the patient suffers from a platelet-related bleeding problem or disorder of fibrin formation. With rare exceptions (Fanconi's anemia, Wiskott-Aldrich syndrome, and so on), platelet-related bleeding (either qualitative or quantitative) is acquired so that a history of lifelong bleeding is lacking. Also, the presentation of bleeding is typically muco-

The author wishes to acknowledge the helpful review of Ake Grenvik, M.D., and the secretarial contribution of Miss Barbara A. Burgman in the preparation of this manuscript.

sal in origin, including the skin, mucous membranes, epistaxis, or gastrointestinal bleeding. When bleeding in the muscle and joints is the presentation, a defect in the fibrin-forming mechanism should be suspected. With the exception of the rare acquired factor inhibitors, these bleeding disorders are most often present from a young age.

Quantitative Platelet Disorders

Patients are thrombocytopenic for one of two reasons. Either they are not producing platelets or they are destroying them at a rate faster than they can compensate for. Thus, a bone marrow examination to assess the presence of megakaryocytes is often required. Thrombocytopenia and an otherwise normal marrow with "increased" megakaryocytes suggest a problem of increased platelet destruction, as the normal bone marrow can boost platelet production tenfold, whereas a reduction or absence in the marrow of the megakaryocyte is often associated with bone marrow pathology (tumor infiltration, leukemia, aplasia, myelodysplasia, granulomas, fibrosis, or even thiazide diuretics, ethanol, megaloblastic anemia from B_{12} or folate deficiency, or even severe iron deficiency).

When increased platelet destruction is suspected, this is often caused by drugs, thrombotic thrombocytopenic purpura (TTP), hypersplenism in the setting of splenomegaly, DIC (disseminated intravascular coagulation), or immune mechanisms. The most common immune mechanism is idiopathic [autoimmune] thrombocytopenic purpura (ITP). ITP has two basic forms, an acute form most often seen in children, which is usually associated with a viral illness and spontaneously remits; and a chronic, more insidious form, usually seen in adults. In adults, the treatments tried are numerous, including splenectomy, steroids, plasmapheresis, and the use of gamma globulin infusions. This last modality is often used to raise the platelet count transiently in patients with ITP before surgery. The currently recommended dose of IGG is 400 mg/kg body weight daily for 5 days. This can be expected to raise the platelet count in two thirds of patients for a few days to a few weeks.

Qualitative Platelet Defects

Platelet dysfunction will present with bleeding similar to thrombocytopenic bleeding (i.e., predominantly skin and mucous membrane bleeding). Functional platelet defects include congenital diseases such as (1) Glanzmann's thrombasthenia and the Bernard-Soulier syndrome, in which the absence of glycoprotein in the platelet membrane prevents platelet adhesion to connective tissue, their aggregation, and thus white thrombus production; (2) storage pool defects in which platelet storage pools are deficient in various substances (like adenosine diphosphate) necessary to propagate platelet aggregation; and (3) von Willebrand's disease, which is not a primary platelet disorder but a defect of the von Willebrand Factor (part of the factor VIII molecule) necessary for platelet adhesion. The most common clinical platelet dysfunctions seen in critical care are associated with various drugs that inhibit normal platelet function. Leading the list is aspirin, other nonsteroidal anti-inflammatories, and several antibiotics including the β-lactams. A clinically significant but poorly understood acquired platelet dysfunction is associated with uremia. DDAVP (1-deamino-(8-D-arginine)-vasopressin) in a dose of 0.3 μg/kg can be tried acutely while dialysis is considered. This drug, in the same dose, is often used in certain forms of von Willebrand's disease to boost Factor VIII levels temporarily for surgery.

Disorders of the Coagulation System

Normal Coagulation System

By international convention, the clotting proteins have been assigned roman numerals and the activated counterpart with the subscript a. Despite this attempt at standardization, several of the clotting factors are still referred to by their names. For example, Factor II is often referred to as prothrombin, Factor IIa is thrombin, and Factor I is fibrinogen. Although multiple interactions are known about the coagulation cascade in vivo, this elegant system can be conceptualized in a fairly simplistic way. Remembering that normal coagulation requires ionized calcium, appropriate temperature (clotting deteriorates as temperature falls), interaction of tissue factors, natural anticoagulants such as proteins S and C, and antithrombin III and functional platelets, we can simplify the coagulation system and conceptualize it in a clinically relevant form. This system can be divided into two pathways, intrinsic and extrinsic. The intrinsic system operates using components found only within the circulation, whereas the extrinsic system requires tissue factors in addition to coagulation factors. The following schematic illustration is a simplified representation of this interaction between the clotting factors.

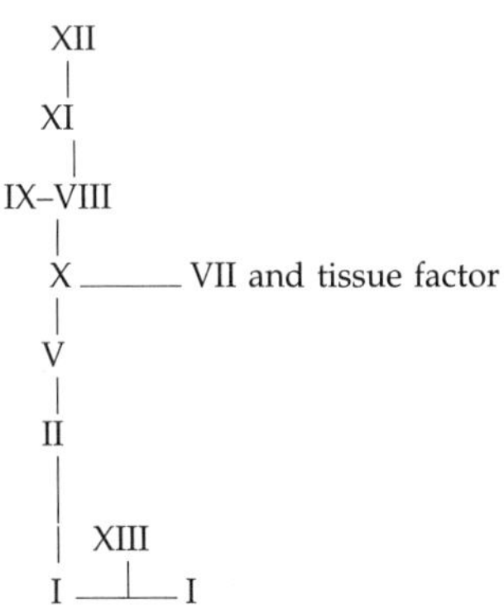

Factors XII, XI, IX, and VIII are the factors exclusively related to the intrinsic pathway. Factor VII is exclusively related to the extrinsic pathway. Factors X, V, II, I, and XIII make up the common pathway. Thus, conceptually, a cascade is produced by which Factor XII, after its activation, activates

Factor XI, which activates Factors IX and VIII, which in turn activate Factor X, and so on. Additionally, activated Factor VII can also activate Factor X. This illustration also has the benefit of helping the clinician interpret the results of two commonly used coagulation tests, the prothrombin time (PT) and the activated partial thromboplastin time (aPTT). The PT tests the adequacy of the extrinsic and common pathway, whereas the aPTT tests the adequacy of the intrinsic and common pathway. The three possible abnormal results of these two tests (PT increased, aPTT normal; PT increased, aPTT increased; PT normal, aPTT increased) can be quickly interpreted so the potential cause might more easily be identified.

When the PT is increased and the aPTT is normal, a defect or inhibitor must involve Factor VII alone. When both the PT and aPTT are increased, the defect or inhibitor must at least involve one or more of the factors of the common pathway (X, V, II, I). Factor XIII deficiency is not associated with a prolonged PT or aPTT. When the PT is normal and the aPTT is increased, then the deficit or inhibition involves one or more of the intrinsic pathway components (XII, XI, IX, VIII). It is also important to remember that the vitamin K–dependent factors (II, VII, IX, X) are involved in all three pathways (i.e., II and X, common; VII, extrinsic; IX, intrinsic). It is thus easy to see that heparin (acting as the cofactor of antithrombin III and thus inhibiting the activation of both Factors II and X) would prolong both the PT and aPTT, as could warfarin through its effect on the vitamin K–dependent factors. Additionally, a patient with a lifelong history of bleeding and a normal PT and prolonged aPTT would in all likelihood have Factor VIII deficiency (hemophilia A), or Factor IX deficiency (hemophilia B), or Factor XI deficiency (hemophilia C), or perhaps von Willebrand's disease.

A patient with Factor XII deficiency (Hageman Factor) will not have a clinical history or problem with bleeding despite the prolonged aPTT. A patient with Factor XIII deficiency will have a bleeding diathesis but normal PT and aPTT. Hemophilia A and B are both transmitted via the sex-linked recessive mode of inheritance. Thus, females born to a hemophilic father will be carriers and the males born to a carrier will have a 50% chance of having the disease. The other congenital coagulation deficiencies affect males and females equally. It is also important to remember that 25% to 30% of cases of hemophilia A and 20% of cases of hemophilia B appear without a known family history and thus likely represent gene mutations.

Hemophilia A can be a disease with a broad range of severity depending on the ability to produce some Factor VIII. For example, mild hemophilia may be present with an aPTT at the upper limit of normal, a Factor VIII level of 25% of normal, and no clinical symptoms until trauma or unplanned surgical stress of the coagulation system occurs. At the other end of the spectrum is the severe hemophiliac with less than 1% Factor VIII levels and a significantly prolonged aPTT. Here, symptoms of bleeding are likely to have been present from a few months of age, with a progressive and deforming arthritis due to recurrent hemarthrosis.

Unfortunately, specific factor assays are not universally available so that critical care physicians, when confronted with the bleeding patient, must act on limited information. These generalizations and some additional ones to be reviewed should be adequate for acute stabilization.

Liver Disease

The liver is the site of synthesis of all the procoagulants, with the likely exceptions of Factor VIII_c (Factor VIII:coagulant). The first factors to be affected in liver disease are the vitamin K–dependent factors (II, VII, IX, and X), followed by Factors V, XI, and XII. Cholestasis, malabsorption, and broad-spectrum antibiotics will further suppress the synthesis of the vitamin K–dependent factors. It is for this reason that vitamin K_1 is administered (usually in a dose of 5 to 10 mg IV) in an effort to reverse some or all of the coagulopathy. Fibrinogen synthesis remains normal until end-stage liver disease is present. Thus, a low level of fibrinogen (Factor I) in severe liver disease (in the absence of DIC) is an ominous prognostic sign. Acquired dysfibrinogenemia is a problem seen in patients with cirrhosis or hepatoma. This abnormal protein converts to fibrin monomers normally but polymerizes slowly and inefficiently. Since the PT and aPTT results depend on the speed of appearance of visible fibrin clot, these results will be prolonged, which might confuse the clinical picture. Identification of dysfibrinogen is made using special testing techniques.

Besides the coagulopathies directly related to the liver's synthetic function, several other problems can be present. Thrombocytopenia may be due to hypersplenism secondary to significant portal hypertension or folate deficiency. Acute ethanol intoxication has direct toxic effects on the megalokaryocyte that can lead to reversible thrombocytopenia. Finally, the diseased liver will not be able to clear activated clotting factors normally, perhaps leading to DIC.

Disseminated Intravascular Coagulation

DIC is a hematologic complication associated with a wide variety of diseases and clinical situations, thus essentially guaranteeing all practitioners exposure to it. In severe cases, fibrin is deposited in the microcirculation, and clotting factors and platelets are consumed in excess of the liver's and bone marrow's ability to compensate (the intact liver can increase the synthesis of fibrinogen fivefold whereas the bone marrow can increase platelet production tenfold). The clinical presentation is bleeding from multiple sites. In mild cases, there is such slow degradation of fibrinogen and other clotting factors and platelet consumption that the liver and bone marrow are able to compensate; in this case, the clinical presentation is large vessel clotting. This is seen in the chronic DIC state associated with various malignancies, particularly the mucus-secreting adenocarcinomas.

It needs to be emphasized that although DIC often requires treatment, it is the underlying disease or condition that must be corrected before one can expect the DIC to abate. DIC has been reported with an extraordinarily broad spectrum of disease, from obstetric problems (e.g., amniotic fluid embolism) to major transfusion reactions, sepsis, various malignancies, and traumatic injury. A listing of diseases associated with DIC appears in Table 9–1.

Pathogenesis

This will vary to some extent, depending on the specific underlying cause. In general, the cause is the presence in the circulation of a thromboplastic material. In DIC associated with massive trauma or large areas of tissue necrosis, the availability of the tissue factor to activate directly the extrinsic pathway of clotting is the likely explanation. Tissue factor can be synthesized by mononuclear and endothelial cells and can activate clotting. This is the suspected mechanism in the presence of endotoxemia and numerous other inflammatory states, in which cytokines such as interleukin-1 and tumor necrosis factor (TNF) are secreted. In major transfusion reactions, DIC is caused by the release of thromboplastin-like substances into the circulation from the red blood cells. The secretion of certain proteases in promyelocytic leukemia or mucus-secreting adenocarcinomas is also a cause of DIC. These proteases directly activate factor X, thus initiating clotting via the common pathway. By contrast, in severe liver disease, the cause might be the inability of the damaged liver to clear various activated proteases.

Diagnosis and Clinical Features

As might be expected from the preceding discussion, the clinical features attributable to DIC vary from the acute and obvious (an acutely ill patient bleeding from multiple sites) to the chronic and subtle (a patient with a solid tumor and migratory thrombophlebitis). The laboratory diagnosis in the uncompensated form includes findings of a combination of low fibrinogen level, prolonged PT and aPTT, and thrombocytopenia with immunoassay evidence of fibrinogen-fibrin split products. In the chronic form, all these values may be normal except for the demonstration of high levels of fibrinogen-fibrin split products in the circulation. Additionally, soluble fibrin complexes in plasma and soluble intermediaries between fibrinogen and fibrin can be demonstrated using the addition of protamine sulfate or ethanol, which causes these intermediate compounds to gel. False-positive results in low titer and negative results occur, but strongly positive results confirm the diagnosis. Occasionally, large aortic aneurysms and giant hemangiomas (Kasabach-Merritt syndrome) can cause high levels of fibrinogen-fibrin split products, as can various acute and chronic renal glomerular disorders.

Treatment

The therapy of DIC remains controversial. As previously mentioned, everyone agrees that the underlying cause of the

Table 9–1. DISEASES ASSOCIATED WITH DISSEMINATED INTRAVASCULAR COAGULATION

Category	Clinical Situation
Obstetric	Abruptio placentae
	Amniotic fluid embolus
	Dead fetus syndrome
	Eclampsia (pre-eclampsia)
	Placenta previa
	Placenta accreta
	Abortion (hypertonic saline solution)
	Hydatid mole
	Extrauterine pregnancy
	Forceps delivery
	"Normal" delivery
Tissue trauma	Major surgery
	Major trauma or burns
	Fat embolus
	Transplant rejection
	Heat stroke
Hemolytic process	Transfusion of mismatched blood
	Drowning
	Acute hemolysis secondary to infection
	Immune hemolysis
	Acid ingestion
Malignancy	Solid tumors
	Leukemia
	Lymphoma
Snakebite	
Cardiovascular system	Myocardial infarction (usually with cardiogenic shock)
	Circulatory collapse of any cause
	Severe progressive stroke
	Aortic aneurysm
	Kasabach-Merritt syndrome
Chronic liver disease	
Infection:	
Bacterial	Gram-negative
	Meningococcal septicemia
	Pneumococcal septicemia
Rickettsial	Rocky Mountain spotted fever
Viral	Hemorrhagic smallpox
	Hemorrhagic fever
Mycotic	Acute histoplasmosis
Parasitic	Malaria (particularly falciparum)
Miscellaneous	Acute and chronic renal disease
	Collagen vascular disease
	Hemolytic uremic syndrome
	Purpura fulminans
	Acute pancreatitis
	Allergic vasculitis
	Amyloidosis
	Polycythemia rubra vera
	Thrombocythemia
	Ulcerative colitis

DIC (sepsis, obstetric problem) needs to be treated. Since the 1960s the therapy of DIC has swung between factor (cryoprecipitate, fresh-frozen plasma, platelets) replacement and full-dose heparin therapy or some combination of both. Presently, with the exception of certain very specific diseases (e.g., meningococcal septicemia and the Waterhouse-Friderichsen syndrome) in which heparin by continuous infusion has been suggested to be beneficial, most physicians treat the DIC component of the illness with coagulation factor and platelet replacement. No data support the use of epsilon-aminocaproic acid (EACA) in DIC states. The heparin dosage ranges from 150 to 600 U · kg^{-1} · day^{-1} by continuous infusion.

Disseminated Intravascular Coagulation Versus Primary Fibrinogenolysis

There have been many reports of a pathologic state of blood clotting and subsequent clot lysis. This has been referred to as primary fibrinolysis and is felt to be caused by activation of the plasmin system. The plasminogen-plasmin system is the system for clot dissolution. However, most authorities question the separate existence of this pathologic state and view this as an activation of the fibrinolytic system in the setting of DIC—i.e., activation of the primary physiologic repair mechanism.

Diagnosis and Treatment of Venous Thromboembolism

Pulmonary embolism continues to be the commonest preventable cause of hospital death in the United States. Most patients who die of pulmonary emboli die within the first 2 hours of the event. Conceptually, therefore, the reason to treat pulmonary emboli is the effort to prevent the next one.

Pathophysiology

Venous thrombi are predominantly composed of fibrin and red blood cells, with a variable platelet and leukocyte composition. The factors that predispose to the development of thrombus include venous stasis, activation of blood coagulation, and vascular damage. The counterbalancing factors include the circulating natural inhibitors (antithrombin III, α_2-macroglobulin, alpha$_1$-antitrypsin, and activated protein C), hepatic reticuloendothelial clearance and metabolism of activated clotting factors, the plasminogen system for fibrin degradation, and leukocyte digestion of fibrin.

Clinical risk factors associated with an increased risk of venous thromboembolism include surgical and nonsurgical trauma, prior venous thromboembolism, immobilization, malignancy, heart disease (particularly congestive heart failure), leg paralysis, obesity, exogenous estrogen use, and parturition. Inherited and acquired abnormalities increasing thrombosis risk include protein S or C deficiency, antithrombin III deficiency, dysfibrinogenemia, and heparin-induced thrombocytopenia.

Ninety per cent of pulmonary emboli arise in the deep

veins of the leg proximal to the popliteal vein. Other infrequent sources of pulmonary emboli include the pelvic, inferior vena caval, and renal veins. The right ventricle or axillary veins are rare sources of pulmonary emboli.

Fifty to seventy per cent of patients with demonstrated pulmonary emboli have detectable deep venous thrombosis of the leg at the time of presentation.

Clinical Features

The prognosis and clinical features of pulmonary embolism depend on the size of the embolus and the cardiorespiratory reserve of the patient. Thus, the clinical presentation of pulmonary emboli can be divided into several overlapping syndromes, including (1) development of dyspnea and tachypnea without other manifestations; (2) pleuritic chest pain, cough, and hemoptysis, with pulmonary infiltrate and pleural effusion on chest x-ray film; (3) right ventricular failure; (4) cardiovascular collapse with hypotension, syncope, and coma (most often with massive emboli); and (5) less common and quite nonspecific features such as confusion and coma, fever, wheezing, resistant heart failure, or unexplained arrhythmia. However, multiple studies have shown that in over half of patients thought on clinical grounds to have pulmonary emboli, the diagnosis cannot be confirmed using objective testing. Thus, objective confirmation of pulmonary emboli is required to make the diagnosis.

The clinical features of venous thrombosis of the leg can include pain, tenderness and swelling, a palpable cord, discoloration, venous distention, and cyanosis. However, the signs of thrombosis may be minimal in the setting of extensive thrombi, or clinical features may be quite significant but due to some other cause. Thus, some form of objective testing is required to establish the diagnosis of venous thrombosis.

Objective Tests for Venous Thrombosis

The best available studies (i.e., highest specificity and sensitivity) for the diagnosis of venous thrombosis include the noninvasive studies of impedance plethysmography (IPG) and ultrasonography (B-mode, duplex, and color-flow technology). The invasive standard is contrast venography.

VENOGRAPHY

This is the standard objective invasive method used in the diagnosis of venous thrombosis. However, it is critical to remember the difficulties associated with the test, its interpretation, and its potential side effects (e.g., 1% to 2% deep or superficial venous thrombosis). If for technical reasons a segment of the venous system does not fill, this could be interpreted as a positive test in error. The common femoral, external iliac, and common iliac veins may not be adequately filled by ascending venography, thus potentially leading to an inaccurate diagnosis. Occasionally, femoral venography is required for further evaluation. The only clear evidence of thrombosis is an intraluminal filling defect that is constant and seen in multiple projections. Besides the pitfall of interpretation, side effects can occur as previously mentioned. Other side effects include hypersensitivity reactions to the dye, necrosis of skin caused by dye extravasation, and possible renal insufficiency, particularly when underlying renal impairment is present.

Impedance Plethysmography

IPG is sensitive and specific for proximal venous thrombosis in symptomatic patients, but it is insensitive to calf vein thrombosis. Thus, in patients clinically suspected of having proximal thrombosis, a positive IPG can be used to make a therapeutic decision in the absence of conditions associated with a false-positive result. These conditions include severe congestive heart failure, constrictive pericarditis, severe arterial insufficiency, hypotension, and external venous compression. Thus reduction of inflow or outflow from the leg will compromise the results of the study. Also, patients who have casts or who cannot be positioned because of immobilization or pain cannot be studied with this technique. A normal IPG excludes proximal thrombosis but does not exclude calf vein thrombosis. This can be overcome by serial study. This is reasonable because, in terms of the leg, only proximal thrombosis is associated with embolus risk, and the distal (calf) thrombosis propagating into the proximal system will be discovered by the serial IPG. Thus, from clinical study, the following conclusions can be drawn: (1) a positive result on IPG is highly predictive of acute proximal thrombosis with a positive predictive value of greater than 90%, and (2) withholding anticoagulation is safe in symptomatic patients with negative IPG results serially over 10 to 14 days.

Unfortunately, IPG lacks sensitivity in the detection of asymptomatic thrombosis in patients who have had total hip replacement or significant trauma. In such circumstances, contrast venography is usually required.

Ultrasonography

As the technique of real time, B-mode ultrasonography has become more common and refined and the technical improvements of Doppler assessment and color flow have evolved, it will likely supplant IPG as the most popular noninvasive test for the detection of venous thrombosis. Doppler ultrasound and IPG are both highly sensitive and specific in the diagnosis of proximal vein thrombosis in symptomatic patients. Doppler ultrasonography is more sensitive in the detection of symptomatic calf vein thrombosis and more reliable than IPG in detecting proximal venous thrombosis in patients with increased central venous pressure or arterial insufficiency. Also, Doppler ultrasonography can be used in patients with the leg in a cast, immobilized by traction or external fixation, or who have had an amputation.

Objective Tests for Pulmonary Embolism

The two objective tests presently available are ventilation-perfusion lung scans and pulmonary angiography. The ancillary study of chest radiograph, arterial blood gases, and electrocardiogram lacks sensitivity and specificity. These studies are valuable to rule out conditions such as pneumothorax, acute myocardial infarction, or pneumonia.

VENTILATION-PERFUSION LUNG SCAN

A normal perfusion lung scan excludes clinically significant pulmonary embolism. However, an abnormal perfusion scan is nonspecific because of physiologic hypoxic vasoconstriction due to reduced ventilation. Thus, an abnormal perfusion scan can be seen in several clinical situations that are not related to pulmonary embolus. An infiltrate on chest x-ray film corresponding to an area of reduced perfusion might be consistent with pneumonia, atelectasis, or pleural effusion. Reduced perfusion and a normal chest x-ray can be seen in regional ventilation abnormalities such as in chronic obstructive lung disease, acute asthma, mucus plugs, or even bronchitis.

Ventilation imaging was introduced to improve the specificity of an abnormal perfusion scan in an effort to differentiate embolic occlusion from reduced perfusion secondary to reduced ventilation. The basic premise is that segmental or larger perfusion defects that ventilate are caused by pulmonary emboli more than 86% of the time (high-probability scan). Other abnormal results, such as (1) segmental or subsegmental matching ventilation-perfusion defects, (2) subsegmental perfusion defects with ventilation mismatch, and (3) a perfusion defect that corresponds to an area of increased density on a chest radiograph (indeterminate perfusion scan results), are associated with embolus 20% to 40% of the time. These intermediate results, depending on the clinical situation, may require confirmation by pulmonary angiography.

Since 80% of patients with pulmonary embolism have thrombi arising in the lower extremities, a strategy of doing IPG or Doppler ultrasonography in these cases of intermediate probability scan has evolved to increase noninvasive diagnostic accuracy. Proximal venous thrombosis of the leg is shown 10% to 25% of the time in patients with intermediate probability scans, and this then establishes the indication for therapy. The venographic result is negative in 30% of patients with pulmonary emboli documented by angiography. The explanation of this includes thrombus originating from a place other than the leg, complete embolization of the leg thrombus, or an inadequate venogram.

When the ventilation-perfusion lung scan is intermediate and the evaluation of the leg is negative, the only way to establish the diagnosis of pulmonary embolism is by pulmonary arteriography.

PULMONARY ARTERIOGRAPHY

This is the accepted reference standard for the diagnosis of pulmonary embolism. Intraluminal filling defects seen constantly or abrupt termination (cutoff) of contrast in a vessel greater than 2 to 5 mm in diameter confirms the diagnosis. Clinically significant complications of the procedure include hypersensitivity reactions to the dye, contrast-induced renal failure, tachyarrhythmias, endocardial or myocardial injury, cardiac perforation, or cardiac arrest. Side effects occur in 3% to 4% of patients.

Anticoagulant Therapy

The treatment objectives of venous thromboembolism are to prevent death from pulmonary embolism, prevent recurrent episodes of thromboembolism, and prevent the post-phlebitic syndrome.

We will discuss anticoagulation therapy with heparin and warfarin but will not review vena caval filters, embolectomy, or thrombolytic therapy.

HEPARIN

Heparin is a mixture of anionic glycosaminoglycans that inhibits the coagulation pathway via numerous mechanisms. The principal sites of this inhibition include inhibition of Factors X and II. Other sites of inhibition include Factors XII, XI, and IX. This inhibition occurs principally through the interaction of heparin and antithrombin III. Thus, it is important to remember that antithrombin III must be present in order for heparin to work effectively. This is of clinical significance in patients with congenital antithrombin III deficiencies and perhaps in the setting of DIC in which antithrombin III is consumed. Heparin also inhibits platelet function and thus prolongs the bleeding time. Of the available routes for heparin injection (i.e., subcutaneous, intermittent intravenous, and continuous intravenous infusion), continuous infusion is the preferred method for the treatment of acute proximal venous thrombosis or pulmonary embolism. In this setting, the subcutaneous route is associated with a higher incidence of recurrent venous thromboembolism because of inadequate initial anticoagulation. The intermittent intravenous schedule is associated with a higher incidence of clinically significant bleeding.

Heparin dosing is monitored using the aPTT and it has become common practice to maintain the aPTT between 1.5 and 2.5 times the control value. It is critical to monitor heparin dosing because of the wide variability in patient response to the same dose of heparin.

Recent studies suggest that if the aPTT remains below this lower limit (1.5 times control) for longer than 24 hours during therapy, the risk of recurrent thromboembolism is much higher. In the study by Hull and coworkers, 24.5% of patients (13 of 53) with an aPTT response of less than 1.5 times control for 24 hours or longer had recurrent venous thromboembolism compared with only 1.6% (1 of 62 patients) in whom an aPTT greater than 1.5 times control was continuously achieved ($p < 0.001$).

It has been clinical practice to maintain the aPTT at less than 2.5 times control based on observations from retrospective studies and the intuitive belief that the risk of bleeding is greater when this limit is exceeded. In recently designed clinical trials, no clear association between supratherapeutic aPTT result and risk of bleeding could be found. However, those patients with supratherapeutic aPTTs during therapy had the same outcome in regard to the treatment of venous thromboembolism as did those whose aPTT was kept below 2.5 times control but, most importantly, above 1.5 times control. However, a recent study in three university-affiliated hospitals demonstrated that 60% of patients failed to obtain an adequate aPTT ratio within the first 24 hours of treatment and that 30% to 40% continued with subtherapeutic levels over the ensuing 3 to 4 days. Because of this, Hull and colleagues have proposed a nomogram for heparin therapy. This protocol has been proved to function clinically with only 2% of patients having subtherapeutic aPTTs (less than 1.5 times control) for more than 24 hours.

Protocol

1. Heparin bolus: 5000 U IV
2. Continuous-infusion heparin: mix 20,000 U of heparin in 500 ml of dextrose solution. Begin at 42 ml/hr = 1680 U/hr heparin, except in the following categories in which the suggested rate is 31 ml/hr = 1240 U/hr.
   a. Patients having undergone surgery in previous 2 weeks
   b. History of peptic ulcer or gastrointestinal or genitourinary bleeding
   c. Patients with thrombotic stroke in previous 2 weeks
   d. Platelet count less than 150,000
   e. Patients with other high risk of bleeding (e.g., hepatic failure, renal failure, vitamin K deficiency)
3. Adjust heparin dose using the aPTT. The aPTT test is performed in all patients as follows:
   a. preheparin bolus
   b. 4 to 6 hours after starting heparin infusion with adjustment per nomogram (see below)
   c. 4 to 6 hours after first dosage adjustment
   d. then by nomogram for first 24 hours of therapy
   e. thereafter, once daily unless patient is subtherapeutic, in which case the aPTT is repeated 4 to 6 hours after the dose increase

Nomogram for Heparin Titration

(Heparin mixed as in protocol, 20,000 U in 500 ml of fluid equaling 40 U/ml)

aPTT	IV Infusion (Rate change, ml/hr)	Additional Action
≤45	+6	Repeat aPTT in 4–6 hr
46–54	+3	Repeat aPTT in 4–6 hr
55–85	None	None*
86–110	−3	Stop heparin for 1 hr Repeat aPTT 4–6 hr after heparin restarted
>110	−6	Stop heparin 1 hr Repeat aPTT 4–6 hr after heparin restarted

*During the first 24 hours, repeat the aPTT in 4 to 6 hours and thereafter once daily, unless the result is subtherapeutic.

HEPARIN "ANTIDOTE"

The anticoagulant effect of heparin can be immediately neutralized by intravenous protamine sulfate. The neutralizing dose of protamine depends on the route of administration and the time of the heparin dose. A full neutralizing dose of protamine given within minutes of an IV dose of heparin is 1 mg protamine for each 100 U of heparin. Because of the 60-minute plasma half-life of intravenously administered heparin, 50 mg of protamine as a bolus is the usual maximum dose. Protamine is given by slow injection (10 to 30 minutes) because of an occasional hypotensive response. Since protamine is cleared from the blood more quickly than heparin, an additional protamine dose is occasionally required.

ADVERSE EFFECTS

The side effects of heparin include bleeding, hypersensitivity, osteoporosis from long-term use, thrombocytopenia, and arterial thromboembolism. The risk of bleeding is more frequent in patients given intermittent intravenous injection, in patients with underlying hemostatic defects, and in those with predisposing risk factors (e.g., peptic ulcer disease, occult carcinoma) or recent surgery or trauma. Hypersensitivity is uncommon but may present as a skin rash or rarely as anaphylaxis.

Thrombocytopenia as a result of heparin exposure (including heparin used in flush lines) is increasingly being recognized and usually occurs 7 to 10 days after the first exposure, but it can occur earlier in previously treated patients. The incidence appears to be in the 1% to 2% range. It is more common in patients receiving beef lung–derived heparin than in those receiving porcine intestine heparin. Thrombocytopenia can be moderate or severe, but the moderate form is more common. This complication is also seen with low-molecular-weight heparin. The precise mechanism is unknown, but it is probably immune mediated in the severe form.

The most significant complication associated with heparin thrombocytopenia is the rare arterial thromboembolism. This may precede or coincide with the thrombocytopenia and is associated with a high incidence of limb amputation and mortality. Thus, once thrombocytopenia is recognized, all administration of heparin must be stopped. Alternative approaches to anticoagulant therapy include, at that point, vena caval filtration devices or the use of Ancrod, a defibrinogenating extract of snake venom, while oral anticoagulation is started. A heparinoid that does not cross-react with heparin has been used effectively in a few patients with heparin-induced thrombocytopenia.

LOW-MOLECULAR-WEIGHT HEPARIN

LMW heparin is derived from commercially prepared heparin and has a mean molecular weight of 4000 to 5000, compared with unfractionated heparin with a mean molecular weight of 10,000 to 17,000. Because the bioavailability of LMW heparin after subcutaneous injection is high, because it has a longer half-life than unfractionated heparin, and because the anticoagulant response observed with a given dose of LMW heparin is highly correlated with body weight, the drug is used subcutaneously every 12 to 24 hours without laboratory monitoring (i.e., aPTT).

To date, the studies comparing fixed-dose LMW heparin given subcutaneously once or twice daily to an aPTT-adjusted continuous intravenous dose of unfractionated heparin in patients with proximal venous thrombosis have had essentially equivalent results both in terms of prevention of recurrent thrombus and bleeding. Thus, the studies to date support the concept that LMW heparin is as effective and safe as conventional dose-adjusted, continuous intravenous unfractionated heparin in the treatment of proximal venous thrombosis. Heparin-induced thrombocytopenia has also been seen with LMW heparin.

Oral Anticoagulant Therapy

There are two chemical groups of oral anticoagulants but because of fewer nonhemorrhagic side effects, coumarin derivatives are the drugs of choice.

Oral anticoagulants inhibit vitamin K–dependent gamma-carboxylation of Factors II, VII, IX, and X and proteins C and S (natural anticoagulants). Thus, warfarin has the paradoxical effect of both inhibiting the procoagulant vitamin K–dependent factors and at the same time, inhibiting the natural anticoagulant vitamin K–dependent proteins S and C. Of the factors and proteins affected by warfarin, Factor VII and protein C have similar and quite short (4 to 5 hour) half-lives. Thus, the Factor VII level will fall first, and the prothrombin time (measuring the extrinsic clotting system) will prolong first. However, it takes 36 to 72 hours for the peak effect of warfarin and a week or so for equilibrium levels of Factors II, IX, and X to be reached. This equilibrium is not achieved faster by large loading doses of warfarin, and sick patients with potentially impaired liver function or reduced vitamin K stores would be particularly susceptible to warfarin effects. For these reasons, a small daily dose (10 mg) is preferred to initiate warfarin therapy over larger one-time loading doses.

For the reasons just cited, it is important to overlap heparin therapy with warfarin. Despite a rising prothrombin time, the maximum antithrombotic effect of warfarin will not occur until the equilibrium levels of Factors II, IX, and X occur, which is several days after the increase in prothrombin time (Factor VII effect). Additionally, since protein C has a similar half-life to that of Factor VII, early on the warfarin dose has the potential to be thrombogenic. Thus, most authorities recommend a 4 to 5 day overlap even though the prothrombin time is in the therapeutic range earlier.

Dosing Warfarin

Warfarin is administered in an initial dose of 10 mg orally daily for 2 days, then is adjusted daily based on the results of the International Normalized Ratio (INR) (2.0 to 3.0, or prothrombin time ratio using rabbit brain thromboplastin 1.25 to 1.5 times control, as discussed later). As outlined in Chapter 144 of the *Textbook of Critical Care*, heparin therapy is stopped typically on the fourth or fifth day of warfarin therapy. Once the dose is stabilized, the INR is monitored weekly throughout therapy. If factors occur that might interfere or prolong the warfarin effect (other drug therapy), more frequent monitoring will be required.

Monitoring Warfarin Therapy

As mentioned, the prothrombin time is used to measure the effects of warfarin. Only recently has the optimum therapeutic range for the prothrombin time been clinically studied. Additionally, the thromboplastic material used to perform the prothrombin time can give significantly different results. Rabbit brain thromboplastin, used extensively in North America, is much less sensitive to warfarin effects than is the standardized human brain thromboplastin used in the United Kingdom and other parts of Europe. Thus a prothrombin time ratio (observed results divided by control) of 1.5 to 2.0, obtained using rabbit brain thromboplastin, is equivalent to a ratio of 4.0 to 6.0 obtained using human brain thromboplastin. Conversely, a two- or threefold increase obtained using human brain thromboplastin corresponds to a 1.25- to 1.5-fold increase using rabbit brain thromboplastin.

In an effort to standardize the prothrombin time, the World Health Organization has developed an international reference thromboplastin for human brain tissue and recommends that the prothrombin time ratio be expressed in terms of this International Normalized Ratio (INR). For practical clinical purposes, the presently recommended therapeutic range for the prothrombin time is 1.25 to 1.5 times the control using rabbit brain thromboplastin, which corresponds to an INR of 2.0 to 3.0.

Adverse Effects

The major side effect of oral anticoagulant therapy is bleeding. When the INR is well controlled in the 2.0 to 3.0 range, bleeding is usually due to another problem, e.g., surgery, trauma, peptic ulcers, or unrecognized carcinoma. The principal nonhemorrhagic side effect of warfarin is skin necrosis. This is quite rare, is more common in women, and typically involves areas of abundant subcutaneous tissue, such as the buttock, pannus, or breast. The mechanism is uncertain but, as previously discussed, is likely related to depression of protein C levels perhaps causing microvascular thrombi. Because warfarin crosses the placenta and has been associated with fetal malformations, it is contraindicated in pregnancy.

Factors Affecting Oral Anticoagulant Therapy

A large number of drugs affect oral anticoagulant dosing, as is shown in Table 9–2. Additionally, increased sensitivity

Table 9–2. DRUGS THAT INTERACT WITH ORAL ANTICOAGULANTS

Increase Anticoagulant Effect	Decrease Anticoagulant Effect
Allopurinol	Barbiturates
Anabolic steroids	Cholestyramine
Clofibrate	Diuretics
Co-trimoxazole (trimethoprim and sulfamethoxazole)	Estrogen
D-Thyroxine	Glutethimide
Neomycin	Griseofulvin
Nortriptyline	Phenytoin
Phenyramidol	Rifampin
Quinidine	
Salicylate	
Sulfinpyrazone	

to warfarin is seen in patients with liver disease, vitamin K deficiency (e.g., postoperative patients with extended nasogastric suction taking broad-spectrum antibiotics), and those with thyrotoxicosis due to more rapid metabolism of the vitamin K–dependent clotting factors.

WARFARIN "ANTIDOTE"

Besides omitting or reducing the dose of warfarin, the effects of the oral anticoagulant can be reversed in two additional ways, depending on the clinical situation. If bleeding is caused by warfarin excess and is severe, clotting factor concentrates of II, VII, IX, and X or fresh-frozen plasma are used. Vitamin K_1 (5 mg) can be given slowly IV (1 mg/min) if warranted. The slow infusion reduces the risk of anaphylactoid reaction. This will produce a demonstrable effect in the INR in 6 to 8 hours and corrects the INR in 12 to 24 hours. Vitamin K_1 can also be given in small doses (2.5 to 5 mg) subcutaneously or orally in the appropriate clinical situation. The half-life of vitamin K_1 is less than that of warfarin, so additional vitamin K_1 may be needed.

Plasma and Blood Substitutes

The purpose of this summary is to review the available colloid plasma expanders and the ongoing investigations into oxygen-carrying solutions. This is not a review of the crystalloid versus colloid discussion for volume expansion.

The synthetic plasma substitutes available are the dextran solutions and hydroxyethyl starch (HES). The currently available oxygen-carrying solutions under investigation include perfluorochemical (PFC) emulsions and hemoglobin solutions.

Dextran

Two dextran solutions are used in clinical practice, both produced by the conversion of sucrose into glucose polymers. Dextran-70 is a 6% solution with an average molecular weight of 70,000, and dextran-40, or low-molecular-weight dextran, is a 10% solution with an average molecular weight of 40,000. Dextran-40 is excreted more rapidly than dextran-70 but has a higher oncotic effect per gram infused and thus produces a more pronounced plasma volume expansion. The efficacy in this regard is equal or even superior to that of albumin. Since dextran-40 is more rapidly excreted in the urine, specific gravity can become extremely high (i.e., 1.088) and acute renal failure can occur due to sludging and obstruction of renal tubules by this highly viscous filtrate. Thus, particularly in the dehydrated patient, concurrent crystalloid infusion is important, and dextran should be avoided in patients with underlying renal insufficiency.

In addition to its oncotic effects, dextran solutions have antithrombotic effects. These effects are likely mediated by inhibition of platelet and leukocyte antigens as well as improved rheology in the microcirculation. Thus, administration of dextran to patients in shock may offer therapeutic advantage because of the improved microcirculatory blood flow. This effect may be mediated through decreased blood viscosity by hemodilution or by inhibition of red cell and platelet aggregation in the capillaries, which may reduce or prevent intravascular sludging. Because of these effects of dextran, platelet adhesiveness is decreased. Low doses of dextran (less than 1.5 g/kg body weight) are not associated with clinically significant bleeding, but larger doses have been associated with significant bleeding. This limits its use in perioperative or bleeding patients to 1000 to 1500 ml in 24 hours. Also, because of the adherence of dextran to antigens on the red blood cell surface, difficulty with blood cross-matching can be encountered, so the specimen for type and cross-matching needs to be obtained before dextran is given.

Anaphylactic reactions occur in 0.03% to 0.07% of patients and may be severe or even fatal. These usually occur with the first 100 ml infused, so close monitoring is suggested. There are isolated reports of fetal death due to dextran given to the mother before or during delivery.

Low-molecular-weight dextran has also been used effectively as a plasma substitute for priming in extracorporeal circulation and has been studied in the setting of myocardial ischemia, cerebral ischemia, and peripheral vascular disease, and in maintaining vascular graft patency.

Hydroxyethyl Starch (HES)

Starch, the energy storage polysaccharide of plants, is composed of glucose polymers. Modification of the starch molecules by hydroxyethylation, creating HES, makes it more stable in plasma.

The most commonly used HES is hetastarch, which is available as a 6% concentration in physiologic salt solution containing 60 g/L colloid and 154 mEq/L of sodium and chloride. It has an osmolarity of 310 mOsm/L, pH 5.5, and a colloid osmotic pressure of 30 mm Hg.

Hetastarch has a large mean molecular weight (69,000;

range, 10,000 to 100,000). With this wide range of molecular weights, small molecules will be excreted unchanged in the urine while the larger ones will diffuse slowly into the interstitium. In normal subjects, the plasma half-life is 17 hours, but only 50% of the HES is eliminated initially. The remaining HES is eliminated very slowly, and much of the given dose persists in the reticuloendothelial system for weeks after infusion. HES, unlike dextran, is not antigenic, and allergic reactions are extremely uncommon. In one large series, the incidence of reactions to HES was 0.085% compared with 0.011% for albumin infusions. Also, unlike dextran, HES does not interfere with blood cross-matching and has no apparent adverse effect on renal function.

The only clinically important adverse effect of HES infusion appears to be some impairment of coagulation, which seems to be dose related. Low doses have no effect on coagulation, whereas moderate doses (20 ml/kg) may transiently decrease platelet counts, decrease fibrinogen levels, and prolong the prothrombin time and partial thromboplastin time. However, platelet function, including adhesiveness, remains intact. Despite the measurement of these effects, there is no evidence of clinical bleeding problems when a dose of 20 ml/kg is not exceeded. There have been no controlled studies in humans of larger infusions, but in animals given very large doses of HES, significantly increased bleeding has been seen.

A problem of unknown significance with HES infusion is an occasional elevation of serum amylase. It is unclear whether this hyperamylasemia is the result of subclinical pancreatitis or if HES acts as a physiologic stimulant to pancreatic amylase secretion, or if HES causes accumulation of amylase. Levels of serum amylase twice normal have been reported.

Pentastarch, which is a modification of the hetastarch formulation, has a lower mean molecular weight and more homogeneous particle size. These differences allow for more predictable and rapid excretion compared with hetastarch. Pentastarch is available as a 10% solution and has a colloid osmotic pressure of 40 mm Hg.

In comparative studies of fluid therapy, infusing 6% HES solution increases central venous pressure, pulmonary artery occlusion pressure, and cardiac output with the same efficacy as that of 5% albumin infusion.

Both HES and dextran effectively raise colloid osmotic pressure and increase plasma volume, although the increase in plasma volume may be greater and more sustained with high-molecular-weight dextran (dextran-70). Dextrans are more useful agents in decreasing blood viscosity and increasing microvascular blood flow, whereas HES is associated with fewer adverse effects, including a lower incidence of anaphylaxis, fewer bleeding problems, and no adverse renal effects.

Perfluorochemical Emulsions

The fluoridation of hydrocarbons generates a biologically inert liquid with high oxygen solubility. Oxygen dissolves in this liquid and is, therefore, delivered to tissue via simple diffusion. Its use as a blood substitute has been delayed because it requires suspension in an emulsion suitable for intravascular infusion.

Work on the PFC emulsions began with Clark and Gallan in 1965. During the 1970s, Fluosol-DA 20% was developed. This emulsion is 20% PFC by weight along with other additives for improved stability. It must be stored frozen and used within 24 hours of thawing.

The plasma half-life is dose dependent (17 hours at a dose of 20 ml/kg) and because of the molecular size is eliminated unchanged through the airway. Since the accumulation of PFC occurs in the liver and spleen, administration more than once every 6 months is not recommended.

Because oxygen dissolves in PFC emulsions and is not bound as it is to hemoglobin, the amount of oxygen transported depends on the PaO_2. Thus its clinical use requires good lung function and high FiO_2. The advantage of this is the relatively low affinity of the PFC for oxygen, enabling essentially all the dissolved oxygen to be delivered at the tissue level.

PFC emulsions improve peripheral blood flow by volume expansion and by improved microcirculatory flow. Additionally, the size of the PFC emulsion particle (1/70th the size of a red blood cell) allows flow into areas of constricted microcirculation not accessible to red cells. This may increase tissue oxygen concentration by both flow and delivery mechanisms.

Fluosol was first used in the United States in 1979, but limited trials have been performed, largely in anemic and bleeding patients who refuse transfusion on religious grounds. In these small series, some improvement in oxygen delivery was seen.

Several adverse effects of PFC emulsions are noted, including transient leukopenia, elevated liver function test values, increased pulmonary artery pressures, transient hypotension, and even respiratory failure. It appears that one of the additives (poloxamer 188) may be responsible for some of these adverse effects via activation of the complement system.

In addition to these potentially adverse effects, there are several other limitations to PFC's use. Not only is the plasma half-life relatively short but the volume of PFC infused is also limited, thus limiting the amount of oxygen that can be dissolved. To dissolve significant amounts of oxygen in Fluosol, high PaO_2 must be achieved by high FiO_2 and good lung function.

The present and potential therapeutic uses of Fluosol other than as a blood substitute include its use as a coronary artery perfusate during angioplasty, during radiation therapy as a hypoxic enhancer (to improve tissue oxygenation for better radiation-induced cell death), for the acute treatment of myocardial or cerebral ischemia, as a drug delivery solvent, and as a radiologic contrast medium.

Second-generation perfluorocarbon emulsions have been developed and are currently under investigation.

Stroma-Free Hemoglobin

To date, the source of hemoglobin for this line of investigation has been human, bovine, or produced by recombinant DNA technology.

HUMAN HEMOGLOBIN SOLUTIONS

The early attempts to transfuse human hemoglobin solutions were associated with major toxicity due to the presence of red blood cell stroma. In the late 1970s, Rabiner and colleagues described a more purified hemoglobin as stroma-free hemoglobin (SFH). This product, despite its purity, is not completely stroma-free and is also associated with adverse reactions. The other major problem with SFH preparations includes its increased oxygen affinity, with a P_{50} almost half that of fresh blood. The reasons for this increased oxygen affinity include loss of tetrameric hemoglobin, absence of 2,3-diphosphoglycerate (2,3-DPG), and a solution of high pH. Various solutions to this problem have included reacting the hemoglobin with pyridoxal-5′-phosphate, thus increasing the P_{50} significantly, or encapsulating the hemoglobin with 2,3-DPG in liposomes, simulating red cells. Liposome-encapsulated hemoglobin (LEH) has a normal hemoglobin dissociation curve and an increased half-life (16 to 24 hours). Another approach to solve the problem of rapid clearance has been selective polymerization of the hemoglobin molecule. HbXL99α, a hemoglobin derivative produced by specific cross-linking of α subunits, has been shown to have oxygen transport characteristics similar to those of whole blood.

BOVINE HEMOGLOBIN SOLUTIONS

To get around several of the problems associated with human hemoglobin, other sources of hemoglobin have been studied. The principal benefit of a nonhuman hemoglobin source includes more abundant supply, apparent absence of virally transmitted disease, and a lack of a requirement for 2,3-DPG to lower hemoglobin oxygen affinity. Bovine hemoglobin uses chloride ion to lower its oxygen affinity, and the concentration of chloride in human plasma is enough to accomplish this. In 1992, this product was transfused into children with sickle cell anemia without adverse reaction, and additional clinical trials are underway or being planned.

RECOMBINANT HEMOGLOBIN SOLUTION

Human hemoglobin can be synthesized using standard bacterial recombinant DNA technology. Modifications are being investigated to deal with the problems of high oxygen affinity and short half-life. Because of the potentially unlimited supply and absence of disease transmission risk, this is a strong candidate for development as a blood substitute.

ONCOLOGY

Intensive Care of Patients with Cancer

Cancer is the second leading cause of death in the United States, and its mortality rate has significantly increased in the 60 years between 1930 and 1990. The principal reasons for this include improved reporting of cancer cases, improved follow-up, and an increase in absolute incidences of several tumors including melanoma and lung cancer, particularly in women. Additionally, for several reasons, including earlier diagnosis and more effective therapy, survival after diagnosis has significantly increased—in fact, doubled during the last 60 years.

For these reasons and because society's expectations of what can be done for the patient with cancer have increased, most critical care physicians will be involved in some aspect of their acute care. Management issues will result from complications and progression of the disease or complications related to the treatment or some combination of both.

The critical care physician will need to be familiar with the prognosis and survival assessment of an individual case so he or she can best advise and help manage a particular crisis event. As a simple example, we need to understand the significant difference in long-term prognosis for the neutropenic patient undergoing adjuvant chemotherapy for breast cancer versus the patient with metastatic breast cancer who is neutropenic from marrow involvement by tumor. The decisions we make based on patient wishes and grounded in objective data will dictate the degree of support we should recommend. If possible, these are issues best addressed before the crisis. Unfortunately, most of the time critical care physicians are not afforded this luxury.

Emergencies in Patients with Cancer

Over the past few decades, there have been some dramatic advances in cure rates for some malignant diseases. For example, the 5-year survival rate of patients with childhood acute lymphatic leukemia was 4% in 1970 and now exceeds 70%, due in large measure to more active chemotherapy, marrow transplant where indicated, and improved supportive care. It is, of course, in this area of supportive care that critical care has become involved. As implied previously in this review and in Chapter 147 of the *Textbook of Critical Care*, aggressive life support of potentially curable cancer is quite reasonable.

In acute leukemia, death is almost always from uncontrolled bleeding, infection, or both. With bone marrow replacement by the leukemic cell population, adequate numbers of hematopoietic cells (e.g., myeloid and megakaryocytic precursors) are no longer present to maintain sufficient numbers of granulocytes and platelets. A significantly reduced number of these cells is the most common reason for morbid events. Platelet transfusion is what is available to reduce the risk of thrombocytopenic bleeding. Neutropenic fever should be viewed as a true medical emergency.

Bodey, in a retrospective analysis of 410 episodes of *Pseudomonas* bacteremia, reported a 70% mortality rate within 48 hours for granulocytopenic patients who did not receive antibiotics at the onset of fever.

It is the current standard of care to initiate an antibiotic regimen at the first sign of infection in this clinical situation. The antibiotic regimen varies depending on the specific bacterial pathogens isolated and their sensitivities in the specific institution. Typically, however, the coverage is designed to be bacteriocidal toward gram-negative organisms, with a second drug added for synergy against *Pseudomonas*. With the increased use of invasive vascular lines, the antibiotic spectrum needs to cover the gram-positive organisms, specifically *Staphylococcus aureus* and *S. epidermidis*. The most common combination is an aminoglycoside in conjunction with a semisynthetic penicillin. Additionally, invasive fungal infections are an increasing problem, with amphotericin B the best available therapy. Often, amphotericin B must be used, at least initially, in certain situations before fungal infection can be documented.

In this patient population, invasive monitoring (e.g., pulmonary artery, arterial and central venous catheters) carries an increased infection risk, and if coagulopathy (commonly due to significant thrombocytopenia) is present, a bleeding risk might also exist unless specific product replacement is accomplished prior to catheter placement.

In leukemic patients, the need for mechanical ventilation for more than 72 to 96 hours is associated with a 60% to 70% mortality rate. Respiratory failure can be caused by overwhelming pneumonia or generalized sepsis with related ARDS in this immunocompromised population, but it can also be the result of a leukemic pulmonary infiltrate and extensive bleeding due to coagulopathy or secondary to chemotherapy. Acute lung injury in conjunction with bleomycin is an example of chemotherapy-induced lung injury, which presents principally as a diffuse interstitial infiltrate in the setting of cough, dyspnea, and progressive hypoxia. This can be confused with ARDS secondary to other causes. This situation is often steroid responsive. Additionally, a recall pulmonary toxicity has been reported in patients ventilated with FiO_2 usually greater than 35% who have had previous bleomycin chemotherapy. This phenomenon could be particularly important in a patient who has had a surgical procedure under general anesthesia and develops progressive hypoxemia in the setting of previous bleomycin exposure. It is important to remember that infectious pulmonary infiltrates with neutropenia may be scant because of the absence of functional granulocytes.

MALIGNANCIES

In lymphoma or oat cell carcinoma, a large mediastinal mass may cause superior vena caval compression or obstruction. Almost always, the diagnosis can be confirmed rapidly before therapy (radiation or perhaps chemotherapy) begins. In these pathologic settings, the response to treatment is often quite dramatic. The trachea or major bronchi may be involved and even obstructed by localized tumor growths. These can often be palliated with interstitial brachytherapy techniques, external radiation, laser vaporization, or various combinations of these modalities. Occasionally, selective intubation of the uninvolved mainstem bronchus is required for ventilatory support until palliation has been accomplished.

Disseminated intravascular coagulation is often associated with sepsis and can further complicate the thrombocytopenic coagulopathy often already present in the patient with leukemia. Besides treatment for sepsis, judicious coagulation factor and platelet replacement are required. Acute promyelocytic leukemia is associated with the development of DIC, particularly during initial treatment. This is because the granules of the promyelocyte contain thromboplastic material, which, when released by cell death from chemotherapy, initiates intravascular clotting. In this disease, heparin by low-dose continuous infusion (7 to 10 units/kg/hr) is often started before chemotherapy in an effort to prevent DIC. However, careful attention to detail is required since the patient may already be thrombocytopenic from the disease, and the addition of heparin increases the bleeding risk, which can be quite problematic.

Kidney dysfunction can occur for several reasons in the setting of malignancy. Renal parenchymal infiltrate by a solid tumor is rare and usually does not cause significant dysfunction. However, lymphomatous involvement of the retroperitoneal nodes with ureteral obstruction does occur and needs to be considered as a cause of renal dysfunction. Once this obstruction has been relieved, usually by percutaneous nephrostomy or stent placement, a significant postobstructive diuresis can occur. This will require attention to fluid and electrolyte replacement to avoid additional renal damage.

Multiple myeloma, for several reasons, can cause renal dysfunction. If it is related to myeloma protein precipitation in the renal tubules, then it is usually not reversible. However, the renal dysfunction associated with hypercalcemia seen in several malignancies, including myeloma, head and neck and lung squamous cell carcinoma, and hypernephroma, to mention some of the more common, can be reversible once the calcium is lowered and the patient rehydrated. In addition to renal dysfunction, hypercalcemia causes neurologic dysfunction, including obtundation and coma. The standard approach to treatment of hypercalcemia includes vigorous hydration with normal saline solution to increase glomerular filtration and loop of Henle diuretics, such as furosemide, which inhibit calcium reabsorption. Additionally, several other approaches, including calcitonin (80 to 150 units/kg) given at 8- to 12-hour intervals, corticosteroids (hydrocortisone, 100 to 300 mg/day intravenously in divided doses), mithramycin intravenously (25 μg/kg), and diphosphonates, have all been used individually or in combination in an effort to lower calcium in these situations.

Hyperuricemia can also be a cause of renal dysfunction that may be reversible by lowering the uric acid level. This is particularly true when rapid tumor lysis is expected with treatment (like de novo treatment of acute leukemia, lymphoma, oat cell carcinoma of the lung, dysgerminoma, or nonseminomatous carcinoma of the testis). Whenever massive tumor breakdown occurs with therapy, uric acid, phosphorus (and subsequent hypocalcemia from binding to phosphorus), and potassium are released into the circulation in large quantities. If the urate precipitates within the renal parenchyma and leads to acute renal failure, the classic tumor lysis syndrome can develop, which is fatal if not aggressively treated (usually requiring dialysis until renal function returns). This situation can be avoided by advance planning, including hydration and allopurinol (often in higher than usual doses).

The hyperviscosity syndrome, commonly associated with Waldenström's macroglobulinemia or with IgA or occasionally IgG myeloma, is also a potentially treatable (by phoresis) cause of renal and neurologic impairment.

Finally, renal insufficiency may be a direct result of the drug therapy of the malignancy (cisplatin, methyl-CCNU, BCNU, cytokines). Hemorrhagic cystitis can be associated with cyclophosphamide or ifosfamide (if given without the uroprotective mesna).

It is important to remember that patients who have lost significant muscle mass from tumor cachexia will have "falsely low" serum creatine levels. For this reason, measurement of creatinine clearance becomes important when potentially nephrotoxic drugs (i.e., aminoglycosides or cisplatin) are used, as does measurement of drug peak and trough levels.

The central nervous system can be affected directly or indirectly (e.g., through hypercalcemia or hyponatremia). Tumors can involve the parenchyma of the brain or meninges, leading to significant morbidity and mortality. Often corticosteroids (dexamethasone, 16 to 100 mg/day given in divided doses) can offer palliation of increased intracranial pressure while radiation or other therapeutic modalities are tried. Occasionally, solitary metastases are surgically excised in the absence of known systemic disease. As an example, the 2-year survival of surgically excised solitary brain metastases in adenocarcinoma of the lung can be as high as 40%.

Severe hepatic dysfunction rarely occurs with primary or metastatic tumor because 80% of the liver parenchyma must be destroyed before clinically significant hepatic dysfunction (e.g., hepatic encephalopathy) occurs. However, once this does occur, it is usually fatal.

Invasion of the gastrointestinal tract can present as massive gastrointestinal bleeding, as seen with lymphoma. Additionally, when chemotherapy-responsive tumors that involve the gastrointestinal tract are treated, perforation (from tumor necrosis) can occur.

Chemotherapy

A complete review of the mechanisms of action or all toxicities of each chemotherapeutic drug is beyond the scope of this summary. Some important generalizations about drug toxicity by class will be reviewed.

ALKYLATING AGENTS

These agents are considered to be "radiomimetic" (i.e., cellular effects are similar to the effects of ionizing radiation). The alkylating agents form covalent bonds between preformed nucleic acids and interfere with the normal function of the nucleic acids. Nitrogen mustard (mechlorethamine), the prototype alkylating agent used principally in the treatment of Hodgkin's disease, causes reversible myelosuppression as its principal toxicity.

Busulfan (Myleran), used principally in the treatment of chronic myelogenous leukemia, is associated with irreversible interstitial lung fibrosis that develops after months or even years of therapy. When this agent is combined with nitrosoureas, this toxicity can be significantly accelerated.

Cyclophosphamide (Cytoxan) is part of the therapy of many malignant diseases. Respiratory failure on the basis of interstitial fibrosis and severe restrictive physiology is seen occasionally after long exposure to this agent. When ventilatory support is required, high airway pressures increase the risk of barotrauma, and high-frequency jet ventilation has been used as a temporary measure but as expected, the overall prognosis is quite dismal. Cyclophosphamide has also been associated with cardiotoxicity, particularly when combined with anthracyclines or in patients with previous mediastinal radiation. Cyclophosphamide and other alkylating agents can deplete plasma cholinesterase. This might lead to delayed resolution of muscle paralysis after anesthesia if this effect is not considered. An additional, potentially life-threatening complication of cyclophosphamide metabolites is hemorrhagic cystitis and subsequent massive hematuria. This is usually, but not always, prevented by adequate diuresis from fluid administration so that these metabolites do not remain in contact with the bladder wall. The treatment of this, besides support of blood volume, includes cystoscopic electrocoagulation, topical formaldehyde bladder instillation, and rarely cystectomy with ureteral diversion.

Chlorambucil (Leukeran) and melphalan (Alkeran) are oral alkylating agents used in the treatment of various lymphomas, leukemias, and myeloma. Their principal toxicity includes nausea, vomiting, and myelosuppression.

ANTIMETABOLITES

These agents have their maximum effects during active DNA synthesis, particularly during the S (synthesis) phase of the cell cycle. Actively dividing normal cells are the hematopoietic cells and mucosal cells of the gastrointestinal tract (including the oral cavity).

Methotrexate and 5-fluorouracil are the most commonly used antimetabolites in cancer therapy, with activity against a wide range of malignancies. Chronic use of methotrexate has been associated with progressive hepatic dysfunction. Acutely, these agents can cause severe neutropenia, thrombocytopenia, and mucositis. Diarrhea, secondary to the toxic effects of these agents on the gastrointestinal mucosa, can be quite severe with profound volume loss and electrolyte abnormalities. Acute renal failure has also been associated with methotrexate, usually in high doses. Methotrexate rarely causes pulmonary toxicity, manifested by a nondesquamative alveolitis and noncaseating granulomas. Leucovorin (folinic acid) or citrovorum has been used to abrogate some of the acute toxic effects of methotrexate.

Vinca Alkaloids

Vincristine, vinblastine, vindesine, and vinorelbine (Navelbine) are the most common of the vinca alkaloids. Although differing in their bone marrow toxicity (vinblastine causes more myelosuppression than vincristine, for example), these agents are primarily neurotoxic. Severe peripheral neuropathy can be associated with these agents (particularly vincristine). Also, autonomic neuropathy with orthostatic hypotension and severe and prolonged ileus can occur. Generally, the ileus is self-limited and responds to conservative therapy, although occasionally cecal dilatation may require emergency cecostomy or colonoscopic decompression to avoid perforation. Other toxicities of these agents include the syndrome of inappropriate antidiuretic hormone and local tissue necrosis at the site of inadvertent extravasation.

Antineoplastic Antibiotics

The anthracycline derivatives are the most prominent of this group of chemotherapeutic agents. The most common members of this family are doxorubicin (Adriamycin), daunorubicin (Daunomycin), mitoxanthrone, and epirubicin. These agents are used in a wide variety of malignancies and have one of the broadest spectra of activity in the chemotherapeutic armamentarium. Toxicities include myelosuppression, stomatitis, alopecia, tissue necrosis from extravasation, and radiation skin recall. The most significant cumulative toxicity particularly associated with doxorubicin (Adriamycin) is cardiotoxicity in the form of cardiomyopathy. This cardiomyopathy occurs with increasing frequency when a cumulative dose of 550 mg/m^2 is exceeded but with lower cumulative doses when mediastinal irradiation or concurrent cyclophosphamide is used. Cardiac function is typically followed by 2-D echocardiography or electrocardiography-gated radionuclide scans (MUGA) to assess ejection fraction. Electrocardiographic findings are nonspecific.

Treatment of this complication is supportive, using the usual combination of diuretics, digoxin, and afterload reduction. An occasional patient in sustained remission of the underlying malignancy has undergone successful heart transplantation for life-threatening cardiomyopathy. Myelosuppression can be profound and prolonged, particularly when single doses greater than 90 mg/m^2 of Adriamycin are used.

Actinomycin D, an agent used against soft tissue sarcoma, choriocarcinoma, and Ewing's sarcoma, is associated with radiation recall reactions, including radiation pneumonitis and skin recall. Myelosuppression, nausea and vomiting, and vascular necrosis are other toxicities of this agent.

Streptozotocin, an agent used in metastatic carcinoid tumors, is associated with renal failure that is often irreversible.

Bleomycin, an agent used in the treatment of several solid tumors, including non-seminomatous carcinoma of the testis, can cause an interstitial pneumonitis, as previously mentioned. The presentation of this can occur with low cumulative doses (100 mg/m^2), but usually this is not seen until higher cumulative doses are delivered (350 mg/m^2). The typical histology is a mixed alveolar and interstitial infiltrate more prominent at the lung bases. As previously mentioned, there has been a recall-like reaction associated with high inspired oxygen concentration during general anesthesia.

TAXANES

This unique group of antineoplastics causes stabilization of the microtubular apparatus, thus interfering with mitosis. A limited supply of taxol, initially available only from the bark of the yew tree, slowed its clinical development. This problem has been partially solved, and this agent is currently being investigated in Phase II and Phase III treatment studies of several common malignancies (such as ovarian cancer, breast cancer, head and neck cancer, and nonsmall cell carcinoma of the lung). Early reports of occasionally fatal hypersensitivity reactions were ultimately linked to the Cremophor vehicle. Use of premedication with antihistamines, H_2-blockers, and corticosteroids has significantly reduced this problem.

TAMOXIFEN

Tamoxifen, an orally administered antineoplastic drug used in the treatment of breast carcinoma, has been associated with significant hypercalcemia in the presence of bone metastases. This agent is presently under investigation as a chemopreventative drug in women at high risk for breast cancer. There is some question of an increased incidence of endometrial carcinoma with this agent.

CISPLATIN

Cis-diamininedichloroplatinum (cisplatin), used in the treatment of several malignancies, including potentially curable diseases such as diffuse lymphoma and nonseminomatous carcinoma of the testis, is associated with significant nephrotoxicity, particularly when the agent has been given without adequate volume diuresis. Neurotoxicity, including ototoxicity, neuropathy, and seizures, has also been reported with cisplatin. The new platinum analog carboplatin is much less nephrotoxic, but its principal toxicity is myelosuppression with thrombocytopenia as the dose-limiting toxicity.

CYTOKINES

Several cytokines have entered clinical trials. The best known and studied of these is interferon and interleukin-2. Interferon has been associated with cytopenia, neurotoxicity, hepatotoxicity, and common flulike symptoms. Interleukin-2, particularly in high doses used for melanoma and hypernephroma, has been associated with a full-blown capillary leak syndrome, including hemodynamic instability, respiratory distress (occasionally requiring intubation and mechanical ventilation), nephrotoxicity, and severe neurologic dysfunction.

Clinical Trials

There are three generally recognized categories of clinical trials. A Phase I clinical trial relates to questions regarding the toxicity and feasibility of an investigational drug in a group of patients with a variety of malignancies. These patients have typically been heavily pretreated with other therapies. Dose escalation of the investigational drug is studied in a systematic fashion, seeking dose-limiting toxicity.

A Phase II clinical trial evaluates the response, toxicity, and survival of patients with a specific malignancy, given the schedule of the investigational drug established in Phase I.

Finally, a Phase III trial is a larger, often multi-institutional study, designed in a prospective, randomized, controlled fashion, comparing at least two different treatment strategies for a given disease. In this way, questions of clinical efficacy can be answered in a scientific manner.

As conventional chemotherapy has evolved, two concepts have emerged that are important to the critical care physician. First, adjuvant treatment is the treatment of a malignancy with chemotherapy after primary treatment (usually surgery). This is done in the hope of increasing the cure rate for a particular tumor (e.g., breast cancer). In this setting, toxicity of therapy should be treated aggressively because of the potential for long-term good prognosis. This would most commonly be the case in the increasingly aggressive adjuvant treatment of breast cancer in which neutropenic sepsis can be a problem. Second, most malignancies are treated with multiple-agent chemotherapy or combined modalities (e.g., concurrent chemotherapy and radiation therapy). Although efforts are made in protocol design to avoid additive toxicity, this can still be a significant problem.

Radiation Therapy

The principal toxicity of radiation therapy relates to the relative sensitivity of the normal tissues adjacent to the target volume (i.e., tumor being radiated). The effects of ionizing radiation are characterized histologically by diffuse microvascular thrombosis, with necrosis of surrounding tissues. Thus, as an example, prior radiation therapy to the mediastinum is a risk factor for the development of coronary artery disease at a later date.

Radiation pneumonitis is likely the commonest acute radiation effect that might require ICU admission because of the need to treat hypoxia. This can occur any time up to 6 months after treatment with radiation when the radiation therapy includes lung tissue in the treatment volume.

Radiation pneumonitis may develop quite insidiously, manifested simply by increasing cough, which can lead to progressive respiratory failure and permanent functional limitations from interstitial fibrosis. The only therapy of any apparent or potential benefit is the use of steroids and, of course, supportive care.

When the normal tissue included in the target volume involves the bowel, severe malabsorption and diarrhea can occur that can lead to significant fluid and electrolyte abnormalities if not appropriately treated. If the spinal cord receives excessive radiation, transverse myelitis with subsequent potentially devastating neurologic dysfunction such as paraplegia can occur. Additionally, certain chemotherapeutic agents (cyclophosphamide, methotrexate, doxorubicin, actinomycin D, bleomycin, and BCNU) can cause radiation recall reactions in various organs—most commonly the skin, lung, or heart—which can lead to additional toxicity in these organs. The spectrum can range from a simple skin erythema that precisely demarcates the skin port of a radiation treatment to the development of congestive heart failure from doses of doxorubicin below those usually associated with this toxicity.

Hyperthermia

It has been recognized that malignant tissue is much more susceptible to heat damage than is normal tissue. This observation has led to the application, usually locally, of hyperthermia in an effort to increase tumor necrosis. Perfusion techniques to increase temperature, particularly of isolated limbs, have been investigated with limited success. These patients are carefully monitored during the procedure. Besides the local problem of thrombosis due to the vascular access device, hyperthermia-induced hyperventilation can lead to a surprising degree of hypokalemia secondary to respiratory alkalosis. Additionally, increased potassium loss in the urine also occurs. Hyperthermia can also cause a mild degree of disseminated intravascular coagulation.

Indications for Surgical Consultation

As with all facets of critical care, it is often appropriate to involve other medical disciplines in the care of the critically ill oncology patient. Although not meant to be exhaustive, the following examples are used to highlight some of the unique management problems brought about by the disease or its treatment.

Epistaxis can always be a severe problem, particularly when it occurs in the setting of severe thrombocytopenia or from necrosis of a local tumor, such as nasopharyngeal carcinoma. In addition to local measures, including removal of a nasogastric tube, if present, and nasal packing, evaluation of the clotting mechanism, particularly platelet function and number, is required. Platelet transfusion may be required in thrombocytopenic bleeding.

Tumor obstruction of the airway from undiagnosed head and neck cancer, bilateral vocal cord paralysis, tumor involving the trachea, or extrinsic compression from a mediastinal mass (particularly lymphoma) can be extremely challenging. Depending on the situation, standard endotracheal intubation may be technically impossible or worsen the situation of the already compromised airway due to traumatic edema or bleeding. Emergency tracheostomy may be the only way to secure the airway. Additionally, laser fulguration of obstructing intraluminal tumors is a technique for palliation of a compromised airway, particularly involving the trachea or mainstem bronchi.

Hemoptysis or bleeding from the endotracheal tube, particularly in the severely thrombocytopenic patient, can be a terminal event. This bleeding manifestation can also be due to an intraluminal tumor; laser fulguration can offer palliative benefit in this situation.

Airway compression by large mediastinal masses can occur. This becomes a particular problem after general anesthesia has been required for diagnostic biopsy. In this situation, it is very important to know that the patient is fully awake and that the muscle strength has returned before extubation. Occasionally, patients are treated with chemotherapy or radiation before extubation in an effort to relieve compression and edema of the airway. When malignant lymphomas are the cause, the response to initial therapy can be quite dramatic and is certainly worth this extra effort.

Life-threatening hemorrhage from a major vessel of the neck, often in the setting of relapsed head and neck cancer, occasionally requires emergency surgical intervention. Unfortunately, this often occurs with advanced local tumor involvement when the overall prognosis is poor even if the patient survives the acute event. This often leads to ethical and moral dilemmas, particularly when there has been no advance discussion of limits of care with the patient.

Infections, especially wound infections, can have an insidious presentation in patients with malignancies, particularly in the presence of neutropenia or steroid therapy. Often, the characteristic local signs of redness, pain, and heat are not present because of the immunocompromised state—an otherwise innocuous watery discharge from the wound may be the only manifestation of a significant infection. Necrotizing skin and fascial infections, particularly in the immunocompromised neutropenic host, can cause sepsis and development of multiple system organ failure, if not recognized and aggressively treated with broad-spectrum antibiotics and surgical debridement.

Esophageal perforation occurring from tumor, severe protracted vomiting and retching, or instrumentation requires prompt recognition and surgical treatment, when appropriate.

Acute cardiac tamponade from tumor invasion of the pericardium or occasionally radiation-induced pericarditis requires prompt recognition and drainage.

Several chemotherapeutic agents can cause severe chemical cellulitis if local extravasation occurs. This has been a lesser clinical problem because of the improvement in venous access devices used with increasing frequency in oncology. The risk can also be minimized by insisting that potential vesicants be handled and infused by personnel with specific training.

Abdominal Complications

Evaluation of abdominal signs and symptoms has always been a challenge. In malignancy, this challenge is even more acute. The primary malignancy, its metastases, or the effects of therapy (i.e., immunocompromise, particularly neutropenia) cloud the issue. The morbidity and potential mortality of a significant abdominal process (such as interstitial perforation) in a compromised host is much higher. Early recognition and treatment is the best defense. The treatment may be the cause of the abdominal problem, which may be reversible with symptomatic care and withdrawal of the inciting agent. An example would be vincristine- or opiate-induced adynamic ileus.

Because of the difficulties in making an accurate diagnosis and the severity of the underlying disease, positive blood cultures, hyperglycemia, progressive renal dysfunction, hypovolemia, and lactic acidosis are common findings at the time of surgical intervention. The gravity of the clinical situation may necessitate limitation of the surgical procedures to simple drainage, diversion, and decompression.

The diagnostic procedures available are the same as those available in any other patient population, including plain and position abdominal x-ray films, ultrasound, CT scan, and radionuclear scans (e.g., gallium-67 citrate, technetium-99, indium-WBC). If an abscess is found, CT scan or ultrasound examination can be used to guide percutaneous drainage, thus delaying or obviating an open surgical procedure. In experienced hands, laparoscopic abdominal exploration has been used and is helpful in differential diagnosis, which might include painful hepatomegaly from metastases or subcapsular bleeding, mesenteric ischemia, acute cholecystitis, intraperitoneal bleeding, or exudative peritonitis.

The patient with malignant disease and right upper quadrant complaints makes the point of the potential diagnostic conundrum. Here the symptoms might be due to tumor metastases in the liver, massive hepatic bleeding, hepatic abscesses, cholangitis caused by common duct obstruction, or acalculous cholecystitis with gallbladder empyema, necessitating prompt drainage.

Hemorrhagic enteritis caused by such different etiologies as viral infection in immunocompromised patients (herpes virus, CMV), fungal infection (strongyloidiasis or giardiasis), uremic platelet dysfunction, coagulopathy, antimetabolite toxicity (particularly in the presence of granulocytopenia), or tumor necrosis and localized bleeding can create a diagnostic and therapeutic dilemma. If bowel perforation occurs as a result of one of these problems, surgery should not be withheld on the basis of pancytopenia alone, unless the patient has failed to respond to therapy of the underlying malignancy. A conservative nonoperative approach in this circumstance carries a mortality rate approaching 100%.

Colonic pseudo-obstruction, associated with multiple system organ failure, electrolyte imbalance, or renal failure, can result in perforation when cecal dilatation exceeds 10 to 12 cm on plain x-ray films unless colonoscopic decompression or cecostomy is performed.

Acute mesenteric ischemia either caused by local venous or arterial thrombosis or low-flow states (e.g., in congestive heart failure, severe hypovolemia, or cardiac tamponade) occurs more commonly in the elderly. In the acutely ill patient with cancer, additional problems, such as the hypercoagulable state associated with malignancy, sepsis, or hypoperfusion, will increase the incidence of acute mesenteric ischemia. Early recognition and aggressive therapy has led to improved survival and quality of remaining life.

Ethical Dilemmas

The critical care of the patient with cancer focuses on some of the dilemmas of contemporary medicine. Medical technology has advanced significantly in what can be done. For societal and humanistic reasons, we need to focus on what we should do (i.e., what is beneficial to the patient). The possible answers to this much more difficult question will come from the wishes of the involved patients or families, who must be informed of the realistic expectations for survival and quality of life in each clinical situation. Outcome-based research will increasingly find answers to the many difficult questions regarding appropriate treatment of these patients.

CHAPTER 10
Trauma

Gail T. Tominaga, MD • Kenneth Waxman, MD

EPIDEMIOLOGY OF TRAUMA

Injury is to a large extent preventable. The epidemiologic study of trauma leads to an increased understanding of the injury process, identification of potential predictors of its clinical course and outcome, and formulation of effective preventive strategies.

In 1983 Trunkey described a trimodal distribution of trauma death as a function of time after injury. The first peak occurs within the first hour and describes fatal injuries for which provision of immediate medical care is minimally effective. This group accounts for more than half of all trauma deaths. The second peak in mortality occurs at 1 to 4 hours after injury and includes patients for whom immediate definitive medical treatment can be lifesaving. The prevention of deaths in this phase is the primary goal of an effective regional trauma care system. The third peak in trauma mortality occurs 1 to 5 weeks after injury and includes deaths from sepsis and multiple organ failure. Early and optimal critical care for the patients at risk in this third phase reduces the number of patients who die from these causes.

Initial severity scoring for triage purposes emphasized an inventory of the wounds sustained. The Abbreviated Injury Scale assigns severities to individual injuries, ranging from 1 (minor injuries) to 6 (always fatal). The Injury Severity Score (ISS) is an anatomic injury score ranging from 1 to 75. It is calculated by summing the squares of the three highest Abbreviated Injury Scale scores for injuries to different body regions (i.e., head and neck, face, thorax, abdomen, pelvis, extremities, external). The Revised Trauma Score has been shown to be a more reliable predictor of outcome than the ISS. It is based on three physiologic measures—Glasgow Coma Scale score, respiratory rate, and systolic blood pressure. A third calculation, TRISS, has been developed to combine anatomic injury (Injury Severity Score) and physiologic status (Revised Trauma Score). TRISS methodology has been used to predict probability of survival, based on data gathered from a large multicenter study, the Major Trauma Outcome Study, which collected trauma registry data from more than 120 designated trauma centers on injury mechanism, injury diagnosis, injury severity, duration of hospital stay, and clinical outcome. This data base includes more than 120,000 trauma patient records and serves as the principal population data base for developing predictive models of clinical outcome following trauma. The most clinically relevant data for injury incidence, severity, and outcome, however, are those collected at the local hospital level.

The magnitude of trauma's impact on health care and society in the United States is significant. Motor vehicle collisions represent the single most common major injury–producing mechanism. The estimated annual cost to society of motor vehicle–related deaths through lost productivity exceeds that for any other single cause of death. Burns account for some 2 million injuries per year, with almost 6000 burn-related deaths each year. Falls are estimated to occur in 12 million persons annually. An alarming and escalating problem is the sharp increase in urban violence and firearm injury.

INITIAL ASSESSMENT OF THE MULTIPLE TRAUMA PATIENT

The role of the intensive care unit (ICU) in the management of critically injured patients includes continuation of the resuscitation and evaluation initiated in the emergency department and operating room. It is essential that ongoing resuscitation be continuously evaluated and adjusted as needed. Goal-directed physiologic monitoring is necessary to provide early warning of the potential problems with an in-depth review and survey of all organ systems most likely to suffer from direct trauma or secondary injury related to hypoxia, hypoperfusion, or sepsis. To avoid missing injuries and to enhance a positive outcome, assessment should be systematic. The most common injuries and potential complications should be kept in mind, and priorities should be established based on the most life-threatening injuries.

Closed Head Injuries

The initial management of a patient with suspected significant head injury and altered consciousness is tracheal intubation, hyperventilation to an arterial carbon dioxide tension (pCO_2) of 25 to 30 mm Hg, and judicious isotonic fluid administration. If the patient has an abnormal head computed tomographic (CT) scan showing focal or generalized injury as well as a Glasgow Coma Scale of 8 or less without intoxicants, placement of an intracranial pressure monitor should be considered. Neurosurgical consultation is necessary to assess the need for operative intervention. Serial examinations and intracranial pressure monitoring are essential in a severely head-injured patient.

Another dilemma is the choice of sedation and pain control in obtunded and combative patients. Although the importance of the ability to follow the neurologic examination cannot be overemphasized, withholding analgesics for these patients, who often have other significant injuries, can worsen their agitation and increase oxygen demand. Adequate pain control can be accomplished with the use of short-acting narcotics whose effects can be pharmacologically reversed. If the neurologic examination shows deterioration, repeat head CT should be considered.

Spinal Cord Injuries

All trauma patients should be considered to have spinal injuries until proved otherwise. Lateral cervical spine radiography, even when demonstrating all seven vertebrae, has a sensitivity of only 0.85 of detecting significant injury. An anteroposterior (AP) view and an open-mouth odontoid view must be used to rule out more than 99% of cervical bone injuries. Patients who have a cervical spine injury or who are obtunded should be evaluated for concomitant thoracic and lumbar spine injuries. If a spine injury is identified, further diagnostic studies are often indicated. All patients with suspected spine injuries should be immobilized and moved in a manner that prevents flexion, extension, or rotation of the potentially injured areas. Airway manipulations should be performed with in-line stabilization of the cervical spine. Rapid diagnosis is essential. Methylprednisolone therapy within 8 hours of injury has been shown to be of benefit. An initial bolus of 30 mg/kg followed by 5.4 mg/kg/h for 23 hours should be administered.

Because of unopposed parasympathetic outflow, patients with spine injuries may have a low systemic vascular resistance, low blood pressure, and at times, bradycardia. The low systemic vascular resistance places patients at risk for uncontrolled heat loss; thus, attention to temperature is critical, particularly in patients with other injuries. If perfusion is inadequate and hemorrhage from other injuries has been ruled out, sympathomimetic agents, such as dopamine, are usually effective.

Chest Trauma

Chest injuries account for 25% of trauma deaths. Most critical chest injuries can be detected by chest radiography. Rib fractures are the most common thoracic injury. The presence of multiple rib fractures increases the likelihood of other injuries. The most common clinical consequence of rib fractures or penetrating chest trauma that requires intervention is a pneumothorax or a hemothorax. Most patients with these injuries require only the placement of a large-bore (e.g., 38-French) chest tube connected to an underwater seal and collection system. Rarely, operative intervention is required for large or persistent air leaks, which can signal major tracheobronchial injuries. A hemothorax that initially drains more than 1500 mL of blood or continues to drain more than 200 to 300 mL/h may necessitate thoracotomy.

Pulmonary contusion is a major factor in the morbidity and mortality of patients with chest trauma. Although the number of fractures does not correlate with the severity of pulmonary injury, rib, scapular, and sternal fractures are important markers of the magnitude of injury, and their presence should increase the suspicion of underlying injury. The extent of pulmonary contusion may not be apparent on initial chest radiograph. Many patients require intubation and ventilatory support, including increasing levels of positive end-expiratory pressure until oxygen saturation is satisfactory. Fluid resuscitation should not be tempered at the expense of delaying restoration of adequate perfusion.

Another serious chest injury is flail chest. It is defined as "paradoxical ventilatory movement" and requires at least two segmental fractures in each of three adjacent ribs. The emphasis of management is on the underlying pulmonary injury, pulmonary toilet, and pain control. Early recognition of this injury is important.

The spectrum of cardiac injuries ranges from concussion and contusion to rupture of the papillary muscles or of any of the cardiac chambers or septa. The major concern in myocardial contusion is dysrhythmias, most of which occur within 12 hours of injury. Patients at risk should have cardiac monitoring with additional testing modalities (i.e., echocardiography) when clinically indicated. Myocardial contusion leading to left ventricular failure is uncommon but is associated with a high mortality rate.

Abdominal Trauma

Abdominal trauma is the most frequent cause of treatable, early, life-threatening hemorrhage. Patients may have unreliable findings on abdominal examination as a result of intoxicants, head injury, or paraplegia. Diagnostic tests include diagnostic peritoneal lavage (DPL) and abdominal CT scan. A prerequisite for CT is hemodynamic stability. Pain medication is best withheld to prevent obscuring of findings on serial physical examination. Organs commonly injured by blunt trauma include the spleen and the liver. Small bowel and colon injuries are less frequent than are solid viscus injuries, but they are becoming more common with increased use of seatbelts. The evaluation of these injuries can be difficult because CT is neither sensitive nor specific; DPL can also be falsely negative. Intervention requires a high index of suspicion, particularly in patients with seatbelt contusion. Findings after injury of increased abdominal pain, abdominal tenderness, and fever should raise suspicion. Other difficult to detect abdominal injuries include pancreatic and duodenal injuries. Serial examination and a high index of suspicion are essential.

Hypothermia is a major contributor to coagulopathy and mortality in patients with significant intra-abdominal injuries. Corrective measures should be instituted.

The most common urinary tract injury after blunt trauma is renal contusion. Most renal contusions resolve without intervention or sequelae. The most common manifestation is hematuria, but significant injuries can occur in the absence of hematuria. Blood at the urethral meatus, scrotal hematoma, and high-riding prostate are all indications for retrograde urethrography before Foley catheter placement for evaluation for possible urethral disruption. The upper urinary tract can be evaluated by either intravenous pyelography or CT with intravenous contrast.

Orthopedic and Extremity Injuries

Pelvic fractures are a common source of morbidity and mortality. For this reason, an AP view of the pelvis is included in the routine radiographs of blunt trauma patients. Bleeding from pelvic fractures can be massive. Opening the retroperitoneal hematoma from a pelvic fracture should be avoided. Placement of an external fixator can stabilize the bone fragments and decrease blood loss. In patients with persistent bleeding, an arteriogram with embolization of bleeding arteries can be helpful. Patients with open pelvic fractures should be considered for diverting colostomy. Associated genitourinary injury must also be suspected and treated.

Many trauma patients have associated extremity fractures that can have a major impact on outcome. Studies comparing early versus delayed stabilization demonstrate a decrease in the occurrence of adult respiratory distress syndrome (ARDS), fat embolism, pneumonia, the number of days in the ICU and hospital, and the cost for patients having early (within 24 hours of injury) stabilization. If early operative stabilization cannot be accomplished, skeletal traction should be instituted and maintained.

Extremity fractures and dislocations also predispose to vascular injuries. Arteriography is the gold standard for evaluation, but duplex Doppler ultrasound examination can be a good screening modality. If a compartment syndrome is suspected, the compartment pressure should be measured. Fasciotomies should be performed if compartment pressures are elevated (i.e., greater than 25–30 mm Hg). Prolonged compartment syndromes may result in permanent muscle or nerve injury, rhabdomyolysis, or loss of the extremity.

Other Critical Care Issues

Immobilization predisposes patients to deep venous thrombosis (DVT) and pressure ulcers. The use of anticoagulants as prophylaxis for DVT may be contraindicated by the presence of other injuries. Pneumatic compression stockings can be placed on the lower or upper extremities to achieve some systemic fibrinolysis. Prophylactic vena cava filtration may be considered in high-risk trauma patients.

Pressure ulcers can occur early from lying on a backboard. Trauma patients should be taken off the backboard soon after arrival in the ICU, and precautions that include in-line stabilization and logrolling should be instituted until spinal injury can be excluded.

Infections often occur in trauma patients. Invasive devices are widely used and often placed in a nonelective and less-than-sterile fashion. All central lines placed in the emergency department should be replaced or removed within the first 24 hours. Other causes of infectious processes include pneumonia, urinary tract infection, sinusitis, intra-abdominal abscesses, and acalculous cholecystitis. Multiple organ failure may be the ultimate expression of infectious complications. The development of multiple organ failure is associated with a high mortality rate and should prompt a search for occult infection.

PREOPERATIVE ASSESSMENT OF CRITICALLY ILL PATIENTS

Complete physiologic assessment of critically ill trauma patients before surgical intervention is frequently not possible because of the urgency of the situation. Trauma patients represent an entirely different spectrum of preoperative problems than do patients undergoing elective surgery. Assessment of any patient begins with a complete history and a physical examination. Monitoring, laboratory tests, and therapeutic interventions are performed as time and patient condition permit. Optimally, a full laboratory profile includes a complete blood count, electrolytes, acid-base status, magnesium, calcium, glucose, and a clotting profile that includes a bleeding time. Routine chest radiography should be performed. Early optimization of the cardiovascular system, especially of oxygen delivery and volume status, appears to be helpful in preventing postoperative mortality and multiple organ failure.

The American Society of Anesthesiologists risk assessment criteria have withstood the test of time as an easy classification system. Most critically ill trauma patients are either class IV-E or V-E. Another system has been proposed by the American College of Surgeons. Class I patients require immediate surgery for survival. The prime concern in this group is to preserve life. Preoperative monitoring takes a secondary position to resuscitation when the source of bleeding must be controlled. Class II patients require urgent operation. In these cases, optimizing a patient preoperatively can protect him or her during the surgical procedure and decrease the incidence of postoperative complications. Class III patients include patients who are critically ill before a relatively elective procedure. In these patients, elective admission to the ICU to correct reparable defects and to optimize cardiovascular function can decrease postoperative morbidity significantly.

Cardiovascular System

The most widely accepted risk for a major postoperative cardiac event is recent myocardial infarction. The definition of *recent* and the results of surgery in these patients have changed significantly since the mid-1970s. In 1972, a large series showed a 20% incidence of perioperative myocardial infarction if surgery was performed within 3 months of a myocardial infarction, with a 69% mortality rate among these patients. The incidence dropped to 11% at 6 months and to 6% after 6 months. In 1983, Rao showed that careful preoperative monitoring and correction of the existing cardiac problems could significantly lower postoperative cardiovascular morbidity and mortality.

Several studies have demonstrated that optimization of oxygen delivery and utilization in high-risk patients can decrease mortality and the occurrence of multiple organ failure. Furthermore, the inability to optimize these parameters is a poor prognostic sign that can preclude operative intervention.

Pulmonary Evaluations

The evaluation of pulmonary risk should encompass both chronic risk factors and those acutely related to the underlying disease process. Factors such as asthma and other bronchoreactive diseases can be controlled preoperatively. Risk factors include tobacco use, dyspnea on exertion, asthma, chronic obstructive pulmonary disease (COPD), environmental exposure to pollutants, neuromuscular disease, and morbid obesity with hypoventilation. Routine physical examination can reveal increased AP chest diameter, expiratory wheezes, hyperresonance, and other stigmata of COPD. The most important tests are chest radiography and pulmonary function screening tests. A forced vital capacity less than 50% of predicted value, a forced expiratory volume in 1 second (FEV_1) of 0.8 to 1 L (or less than 60% of predicted value), or an abnormal ratio of forced vital capacity to FEV_1 is a predictor of increased morbidity and mortality. Arterial blood gas analysis is helpful to determine baseline values.

Acute pulmonary problems occur in patients sustaining pulmonary contusion, thoracic wall trauma, and acute bronchial obstruction with resultant atelectasis and pneumonia, as well as in those who require preoperative mechanical ventilation. The liberal use of perioperative therapeutic bronchoscopy, optimizing positive end-expiratory pressure, adequate pain relief, and vigorous pulmonary toilet help to minimize the occurrence of major complications.

Preoperative Nutritional Status

Most trauma patients admitted to the emergency department are nutritionally replete before injury; however, a large percentage of critically ill patients requiring emergent surgery have nutritional deficits. Providing alimentary nutrition for critically ill patients in the ICU by enteral or parenteral route has an impact on wound healing, infectious complications, and nitrogen balance. Eliminating the problems of central vein hyperalimentation through the use of early enteral feeding has been shown to decrease the rate of infectious complications in stressed patients.

Renal and Electrolyte Status

Electrolyte status must be normalized preoperatively. Hypokalemia with arrhythmias or a potassium level below 3.0 mEq/L should be treated with administration of potassium chloride solution at a rate of 20 to 40 mEq/h with arrhythmia monitoring. Hyperkalemia with rhythm disturbances or a potassium level greater than 5.5 mEq/L indicates the need for urgent therapy with bicarbonate, insulin, glucose, and calcium with concomitant administration of binding agents such as sodium polystyrene sulfonate (Kayexalate) orally or by enema. Beta agonist inhalants (e.g., albuterol) also cause a transitory decrease in potassium levels and can be used for the acute treatment of hyperkalemia. Hyponatremia with a sodium level less than 120 mEq/L should be treated with fluid restriction and diuretics if time allows. If the patient has symptoms or requires emergent surgery, a 3% sodium chloride solution can be carefully administered to correct the problem. Acid-base abnormalities amenable to therapy should be corrected, as should magnesium and calcium depletion.

Patients in acute or chronic renal failure should undergo dialysis within the 24 hours preoperatively. Cardiovascular monitoring is essential to the determination of volume status in this patient group. Correction of anemia with blood and blood products should be undertaken preoperatively and intraoperatively.

Neurologic Status

A full mental status evaluation and neurologic examination should be undertaken before surgery. If a focal process or evidence of increased intracranial pressure is discovered, a head CT scan may be warranted. Lumbar puncture should be performed for suspected meningitis once cerebral edema has been ruled out.

Obesity

Morbidly obese patients, especially those with hypoventilation syndrome or pulmonary hypertension, are at high risk because of problems unique to their obese state. Invasive cardiopulmonary monitoring should be performed in morbidly obese patients with sleep apnea, hyperventilation, or hypoventilation syndrome, and in those with pulmonary hypertension and hypoxia. Frequently, this population is fluid overloaded, and vigorous diuresis is necessary preoperatively. Cardiac index is frequently elevated preoperatively; however, surgery appears to reduce ventricular performance in obese patients more than in nonobese patients.

Age

The overall perioperative mortality rate for elective surgical procedures is 0.5% if no concomitant medical conditions are present. Age greater than 70 years raises this rate to 1.25% to 2.5%.

PHYSIOLOGIC RESPONSE TO INJURY

Critical illness that can follow complicated trauma or surgery is to a large extent mediated by exaggeration and imbalance of physiologic compensations that normally occur. The normal metabolic response to trauma can be divided into two phases, an ebb phase and a flow phase. The ebb phase occurs during the first several hours after injury and is characterized by hypovolemia, low blood flow, and the initial compensatory physiologic reactions to trauma and shock. Once resuscitation is complete and perfusion is reestablished, the flow phase begins. It is characterized by a hyperdynamic stress response, fluid retention and edema, catabolism, and hypermetabolism. This catabolic stage can last for days or weeks, depending on the severity of injury. Once volume deficits have been eliminated, wounds have closed, and infection has been controlled, the anabolic stage begins. This is characterized by a return to normal hemodynamics, diuresis, reaccumulation of protein and body fat, and restoration of body function.

Stimuli That Initiate the Physiologic Responses to Trauma

The stress response is initiated not only by injury but also by pain, acute blood loss, shock, hypoxia, acidosis, hypothermia, and the wound itself. Psychologic stressors such as fear also activate centrally mediated responses to trauma. The stress response is mediated by the central nervous system, circulating hormones (e.g., cortisol, glucagon, epinephrine), substances acting both locally and systemically produced in response to local inflammation, and activated circulating cells. The physiologic response and duration are proportionate to the magnitude of injury. Anesthesia diminishes the perception of injury and may diminish the magnitude of the stress response to injury.

Mediators of the Responses to Trauma

Activation of the sympathetic nervous system triggers the release of epinephrine and norepinephrine. Catecholamines exert a multitude of effects, including an increase in blood pressure and heart rate, improvement in cardiac contractility, an increase in minute ventilation, and vasoconstriction throughout the arterial and venous circulation. Catecholamines also affect pancreatic hormone release and glucose, amino acid, and fat metabolism. Prolonged and excessive stimulation of the sympathoadrenal axis can lead to adverse physiologic effects. An immediate effect of an increase in sympathetic tone is the redistribution of intravascular volume from the venous capacitance vessels, which increases central blood volume; the vasoconstricting effects on postcapillary venules may subsequently result in an increase in intraluminal capillary pressure. This contributes to loss of intravascular volume, intravascular hypovolemia, and edema formation.

Activation of the hypothalamic-pituitary-adrenal axis triggers the release of adrenocorticotropic hormone (ACTH) and cortisol. The degree of hypercortisolism parallels the degree of injury and classically has been used as a marker for the degree of stress response. The effects of circulating glucocorticoid include sodium retention, insulin resistance, gluconeogenesis, lipolysis, and protein catabolism. Cortisol causes demargination of leukocytes and also inhibits the activity of phospholipase A, thereby down-regulating prostaglandin synthesis. The elevation of cortisol levels enhances the catabolic effects of tumor necrosis factor and interleukin-6 (IL-6).

Antidiuretic hormone is released in response to decreased blood volume and decreased pressure. It is a potent vasoconstrictor and has a pressor effect. It also acts on renal collecting ducts to promote reabsorption of water, causing water retention.

After trauma, when blood flow through the kidneys is decreased, the juxtaglomerular cells secrete renin. Renin enzymatically cleaves a protein precursor to form angiotensin I, which is further cleaved to form angiotensin II. Angiotensin II is an extremely potent vasoconstrictor and has significant pressor effects. It also acts directly on the kidney to induce a decrease in salt and water excretion.

Endogenous opioids are released from the pituitary gland as part of the initial stress response in an amount equimolar to ACTH. Endorphins are released into the circulation from the adrenal glands in response to sympathetic stimulation. Endogenous opioids modulate catecholamine release from the adrenal medulla and may exert inhibitory feedback on pituitary activation and decrease ACTH release. Beta-endorphin directly increases the secretion of insulin. The opioids may be important as counter-regulatory inhibitors of the stress response in addition to minimizing pain. Endogenous opioids may also modulate normal neutrophil and lymphocyte function and activate neutrophils. Endorphins have also been implicated as mediators that may worsen brain injury.

Important mediator substances arise from sites of tissue injury and cause both local and systemic effects. An important initiating factor for the production of local mediators is endothelial disruption at sites of injury and ischemia. This activates Hageman factor (Factor XII), which then initiates coagulation by means of the intrinsic pathway. Protein clotting activation in turn activates the kinin and plasmin systems. Activated Hageman factor also triggers activation of the complement cascade, which initiates inflammation. The arachidonic acid cascade is activated by injury, ischemia, and endothelial disruption. A byproduct of arachidonic acid release from the cell membrane is platelet-activating factor, which is a potent stimulator of platelet and neutrophil activation. Activation of neutrophils by platelet-activating factor further contributes to tissue injury and inflammation.

Activation of coagulation and inflammation at sites of injury is an essential component of healing and recovery. These local processes can also amplify into systemic responses after major trauma. Activation of monocytes and macrophages, with the resultant activation of cytokine cascades, helps to mediate many of the systemic, immunologic, and metabolic effects after trauma.

Reperfusion injury may be another important mediator after shock and trauma. Ischemic tissues release toxic oxygen radicals on reperfusion, which can initiate both local and systemic tissue injury.

The gut can play a central role in the elaboration of mediators. Gut ischemia may lead to the direct elaboration of inflammatory and reperfusion products.

Physiologic Responses

Following trauma or major operation, patients are typically febrile, hypertensive, tachycardic, and tachypneic. Sympathetic stimulation and high levels of circulating catecholamines cause tachycardia that typically persists even after hypovolemia has been corrected and pain controlled. The return of heart rate toward normal often correlates with the onset of the anabolic phase of the flow period. Increased minute ventilation, reflected by the presence of tachypnea and an increase in tidal volume, is also an expected response to injury or major operation. It is driven by increased catecholamines and sympathetic tone as well as by increased oxygen consumption and carbon dioxide (CO_2) production following trauma. Urine output is often diminished early after trauma or operation because of hypovolemia, a decrease in renal blood flow, and a hormonal milieu that leads to sodium and water reabsorption. Several opposing factors tend to increase urine output. Hence, urine output may not accurately reflect the intravascular volume.

The initial responses to trauma contribute to the preservation of body fluids. Vasoconstriction with sodium and water retention occurs. With severe and prolonged trauma and stress, marked disturbances of the distribution of body water occur; there is a flux of salt and water from the intravascular space into the interstitial space. This results in intravascular hypovolemia as well as edema. Edema soon becomes generalized and is present within tissues distant from the injury. The magnitude of edema formation tends to be proportionate to the severity of injury and is progressive as long as the stress state persists. The more edema progresses, the greater the amounts of fluid that are required to maintain intravascular volume because the volume of distribution of salt and water into the interstitium increases.

The initial stress response tends to maintain blood pressure by vasoconstriction, even if circulating blood volume is significantly decreased. Heart rate and cardiac contractility are increased, which tends to maintain cardiac output. The combination of blood loss and fluid shifts from the intravascular into the interstitial spaces often results in decreased preload, such that cardiac output is decreased in the hours after trauma. As bleeding is controlled and resuscitation restores intravascular volume, cardiac output reaches supernormal levels and a hyperdynamic circulatory state is reached. This state is characterized by rapid heart rate, increased blood pressure, and increased cardiac output. The intensity of this hyperdynamic state and its duration are generally proportionate to the severity of shock and trauma or the magnitude of operation.

Microcirculatory blood flow may be markedly altered early after trauma secondary to intense vasoconstriction and capillary endothelial adherence of circulating cells. This then leads to a decrease in tissue perfusion in certain areas. Edema formation also contributes to impaired oxygen transport.

Following trauma, energy demands increase to supernormal levels. This hypermetabolic state is closely related to the hyperdynamic circulatory state. The high metabolic demands require increased oxygen delivery and oxygen consumption as well as increased minute ventilation secondary to the resultant increased CO_2 production. Inflammatory substances, such as cytokines (TNF, IL-1, IL-6), are important mediators of the post-traumatic hypermetabolic state.

Following severe trauma, marked alterations of protein metabolism occur. Total-body catabolism is increased, particularly within skeletal muscle. To a lesser extent, total-body protein synthesis is also increased, especially hepatic synthesis of acute-phase proteins. Following severe injury, protein breakdown results in a significant loss of muscle mass and may progress to the loss of visceral protein mass as well. The wound appears to be spared to some extent. A high rate of protein breakdown persists for the duration of the stress response, regardless of nutritional support.

The stress hormones cortisol, glucagon, and epinephrine increase the breakdown of glycogen to glucose, which rapidly depletes glycogen stores after injury. Glucose is also produced by gluconeogenesis from alanine and other amino acids released by skeletal muscle breakdown. The net effect of increased glucose production is to increase extracellular glucose concentrations. The increase in glucose provides energy for wounds and the inflammatory process.

Insulin levels are initially low after injury but subsequently increase to normal or supernormal levels. After severe injury, however, hyperglycemia persists. This insulin resistance may be due primarily to the persistent elevation of glucagon, cortisol, and epinephrine levels.

The stress response results in mobilization of fat into free fatty acids; however, there are limitations to this effect. Following injury, fat is oxidized at an accelerated rate and fatty acid synthesis is inhibited. Hence, fatty acids are released into the circulation and become available as energy substrates.

Important changes in coagulation occur following injury, including activation of both clotting and fibrinolytic systems. Early after major trauma, clotting is often impaired. Simultaneously, injured tissues release tissue thromboplastin, activating the extrinsic coagulation system. Activation of the protein clotting system also activates the kinin and plasmin systems, which in turn activates the complement cascade. These processes are amplified further by platelets, monocytes, macrophages, and neutrophils.

Leukocytosis is usually found following trauma. Granulocytosis, monocytosis, and lymphopenia are usually seen. This pattern mimics that of sepsis, but it often occurs without infection. In severe trauma, capillary adherence of neutrophils may predominate, and leukopenia may be seen.

Following trauma, the immune response is markedly altered. The extent of immune disturbance is proportionate to the magnitude of injury or operation. Abnormalities seen include a decrease in antibody response, a decrease in neutrophil chemotaxis, a decrease in delayed-type hypersensitivity, an increase in serum immunosuppressive factors, a decrease in fibronectin levels, and a reduction in serum opsonic activity.

Anabolic Phase of the Flow Cycle

The onset of the recovery phase is heralded by a sense of well-being. Catecholamine and cortisol levels return to normal. Temperature, heart rate, and blood pressure normalize. Respiratory demands decrease. Urine output increases with negative fluid balances and resolution of generalized edema. Metabolic demands decrease, gut function improves, and appetite returns. The anabolic phase of recovery generally takes longer than the acute injury and catabolic phases, and thus may last many days or weeks.

ANESTHESIA IN THE HIGH-RISK PATIENT

Anesthesia carries serious risks in patients who have suffered trauma or who are critically ill. These patients may have life-threatening injuries that are not diagnosed when anesthesia is administered. In addition, although their intravascular volume status is often unknown, they are often hypovolemic.

Preoperative Evaluation

Medical histories are incomplete or nonexistent. Important points in the patient's history include nature and extent of all injuries; vital signs and level of consciousness; adequacy of the airway, ventilation, and circulation; medications taken; all chronic medical problems; surgery and anesthesia history; use of alcohol, tobacco, or recreational drugs; and relevant family history, especially malignant hyperthermia.

The physical examination of the acute trauma victim is heavily influenced by urgency and available time. The assessment should begin with the ABCs (airway, breathing, circulation). Supplemental oxygen should be administered by mask, and clinical evidence of shock should be ascertained.

When time permits, all trauma patients should undergo lateral cervical spine and AP chest radiography, hemoglobin measurement, and electrocardiography (ECG). Emergency surgery must not be delayed while awaiting the results of these tests, however.

Preparation

The operating suite should be warmed and the high-volume fluid warmers set up in advance. The anesthesia machine and ventilator, as well as monitors and anesthesia supply cart, must be checked before the patient enters the room. Rapid induction agents, muscle relaxants, and pressors should be prepared. Airway equipment and emergency drugs should be located on top of the supply cart in an organized fashion.

Preoperative preparation of critically ill patients should concentrate on ensuring adequate oxygenation and perfusion. In head-injured patients, prevention of increased intracranial pressure also assumes a high priority. If there is any question about either oxygenation or intracranial pressure, the trachea should be intubated and mechanical ventilation instituted before the patient comes to the operating room. Cervical spine precautions should be continued in all trauma patients unless the spine has been cleared by both radiographic and neurologic examination.

Adequate intravenous access should be established before the patient comes to the operating suite. In the adult trauma patient, this implies a minimum of two 16-gauge or larger peripheral cannulas placed in noninjured extremities. For patients with undiagnosed thoracic or abdominal injuries, one or more central cannulas of the "introducer" type are recommended. An intra-arterial cannula should also be inserted for craniotomy or thoracotomy.

Sedative or analgesic premedication should be used with extreme caution, particularly in the trauma setting. No sedative or analgesic drugs should be given to a nonintubated patient whose neurologic, respiratory, or hemodynamic status may be unstable. All trauma patients should be treated as if they have a full stomach. Emptying the stomach by means of a nasogastric tube may be helpful.

Monitoring

Noninvasive monitors that should be used in every patient include ECG, sphygmomanometer, pulse oximeter, capnograph, core temperature probe, and stethoscope. The combination of leads II and V_5 is probably the most sensitive for cardiac ischemia detection; however, the onset of ST changes can occur 10 minutes after the beginning of wall motion abnormalities following partial coronary occlusion. Automated sphygmomanometers are least reliable during hypovolemic shock. The manual sphygmomanometer is still the best alternative to an arterial cannula in these patients. Transcutaneous oxygen is useful in this setting; the restoration of transcutaneous oxygen to its normal value of roughly 80% of PaO_2 is one indication of adequate volume resuscitation.

A urinary catheter should be placed in all significantly injured trauma patients. Measurement of urine volume every 15 to 30 minutes provides an important indication of both volume status and renal function. In addition, the appearance of hematuria or hemoglobinuria can warn of genitourinary injury or transfusion reaction.

An arterial cannula should be placed in any patient with hemodynamic instability or questionable oxygen or ventilation status. Central venous pressure monitoring should be considered in patients who are hemodynamically unstable or who may have significant hemorrhage. Perioperative pulmonary artery catheterization should be considered in patients with massive trauma, multiple organ failure, or underlying cardiopulmonary disorders. Continuous intracranial pressure monitoring should be considered in patients with closed head injury and altered mental status.

Airway Management

Trauma patients are often hypovolemic; hence, they may not tolerate a rapid-sequence induction to secure the airway quickly. In addition, their injuries or their anatomy may make intubation difficult by direct laryngoscopy. Despite the risk of aspiration or spinal cord injury, the avoidance of hypoxemia takes the highest priority at all times.

Indications for obtaining a secured airway early include poor ventilation or oxygenation, decreased or changing mental status, signs of developing airway obstruction, possible airway burns, shock, and combativeness requiring sedation. Orotracheal intubation under direct laryngoscopy is the method of first choice. Manual cervical spine stabilization should be maintained, and cricoid pressure (Sellick's maneuver) should be applied during both intubation and mask ventilation. If orotracheal intubation is not possible and an immediate airway is needed, either transtracheal ventilation or emergency cricothyroidotomy should be performed without delay. Using a 14-gauge intravenous cannula inserted through the cricoid membrane and a source of oxygen at 30 to 50 psi, transtracheal ventilation can maintain both adequate oxygenation and ventilation in most patients. In the less emergent setting of a breathing patient who needs a secured airway, several intubation techniques can be considered. Options include blind nasal, fiberoptic-assisted, retrograde, and blind oral intubation using an intubating stylet.

Time permitting, the patient should breath 100% oxygen by mask for at least 2 minutes before intubation or induction of anesthesia. After intubation, positive-pressure ventilation with 100% oxygen should be maintained. Anesthetics or muscle relaxants must be used with caution in critically ill patients. Drugs may be required to facilitate intubation in the alert or uncooperative patient, or they may be indicated to prevent dangerous increases in intracranial pressure in head-injured patients. If a hypnotic agent must be used, the method of choice is rapid-sequence induction, in which the hypnotic and succinylcholine are given as a rapid intravenous bolus while cricoid pressure is maintained until the airway is secured. Rapid sequence minimizes the risk of pulmonary aspiration, but it entails hemodynamic changes that may not be tolerated by the hypovolemic patient. Alternatives in moderately hypovolemic patients include lower dose thiopental (1 to 2 mg/kg IV), etomidate (0.2 to 0.3 mg/kg IV), and ketamine (1 to 2 mg/kg IV). Ketamine is contraindicated in head-injured patients because of its potential to increase intracranial pressure. However, patients with clinical signs of shock should receive none of these hypnotic drugs. Intubation should be performed with a muscle relaxant alone or combined with a small dose of narcotic (fentanyl, 1–3 μg/kg). All drugs to facilitate intubation should be given intravenously if possible. If venous access is not available, ketamine and succinylcholine can be given intramuscularly.

Induction and Maintenance of Anesthesia

Standard rapid-sequence induction with thiopental, 4 to 5 mg/kg, and succinylcholine, 1 mg/kg, is usually not tolerated in a hypovolemic patient. Although succinylcholine remains the muscle relaxant that achieves good intubating conditions most rapidly, its side effects must be understood. Succinylcholine can cause dysrhythmias, including asystole, ventricular tachycardia, and fibrillation. Its potassium-releasing property contraindicates succinylcholine use in patients with severe burns or crush injuries more than 24 hours old, highly elevated serum potassium, denervating diseases, serious intra-abdominal infections, or myotonic dystrophy.

Once the patient is intubated, volatile agents, nitrous oxide, or narcotics can be used for maintenance anesthesia. Trauma patients often exhibit a golden period of 1 to 2 hours, followed by rapid decompensation. Moderately hypovolemic patients often cannot tolerate volatile anesthetic agents; maintenance should involve either a nitrous-narcotic technique or a narcotic alone until intravascular volume is restored. Benzodiazepines (e.g., diazepam, midazolam) can be used for their amnestic effects, but these can also worsen hypotension and must be given with caution.

Regional anesthesia is an option in patients provided they are not hypovolemic and do not have significant ongoing hemorrhage, they are alert and cooperative, and coagulopathy is not present.

Fluid Management

Anesthetic agents change the "functional" volume status by increasing intravascular capacity. In addition to the volume monitors previously discussed, increased alveolar dead space or "wasted ventilation" is an indicator of hypovolemia. Arterial blood gas analysis will reveal metabolic acidosis when significant hypovolemia persists.

Fluid therapy requires adequate vascular access. All resuscitation fluids should be warmed to 37°C. Pressurization devices should be available for large-bore intravenous rapid infusion. A satisfactory fluid-warming and infusion system should be capable of giving one unit of blood (450 mL) in less than 2 minutes. The first priority of fluid resuscitation is restoration of circulating volume. After volume status has been stabilized, the second priority is the restoration of blood oxygen-carrying capacity followed by the normalization of coagulation status.

The most common coagulopathy in trauma patients is dilutional thrombocytopenia. The decision to transfuse platelets should be based on a measured thrombocytopenia in the presence of abnormal bleeding. The platelet count should be kept above 70,000 in the operating room. Deficiencies of fibrinogen or other coagulation factors usually appear later than does thrombocytopenia. Replacement therapy should be guided by measured values of prothrombin and partial thromboplastin time (PTT).

Perioperative Disseminated Intravascular Coagulation

Disseminated intravascular coagulation (DIC) is the generalized activation of the coagulation cascade, causing rapid consumption of platelets, fibrinogen, and Factors V and VIII. This results in diffuse, uncontrollable bleeding from the entire surgical field. Intravascular fibrin formation activates the fibrinolytic system, causing an elevation in fibrin-split products, which in turn produces platelet dysfunction. The diagnosis of DIC is confirmed by clinical evidence of bleeding accompanied by a decreased platelet count, decreased fibrinogen level, positive fibrin-split products, and abnormal activated PTT. Patients at risk include those with vascular endothelial damage resulting from burns, trauma, extensive surgery, or shock. In addition, obstetric complications (amniotic fluid embolism, fetal demise, placental abruption) and sepsis can cause DIC. Therapy is aimed first at the underlying cause. The second step is replacement of consumed blood constituents, primarily platelets, fibrinogen, and Factors V and VIII. The goal of replacement therapy is to maintain a platelet count of at least 100,000/mm^3, a normal activated PTT, and a fibrinogen level of at least 200 mg/dL.

Perioperative Hypothermia

General anesthesia lowers the threshold temperature at which hypothermic corrective responses begin. Anesthesia also reduces cutaneous vasoconstriction, which normally helps to conserve heat, and muscle relaxants block the shivering response. Given the dangers of hypothermia in critically ill trauma patients, every attempt at prevention must be made. The operating room should be kept warm, respired gases should be warmed and humidified, all replacement fluids should be warmed, and a warming blanket should be placed between the patient and the operating table. Plastic wrapping can also be placed around the head to decrease convective heat loss, and warmed air blankets can be placed on all parts of the body not in the operative field.

Pulmonary Aspiration

Pulmonary aspiration of gastric contents is responsible for up to 20% of all anesthesia-related deaths. The risk of aspiration is greatest when the airway is unprotected and the patient is obtunded. The pathophysiology of aspiration depends on the nature and volume of the aspirate. Nonacid liquids (pH>2.5) cause less damage than acid liquids; nonparticulate liquids cause less pulmonary damage than particulate matter. Acid particulate is the most damaging aspirate, causing severe hemorrhagic pulmonary edema and alveolar septal necrosis. Severe hypoxemia and hypercarbia are combined with systemic hypotension and pulmonary hypertension.

Clinical signs of aspiration include vomitus in the oropharynx, wheezing, cyanosis, coughing, hypoxemia, pulmonary edema, and hypotension. Chest radiographs may show changes only after several hours. Diffuse bilateral infiltrates can indicate significant aspiration. The most suggestive sign is sudden hypoxemia with no other explanation.

Prevention of aspiration is important. Prophylactic antacids to increase gastric pH are appropriate, but particulate antacids should never be used. After securing the airway, a nasogastric tube should be used to empty the stomach as much as possible before extubation.

Bronchoscopy is indicated if significant solid material has been aspirated. Very mild aspiration may require supplemental oxygen and monitoring of arterial blood gases. If the patient is hypoxic despite an FIO_2 of 0.5, continuous positive airway pressure may be indicated. Patients with severely impaired compliance may also require mechanical ventilation to maintain acceptable blood gas values. Prophylactic antibiotics are not indicated for most aspirations. Antibiotic use should be reserved for secondary bacterial pneumonia or suspected feculent aspiration. Steroid therapy is not recommended.

INTRAOPERATIVE AND POSTOPERATIVE TRANSFUSION THERAPY

A continuous and adequate supply of oxygen to tissues is a prerequisite for human survival. Independent of etiologic mechanisms, all forms of the shock syndrome are characterized by inadequate oxygen delivery to tissues, often associated with impaired oxygen utilization.

Oxygen Delivery System

The transfer of oxygen from the alveolus in the lung to the intracellular mitochondria is quite complex. The relation between saturation and oxygen content is shown in the following equation, where Cao_2 is arterial oxygen content, Sao_2 is arterial oxygen saturation, Pao_2 is partial pressure of oxygen in arterial blood, and Hb is hemoglobin in grams per deciliter:

$$Cao_2 = Hb \times 1.34 \times Sao_2 + Pao_2 \times 0.0031.$$

The delivery of oxygen (Do_2) is most dependent on hemodynamics because it is defined as the product of flow, cardiac output, and arterial oxygen content. Oxygen consumption is the product of cardiac output and the arteriovenous oxygen content difference. Like Do_2 it is subject to measurement error in each of the variables and is sensitive to regional flow distribution and metabolic activity.

The oxygen extraction ratio (OER) is defined as the ratio of global oxygen consumption and global Do_2. Normally between 0.25 and 0.30, the OER, when increased, most likely reflects poor flow with increased extraction, whereas values below 0.25 generally indicate high flow and poor extraction, or tissue inability to consume and use oxygen.

Another factor influencing Do_2 is the position of the oxyhemoglobin dissociation curve, which is regulated primarily by intraerythrocytic 2,3-diphosphoglyceric acid and plasma pH. The normal P_{50} (the oxygen tension at which hemoglobin is 50% saturated) is 27.5 ± 1.0 mm Hg.

When Vo_2 is plotted against Do_2, there appears to be a critical level of Do_2 below which tissue is deprived of oxygen. Further decreases in Do_2 significantly decrease Vo_2 in a nearly linear fashion; Vo_2 is said to be flow dependent. The point at which Vo_2 changes from flow dependent to flow independent is called the critical Do_2 point and has implications for transfusion therapy. Below this critical Do_2, the OER begins to increase exponentially, reflecting a decrease in Do_2.

Responses to Decreased Oxygen Delivery

When the state of decreased Do_2 is present, physiologic compensation occurs at many levels. Intracellularly, less energy is produced from glucose consumption, with resulting intracellular acidosis producing cellular dysfunction initially, which can progress to tissue and organ failure. Unreversed, this leads to cell death.

Lactic acidosis can often be detected at the point of critical Do_2, where the OER increases and the Do_2 decreases. This point could be considered a possible transfusion trigger. Global compensatory mechanisms for a decreased Do_2 exist. Any acute decrease in concentration or intravascular volume increases cardiac output as compensation. This relation is generally linear over the clinically relevant range, assuming that intercurrent disease, age, and pharmacologic agents do not prevent the homeostatic mechanisms from being activated. Interventions that increase cardiac output can be used to improve Do_2 without reverting to red blood cell (RBC) transfusion provided the patient has sufficient cardiac reserve. The limitation is the ability of the heart to meet the increased demands. If the heart has limited reserves and cannot provide adequate Do_2, it may be more appropriate to transfuse RBCs early.

Transfusion Trigger

An absolute value for a transfusion trigger does not exist. The transfusion trigger is a dynamic variable, governed by many factors, including cardiovascular status, vascular volume, and hemoglobin concentration. A patient with adequate global Do_2, flow-independent oxygen consumption, a normal OER, and no lactic acidosis has no obvious indication for an RBC transfusion.

Products and Techniques for Effecting Increased Oxygen Delivery

Any intervention that increases cardiac output, by definition, increases Do_2. Thus, agents used to increase preload, contractility, or afterload can be used to augment Do_2, up to a point. Transfusion of RBCs is another method of increasing Do_2 and may be the best and most appropriate treatment in specific situations.

Risks of Transfusion of Red Blood Cells

Because of great concern about the transmission of infectious disease by RBC transfusion, newer concepts of transfusion triggers and indications for transfusion are evolving. Withholding a transfusion until it is absolutely indicated would be reasonable if the point of necessity could be easily identified. Unfortunately, this point is not readily apparent outside the areas of sophisticated monitoring.

The most commonly transmitted viral agent associated with blood transfusion is cytomegalovirus. Although this infection is rarely of clinical significance, a patient with immune system compromise is more likely to show signs of cytomegalovirus infection if it is present.

Dilutional coagulopathy and DIC may be technique specific. The coagulopathy of massive transfusion is dilutional; it requires treatment only if symptomatic. The appropriate initial therapy is transfusion of platelets, followed by replacement of clotting factors when necessary.

Transfusion therapy can also cause hypothermia; hence, warming of blood is desirable. Hypothermia is related to bleeding; the coagulation system is thermodynamically regulated. The coagulopathy induced by hypothermia is believed to be related primarily to platelet dysfunction.

Transfused bank blood also has a significant concentration of potassium (20–50 mEq/L) as a result of RBC lysis during storage. An excess of citrate (the primary anticoagulant of stored blood) can bind serum calcium, inducing cardiac dysfunction. This is not a problem if the RBC infusion rate is less than 100 mL/min.

An area of recent concern is an apparent immune suppressive effect of transfusion therapy. The induced immune suppression is related to the volume of allogeneic blood infused. The mechanisms proposed implicate both cellular and plasma components of blood. Changes in suppressor T cell function, cytokine production, monocyte function, and natural killer cell function are postulated. It is generally assumed there is an increased risk of infection after allogeneic transfusion.

Red Blood Cell Transfusion Options

The options for RBC transfusion late in the 20th century are many. The RBC options for use in emergency situations are more limited. Homologous RBCs are likely to be used in urgent and emergency situations. Various forms of homologous blood are available: whole blood, packed RBCs (PRBCs), leukocyte-free RBCs, adenine-stored RBCs, washed PRBCs, frozen PRBCs, and rejuvenated frozen PRBCs. The differences in terms of oxygen-carrying capacity are relatively small. The main differences are in the quantity of non-RBC material infused, which could lead to undesirable side effects. Factors that influence oxygen availability changes in P_{50} are related to length of storage and type of storage solution, preservatives, and anticoagulant used. Washing RBCs and depleting them of white blood cells are techniques used to decrease the incidence of allergic transfusion reactions.

Various forms of autotransfusion are available for use, including preoperative autologous blood donation with or without erythropoietin augmentation, intraoperative and postoperative cell salvage, and intraoperative hemodilution. Autologous blood is perceived to be safest, at least with respect to transmission of infectious disease. Whether autologous transfusion is safe relative to placing the immune system or host defense mechanism at risk is less well defined. Transfusion of aged, dysfunctional RBCs may lead to immunocompromise whether cells are homologous or autologous.

Transfusion in Emergency and Urgent Resuscitation Situations

Acute massive hemorrhage of 30% or more of the circulating blood volume requires blood transfusion as part of the resuscitation effort.

Type-specific, uncrossmatched PRBCs are preferred in an emergency. Typing of blood is relatively rapid (5–7 minutes). Type-specific uncrossmatched blood can cause a transfusion reaction in previously transfused patients and multiparous women.

Type O RBCs can theoretically be administered without fear of a major ABO incompatibility reaction. Type O, Rh-negative blood is the universal donor. After receiving large quantities of universal RBCs, patients with type A, B, or AB blood may have transfusion reactions when they receive subsequently administered RBCs typed and crossmatched to their initial, pre–universal donor transfusion specimen.

In men and women beyond the childbearing age, in whom antibody formation is less of a problem, type O, Rh-positive blood is another universal donor. Rh-negative multiparous women and previously transfused Rh-negative patients are at increased risk. About 70% of Rh-negative individuals who receive Rh-positive RBCs acquire anti-D antibodies. Type O, Rh-positive blood should be considered the third option after type-specific uncrossmatched and type O, Rh-negative blood for emergency RBC replacement.

Applications of the Options for Red Blood Cell Transfusion

Autologous blood is safe with respect to transmission of infectious disease and transfusion reaction. Acute normovolemic hemodilution is an excellent technique for elective surgical procedures and some urgent cases. The risk of transmission of infectious disease is minimized, and other forms of transfusion reactions should be eliminated. When acute normovolemic hemodilution is used in combination with predeposit autologous and RBC salvage, it is possible to acquire six to eight units of a patient's blood for use in a single perioperative period.

Intraoperative RBC salvage is a major advance. Washing the RBCs effectively eliminates some complications, especially coagulopathy. The general risks of cell salvage techniques are the potential induction of coagulopathy, overdilution, infusion of excessive anticoagulant, and the possible infusion of cell fragments, proteins, protein fragments, and other debris that could have toxic consequences on many key host systems.

Allogeneic Transfusion Options

Traditional transfusion for nearly a century has been allogeneic—that is, homologous—RBCs evolving from whole blood to mostly, if not exclusively, PRBCs. RBCs typed and crossmatched to a recipient are the first line of allogeneic units generally available. The directed-donor option has gained popularity. Blood collected through directed donation is fully processed and tested before release. Some centers irradiate the blood before use.

A Look at the Future

A number of hemoglobin-based solutions are in various phases of clinical testing. At this time, there are at least 11 modifiers or families of modifiers and 4 or 5 cross-linkers for hemoglobin being explored. These oxygen-carrying RBC substitutes may play a major role in augmenting Do_2 in the future.

INTRAOPERATIVE HEMOSTASIS

It is imperative to control exsanguinating hemorrhage and to restore circulatory intravascular volume as rapidly as possible intraoperatively. Techniques and materials to achieve intraoperative hemostasis include manual compression; mechanical tamponade; sutures, clips, and ligatures; clamps and shunts; thermal and laser energy; hemostatic agents; and tissue adhesives.

Manual Compression

The simplest method for rapidly controlling hemorrhage from an isolated bleeding point is digital compression. Manual compression techniques rely on reduction in blood flow to the bleeding area, which allows clotting to proceed.

Mechanical Tamponade

Mechanical tamponade, in its simple form, consists of applying pads and packs to a bleeding site with sufficient pressure to slow or halt hemorrhage and to enable blood clots to form. Most cases of intra-abdominal organ bleeding can be initially controlled by temporary packing to allow time to correct hypovolemia, acidosis, hypothermia, and cardiac arrhythmias. The use of compression packing can also be used for extended periods postoperatively, if necessary. Another option available is the use of a pedicle flap of greater omentum, which can be sutured in place for mild to moderate bleeding tamponade of hepatic, splenic, and other intra-abdominal injuries.

Mechanical tamponade has also been applied externally in patients experiencing exsanguination from pelvic fractures as an alternative to surgical exploration. Mechanical tamponade by the abdominal wall often occurs naturally with massive hemoperitoneum in the trauma patient with a tense, distended abdomen.

Sutures, Clips, and Ligatures

The individual ligature is a permanent method for establishing complete hemostasis of a single bleeding vessel. Nonabsorbable sutures are resistant to enzymatic digestion or hydrolysis, whereas absorbable sutures are not. Monofilament or absorbable sutures are usually recommended for use in potentially infected wounds.

Metallic clips and staples have been used to achieve rapid control of hemorrhage and to provide hemostasis in an otherwise inaccessible area. Staplers may not be suitable to control bleeding from large blood vessels and internal organs.

Clamps and Shunts

The temporary clamping of blood vessels to effect hemostasis is basically a form of mechanical tamponade. Varying degrees of intimal damage can occur when major blood vessels are temporarily clamped, even with atraumatic clamps. Only the least amount of pressure required to occlude flow should be applied. Temporary intravascular shunts are valuable in surgery involving critical vessels.

Thermal and Laser Energy

Electrocautery devices convert electrical energy into thermal energy. By concentrating a large amount of current into a small area, a high-current density generates a high resistance and intense heat. As the current spreads out through the tissues, resistance and heat production decrease. The degree of coagulation or cutting is determined by the waveform of the current.

Direct cooling increases blood viscosity and produces vasoconstriction, resulting in hemostasis. Cryogenic surgery uses localized extreme cooling to −200°C.

The laser has also been used for hemostasis. It converts light energy into thermal energy, which in turn vaporizes tissue water.

Hemostatic Agents

Most solid hemostatic agents work by providing a scaffold or network of interstices that entrap platelets and blood components, which provide for organization of clot. Platelets are probably more important than the soluble clotting factors in the hemostatic reaction. Liquid hemostatic agents, such as epinephrine and thrombin, act by vasoconstriction and stimulation of the clotting cascade.

Gelatin foam, made from denatured animal gelatin, is available as a sponge. Its effects are mainly related to direct contact between blood and sponge by the pressure exerted on the wound surface.

Oxidized regenerated cellulose and microfibrillar collagen work by aggregating platelets in thrombi contained within their interstices and are thus effective in the presence of heparin. Oxidized regenerated cellulose is available as a sheet, whereas microfibrillar collagen is available in powder and nonwoven web forms. Both substances stimulate a chronic inflammatory response and require phagocytosis to be removed from the body.

Hemostatic agents left in contaminated wounds potentiate infection. Oxidized cellulose is superior to gelatin sponge and microfibrillar collagen in resisting infection.

Tissue Adhesives

Tissue adhesives are synthetic or natural chemicals used to glue bleeding sites. Highly concentrated human fibrinogen in conjunction with thrombin, Factor XIII, and calcium chloride results in the formation of a natural fibrin glue that lacks significant tissue reactivity or toxicity. Although not yet available for commercial use in the United States, this adhesive has been found to be extremely effective in establishing parenchymal organ hemostasis. Fibrin glue has been found to be significantly superior to oxidized cellulose in establishing complete hemostasis and preventing recurrent bleeding postoperatively. Methods for preparing autologous fibrin glue have been devised, but its tensile strength is inferior to that of nonautologous, highly concentrated fibrinogen mixtures.

THORACIC INJURIES

Chest injuries are directly responsible for over 25% of trauma deaths. Patients with chest trauma who are in shock or respiratory distress when first seen in the hospital have a particularly high mortality rate.

Massive Subcutaneous Emphysema

Subcutaneous emphysema is usually caused by injuries to lung parenchyma. It can also be caused by injury to the esophagus or pharynx. For patients placed on positive-pressure ventilation, it is prudent to assume that there is an underlying pneumothorax.

Injury to the Chest Wall

Probing of chest wounds to determine their depth or direction is not advised. Underlying pneumothorax and hemothorax should be identified and treated promptly. Open, sucking chest wounds occur when the chest wound is two thirds the cross-sectional area of the upper airway. Air preferentially enters the chest through the wound rather than through the tracheobronchial tree. Management of such wounds includes placement of a sterile, airtight dressing and tube thoracostomy.

Rib Fractures

Pain and localized tenderness over the ribs after chest trauma implies the presence of rib fractures. Up to 40% of rib fractures may not be visible radiographically until 7 to 14 days after injury. In the presence of suspected rib fractures, identification of associated complications (pneumothorax, hemothorax) is the goal. An upright posteroanterior chest radiograph has the greatest yield in detecting fractures and associated injuries or complications. Delayed pneumothorax or hemothorax occasionally develops more than 6 to 12 hours after initial injury. Radiographic rib series are unnecessary. Once associated injuries are ruled out, pain control becomes the mainstay of treatment. Intercostal nerve blocks or epidural analgesia is often effective for severe pain.

Fractures of the first or second rib require significant blunt force trauma. Fractures of the first rib are associated with higher mortality rates (15–30%) than are fractures of the other ribs because of the frequently severe associated injuries.

Increased morbidity and mortality rates are seen in patients with three or more rib fractures. Intra-abdominal bleeding must be suspected in the presence of fractures of rib 9, 10, or 11 associated with hypotension. Rib fractures in the pediatric patient denote significant blunt chest trauma, and the presence of associated injuries must be investigated.

Flail Chest

Flail chest is defined as segmental rib fractures of three or more adjacent ribs. Although the flail segment increases the work of breathing, the main cause of the hypoxemia in patients with flail chest is the underlying lung contusion. Lung changes and the flail tend to get worse during the 24 to 48 hours after injury. Treatment is supportive, with early ventilatory assistance. Indications for early ventilatory assistance with flail chest include shock, three or more associated injuries, severe head injury, previous severe pulmonary disease, fracture of eight or more ribs, and age greater than 65 years. Operative stabilization of the chest wall is rarely indicated. Death in patients with flail chest is due primarily to associated injuries.

Sternal Fractures

Sternal fractures are associated with flail chest or other severe injuries, including myocardial contusions, in up to 50% to 60% of patients.

Traumatic Asphyxia

Sudden severe crushing of the chest, especially by heavy weights, can result in traumatic asphyxia. This entity includes subconjunctival hemorrhage plus petechiae, edema, and cyanosis of the head, neck, and upper extremities. Associated neurologic impairment, if present, is usually temporary. Long-term morbidity is due to associated injuries.

Injuries to the Lungs

The main pathologic change in pulmonary contusion is capillary damage, resulting in increased interstitial and intra-alveolar fluid, which causes a progressive decrease in lung compliance and an increase in physiologic shunting and hypoxemia for at least 24 to 48 hours. In general, the chest radiographic changes lag at least 24 hours behind the arterial blood gas changes. Treatment involves the maintenance of adequate ventilation. Chest physiotherapy, intercostal nerve or epidural blocks, and nasotracheal suction should be used as needed. Ventilatory assistance occasionally is required. Survival is determined primarily by the associated injuries and the patient's age. In severe cases of unilateral lung injury unresponsive to conventional mechanical ventilation, synchronous independent lung ventilation may be beneficial.

Systemic air embolism can occur in the presence of bronchial injury. High ventilatory pressures may force air from an injured bronchus into an adjacent open pulmonary vein, producing air emboli. The diagnosis should be suspected in any patient with penetrating chest trauma who develops arrhythmias or sudden death. If systemic air embolism occurs, the patient should be turned onto the left side and the head lowered. In the absence of a prompt response to nonoperative therapy, a thoracotomy should be performed to clamp the injured area of lung and then aspirate air from the heart and aorta. Open-heart massage with clamping of the ascending aorta or cardiopulmonary bypass may be required.

Intrabronchial bleeding is poorly tolerated and can rapidly cause death by flooding alveoli. Severe hypoxemia occurs. The noninvolved lung must be kept free of blood; nasotracheal suction and bronchoscopy should be used if needed. If the bleeding is severe, a double-lumen endotracheal tube should be used to confine bleeding.

Blood in the pleural cavity should be removed as completely and rapidly as possible. A hemothorax can restrict ventilation and venous return. In addition, the clots release fibrinolytic and fibrinogenolytic substances that act as anticoagulants and that contribute to continued intrathoracic bleeding. Most patients (85–90%) can be treated by placement of a large (32- to 40-French) chest tube. The high concentration of thromboplastin and the low arterial pressures combine to reduce bleeding from torn lung parenchyma. If significant intrathoracic bleeding continues, severe lung injuries or major vessel damage may be present. Indications for thoracotomy include unstable vital signs, chest tube drainage greater than 1500 to 2000 mL, chest tube drainage exceeding 200 to 300 mL/h for more than 3 hours, and the chest remaining more than half full of blood on chest radiography. In patients with massive bleeding into the chest, autotransfusion should be considered. Most hemothoraces completely resorb spontaneously within 3 to 4 weeks. A retained hemothorax should be evacuated if it occupies more than a third of one hemithorax, causes atelectasis of a lobe or two or more segments, or is associated with spiking fever exceeding 101°F. In selected cases, early thoracoscopic drainage is indicated.

A pneumothorax occurs when air collects within the pleural cavity. This reduces vital capacity and increases intrathoracic pressure, thereby decreasing minute ventilation and venous return to the heart. Physical examination and chest radiography are used for diagnosis. An occult pneumothorax is a small pneumothorax not apparent on chest radiographs but seen on CT scans. A tension pneumothorax occurs when there is significant decrease in venous return and is associated with respiratory distress, decreased breath sounds, and contralateral tracheal deviation. Insertion of a large needle into the involved side can confirm the diagnosis and provide temporary relief of symptoms; this should be followed by tube thoracostomy. Treatment of a simple pneumothorax is chest tube placement (24- to 28-French) in the anterior second intercostal space along the midclavicular line. Occasionally, aspiration of a pneumothorax can be performed. Once placed, the chest tube can be removed when the drainage decreases to less than 100 mL over 24 hours and no air leak is present. An air leak usually stops within 24 to 48 hours if the lung is completely expanded and the visceral and parietal pleura are in contact. The persistence of an air leak and pneumothorax despite two well-placed chest tubes attached to 20 to 30 cm H_2O suction is generally due to occlusion of bronchi with secretions or foreign body, tear of a larger bronchi, or large tear of the lung parenchyma. Under such circumstances, emergency bronchoscopy should be performed to identify any damage to the tracheobronchial tree.

Occasionally after trauma, an airspace without a bronchial or pleural connection develops within the injured lung parenchyma. This can cause cough, chest pain, leukocytosis, and low-grade fever. Most of these resolve spontaneously within a few weeks or months. If they enlarge or become infected, resection or drainage may be required.

Pneumomediastinum should be suspected in the presence of a crunching sound (Hamman's sign) over the heart during systole. The presence of pneumomediastinum should warrant a close investigation of injury to the airways or the digestive tract. Rarely, a tension pneumopericardium develops in newborns or older individuals.

Tracheobronchial Injuries

Most blunt injuries to bronchi are due to rapid deceleration and shearing of mobile bronchi from relatively fixed proximal structures. Forced expiration against a closed glottis or compression against the vertebral column can also play a role. Injuries to the trachea or major bronchi should be suspected if there is a persistent pneumothorax with a continuing large air leak. On bronchoscopy, the usual injury is a transverse tear in a mainstem bronchus or at the origin of an upper lobe bronchus. The characteristic tracheal injury is a vertical tear in the membranous portion near its attachment to the tracheal cartilages.

If the lung expands and the air leak stops, partial lacerations of the bronchi involving more than a third of the circumference may be missed initially; they often result in repeated pulmonary infections or severe bronchial stenosis. Low tracheal and major bronchial lacerations require thoracotomy and direct repair as soon as feasible.

Penetrating Cardiac Trauma

Most patients who reach the hospital alive after penetrating cardiac trauma have relatively small cardiac injuries, and a pericardial tamponade is often present to help stop the bleeding from the heart. Pericardial tamponade after penetrating trauma can be delayed for weeks or months.

All patients in shock with a penetrating chest wound between the midclavicular line on the right and midaxillary line on the left should be considered to have a cardiac injury until proved otherwise. Beck's triad (distended neck veins, decreased blood pressure, and muffled heart tones) may be deceptive. Pulsus paradoxus, a drop in systolic blood pressure of more than 10 to 15 mm Hg during normal inspiration, should suggest tamponade. The quickest way to correct hypotension caused by pericardial tamponade is to increase preload by rapid infusion of intravenous fluids.

Chest radiographs are of little help in diagnosing cardiac injury except in the unusual case with intrapericardial air. Echocardiography can be helpful in diagnosing the presence of pericardial blood. A subxiphoid pericardial window or pericardiocentesis can also be used for diagnosis. If blood is found, a median sternotomy with cardiac repair should be performed, but at least 25% of patients with acute tamponade have normal pericardiocentesis results. Therefore, if there is strong suspicion of tamponade in a stable patient but the pericardiocentesis is negative, thoracotomy should be performed promptly.

Thoracotomy

Prompt thoracotomy to relieve pericardial tamponade and repair the heart wound, preferably in the operating room, is the treatment of choice for cardiac wounds causing bleeding and tamponade. Performance of a thoracotomy for penetrating cardiac injuries in the emergency department is recommended for patients who are clinically dead on arrival but who had some signs of life in transit and for patients who are deteriorating and who have no measurable blood pressure. Emergency department thoracotomies for patients with no signs of life at the scene or within 5 minutes of arrival in the hospital are futile.

Ligation of the cut ends of lacerated coronary arteries is the treatment of choice for small vessels. If arrhythmia, myocardial infarction, or impaired hemodynamic function develops, an aortocoronary bypass with coronary artery bypass grafting should be performed.

Injuries to the great arteries in the chest are uncommon in patients who reach the hospital alive. Diagnosis is difficult, and a high index of suspicion and arteriography are often required.

Blunt Cardiac Trauma

Cardiac trauma is the most frequent unsuspected visceral injury responsible for death in fatally injured accident victims. A tachycardia that is out of proportion to the degree of trauma or blood loss may be the first tip to the diagnosis. Helpful physical signs include a friction rub and abnormal heart sounds. Arrhythmias may develop up to 72 hours after injury. Significant arrhythmia developing after 24 hours, however, is uncommon. Diagnosis is often difficult. Serum glutamic oxaloacetic transaminase, lactate dehydrogenase, and creatine phosphokinase levels are not diagnostically helpful. If myocardial contusion is suspected, patients should be admitted and monitored for early detection and treatment of complications, namely arrhythmias and congestive heart failure.

Pericardial injury should be suspected if there is ECG or other evidence of myocardial damage. A normal ECG, however, does not rule out traumatic pericarditis. Echocardiography may be helpful. Tamponade resulting from effusion can occur within minutes or as late as months after injury. Retained pericardial blood can also cause later constrictive pericarditis.

Shock not responding promptly to fluid replacement or transfusions after blunt trauma may represent pericardial tamponade from a ruptured cardiac chamber. In patients who reach the hospital alive, the injury is usually a tear in the superior or inferior vena cava at its junction with the atrium.

Septal defects after blunt chest trauma are rare. The muscular interventricular septum near the apex is particularly susceptible to perforation after blunt trauma. The triad of chest trauma, systolic murmur, and an infarct pattern on ECG should suggest an interventricular septal defect. Although small, traumatic ventricular septal defects may close spontaneously, surgical repair, preferably 6 to 8 weeks after trauma, is the treatment of choice. The presence of poorly controlled congestive heart failure requires earlier operation.

Rupture of the aortic valve is the most common valvular lesion in patients who survive nonpenetrating cardiac injury. Blunt trauma rarely may also lacerate a papillary muscle or the chordae tendineae of the mitral valve. The prognosis for traumatic rupture of a mitral papillary muscle or mitral valve leaflet is grave, and death usually occurs within a few hours or days after injury. The tricuspid valve is rarely involved in blunt trauma.

Traumatic Rupture of the Aorta

Traumatic rupture of the aorta (TRA) causes death within minutes of injury in 80% to 90% of patients. Of patients who survive at least 1 hour and are not treated, 30% die within 6 minutes, 40% within 24 hours, 72% within 8 days, 83% within 3 weeks, and 90% within 10 weeks. The most common site of injury is just distal to the left subclavian artery. The next most common site of thoracic great vessel injury is the innominate artery at its origin or the left subclavian artery at the first rib. Tears in the lower descending aorta are rare.

One third of patients with TRA have little or no external

evidence of chest trauma. The diagnosis must be suspected in any patient involved in a high-speed motor vehicle accident. Clinical findings that suggest TRA include (1) a systolic murmur over the precordium or the back, (2) voice change secondary to pressure on the left recurrent laryngeal nerve, (3) hypertension in the upper extremities, and (4) weak pulses in the lower extremities. The most frequent radiologic finding with TRA is widening of the superior mediastinum adjacent to the aortic knob. The most accurate chest radiographic signs of TRA include deviation of the esophagus to the right and blurred or obscured aortic knob. Other radiologic findings include apical cap, downward displacement of the left mainstem bronchus, obliteration of the aortopulmonary window, first or second rib fracture, and displacement of the right paraspinous interface. Many patients with TRA have normal initial chest radiographs.

If TRA is suspected because of the mechanism of injury or chest radiographic findings, an aortogram should be performed. It is also important to avoid hypertension or excessive gagging or straining. If the patient is in shock or has a large or rapidly expanding mediastinal hematoma, the patient should be taken directly to the operating room without aortography. Other studies that have been used include thoracic CT scans and transesophageal ultrasonography. At this time, however, the aortogram is the gold standard for diagnosis of thoracic aortic injuries.

Many patients with TRA have multiple injuries and are at extremely high risk for emergency repair. By carefully controlling blood pressure, using α- or β-blockers as needed, surgery can be delayed until conditions are optimal. Two methods of aortic repair have been used: (1) the "clamp and sew" technique, and (2) the use of external shunts or cardiopulmonary bypass. The usual circuit used for partial bypass is from the femoral vein to the femoral artery. This requires an oxygenator and heparin. Use of a special vortex (Bio-Medicus) bypass pump with catheters in the left atrium and femoral artery may be particularly helpful and safe because neither an oxygenator nor heparin is required. An alternative to cardiopulmonary bypass is a shunt to divert blood around the involved aorta.

Esophageal Injuries

Lacerations of the esophagus occur most frequently during endoscopic biopsy or dilation. Swallowed foreign bodies can also cause injury. External trauma is a rare cause of esophageal injury.

If esophageal injury is suspected, esophagogram and esophagoscopy should be performed. Bronchoscopy should also be performed to rule out associated tracheobronchial injuries. If treatment is delayed beyond 24 hours, primary closure of a torn esophagus is not advisable. Continuous complete drainage of the stomach and mediastinum is necessary. The mortality rate of esophageal injuries is 5% to 25% for patients treated definitively within 12 hours and 25% to 66% or higher for those treated after 24 hours.

Thoracic Duct Injuries

Chylothorax is usually the result of thoracic surgery or penetrating trauma. Injuries to the thoracic duct usually cause a right chylothorax. Thoracic duct leakage in the chest can result in the loss of 1500 to 2500 mL/d of a clear or milky white odorless fluid that contains lymphocytes and fat globules or chylomicrons with minimal cholesterol.

Adequate drainage of the pleural cavity with a chest tube for several days usually results in spontaneous fistula closure. If the fistula persists and is large, intravenous hyperalimentation with nasogastric suction can reduce the amount of chyle draining, thereby preventing protein malnutrition. If the patient is allowed to eat, medium-chain triglycerides are the preferred source of fat.

ABDOMINAL AND PELVIC TRAUMA

Abdominal and pelvic trauma accounts for 10% of trauma deaths. Intraperitoneal penetration occurs in 90% of gunshot wounds to the abdomen, and 30% to 40% of stab wounds. Overall mortality rates from intra-abdominal injuries are 5% for gunshot wounds and 2% for stab wounds. Blunt trauma leads to abdominal operative intervention 10% of the time in the civilian population.

Anatomy

Penetrating injuries that occur below the fourth intercostal interspace anteriorly, the fifth interspace in the midaxillary line, and the sixth interspace posteriorly or below the tip of the scapula have the possibility of entering the abdomen. The lower extent of the pelvis is the perineal area, which anteriorly extends to the inguinal ligament attachments at the anterosuperior iliac spine. The lateral border of the abdomen lies at the level of the anterior axillary line.

Mechanism of Injury

Motor vehicle accidents account for 50% of blunt abdominal injuries; other causes include falls, assaults, contact sports, and crush injuries. The severity of injury is related to the offending agent and the amount of energy produced and dissipated. A rapid deceleration injury can cause a shearing effect, leading to avulsion of solid viscera with hemoperitoneum. Lap belt restraints can cause sudden elevation in intra-abdominal pressure, leading to hollow viscus rupture or mesenteric tear. In blunt trauma, the incidence of specific organ injury is as follows: spleen, 25% to 35%; liver, 15% to 25%; kidneys, 10% to 15%; and retroperitoneal hematoma, 10% to 15%. In penetrating abdominal trauma, the incidence of specific injuries is as follows: small bowel, 30% to 35%; mesentery and omentum, 15% to 20%; liver, 15% to 20%; colon, 10%; and diaphragm, 10%.

Regardless of the mechanism of injury, an adequate history is crucial to provide insight as to what might be injured.

In penetrating injuries, the identification of entry and exit sites can give a rough idea of injuries sustained; however, bullets do not travel in straight lines.

Major blunt abdominal trauma resulting from child abuse can be lethal, with reported mortality rates of up to 50%. Suspicion should peak when continued injury lacks explanation, stories appear to be changing, unexplained or inappropriate blame is assigned to another individual, a discrepancy exists between history and physical examination, the injury pattern delays child development, or there is an obvious delay in seeking healthcare.

Initial Approach

The initial approach to all victims of injury is the same, with airway, breathing, circulation, and resuscitation being performed concurrently. A history should be obtained, including medical and surgical history, present medications, drug or alcohol abuse, and allergies. Unfortunately, the physical examination can be misleading, since 23% to 36% of patients with intraperitoneal injuries lack significant findings.

The physical examination is a continuous process and should be repeated periodically during the work-up. Interpretation of the abdominal examination in a paralyzed or intoxicated patient or in a patient euphoric from illicit drug use also is unreliable. The physical findings most associated with internal injuries in blunt trauma include abdominal tenderness and guarding in up to 75% of patients. Peritoneal signs of rebound, rigidity, and tenderness occur in only 28% of patients with significant intra-abdominal injuries. Significant findings on physical examination are absent or misleading in up to 45% of patients with intraperitoneal injury. During the physical examination, a nasogastric tube should be placed if there is no obvious maxillofacial injury, bleeding diathesis, or other contraindications; otherwise, an orogastric tube is necessary. A rectal examination should be performed to evaluate whether the prostate is high-riding and whether there is rectal bleeding. When the results of rectal examination are normal and there is no blood at the urethral meatus and no evidence of a scrotal hematoma, a Foley catheter is placed and a urinalysis obtained.

The likelihood of abdominal injury is heightened when three or more of the following clinical indications exist: gross hematuria, lap belt injury, bicycle injury, abdominal tenderness, or trauma score of 12 or less.

Diagnostic Modalities

After blunt abdominal trauma, urgent celiotomy is indicated in patients with abdominal distention, hypotension, overt peritonitis, or signs of visceral injury.

DPL is a useful test in the evaluation of victims with abdominal trauma. Commonly used criteria include an RBC count of more than 100,000 cells/μL, a WBC count of greater than 500 cells/μL, an elevated amylase level, and the presence of bile or other intra-abdominal debris. When DPL amylase and alkaline phosphatase levels are elevated in patients with histories consistent with possible small bowel injury, laparotomy should be strongly considered. Before the DPL catheter is placed, bladder and gastric decompression should be accomplished. If lavage fluid drains from the Foley catheter, the gastric tube, or a chest tube, the patient needs to undergo prompt laparotomy. DPL has an accuracy rate of greater than 98% and false-positive and false-negative rates of less than 4%.

Another useful diagnostic test for victims of blunt trauma is abdominal and pelvic CT. CT is relatively noninvasive, identifies specific organ injury and function, and allows for evaluation of the retroperitoneum. Generally, intravenous and oral contrast media are administered to a hemodynamically stable patient. The use of CT can decrease the nontherapeutic laparotomy rate from 25% to 6%. One limitation of CT is the inability to evaluate bowel perforation, which occurs in up to 4% of major blunt abdominal trauma. Disadvantages of CT include the necessity for specialized personnel and equipment, time to perform (20–30 minutes), movement of the patient out of the resuscitation bay, limitation to patient access, increased cost over DPL, and user-dependent interpretation.

DPL and CT scanning can be complementary. DPL and CT are associated with unnecessary laparotomy rates of 15.5% and 0.8%, respectively, and inappropriate observation rates of 1.7% and 6.9%, respectively. DPL is not as specific as CT, but both have a sensitivity of 99%. CT accuracy is 98%, whereas DPL accuracy is 92%. Both studies can be done in a serial manner. Because CT is not portable, DPL is attractive for patients who are undergoing extensive monitoring procedures in the ICU.

Ultrasonography is being used increasingly for the evaluation of blunt abdominal trauma. Accuracy approaches 100%, sensitivity 84%, and specificity 98%. About 70 mL of intraperitoneal blood is necessary for visualization on ultrasonography, which has a 20% to 25% incidence of failure to detect spleen or liver injury.

Abdominal and pelvic angiography for abdominal and pelvic trauma aids in identifying and controlling arterial bleeding from pelvic fractures and, on rare occasion, intra-abdominal visceral bleeding.

The usefulness of laparoscopy for trauma is not established but is being evaluated in many centers.

A more direct approach is used in penetrating trauma. Mandatory exploratory laparotomy for all abdominal stab wounds is no longer universally practiced. Frequently, treatment involves local exploration in the emergency department with the potential for discharge if the peritoneal cavity is not violated. Penetration into the abdominal cavity can be evaluated by DPL, although the RBC count needed to lead one to laparotomy is debatable. Rather, careful initial and repeated clinical examination should be used.

Posterior stab wounds are more difficult to explore locally. CT scanning is 89% sensitive, 98% specific, and 96% accurate in evaluating stab wounds to the back.

For the most part, gunshot wounds to the abdomen are explored.

Antibiotics

Major trauma increases neutrophil adherence, decreases chemotaxis, impairs phagocytosis, and decreases bactericidal activity. Injury leads to fibronectin deficiency, decreases in levels of complement and immunoglobulins, and decreases in cell-mediated immunity. All this promotes infection. Surgical wounds are defined as clean, clean contaminated, or contaminated, with infection rates of 3.2%, 8.1%, and 24.6%, respectively.

Subcutaneous wound infections are treated by opening the wound, irrigating, débriding, and packing. Surrounding cellulitis, subfascial infection, or the use of prosthetic material dictates the need for antibiotics. The most common offending organism is *Staphylococcus aureus*.

Fever occurs in about 50% of patients sustaining significant intra-abdominal injury and may not correlate with infection. Intra-abdominal abscess formation tends to manifest 7 to 10 days postoperatively.

The incidence of postinjury infection is 24% in major penetrating injuries. Single antibiotics such as the cephalosporins have equivalent or better results in preventing intra-abdominal abscesses and wound infection than do antibiotic combinations. Risk factors for the development of infection include perioperative shock, massive blood transfusion, high severity of injury, left-sided colon injury with colostomy, more than one intra-abdominal organ injury, old age, presence of immunosuppression, and a catabolic nutritional state. Abdominal trauma with associated open fractures increases the risk of infection.

Stomach

Injuries to the stomach are more common with penetrating injuries than blunt injuries (7–20% versus 0.4–1.7%). Blunt gastric injury is most frequently due to a sudden and acute increase in intraluminal pressure secondary to a direct blow to the full stomach. Perforation usually occurs along the anterior greater curvature of the stomach. Signs of peritoneal irritation or shock are present in 50% to 80% of patients with blunt gastric rupture. Free abdominal air is found in less than 66% of patients. Blood in the nasogastric tube is an ominous sign.

Duodenum

Duodenal injuries are frequently difficult to recognize. A high index of suspicion is required, because diagnostic delay significantly increases mortality. Penetrating wounds account for most injuries to the duodenum. Blunt trauma leads to duodenal rupture by crushing, bursting, or shearing effects. Early mortality is secondary to hypovolemic hemorrhagic shock, whereas late mortality is related to associated injuries or sepsis. Hyperamylasemia is present in 50% of patients with duodenal injury.

Plain radiographs rarely show intraperitoneal, retroperitoneal, or intrabiliary air. Obliteration of the right psoas margin, right scoliosis, and retroperitoneal air around the kidney suggest duodenal injury. A water-soluble upper gastrointestinal study with the patient in the right lateral decubitus position may show the injury. CT scanning may not reveal the injury.

Treatment of duodenal injury is surgical. Postoperative care involves resuscitation and gastrointestinal decompression with suction until bowel function returns. Duodenal fistulization occurs in up to 14% of patients. Nutritional support is essential. Operative intervention should be considered in patients with duodenal fistula.

Small Bowel

The small bowel is the intra-abdominal organ most commonly injured by penetrating trauma and the third most common organ injured by blunt abdominal trauma. Blunt abdominal trauma in children can lead to an intramural hematoma of the small bowel, which is compressed between the abdominal wall and the vertebrae. Under these circumstances, the diagnosis can be made from an upper gastrointestinal series.

The neutral pH and low bacterial count of the succus entericus provoke only a minimal inflammatory response initially. Blood serology and plain radiographs are generally not helpful. CT scanning misses intestinal injury, because findings are subtle or nonspecific. The presence of gastrointestinal contents on DPL makes this test useful.

Operative intervention is mandatory for small bowel perforation. Perioperative antibiotics are administered, nasogastric decompression is undertaken, and once hemodynamic stability is established, the patient is taken to the operating room. Resectional therapy or primary repair can be performed. Signs and symptoms of postoperative small bowel leakage are fever, tachycardia, leukocytosis, peritonitis, and external fistulization. The presence of multiple organ failure or persistent fever after abdominal surgery with temperature spikes and tachycardia should lead one to consider performing CT to look for an abdominal abscess. Abscess can be drained by percutaneous, radiographically guided, or operative techniques.

Colon

The colon is injured in less than 5% of all blunt abdominal trauma victims and in 15% of victims with penetrating trauma. Diagnosis is difficult because physical findings may be delayed, CT scanning can miss injuries, and DPL may not pick up retroperitoneal colon injury. Risk factors for infection from colon injury include old age, two to four units of blood transfused, two or more associated injuries, injury to the spleen, shock, and significant contamination. Wound infection frequently occurs in the presence of gross contamination; the wound should be left open or delayed primary closure considered.

The presence of fever and leukocytosis 5 days after operation may be related to a leak resulting from the colon repair. The presence of peritonitis dictates the need for another laparotomy. The presence of a retained foreign body (i.e., bullet) that has gone through the colon increases the likelihood of an associated abscess, necessitating operation to remove the foreign body and drain the abscess.

Liver

Hepatic injury occurs in 15% to 20% of blunt abdominal trauma, 40% of abdominal stab wounds, and 30% of abdominal gunshot wounds. In hemodynamically stable patients, CT scanning provides quantitative and qualitative information about the liver and other intra-abdominal organs. Unstable patients, however, should undergo DPL in the emergency department or the ICU when there is concern of intra-abdominal hemorrhage. On rare occasions, embolization of hepatic bleeding is required.

Hemodynamically stable patients with grade I to III injury can be treated nonoperatively with initial bed rest and gastric decompression in the presence of an ileus. The continuing need for transfusion (more than two to four units within 24 hours), a deterioration in vital signs in a patient with isolated liver injury, an increase in abdominal tenderness with signs of peritonitis, or a worsening CT scan dictates laparotomy. Grade IV, V, and VI injuries usually require prompt laparotomy. Correction of hypothermia, metabolic acidosis, and coagulopathy is imperative in control of bleeding from the liver.

The rate of intra-abdominal infection depends on the magnitude of injury and the success of repair, varying between 1.9% and 17%. Drainage should be considered in severe injury using a closed-suction system. Factors associated with intra-abdominal abscess formation from hepatic injury include severity of injury, type of drainage, transfusion of more than six units of blood, and the presence of three or more organ injuries. Continued, ongoing evaluation is necessary if pyrexia persists after the third postoperative day. Persistent pyrexia may be due to reabsorbed, devitalized hepatic parenchyma in patients who underwent débridement, placement of deep parenchymal sutures, or selective vascular ligation of liver structures. In most instances, these high temperatures resolve within 5 days of initial operation.

Hemobilia may manifest itself with jaundice or gastrointestinal bleeding days to weeks after injury. Arterial embolization angiographically is the initial procedure of choice. Bleeding that occurs several days to weeks after injury may be secondary to erosion of a drain into the liver or vascular bleeding.

Biliary fistulas occur in up to 10% of patients with major hepatic injury. Most close within weeks if there is no distal biliary obstruction. A persistent fistula should be evaluated with fistulography or endoscopic retrograde cholangiopancreatography. Major intrahepatic duct or common bile duct involvement mandates operative intervention with resection or reconstruction.

With major hepatic injury, gluconeogenesis is impaired and hypoglycemia is seen in 4% of patients. Glucose levels should be monitored and early nutritional support should be instituted.

Necrosis or occlusion of venous outflow may occur after major hepatic injury. Angiography or radionuclide scanning may further define the problem. The overall mortality rate of 10% to 15% in hepatic injuries is due to shock or transfusion-related coagulopathy perioperatively.

Spleen

Preservation of the spleen, when possible, is a therapeutic goal. The spleen is an important immunologic organ. With splenectomy, there is a decrease in IgM levels, and the greatest reduction in bacterial clearance occurs with encapsulated gram-positive bacteria.

Diagnosing splenic injury by physical examination alone is 65% accurate. Findings include left upper quadrant tenderness or referred left shoulder pain, known as Kehr's sign. The presence of left lower rib fractures in blunt trauma should raise the possibility of splenic injury. Hematocrit decreases may be delayed, even with massive splenic injury. In unstable patients, DPL remains the standard for diagnosing intra-abdominal injuries. CT, however, is more specific and may be preferred in stable patients.

Conservative management is an alternative approach for splenic injury. The best candidates are those younger than 55 years with a grade I to III injury, no other major concomitant injuries, and no abnormal mental status changes precluding continued abdominal assessment. If, however, the patient becomes unstable after volume replacement, has other associated abdominal injuries, cannot be evaluated, or has an equivocal abdominal examination, laparotomy with possible splenic salvage should be considered. Nonoperative therapy is successful in 90% of children. Nonoperative management should be abandoned when blood requirements exceed 20 mL/kg or approximately 30% blood volume. In adults, laparotomy should be performed if more than two units of blood are transfused within 24 hours for an isolated splenic injury. The incidence of delayed splenic rupture is less than 1%.

Splenectomy is indicated in unstable patients, patients with continued blood loss, or patients with grade V splenic injury. Reactive thrombocytosis occurs 2 to 10 days after splenectomy and resolves in 2 to 12 weeks. When platelet counts exceed 1.5 million, the use of antiplatelet agents should be considered.

Overwhelming postsplenectomy sepsis (OPSI) can occur following splenectomy. The mortality rate for trauma-related splenectomized children is 0.56%. The risk of lethal OPSI in a 4-year-old child is 2.5 times that of an older child; the risk in adults is low. OPSI has a rapid onset, with a 12- to 18-hour prodrome of sore throat, fever, and malaise rapidly progressing to headache, vomiting, worsening fever, and, within hours, convulsion, coma, and death. The predominant organism is *Pneumococcus*. Pneumovax should be administered to patients, generally during their first outpatient visit. Penicillin should be used prophylactically when an invasive procedure or dental work is performed.

Pancreas

Associated injuries are seen in 90% of patients with pancreatic injuries. Two thirds of pancreatic injuries are penetrating and one third are blunt. In blunt trauma, 60% of pancreatic injuries are due to the impact of the steering wheel on the upper epigastric region during an automobile accident. Only 8% of patients with blunt abdominal injuries with hyperamylasemia have pancreatic injuries, and 40% with pancreatic injury have normal initial serum amylase values. Endoscopic retrograde cholangiopancreatography (ERCP) can help in delineating pancreatic ductal injuries.

Excision of over 90% of pancreatic substance is required before deficiency is seen, because there is hypertrophy and increased physiologic activity of the remaining islet cells after resection.

Pancreatic injuries are identified primarily at the time of laparotomy for hemorrhage and other associated injuries. Mortality rates can be as high as 10% to 25%, and morbidity rates as high as 30% to 40%. Contusions and simple lacerations are treated with closed-suction drainage. Distal pancreatectomy or pancreatic-enteric reconstruction is considered for ductal injuries or transection.

Enteral feedings distal to an anastomosis should be instituted shortly after surgery. Somatostatin can be given to decrease pancreatic exocrine secretions. High-output fistulas (>500 mL/d) may require surgical intervention. A low-fat, high-pH elemental feeding leads to less pancreatic stimulation.

Pancreatic abscess occurs in less than 5% of injuries; surgical débridement is required. Secondary hemorrhage requiring blood transfusion occurs in up to 10% of pancreatic injuries. In such cases, reoperation should be considered.

Post-traumatic pseudocysts occur in less than 5% of patients, usually weeks after injury. Those communicating with the pancreatic duct require operative intervention. Children are prone to development of traumatic pancreatitis and pseudocysts, which are treated conservatively. Postoperative pancreatitis is seen in up to 13% of patients, but it rarely progresses to hemorrhagic pancreatitis.

Genitourinary Tract

Evaluation for genitourinary tract injuries by clinical examination is unreliable. In the absence of symptoms or shock, a urinary dipstick serves as a reliable screen for hematuria. The urinalysis RBC count that correlates with significant renal injury is debatable, but there may be no RBCs present with total ureteral transection. In blunt trauma, blood at the urethral meatus, scrotal hematoma, or a high-floating prostate on rectal examination suggests urethral injury, and urethrography should be performed before Foley catheter placement. Once a Foley catheter is placed, cystography with 300 mL contrast should be performed to determine whether a bladder injury exists. Extraperitoneal bladder perforation is treated conservatively with bladder decompression through suprapubic cystostomy or Foley catheter.

CT scanning with contrast has replaced intravenous pyelography in screening for renal and ureteral injuries. Renal vascular injury needs to be repaired operatively within 6 hours. Intraperitoneal renal injury, caliceal renal injury, ureteral transection, and intraperitoneal bladder perforation are repaired urgently by laparotomy.

If nephrectomy is required, mild elevation of creatinine level is seen for 48 hours.

Pelvic Fractures

Massive pelvic fracture has a mortality rate of up to 50% and a complication rate of 74%. The incidence of vascular injuries with high-energy pelvic fractures is significant; early intervention is crucial. Temporary stabilization can be obtained using pneumatic antishock garments. An external fixator can be applied quickly at any time, although not all pelvic fractures respond to external fixation. Percutaneous transcatheter arterial embolization has been used when transfusion of four or more units of blood is required within 48 hours in a patient with an unstable pelvic fracture and a negative or borderline DPL or a patient with a large pelvic retroperitoneal hematoma.

Penetrating pelvic injuries and continued hemorrhage refractive to external fixation and embolization require laparotomy. Frequently, oozing from the pelvic venous plexus is refractive to pressure, hemostatic agents, packing, and even bilateral internal iliac artery ligation. On rare occasion, packs are left in the abdomen for 48 hours. Internal fixation can be used, depending on the clinical status of the patient.

Most patients with pelvic fractures are treated conservatively with bed rest or unilateral non–weight bearing for about 6 weeks. Pelvic fractures and bed rest are risk factors for DVT and pulmonary embolus. Early DVT prophylaxis should be instituted; measures include pneumatic compression stockings and use of heparin (or low-molecular-weight heparin), aspirin, or other anticoagulants. Early mobilization is ideal if possible. Continued resuscitation and repeated angiography may be needed if extraperitoneal bleeding persists. Rarely, hemicorporectomy is required for hemorrhage control.

Pregnant Patient

Trauma complicates about 6% of all pregnancies. The management priority is the mother—that is, the mother should be stabilized before the fetus. The physiologic changes during pregnancy need to be considered when evaluating a pregnant trauma patient. Blood volume steadily increases by the 28th week to 49% to 50% above normal. A smaller increase in RBC mass occurs in relation to plasma volume, resulting in the physiologic anemia of pregnancy. Thus, significant blood loss may not be recognized in pregnant patients because of delay in hypotension.

By the end of the first trimester, cardiac output increases by 30%, heart rate increases by 15 to 20 beats per minute, and blood pressure may drop 10 to 15 mm Hg. Positioning of the pregnant patient is crucial because after 20 weeks' gestation, the uterus can occlude the inferior vena cava, thus decreasing cardiac output. By positioning the patient in the left lateral position, pressure is taken off the inferior vena cava.

During pregnancy, a chronic state of compensated respiratory alkalosis exists and buffering capacity is decreased, which can aggravate the acidosis of shock.

As a result of decreased gastric motility and decreased gastroesophageal sphincter tone, vomiting and delayed gastric emptying can occur in pregnant patients. Thus, gastric decompression with suction should be performed early.

A complete blood count, screening for blood type and antibodies, and the Kleihauer-Betke stain are required in most patients. If the mother is Rh-negative, Rh immunoglobulin should be administered. A leukocytosis of 20,000 cells/μL with normal differential count occurs by term. An increase in coagulation Factors VII, VIII, and IX and in plasma fibrinogen, coupled with a decrease in plasminogen activator, promotes clotting. Thus, DVT prophylaxis should be instituted early. Abruptio placentae can release thromboplastic substances and initiate fulminant intravascular coagulation.

Radiation exposure to the mother of 0.05 Gy or less is considered safe, with teratogenic risks being greatest during organogenesis, the second through eighth weeks after conception. About 30% of the dose absorbed by the mother is transmitted to the fetus.

Continuous fetal monitoring should be used in the ICU. Vaginal bleeding may be an indication of placental separation secondary to direct injury or of vaginal or uterine injury secondary to pelvic fractures. Fetal demise is associated with direct uteroplacental fetal injury, maternal shock, pelvic fracture, maternal severe head injury, and hypoxia. Continued, thorough evaluation of mother and fetus is mandatory.

Postoperative Complications and Reoperation in Abdominal and Pelvic Trauma

Complications are minimized by taking patients with obvious intra-abdominal injuries directly to the operating room and continuing resuscitation in concert with laparotomy. When persistent hypotension, tachycardia, abdominal distention, or bloody drainage from abdominal drain sites exists in a noncoagulopathic normothermic patient, reoperation should urgently be performed.

On occasion, abdominal or pelvic injuries are missed with early signs of hypovolemic hemorrhagic shock. A hollow viscus injury can be missed and may not be evident until 5 days after laparotomy. Early development of adult respiratory distress syndrome or deterioration in a patient's status can also suggest missed intra-abdominal injury or ongoing intra-abdominal catastrophe.

MANAGEMENT OF HEAD TRAUMA

The aims of ICU management for patients with brain trauma are two: (1) to detect and treat the complications of the primary injury that can cause delayed brain damage, and (2) to provide the optimal conditions for natural recovery of brain function. No specific pharmacologic therapy has been conclusively shown to improve outcome after traumatic brain injury.

Causes of Brain Damage Due to Cerebral Trauma

Shear forces due to postimpact acceleration–deceleration events are particularly harmful to the brain because of its soft consistency, mobility within the closed skull, and lack of fibrous tissue restraint. Primary impact damage causes focal cerebral contusions. Tensile damage to axons in both gray and white matter causes both reversible and nonreversible ultrastructural changes, which can lead to diffuse axonal injury. When this process is widespread, it carries a particularly poor prognosis.

Intracranial hematomas occur in about 30% to 40% of severely head-injured patients. Although most intracranial hematomas develop within the first hour after impact, they can occur hours and occasionally even days after the injury in a significant number of patients, particularly those with early post-traumatic hypotension and coagulation disorders.

Secondary Intracranial Damage and Delayed Damage

Hypoxic-ischemic brain damage is widespread in 80% to 90% of patients who die after head injury. In most patients, it is focal, occurring in relation to contusions and hematomas. Secondary damage can be caused by metabolic changes, by raising intracranial pressure, and, most significantly, by extracranial events such as hypoxemia and hypotension.

After impact, massive ion flux occurs across neuronal and astrocytic membranes, followed by anaerobic glycolysis leading to marked cerebral acidosis. This can produce astrocytic swelling, an increase in brain stiffness, whole brain swelling, and increased intracranial pressure in some circumstances. Calcium flux into neurons may occur after brain trauma because of release of excitatory amino acids, and this can cause early or late damage to intracellular systems. Delayed damage to neurons, astrocytes, and endothelial cells of the microvasculature can result from free radical generation.

Within the first few hours of injury, 30% of severely head-injured patients have sufficiently low cerebral blood flow to cause failure of aerobic neuronal and astrocytic metabolism. This leads to cessation of ionic and neurotransmitter homeostasis and consequent cell swelling. In addition, the blood-brain barrier becomes permeable to small molecules in the region of focal cerebral contusions after head injury. This process is maximum several days after the injury.

Cerebrovascular autoregulatory capacity is lost for up to several days in severely head-injured patients. Thus, head-injured patients are predisposed to ischemic brain damage at levels of mean arterial blood pressure that would be satisfactory in a normal individual.

High intracranial pressure can jeopardize perfusion of the whole brain. Prolonged periods of reduced cerebral perfusion pressure, even at 50 to 60 mm Hg, have an adverse effect on prognosis.

Metabolic factors that cause delayed damage include systemic hypoxemia, hyperglycemia, and hyperthermia. Some evidence suggests that brain temperature rises 1° to 2°C higher than body core temperature after severe head injury. Preliminary data suggest that moderate hypothermia (32°C) is beneficial for outcome.

Initial Management of Head-Injured Patients

Significant brain injuries are followed by periods of apnea, the duration of which increases with the severity of the injury. Because of this, as many as 30% of head-injured patients are hypoxic by the time they reach the hospital. Therefore, the first priority is to establish and maintain adequate cerebral oxygenation and perfusion. Specific concerns in head-injured patients include early intubation, oxygenation and ventilation, and maintenance of blood pressure by rapid infusion of fluids to achieve adequate central venous pressure. Continuous pulse oximetry and early blood gas analysis should be performed. Chest and cervical spine radiographs are mandatory for all head-injured patients who are unable to speak or obey commands.

CT scanning should be delayed until adequate blood pressure (mean arterial pressure >80 mm Hg) and cerebral oxygenation have been achieved. CT scanning can diagnose intracranial hematomas and give useful information about the presence or absence of raised intracranial pressure. Effacement of basal cisterns is almost always present when this pressure exceeds 20 mm Hg. The prognosis is most favorable when hematomas are diagnosed by CT scan and removed before they can cause neurologic deterioration. In circumstances of smaller intracranial lesions, intracranial pressure monitoring, together with subsequent CT scanning at intervals, can assist the neurosurgeon in determining which patients require surgical evacuation of their mass lesions.

Once diagnosed, the hematoma must be evacuated as rapidly as possible, but hypotension during the procedure must also be prevented, especially at the moment the dura is opened. This is best achieved by administration of 20% mannitol (1 g or 5 mL/kg), given as rapidly as possible, as soon as an intracranial hematoma is diagnosed on CT. Bleeding at the time of hematoma evacuation must be anticipated, and sufficient transfusion should be given to maintain a normal circulating blood volume.

Immediate abdominal or thoracic surgery may be necessary to achieve hemodynamic stability before the CT scan can be obtained. Under these circumstances, if pupil dilation develops, an intraoperative ventricular tap can be performed to facilitate intracranial pressure measurement. A ventriculogram, using 2 to 5 mL of air, can be performed using an AP skull radiograph to detect midline shift and mass effect. Exploratory burr holes can be drilled during the same surgery, if needed.

Monitoring of Head-Injured Patients

Monitoring is aimed at early detection of cerebral hemodynamic, systemic, or metabolic changes that can induce secondary brain damage. Careful hourly evaluation of pupils, motor responses, and hemodynamic parameters still constitutes the mainstay of ICU management.

Continuous monitoring of blood pressure and arterial oxygen saturation is mandatory for optimal hemodynamic management. In addition, end-tidal CO_2 and core temperature should be monitored.

Various intracranial pressure monitors are available, and placement should be considered in patients with an abnormal head CT scan as well as Glascow Coma Scores of 8 or less. Intracranial pressure can be monitored using an intraventricular catheter, which allows therapeutic cerebrospinal fluid drainage when pressure is high. Fiberoptic sensors are available for intraparenchymal or intraventricular use. Extradural and subdural sensors are generally regarded as highly inaccurate, particularly when the pressure is high. By measuring intracranial pressure, cerebral perfusion pressure can be determined by the following formula: cerebral perfusion pressure equals mean arterial pressure minus intracranial pressure (CPP = MAP − ICP). The cerebral perfusion pressure should be kept at levels of 70 mm Hg or greater in severely head-injured patients.

Laser-assisted spectrophotometric techniques allow continuous measurement of venous oxygen saturation, using fine-bore catheters. These catheters can be placed within the jugular bulb, thus allowing continuous monitoring of cerebral arteriovenous oxygen differences. Continuous jugular oxygen saturation techniques are particularly valuable in detecting brain ischemia due to poor brain perfusion. Their main value may be in guiding hyperventilation therapy in patients in whom high intracranial pressure is suspected to be due to cerebral hyperemia. They are also useful for confirming the diagnosis of cerebral hyperemia and assessing its response to hyperventilation and drug therapy.

Arterial blood gas analysis is mandatory to guide respiratory therapy, and measurements of serum osmolarity may be required every 6 hours in patients receiving mannitol therapy for raised intracranial pressure. Blood glucose, urea, and electrolyte values also require frequent evaluation. Hyperglycemia should be cautiously treated with low-dose insulin, as needed, to maintain normoglycemia.

Adequate circulating volumes should be maintained using central venous pressure monitoring, with optimal pressure being 6 to 12 cm H_2O in paralyzed ventilated patients. A minimum fluid volume of 3 L/d should be maintained, but some patients require considerably larger volumes to maintain adequate cerebral perfusion pressures. Some patients with severe head injuries require placement of a pulmonary artery catheter to aid in titration of fluid therapy.

Management of High Intracranial Pressure

When the intracranial pressure exceeds 20 mm Hg for more than a few minutes at a time, action must be taken. Once hypercapnia and excessive end-tidal airway pressures have been excluded, the first stage of management is to exclude a new mass lesion or enlargement of a preexisting cerebral contusion. CT scanning must be performed urgently. When a significant mass lesion is present, the optimal form of management may be surgical. If no operable lesion is found, a trial of medical management should be instituted.

Elevation of the head of the bed aids in cerebral venous drainage and may aid in intracranial pressure control. Sedation may be required to control agitation associated with elevated intracranial pressure. Mannitol can be administered in repeated bolus doses until the serum osmolarity approaches 320 mOsm/L. When ventricular drainage is possible, this measure should be used intermittently, with alternating periods of drainage and pressure monitoring. Hyperventilation to P_{CO_2} of 30 mm Hg can help decrease intracranial pressure. If these measures fail, moderate hypothermia should be induced, the patient being cooled with a cooling blanket, ice packs, and neuromuscular paralysis until the core temperature is around 32°C.

As a last resort to manage intracranial pressure, barbiturate therapy can be used. Pentobarbital is usually administered (5–10 mg/kg bolus) until the electroencephalogram (EEG) shows burst suppression. Further intermittent intravenous doses can be given to maintain blood levels between 3.0 and 4.5 mg/dL. Prophylactic administration of barbiturates, however, has been shown to be ineffective in improving outcome after severe head injury.

Conventional steroids have no place in the management of head injury.

Intensive Care Management

Head injury alone increases nitrogen loss and body mass catabolism. This is further exacerbated when multiple injuries are present. Therefore, it is important to provide nutritional support early. Enteral feeding is preferred.

The aims of respiratory therapy in head-injured patients are to maintain optimal oxygenation of the injured brain and to control P_{CO_2} and thus influence cerebral blood flow and intracranial pressure. In patients who retain the cerebrovascular CO_2 response, a reduction in intracranial pressure of 1.3 mm Hg can be achieved for each mm Hg of P_{CO_2} reduction. When the cerebrovascular responses are compromised, however, this is less predictable.

Neuroprotective Drugs

Laboratory studies have yielded a number of potent neuroprotective compounds that are capable of reducing ischemic brain damage due to focal and global cerebral ischemic events. Large-scale phase III efficacy studies are now under way with free radical–scavenging compounds, glutamate antagonists, and calcium channel blockers.

ACUTE SPINAL CORD TRAUMA

Spinal Cord Injury

Acute spinal cord neuronal damage is due to two types of injury. First is the direct mechanical injury from the traumatic impact. Secondary injury results from the vascular and chemical processes set in motion by the initial impact. Attempts to resuscitate the human spinal cord after injury have been disappointing. The most consistent early change is in spinal cord blood flow.

Spinal cord blood flow is maintained over a wide blood pressure range, 60 to 120 mm Hg, by autoregulation. After spinal cord injury, autoregulation is altered or completely lost.

Clinical Patterns of Spinal Cord Injury

In complete spinal cord injury, total paralysis and loss of sensation result from the complete interruption of the ascending and descending pathways below the level of the lesion. High cervical lesions with brain stem damage to level C-1 are termed *pentaplegia*. These patients have paralysis of the lower cranial nerves and accessory muscles, as well as sensory and motor loss in the arms and legs. Non-breathing quadriplegics may have functional levels at C-2 to C-3, which leaves face and neck sensation intact and allows control of the sternocleidomastoid, trapezius, and accessory muscles. Quadriplegia involves motor and sensory loss in the extremities (injury of C-4 to C-8), and paraplegia involves loss of function in the legs only (injury of T-1 to S-1). Perineal paraplegia involves loss of sacral roots S-2 to S-5, causing bowel, bladder, and sexual dysfunction.

An incomplete injury results in preservation of some of the sensory or motor fibers below the lesion. Various incomplete symptom complexes have been delineated. The anterior cord syndrome is characterized by paralysis with hypesthesia and hypalgesia below the level of injury with preservation of light touch, position, and vibration sense. In central cord syndrome, a disproportionate degree of motor paralysis in the upper extremities is seen compared with that in the lower extremities.

Brown-Séquard syndrome is a lesion of the lateral half of the spinal cord and is manifested by ipsilateral paresis and contralateral loss of pain and temperature sensation. The cauda equina syndrome involves peripheral nerves instead of the spinal cord directly. When complete, it includes paralysis of the lower extremities, sensory loss, and bowel and bladder dysfunction. When incomplete, symptoms can include sciatica, numbness, and patchy sensation or bowel and bladder dysfunction with saddle anesthesia. The prognosis for recovery from this syndrome compared with spinal cord syndromes appears to be better.

A specialized form of incomplete lesion is sacral sparing. The lesion appears to be complete except for the presence of function in the sacral area, such as rectal tone, perianal sensation, or deep touch. Prognosis is often more favorable with this condition.

Physiologic Disturbances

Pulmonary complications are a major cause of morbidity and mortality after acute spinal cord injury. Damage to cord segments C-3 to C-5 involves the phrenic nerve nuclei; when the lesion is above C-4, voluntary diaphragmatic respiration mediated by the phrenic nerve is not possible. Although low-level cervical quadriplegics have intact phrenic nerve nuclei, they lack the intercostal muscle activity necessary to stabilize the rib cage, and diaphragmatic contraction can result in a paradoxical inward motion of the upper thorax during inspiration. Abdominal muscle dysfunction also occurs, leading to the inability to achieve normal residual volumes during expiration.

A reduction in vital capacity occurs 1 to 5 days after cervical spinal cord injury and gradually improves over time. Quadriplegic patients also have a reduction in total lung capacity, expiratory reserve volume, and forced expiratory flow rates, with an increase in residual volume and the work of breathing. As a result of these alterations, retention of secretions, atelectasis, increased ventilation-perfusion mismatch, and poor ability to sigh and cough occur. Unlike the effect in noninjured patients, a change in body position in quadriplegic patients, from upright to supine, may improve ventilatory function. In addition to the altered ventilatory function intrinsic to patients with spinal cord injuries, other insults also compromise ventilation. Gastric atony secondary to spinal shock can cause a large gastric bubble that limits diaphragmatic excursion and increases the risk of aspiration. Aspiration is a particular risk in patients who have depressed consciousness due to associated head injury. Pulmonary embolism secondary to DVT can occur as a consequence of bed rest, immobilization, and muscle paralysis. Pulmonary edema attributed to autonomic dysfunction at the time of injury (neurogenic pulmonary edema) has also been noted.

Spinal cord injury is characterized by autonomic dysfunction that interferes with maintenance of cardiovascular stability. Loss of sympathetic innervation to the heart at T-1 through T-4 cord levels leaves the parasympathetic cardiac innervation by means of the vagus unopposed, resulting in bradycardia. Elimination of sympathetic arterial tone results in hypotension. Cellular damage to the myocardium also contributes to cardiovascular instability.

Bradycardia is most frequently associated with spinal cord

injury in patients with complete injury at the cervical level. It generally resolves by 3 to 5 weeks after injury. Bradycardia is a frequent occurrence with suctioning or changes in body position. Treatment of bradycardic episodes is with vagolytic therapy (atropine, propantheline bromide) and, if associated with tracheal suctioning, increased ventilation and oxygenation. Symptomatic bradycardia unresponsive to medical measures may require cardiac pacing.

Body temperature can decrease or increase as a result of the loss of the ability to sweat in hot environments or vasoconstrict in cooler environments. Thus, hypothermia and hyperthermia are common.

About half of all patients with traumatic spinal cord injuries sustain other injuries. The possibility of concomitant head injury and spinal cord injury should always be considered. The diagnosis of intra-abdominal injuries, which occur in 5% of patients sustaining blunt cervical injury, can be particularly difficult. Acute cervical spinal cord injury masks the typical signs of blood loss due to abdominal injury.

The syndrome of spinal shock is characterized by the absence of all cutaneous and tendon reflexes below the level of the lesion. Patients exhibit flaccid paralysis and evidence of interruption of sympathetic pathways, including bradycardia, hypotension, and decreased systemic vascular resistance. Sympathetic interruption associated with spinal shock also leads to gastric atony, dilation, and ileus, which require nasogastric suctioning, and bladder atony, which requires indwelling or intermittent catheterization. The duration of areflexia varies but is usually 3 to 6 weeks in adults.

Assessment of Patients with Spinal Cord Injuries

A thorough evaluation is important for patients with spinal cord injuries. Basic considerations are spinal stability, time since the neural injury, level of spinal injury, and degree of neural injury.

The degree of spinal instability is important, since neurologic injury can be aggravated by improper management. In some acute cases, muscle spasm partially splints the bony instability, protecting the patient until anesthesia or muscle relaxants eliminate that effect.

During the acute phase, associated injuries and the presence of a full stomach warrant attention in addition to the spinal injury. After 24 hours, the possibility of excessive potassium release after the administration of succinylcholine must be considered. It is prudent to avoid succinylcholine for 1 year after spinal cord injury when denervation of muscle has occurred.

As the time after injury progresses into the phase of chronic spinal injury, uncontrolled spinal reflexes can pose problems. Muscle spasms can occur as a result of hyperactive spinal reflexes controlling muscle tone. Hyperreflexia may also be due to autonomic vascular reflexes. Usually beginning 2 to 3 weeks after injury, afferent impulses to the spinal cord can elicit unchecked sympathetic efferent activity. The afferent stimulation is typically due to distention or manipulation of hollow organs, although it can be elicited by other sensory stimulation. "Autonomic hypertension" may result and may be accompanied by headache and nasal stuffiness, as well as vague feelings of discomfort. Intravenous agents such as ganglionic blockers, direct-acting vasodilating agents, or β- and α/β-blockers can be titrated to correct the blood pressure until the inciting problem is corrected.

Chronic spinal injury is associated with problems seen in other chronically debilitated patients. Gastric erosions can be aggravated by steroids. Hypercalcemia can occur in cervical injury and is most common in adolescent boys with high cervical lesions 1 to 12 weeks after injury. This may be manifested as early as 10 days after injury and can lead to cardiac conduction defects.

Bowel and bladder problems are common. Urinary tract infection can cause systemic derangements. Chronically, recurrent infections can cause pyelonephritis and renal insufficiency. These and other chronic infections can cause amyloidosis, leading to organ dysfunction. Bowel problems tend to be more significant if a bowel regimen is not optimal.

Problems Relating to the Level of Injury

Patients with injury of the lumbar cord face further concerns because of the loss of neural control of the legs. Loss of sympathetic tone causes passive heat loss and gain through the skin surface. Chronically, reflex muscle spasms can make management difficult. The loss of muscle tone leads to flexion contractures and fixed deformities that make nursing care difficult. Finally, decubitus ulcers over the buttocks can lead to chronic infection.

Injury in the thoracic column is attended by a loss of pulmonary reserve for coughing and clearing secretions. The loss of abdominal and intercostal musculature, as well as gastric distention, contributes to increased pulmonary morbidity. When the level of injury is above T-7, autonomic reflexes in chronic cases can lead to hypertensive episodes. In injuries in the high thoracic region (T-1 to T-4), the loss of sympathetic tone of the heart can cause bradycardia because of the relative imbalance of sympathetic and vagal influences. Treatment is with vagolytic therapy.

Injuries in the cervical region can cause ventilatory difficulty that requires ventilatory support and intubation. Acutely, neck instability places the spinal cord at risk for injury with neck manipulation. This risk attends instabilities as low as T-4 and as high as the odontoid. Only one third of all cervical fractures are associated with posterior ligamentous injury, in which the spine is more unstable when flexed than when extended. Stabilization devices, such as a halo brace, may be needed.

In the midcervical region, the loss of arm musculature causes further loss of tone in the vascular beds, leading to increased heat exchange with the environment and lack of cardiovascular reserves. Hypotension and cardiac arrest have been reported with position change. Lesions in the high cervical region can cause marked impairment of ventilation, because innervation of the diaphragm by means of the phrenic nerve is impaired by injury or edema from lower levels.

Pulmonary Management

Various methods are available for securing the airway when intubation is necessary. If time allows, awake intubation permits continuous assessment of neurologic function and may preclude the use of succinylcholine. For patients with unstable cervical lesions, direct laryngoscopy is not the method of choice because extension can cause further spinal injury. Direct laryngoscopy with axial traction is a safe alternative in an acute situation. The assistant should apply traction of 5 to 10 lb at the mastoid area, pulling while the head and neck are kept aligned. For unstable C-1 and C-2 lesions, stabilization of the head to minimize motion and extension is preferable.

Aggressive chest physiotherapy is required to maintain pulmonary function. This therapy includes incentive spirometry, aerosol therapy, percussion and vibration, limited postural drainage, frequent changes in position, warm mist humidification of oxygen-enriched air, and avoidance of anticholinergics.

If respiratory function continues to deteriorate despite aggressive chest physiotherapy, intubation and ventilation should not be delayed. Once the decision is made to ventilate a patient, ventilator settings should provide close to full respiratory support, requiring only relatively modest respiratory work by the patient. Weaning parameters of forced vital capacity, negative inspiratory force, and oxygenation index should be routinely checked while the patient is being weaned from the ventilator. Satisfaction of weaning parameters often occurs 10 to 21 days after injury. Because of possible laryngeal incompetence, enteral feedings are suspended in the periextubation period. For patients with high quadriplegia, a permanent tracheostomy or electrical stimulation of the phrenic nerve is required.

Drug Therapy

Treatment strategies for spinal cord injury have focused largely on reducing the degree of secondary injury or attempting to promote regeneration of the damaged neurons. Animal experiments support the concept that motor function can recover to normal levels with as few as 4% to 6% of the cortical neurons having connection to the cord. If the axonal survival rate exceeds 6%, full motor function is possible. Because the gray matter may be more sensitive to injury than white matter, strategies to improve spinal injury outcome may revolve around improving gray matter viability. Unfortunately, a major disparity exists between experimental spinal cord injury and clinical human injury with respect to treatment success.

Methylprednisolone is considered routine in spinal injury. In a multicenter, randomized, placebo-controlled trial of the drug in acute spinal cord injury, 162 patients received methylprednisolone, 30 mg/kg, followed by a continuous infusion of 5.4 mg/kg/h for 23 hours. Improvement in motor neurologic scores was noted at 6 weeks, 6 months, and 1 year in patients with complete as well as incomplete lesions, provided the drug therapy was instituted within 8 hours of injury.

The neuroprotective effects of steroids have been determined not to depend on steroid receptors. The mechanism probably is inhibition of lipid peroxidation. Compounds with steroid nuclei but without glucocorticoid effects have now been synthesized (21-aminosteroids). Tirilazad (U-74f006F) is currently in phase II clinical trials. Also under investigation are gangliosides.

CRITICAL CARE OF WOUNDS AND WOUNDED PATIENTS

Healing is an amazingly complex collection of normal coping processes that is easily and commonly impaired and falls short of its full potential unless actively supported.

Nature of Repair

Healing follows disruption of the normal extracellular environment in which local perfusion is interrupted and, as a consequence, coagulation and inflammation are recruited. Eventually, healing forms a new circulation and with it a new extracellular matrix made mainly of collagen and proteoglycans. The end of normal wound healing coincides with restoration of a normal extracellular environment.

The first stimulus to wound healing is activation of tissue complement, which attracts polymorphonuclear leukocytes to defend against infection. The next stimulus is the activation of Hageman factor, activating the coagulation process. Thrombin causes platelets to release various platelet-derived growth factors, all of which stimulate fibroblast replication. Polymerization of fibrinogen to fibrin is followed by fibrinolysis and release of peptides that are chemotactic mainly to monocytes. Fibrin itself activates monocytes to release cytokines. Plasmin, which digests fibrin, also digests basement membranes of vessels, an event essential to angiogenesis. Next follows a complex array of proteolytic events in which preexisting matrix is digested.

The initial cellular reaction is composed of polymorphonuclear leukocytes. A few days later, macrophages predominate and contribute mainly to resistance to infection and matrix digestion. Macrophages, with some help from lymphocytes, release a number of growth factors and cytokines when stimulated by injured tissue, fibrin, foreign bodies, and low oxygen and high lactate concentrations found in wounds. These substances then stimulate growth and migration of fibroblasts and endothelial cells. This local environment begins to encourage cell growth as well as to attract inflammatory cells, new fibroblasts, and endothelial cells into the area. Granulocytes and macrophages are activated, or primed, on entering the wound space. This causes rapid conversion of molecular (dissolved) oxygen to superoxide.

The critical enzyme in this set of reactions is an NADPH-linked oxygenase. This is a central event in healing and accomplishes three important steps: (1) it contributes superoxide, which is essential to intraleukocytic bacterial killing; (2) it consumes oxygen, and the resulting hypoxia later limits new matrix formation; and, (3) it produces lactate and stimulates collagen synthesis and angiogenesis. Macrophages and granulocytes also release proteolysins, including collagenases. These aid in débridement of denatured tissue and remodeling of the new scar tissue, and they assist angiogenesis.

After a few days, fibroblasts migrate in and multiply. They synthesize and deposit collagen and proteoglycans, which eventually connect the edges of the wound and give it strength. Fibroblast replication rates are proportional to oxygen availability. The optimal tissue partial pressure of oxygen (po_2) is 50 mm Hg. New vessels, in the form of blind-ended capillaries, emerge from normal tissue and move toward the wound space, leaving behind a maturing circulation. All new vessels start as endothelial cell buds from venules that follow the lead of macrophages and fibroblasts. Neovascularization follows the steep oxygen gradient that characterizes wounds. The major angiogenic stimulus in wounds is derived from macrophages.

By the end of the third or fourth day, full-thickness wounds have a characteristic cellular architecture; from top to bottom, this includes a layer of macrophages surrounding the wound space, a layer of immature fibroblasts, a layer of replicating fibroblasts, then mature fibroblasts and the earliest visible traces of scar collagen. The wound advances into the wound space, drawn inward by products of activated macrophages. Dead spaces heal until filled.

Regeneration of connective tissue is the next step. Fibroblasts release the collagen monomers into the extracellular space, where they polymerize and eventually glue the sides of the wound together. The synthesis of collagen monomers requires molecular oxygen, ferrous iron, ascorbic acid, and oxoglutarate. The major stimulus for collagen formation is closely related to the low oxidation-reduction potential in the healing area. This low potential is due largely to the high lactate concentration that is contributed by leukocytes during aerobic glycolysis. Lactate dihydroascorbate, the reduced form of ascorbate, stimulates the formation of collagen-synthesizing enzymes and collagen synthesis in aerobic fibroblast cultures. The mechanism for collagen synthesis and deposition relies on a low NAD^+; however, collagen deposition depends on po_2. The paradox is resolved by the fact that the low NAD^+ is a direct consequence of the lactate released aerobically by leukocytes. When po_2 is elevated, little effect on either po_2 or lactate is seen in the wound space. A larger effect on po_2 is observed in the zone of collagen synthesis. Collagen deposition is a function of po_2 throughout the clinical range and higher. Other requirements for collagen synthesis are amino acids for its structure, glucose to meet the energy needs of protein synthesis, and ascorbate to transfer oxygen for proline and lysine hydroxylation; sulfated amino acids, iron, lysine, and vitamin A are also required. In addition, arginine in high doses markedly stimulates collagen deposition.

Collagen turns over rapidly in wounds and areas of inflammation. Lytic mechanisms consist of collagenases, lysosomal enzymes, and the plasmin/plasminogen system. Wound edge fusion depends on net collagen synthesis and deposition. Collagen synthesis consumes energy and nutrients and depends heavily on vascular resources, but collagen lysis uses few if any vital resources and is activated by ischemia.

The epithelia that eventually cover the surfaces of wounds are led largely by growth factors released by their own stem cells. As epithelium advances over healing wounds, the underlying connective tissue contracts and mitotic and synthetic activity in the deeper tissue begins to recede. Epithelization is easily hindered, especially in zinc and vitamin A deficiencies and during anti-inflammatory steroid therapy. Epithelization is also oxygen dependent.

Wound Infection and Immunity

The incidence of wound infection is inversely proportional to the vascularity of the wounded tissue. Resistance to infection is one of the most important contributions of rapid repair and healing. Leukocytes phagocytose bacteria nonoxidatively. Phagocytosis also activates the oxidative killing system. The size of the oxygen radical pool is determined by the rate at which oxygen is converted to superoxide by the NADPH-linked oxygenase. Bacterial killing capacity is limited by pO_2; thus, bacterial killing is seriously impaired in the oxygen-starved environment of wounds.

Killing capacity is also limited by pH. If extracellular pH is low, the pH of the phagosome is similarly low, and this limits superoxide production. Hypoxia also potentiates infection. Hypoxia stimulates tumor necrosis factor and interleukin-1 (IL-1) secretion by leukocytes in culture. Useful therapeutic options are reperfusion and reoxygenation as well as débridement of ischemic tissue.

Physiology of Reparative Tissue

When tissue is divided sharply, an ischemic zone about twice the intercapillary distance is created by the injury and hemostasis. Capillary pO_2, which is the driving force to diffusion, becomes the major limiting determinant of oxygen delivery. Removal of CO_2, lactate, and H^+ is seriously impeded.

The importance of pO_2 and the relative lack of importance of hemoglobin and total oxygen delivery to wounds are emphasized by two points. First, the rates of three enzymes that are vital to wounds, prolyl and lysyl hydroxylases and the NADPH-linked oxygenase of leukocytes, depend on pO_2 throughout the range of 0 to 200 mm Hg. Second, wounds use relatively little oxygen at a constant rate. Hence, it is clinically advantageous to maintain a high pO_2 in wounded tissue. Perfusion must also be adequate. The way to maintain a high local pO_2 is to maintain a high flow of blood at a high pO_2 and keep the extraction ratio as low as possible. In addition, local vasoconstriction mediated by the sympathetic nervous system, hypothermia, smoking, and drugs is an obstacle to maintaining the high tissue pO_2 necessary for prompt repair and prevention of infection.

The nature of a wound affects its oxygen economy. The more severe the wound, the lower the oxygen supply in relation to demand. pO_2 decreases in all wounds during the first few days as inflammation develops and fibroblasts accumulate.

Intensive Care of Wounded Patients

Measures to avert peripheral vasoconstriction and boost peripheral flow should be instituted. These include maintaining a high cardiac output, usually by keeping optimal blood volume, avoiding pain, and preventing chilling and fear.

Fluid infusion rates in postoperative patients have been linked to peripheral tissue pO_2. This measure has often shown the need to give more fluid than otherwise seems necessary. In these instances, pulmonary artery monitoring may be necessary. When tissue oxygenation normalizes, fluid replacement can be safely reduced. Overall, present ICU methods are not directed to peripheral wound perfusion and pO_2. When healing and tissue infections are a problem, one should consider measuring peripheral tissue pO_2.

Anemic Patients

Wound healing in anemic patients is rarely improved by blood transfusion unless anemia is very severe (i.e., hematocrit $<15\%$) or cardiac output cannot compensate normally. Correcting circulating blood volume deficits is more important than correcting anemia. Considerations of wound healing should not be used as an indication for transfusion unless hematocrit falls below 20% or cardiac or brain function is threatened by critical stenoses in major feeding vessels.

Antibiotic Therapy

Normal tissues are saturated by antibiotics in minutes; peak antibiotic concentrations, however, are not reached in wound tissue until 1.5 hours after intravenous bolus doses and 4 to 6 hours after starting a constant infusion.

Nutrition

Nutrition affects both healing and immunity to infection. Unfortunately, the relations are vague. Calorie and protein needs are governed by the extent of injury and infection. Vitamins A and D, riboflavin, niacin, pyridoxal and ascorbic acid, zinc, copper, manganese, iron, methionine or cysteine, and lysine are all essential for wound healing. Glutamine and arginine are particularly important. Arginine in large doses enhances collagen deposition even in normal volunteers. Hence, early resumption of enteral feeding is highly desirable.

The wound suppressive effects of anti-inflammatory steroids can be counteracted through the use of vitamin A (10,000–15,000 U/d for 1 week), zinc (50–100 mg/d for 1 week), and ascorbic acid (1 g/d).

ACUTE PAIN IN THE INTENSIVE CARE UNIT

The International Association for the Study of Pain defines pain as an "unpleasant sensory and emotional experience associated with actual or potential tissue damage." Pain can accelerate catecholamine release, which in turn increases systemic vascular resistance, increases cardiac stroke work, and worsens myocardial oxygen supply/demand ratios. Therefore, it is beneficial, both psychologically and physiologically, to treat pain.

Pain Pathways and Mechanisms

Painful impulses are known to stimulate peripheral pain receptors, known as nociceptors, that transmit impulses by means of specialized peripheral afferent pain fibers to the spinal cord and into the brain. Subsequently, mechanisms are activated to prevent injury to minimize perceived pain. Chemical modulation of pain transmission occurs through several neurotransmitter-receptor systems that have been shown to affect spinal processing of nociceptive input.

Traditional Acute Pain Treatment Regimens

Several studies have demonstrated the ineffectiveness of intramuscular opioids administered as needed. Caregivers often underestimate the amount of analgesia required. In addition, the choice of medications may be incorrect. For example, paralyzing agents have been used for analgesia and sedation in critically ill patients who are ventilator dependent, when paralyzing agents have no anxiolytic properties and should be administered only concomitantly with appropriate pain and anxiety control.

Intermittent administration of systemic opiates is an effective method of postoperative pain control. Opioid analgesics act on multiple opiate receptors in the central nervous system, spinal cord, and peripheral nervous system. Drugs acting at opioid receptors are divided into agonists, agonist-antagonists, and partial agonists. Analgesia is most profound with pure opioid agonists. Opiate side effects parallel the amount of agonist activity, however, and are diminished with accompanying antagonism.

The side effects of opiates, most notably respiratory depression and hypotension, are the limiting factor in their use. Other side effects with systemic narcotics include nausea, vomiting, pruritus, urinary retention, and gastrointestinal dysfunction.

Patient-Controlled Analgesia

Patient-controlled analgesia (PCA) with parenteral medications consists of a set dosage of drug given at a preset lockout interval by patient demand, with or without an accompanying continuous infusion. With continuous intravenous infusions or PCA dosing of opioids, a more consistent opioid plasma concentration is achieved. The incidence of opiate side effects with PCA does not appear to be any different than with other methods of narcotic administration. PCA has demonstrated outcome advantages in terms of decreased confusion, restoration of pulmonary function, fewer pulmonary complications, shorter time to ambulation, and shortened hospital stay.

Central Neural Blockade

The administration of local anesthetics in the intrathecal or epidural space is associated with dramatic cardiovascular side effects that accompany the superior analgesia that the drugs provide. In the late 1970s, intraspinal opiate use gained popularity because of the superior analgesia provided segmentally with greater cardiovascular stability. The most troubling side effect is the occurrence of late respiratory depression. Various drug combinations have been proposed, including opiate analgesics that are more lipid soluble, agonist-antagonist narcotics, combinations of narcotics and local anesthetics, and non-narcotic analgesics such as the $alpha_2$ agonist clonidine. Epidural catheters are now available for continuous or repeated dosing.

Epidural local anesthesia for postoperative pain has been used for abdominal, thoracic, and orthopedic surgeries, and has been associated with shorter time to ambulation, decreased hospital stay, and lower incidence of pulmonary complications in selected patients. The side effects of cardiovascular instability and motor weakness prohibit its use in many patients, however.

Spinal Opiate Analgesia

Spinal opiate analgesia refers to either intrathecal or epidural administration of a narcotic analgesic. Commonly used opiate analgesics include morphine, meperidine, fentanyl, and sufentanil. Management differences are related to physicochemical properties of the drug selected, catheter placement, and dosing guidelines. Nonopiate analgesics and opiate agonist-antagonists have also been used with varying degrees of success. Analgesia with spinal opiates has decreased the time needed for mechanical ventilation, ICU stay, and hospital stay.

Morphine is the standard to which all other spinal analgesics are compared. Epidural morphine administration demonstrates analgesia superior to that of conventionally administered parenteral narcotics. Morphine is the least lipid-soluble spinal opiate of those commonly used. Its onset of action is 45 to 60 minutes. It can be administered in the low lumbar region for high abdominal or thoracic procedures. Side effects include nausea and vomiting (30–40%), pruritus (10–90%), urinary retention (5–40%), and early and late (up to 24 hours) respiratory depression. The incidence and severity of side effects appear to be greater than those of more lipid-soluble opiates. Pruritus usually responds to diphenhydramine.

Meperidine has a greater lipid solubility, quicker onset of action (15–30 minutes), lower degree of cephalad spread (potentially fewer side effects), and a shorter duration of action (4–6 hours). Meperidine also has the advantage of possessing local anesthetic properties and is the only opiate to have been used as a sole anesthetic when given intrathecally.

Fentanyl is a synthetic opioid agonist that contains the same chemical nucleus as morphine. Fentanyl is 100-fold more potent than morphine and 500-fold more lipid soluble. This gives fentanyl a rapid onset of analgesia, a short duration of action, and minimal cephalad migration. Larger doses must be administered through a lumbar epidural catheter to provide analgesia for upper abdominal and thoracic surgery (100–200 μg). Fentanyl is an ideal drug for use in continuous infusion through an epidural catheter; an infusion of 0.5 to 1.0 μg/kg/h is used for postoperative pain.

Sufentanil is a synthetic opiate that is five to seven times as potent as fentanyl when given systemically and twice as potent as fentanyl when given in the epidural space. Its lipid solubility is twice that of fentanyl. It has a short onset of action (<15 minutes), and a duration of action that is longer than that of fentanyl (4–6 hours). Boluses of 30 to 50 μg for upper abdominal or thoracic surgery and 15 to 30 μg for peripheral operations are required for analgesia. Epidural infusion rates of 0.15 to 0.30 μg/kg/h are sufficient when a dilute 1-μg/mL solution is used.

Problems arising from spinal opiate side effects and systemic absorption have led to the use of narcotic–local anesthetic combinations. Addition of local anesthetics to spinal opiate infusions or boluses can enhance analgesia without clinical signs of local anesthetic blockade. The benefit in superior analgesia and decreased spinal opiate requirements may come at the expense of the potentially deleterious local anesthetic side effects of hypotension, motor weakness, and inability to ambulate.

Regional Blockade

If the use of systemic opioids is to be avoided, regional anesthetic techniques can provide excellent analgesia and help maintain patients' mental status.

Local infiltration is the simplest method for providing extended wound analgesia. Bupivacaine 0.25% is the preferred local anesthetic. Epinephrine-containing local anesthetics should be avoided because of the theoretic risks of delayed wound healing.

Intravenous regional techniques are extremely useful for manipulation of limb fractures and for simple surgical procedures. The procedure involves placement of a double tourniquet on the proximal extremity and the intravenous administration of large volumes of dilute local anesthetic distally (40–50 mL of 0.5% lidocaine). Systemic levels of local anesthetic can result from its inadvertent release or from tourniquet leakage.

Peripheral nerve blockade produces effective, long-lasting analgesia with a minimum of side effects. With the use of a long-acting local anesthetic such as bupivacaine, analgesia can last up to 24 hours.

Intercostal blockade is simple and effective and has been used extensively to provide pain relief for patients with fractured ribs or blunt trauma, or who have undergone upper abdominal and thoracic surgery. Intercostal blockade has advantages over interpleural and thoracic epidural blockades in that it is technically easier to perform and is not associated with hypotension, motor weakness, or urinary retention. Disadvantages include the need for multiple injection sites (for multiple levels), frequent repeated injections, risk of pneumothorax, and risk of accumulation of significant systemic levels of local anesthetic. Continuous intercostal analgesia provided by indwelling catheters eliminates the need for multiple injections and frequent repeated injections.

Administration of local anesthetic through a percutaneous catheter placed between the visceral and parietal pleura provides good unilateral thoracic dermatomal analgesia. The mechanism of action of interpleural analgesia is still uncertain. Contraindications to this block include a recent thoracic infection with pleuritis and fibrosis of the pleura. The degree of sensory anesthesia obtained with interpleural block is inconsistent.

Multiple nerve blocks have applications in acute pain management of postoperative, post-traumatic, or critically ill patients. Femoral nerve blockade has been used to provide analgesia and muscle relaxation for femoral fractures and after total-knee arthroplasty. Brachial plexus blockade can be performed by means of the axillary, infraclavicular, interscalene, and supraclavicular routes. This is useful after reimplantation procedures or vascular injuries that result in diminished blood flow and vasospasm. The prolonged blockade permits improved blood flow to the area of injury. Ilioinguinal-iliohypogastric nerve blocks are helpful after inguinal hernia repair. A wrist block can be performed by blocking the median, radial, and ulnar nerves at the wrist. An ankle block requires blockade of the tibial, sural, saphenous, and superficial and deep peroneal nerves. Psoas compartment lumbar plexus blockade is another alternative for lower-extremity analgesia.

Special Cases

In the acute phase of trauma, immediate attention must be given to stabilization of the respiratory and cardiovascular status. Treatment of pain is appropriately deferred until the patient is stabilized and the injuries are investigated and diagnosed. Acute pain from trauma results in profound sustained catecholamine release that may support the blood pressure and cardiac output in a patient who has sustained large blood losses. Once respiratory and volume status have been restored, the slow titration of intravenously administered opioids for pain management is appropriate. In the patient with altered mental status, systemic opioids should be used cautiously, and regional analgesic methods should be considered.

Burn patients should be treated with intravenous opioids once the airway is secured and hemodynamic status is stabilized. Constant pain from the burn injury occurs at rest and should be managed with around-the-clock opioids. Burn treatment (i.e., dressing changes, hydrotherapy) should take place with additional opioids alone or in combination with anxiolytics or dissociative anesthesia. Fentanyl, 1–6 μg/kg, is often used with midazolam, 0.08 mg/kg, in divided doses. It is best to avoid intramuscular drugs in burn patients. Ketamine can be titrated using 0.5 to 1.0 mg/kg intravenously. Ketamine should be used with anxiolytics to abate the increased incidence of hallucinations and excitement.

With major organ dysfunction, significant changes can occur in the pharmacokinetic profile of analgesic medication. Volume of distribution, clearance, and excretion are affected by organ failure. Hence, dosages may need to be adjusted in this patient group.

Patients with severe pulmonary conditions who sustain multiple trauma or who undergo thoracic or abdominal procedures are excellent candidates for continuous epidural opiate infusions. Ketorolac and transcutaneous electrical nerve stimulation to supplement opioid use have had good results. Individuals with severely depressed cardiac function who receive intravenous morphine are susceptible to hypotension. Meperidine should be used with caution in these patients because of its vagolytic action. Epidural and intrathecal opioids suppress the catecholamine response to pain more effectively than intravenous opioids, which may be advantageous in these patients.

Risk of analgesic overdose is present in patients with liver disease. If no contraindications to catheter placement exist, spinal opiate therapy is acceptable and provides excellent benefits for patients with hepatic failure. If coagulopathy exists or the surgical site does not permit the use of regional analgesia, intravenous fentanyl administered continuously or by a PCA device can be a safe alternative.

Epidural or intrathecal morphine in renal failure patients offers several advantages over systemic narcotics, including superior analgesia, low dosage requirements, minimal accumulation, and absence of renal toxicity. PCA with fentanyl is a good option in renal failure patients.

Pediatric Patients

Assessment of pediatric pain can be difficult. The mainstay of pediatric pain control is systemic analgesic therapy. Mild to moderate forms of postoperative pain should be treated with nonopiate analgesics such as acetaminophen, 10 to 15 mg/kg orally or 15 to 20 mg/kg rectally every 4 hours, and nonsteroidal anti-inflammatory agents. If pain persists, opioid analgesia may be required. Narcotic analgesics provide excellent relief if given in sufficient amounts at effective intervals. These agents can be given by the oral, rectal, intranasal, transdermal, intravenous, intramuscular, epidural, and intrathecal routes. Intramuscular injections are particularly distressing to pediatric patients. PCA and regional analgesia are suitable alternatives in older children.

MANAGEMENT OF BURNS

Burn injuries are a leading cause of mortality and severe long-term dysfunction, especially in children and young adults. Advances in burn management have resulted in a marked decrease in mortality. Burns that involve 70% to 80% of the body surface area used to be 100% fatal; now mortality rates below 50% have been reported. The major advances have been made in two areas: (1) the rapid and safe removal of burn tissue before the onset of infection and wound closure, and (2) critical care management. The leading cause of death in burn patients is no longer burn wound sepsis but respiratory failure. A persistent immunodeficient state and increased skin and lung colonization by infectious organisms lead to a high risk of continued nosocomial infection. Multisystem organ failure in burn patients has a mortality rate approaching 100% compared with 50% to 70% in the trauma patients who are not burned.

The simplest way to clarify the postburn pathophysiology is to divide the postburn period into three parts: the resuscitation phase (0–36 hours), the postresuscitation period (2–5 days), and the inflammation-infection phase (6 days to wound closure).

Resuscitation Period

Airway and lung dysfunction are of particular concern immediately after a burn. Although clinical evidence of such dysfunction is often delayed in onset, early preventive measures need to be initiated to avoid potentially life-threatening problems. A hypoxic insult, carbon monoxide toxicity, and cyanide toxicity are evident immediately after injury. Maintaining a high index of suspicion is mandatory. Clues to the diagnosis of carbon monoxide toxicity include a measured oxygen saturation of hemoglobin that is lower than predicted by the oxygen tension and the presence of an unexplained increase in anion gap metabolic acidosis. Verification can be done by assessing carboxyhemoglobin level (normal, $<5\%$). The value often underestimates the initial magnitude of the carbon monoxide toxicity. Cyanide poisoning is more difficult to diagnose. Treatment with sodium nitrate, followed by sodium thiosulfate therapy, can be initiated if high cyanide levels are suspected.

Upper airway injury from heat and chemicals in smoke can be detected by direct laryngoscopy; however, risk of subsequent edema cannot be accurately predicted by initial findings. A body burn injury markedly increases the upper airway edema process. Therefore, early elective intubation is indicated when deep facial burns and any evidence of an airway injury exist as well as in large body burns. The pulmonary response to a chemical burn to the lower airway is initially bronchorrhea, bronchoconstriction, small airway closure, and marked ventilation-perfusion mismatch. Atelectasis is also common. Endotracheal intubation is often indicated for pulmonary toilet. Pulmonary dysfunction can also occur with deep burns to the chest wall, which produce a restrictive defect and necessitate chest wall escharotomy.

The massive fluid losses from a skin burn are the result of three processes. The first is the alteration in vascular permeability, which results from heat and vasoactive mediators in burn tissue and which leads to a loss of plasma. The second is a marked increase in negative interstitial forces. The third is a fluid shift into unburned interstitium as a result of burn-induced hypoproteinemia. A component of decreased contractility is also seen in patients with large burns. Estimation of fluid requirements initially is guided by various mathematical formulas. Subsequent replacement is dictated by an ongoing assessment of perfusion. The first 24-hour fluid need is estimated based on the following: 4 mL fluid × percentage of body surface area burned × patient's body weight in kilograms. Half of the result is given in the first 8 hours. Because the fluid losses are ongoing, the rate of tissue edema depends on the rate of fluid infusion. Reliable parameters to follow in a young patient include pulse rate 120 beats per minute or lower, systolic blood pressure 100 mm Hg, urine output 0.5 mL/kg/h, correction of base deficit, and mixed or central venous oxygen saturation exceeding 60%. The risks of infection and thrombotic complications usually preclude the routine use of pulmonary artery catheters. The exception is in elderly patients. Isotonic crystalloid solution, preferably lactated Ringer's solution, is the initial fluid of choice. Protein- or non–protein-containing colloid solutions can be infused immediately if perfusion with crystalloid solution alone is inadequate. The fluids should be infused at a constant rate rather than as a bolus. Hematocrit is often a false indicator of blood volume. RBC mass may be decreased as a result of the damage of RBCs by heat, acute hemolysis, external losses, and other trauma. RBC transfusion is often useful in restoring hemodynamic stability in patients who do not respond to crystalloid and colloid solutions alone.

Coagulopathy manifests as a hypercoagulable state in patients with modest burns and as a consumptive coagulopathy in patients with massive burns. Renal and splanchnic blood flow are more selectively decreased, and levels of antidiuretic hormones, such as aldosterone, are increased.

Wound management is the next priority after addressing airway, pulmonary, and cardiovascular issues. The ideal time for excision is before the onset of wound inflammation (i.e., within the first 5 days after the burn). Heat loss is a major problem in burn patients, and a warm environment is mandatory to avoid hypothermia.

Postresuscitation Period

In general, the ideal time to initiate aggressive wound excision and closure is 2 to 5 days after injury. For this to occur, the patient must be hemodynamically stable. This grace period is short-lived, and once wound colonization, inflammation, and profound hypermetabolism develop, operative risks escalate, especially in the presence of lung or cardiac problems. It is extremely important that operative procedures be kept short (i.e., <2 hours) and that optimal pulmonary support be provided. Early initiation of antibiotic therapy is critical when signs of bacterial tracheobronchitis are observed.

The postresuscitation period is characterized by major fluid shifts in both directions, as well as by a progressive decrease in red blood cell mass in large burns of the body. Losses of plasma into burn tissue and wound surface continue. Losses per hour can be estimated by the following formula: loss in milliliters per hour = (25 + percentage of body surface burned) × body surface area in square meters. Fluid gains include those of resorbing edema. Hypotonic salt solution with added potassium, calories, and protein should be used to replace evaporative and urinary losses. The hematocrit should be maintained above 30%. Rapid clearance of injured cells by the reticuloendothelial system occurs. In addition, RBC production is markedly impaired. Hence, a decreasing hematocrit in the absence of bleeding is typical of a major burn. When wound inflammation begins to evolve after day 3, heart rate increases, reflecting a hyperdynamic state and not necessarily a hypovolemic state. In addition, an osmotic diuresis can develop, making it difficult to assess volume status.

Wound management includes the use of topical antibiotics twice daily, excision of burn tissue, and skin closure. Blood loss from débridement can be substantial, but losses for the same area excised in the first 3 or 4 days are less than half of those seen with excisions after 1 week, when wound hypervascularity develops. All wounds should be considered to be contaminated. Perioperative antibiotic coverage is indicated, usually with a first-generation cephalosporin.

Inflammation-Infection Period

The hypermetabolic response to injury begins 4 or 5 days after injury and peaks at about 7 to 10 days. It is extremely difficult to distinguish burn inflammation–induced hypermetabolism from an infection-induced process. This period is by far the most difficult period for management.

The smoke-injured lung is prone to pneumonia for weeks after injury until the mucociliary border is resolved. Impaired cough, the presence of an endotracheal tube, alterations in consciousness, smoke inhalation, pulmonary congestion with increases in interstitial and alveolar water, and decreased systemic immune function enhance the likelihood of pneumonia development. In addition, the marked increase in metabolic rate results in a concomitant increase in CO_2 production, which increases the work of breathing. Partial ventilatory assistance is often required. Sepsis or inflammation-induced adult respiratory distress syndrome is also prominent during this period. CO_2 production should be reduced by limiting excess carbohydrate intake, controlling temperature, and avoiding the provocation of unnecessary anxiety and pain.

Maintaining adequate fluid replacement for evaporative loss and for blood and plasma loss from débridement is required. Cardiac output is often more than twice normal to supply the increased oxygen demands. Elderly patients with limited cardiac reserve often develop myocardial dysfunction as workload exceeds functional ability. The need for inotropic support is much more common.

Maintenance of adequate nutrition is critical during this period. The ideal route is the gastrointestinal tract.

Nosocomial infection is particularly prevalent during the inflammation-infection period. The burn wound is best managed with topical antibiotics. Vascular catheter sepsis is a major problem that can be controlled only by frequent catheter replacement and by early removal of monitoring lines. Nosocomial pneumonia is common and is diagnosed by an increase in sputum quantity and an increase in white blood cell count and bacteria on Gram staining of a deep sputum sample.

Systemic antibiotics for burn wounds are indicated only if there is evidence of an invasive burn infection. Surface wound cultures are always positive, demonstrating colonization. The wound is colonized and subsequently infected most commonly by *Staphylococcus aureus* within the first week; gram-negative organisms are prevalent beginning in the second week. Wound purulence is a reliable indicator of infection only if the purulence is in the subeschar space. Bacterial analysis of a burn wound biopsy is the most reliable method of diagnosing a burn wound infection. The biopsy must include some underlying viable subcutaneous tissue. Fewer than 10^5 organisms is indicative of colonization, whereas 10^5 or more indicates infection with a high potential for progression to wound sepsis. Gentle daily débridement is the appropriate management during this period for burn tissue not yet excised. A granulation tissue bed then develops; this tissue bed is more resistant to infection and is used as the appropriate bed for a skin graft.

Rehabilitation

Exercise routines, including active and passive range-of-motion exercise of all burned and nonburned areas, are necessary shortly after a patient's admission if permanent loss of function in burned joints is to be avoided.

SMOKE INHALATION INJURY

The leading cause of death in fires is the inhalation of smoke, not burn injury. Smoke injury is also the cause of more than half of the deaths among burn patients. Three postinsult phases can be identified: the early resuscitation phase (0–36 hours), the postresuscitation phase (2–5 days), and the inflammation-infection phase (5 days to lung healing and burn wound closure).

General Pathophysiology

The injury to the lung itself depends on the components of the smoke inhaled, the degree of smoke exposure, and the lung's response to the insult. The injury caused by heat is usually confined to the area above the vocal cords, except in long-term exposure or steam exposure. The gas phase contains a host of toxins, including carbon monoxide, cyanide gas, acids, aldehydes, and oxidants. The vapors are in large part mucous membrane irritants that cause intense bronchorrhea, bronchoconstriction, and airway edema. This process peaks hours after injury. The particulate phase injury depends on the particle size and the patient's breathing pattern. In general, particles larger than 5 μm are cleared by the nasopharynx if the patient is able to breathe nasally. With mouth breathing, most of the larger particles deposit in the larynx, trachea, and large airways. Particles smaller than 5 μm deposit in both large and small airways and in the alveoli. Particles can adhere to the mucosa and perpetuate the local tissue injury.

The degree of smoke exposure depends on the mass of smoke inhaled, the depth of breathing, and the time of exposure. A high carboxyhemoglobin level (>40%) produces an obtunded state and provides evidence of prolonged exposure. This assumes that head injury, drugs, and alcoholism are not present.

The degree of initial and late injury is in large part related to the status of the lung before injury. A lung with any element of reactive airway disease or chronic changes reacts to smoke exposure more intensely than does a healthy lung. Airway and parenchymal injury result from a sequence of pathologic events. First, direct mucosal injury, loss of ciliary activity, and subsequent impairment of particle, mucous, and, later, bacterial clearance occur. Second, bronchial blood flow and bronchial vessel permeability increase; this leads to submucosal edema and vascular engorgement, which narrow airway lumina. Third, tissue destruction, the result of these factors, and a secondary inflammatory response ensue. The result is a slough of mucosa in both large and small airways and a marked increase in mucus production.

After 2 or 3 days, the lung may progress to a state that presents all of the signs and symptoms seen with a large inflammatory focus, including a hyperdynamic state, an increase in oxygen demands, and maldistribution of blood flow.

Early Resuscitation Phase

Inspired air in a fire has a decreased oxygen tension (pO_2) in view of oxygen utilization during combustion. This low fraction of inspired oxygen leads to hypoxia. Treatment involves the immediate administration of high-flow oxygen.

Carbon monoxide toxicity is one of the leading causes of death in fires. Carbon monoxide is a byproduct of combustion and is rapidly transported across the alveolar membrane and preferentially binds with the hemoglobin molecule in place of oxygen. Carbon monoxide shifts the hemoglobin-oxygen curve to the left, impairing oxygen unloading at the tissue level. With prolonged exposure, carbon monoxide can also saturate cells, binding to cytochrome oxidase and thereby further impairing mitochondrial function and adenosine triphosphate (ATP) production. Symptoms of carbon monoxide toxicity are usually not present until the carboxyhemoglobin level exceeds 15%. Initial manifestations are neurologic because of the impairment of cerebral oxygenation. This can lead to progressive and permanent cerebral dysfunction. Major myocardial dysfunction can also develop. The persistence of a metabolic acidosis in a patient with adequate volume resuscitation and cardiac output suggests persistent carbon monoxide or cyanide impairment of oxygen utilization and delivery. Oxygen saturation is less than expected based on the measured PaO_2. Therefore, if a discrepancy exists between the measured PaO_2 and the measured oxygen saturation, carbon monoxide toxicity is present until proved otherwise. A high carboxyhemoglobin level is also indicative of a significant smoke exposure, but a low carboxyhemoglobin level does not always indicate a minimal smoke exposure. Treatment of carbon monoxide toxicity consists of the early displacement of carbon monoxide from hemoglobin by administration of 90% to 100% oxygen. Oxygen administration is required for all patients with major burns until carbon monoxide toxicity can be ruled out or until carboxyhemoglobin levels return to normal. Administration of hyperbaric oxygen (2–3 atm) produces an even more rapid displacement of carbon monoxide and is most useful in patients who have had prolonged exposure.

The burning of synthetic substances, such as polyurethane, produces hydrocyanide, the gaseous form of cyanide. The hydrocyanide binds to the cytochrome system, inhibiting cell metabolism and ATP production. Cyanide toxicity presents in a similar fashion to carbon monoxide toxicity, with profound metabolic acidosis and obtundation in severe cases. Diagnosis is more difficult because cyanide levels are not always readily available or reliable. Normal cyanide levels in smokers are less than 0.1 mg/L. A lethal level is considered to be 1 mg/L. In patients with cyanide poisoning, cardiopulmonary support is usually sufficient treatment, since the liver clears the cyanide from the circulation by means of the enzyme rhodanese. Sodium nitrate, 300 mg intravenously over 5–10 minutes, is used in severe cases, especially in patients in whom the diagnosis is made based on blood levels. Methemoglobin is produced by the nitrite, which in turn binds the cyanide. Thiosulfate is then given to bind the cyanide to form thiocyanate.

Heat produces an immediate injury to the airway mucosa, resulting in edema, erythema, and ulceration. Physiologic alterations do not occur until the edema is sufficient to produce clinical evidence of impaired upper airway patency. This may not occur for 12 to 18 hours. Another compounding injury is any face or neck burn that produces marked anatomic distortion and, in the case of a deep neck burn, external compression on the larynx. A third-degree facial burn may have minimal external edema but massive intraoral edema. The local edema process usually resolves within 5 days. Symptoms of obstruction do not develop until a critical narrowing of the airway is present. Upper airway noise often precedes obstruction. The airway edema and the external burn edema processes have a parallel time course. Inspection of the oropharynx in search of soot or evidence of a heat injury should be performed on every burn victim. Fiberoptic bronchoscopy or laryngoscopy is used to evaluate the pharyngeal and laryngeal mucosa. Unfortunately, the initial examination does not accurately predict the severity of subsequent airway compromise, since the edema is progressive during the first 18 to 24 hours after injury. Treatment includes maintenance of airway patency, protection against aspiration, pulmonary toilet, and positive-pressure ventilation. When in doubt, it is safer to intubate.

Chemical burns to the upper and lower airways are generally more serious than burns produced by heat alone. Alveolar edema is not a major component of the early disease state and is therefore less responsible for the early impairment of gas exchange than are atelectasis and airway closure. The mortality rate for patients with severe inhalation injury alone is 5% to 8%. Early symptoms, bronchospasm with wheezing and bronchorrhea, may not be evident until 24 to 48 hours after injury. Early bronchospasm and bronchiolar edema initiated by the irritant gases cause a marked decrease in lung compliance and an increase in the work of breathing. Diagnostic indications are a history of closed space exposure, physical findings (e.g., soot, presence of symptoms), an increase in carboxyhemoglobin level, direct visualization of injury (with laryngoscopy), fiberoptic bronchoscopy, and indirect visualization (with ventilation-perfusion xenon scanning). Physical findings suggestive of smoke exposure include facial burn, soot in the sputum, dyspnea, coughing, wheezing, and bronchorrhea. Initial treatment of a chemical burn consists of aggressive upper airway maintenance and pulmonary support. Careful and well-monitored fluid resuscitation is necessary. Early endotracheal intubation and positive end-expiratory pressure are frequently necessary. A large endotracheal tube and humidified oxygen are indicated to assist in the clearance of secretions. Elevation of the patient's head and chest 20° to 30° is also helpful. Bronchospasm can be treated with bronchodilators, parenterally or by aerosol. Beginning about 18 to 24 hours postburn, an increase in airway resistance is often due to bronchiolar edema and airway plugging rather than to bronchospasm. The impaired gas exchange often responds to further increases in positive end-expiratory pressure and to bronchodilators. The use of high-dose corticosteroids in the presence of a body burn increases rather than decreases morbidity and mortality of smoke inhalation.

A reduction in chest wall compliance may accompany reductions in pulmonary compliance. The loss of elasticity in the chest wall due to the burn tissue markedly increases the work of breathing required to maintain functional residual capacity and an adequate tidal volume. Symptoms peak at about 10 to 12 hours. The first clinical evidence of the chest wall restrictive defect is often labored breathing followed by a rapid respiratory deterioration. The three main treatment principles are recognition of the problem, control of the tissue edema process, and surgical decompression of chest wall constriction (i.e., escharotomy).

Postresuscitation Phase

The postresuscitation period is often the calm before the storm. Early symptoms are resolving, but the peak tracheobronchial mucosal slough and bronchopneumonia have not yet appeared. With severe injury, the damaged mucosa becomes necrotic 3 or 4 days after injury and begins to slough. The increase in viscous secretions can lead to distal airway obstruction, atelectasis, and a high risk for the rapid development of bronchopneumonia. As airway inflammation increases during the next several days, a diffuse interstitial edema develops. The risk of infection persists for several weeks. The characteristics of the symptom complex are change of sputum from loose to mucopurulent, evidence of necrotic tissue in sputum, increase in the work of breathing, alteration of gas exchange, and visualization of infiltrates on radiography. Chest radiographic findings invariably underestimate the magnitude of the chemical inhalation–induced airway injury. Treatment includes clearance of soot, mucopurulent exudate, and sloughing mucosa. If the injury is severe, early tracheostomy through unburned skin or a previously excised and grafted neck burn significantly improves secretion clearance and helps to more safely secure the airway. Ventilator assistance may be necessary. Postural drainage assists in the removal of airway plugs. Infection surveillance is crucial. Systemic antibiotics are given when a bacterial process becomes evident.

Common pitfalls in management during this period include extubating the patient too soon, underestimating the lower airway injury, failure to provide adequate postanesthetic support, and underestimating the effect of chest wall stiffness on lung function.

Inflammation-Infection Phase

Pulmonary problems remain a major cause of morbidity and mortality during the inflammation-infection phase. Three major processes occur during this period: (1) nosocomial pneumonia, (2) hypermetabolism-induced respiratory fatigue, and (3) adult respiratory distress syndrome. Burn patients with a combination of inhalation injury and a major body burn are at the greatest risk for pneumonia, with an incidence exceeding 50%. Preventive measures are key. Maintenance of adequate oxygen delivery to the burn wound tissue and to other tissue at risk for infection is necessary. Nutritional status must be maintained. Underlying chronic diseases must be controlled. Maintaining an adequate cough mechanism is of utmost importance. Analgesics and sedation must be used carefully. If continued intubation is expected for many weeks, conversion to a tracheostomy within the first several days greatly assists in the clearance of secretions. The tracheostomy should not be placed through burned tissue.

The increase in oxygen consumption and carbon dioxide production during this period requires increased gas exchange relative to that seen in previous periods. In addition, severe catabolism, initiated by the inflammatory response, can lead not only to extremity weakness but also to weakness of the chest wall muscles. Chronic pain and anxiety result in sleep deprivation and fatigue. The major problem during this period is hypercapnia, not hypoxia. The underestimation of increased ventilatory needs can lead to the development of hypercapnia. An increase in Pa_{CO_2} produces an intense catechol release, anxiety, and a further increase in oxygen demands and CO_2 production. Controlling lung edema and infection while maintaining nutrition and adequate rest as well as chest wall exercise is a key component of management. Partial ventilatory support with a tracheostomy may be useful.

Common pitfalls during this period include underestimation of the risks for pneumonia, underestimation of increased ventilatory requirements in the perioperative period, underestimation of the workload of breathing during the hypermetabolic state, and underuse of the tracheostomy.

HYPOTHERMIA AND COLD-RELATED INJURIES

Hypothermia

Hypothermia is defined as a decrease in core body temperature to below 35°C (95°F). The causes of hypothermia may be accidental or iatrogenic. The heat loss responsible for hypothermia occurs in three ways—radiation, conduction, and convection. Radiation implies thermal loss in the form of infrared radiation. Conduction loss occurs as a result of body contact with a colder surface. Convection loss occurs whenever the rate of temperature decrease depends on the flow of environmental air or fluid across a surface, which decreases surface temperature. Many factors besides exposure contribute to or predispose a patient to hypothermia. These include metabolic disease, central nervous system disorders, medications, recreational drug use, mental and psychiatric illness, associated trauma or surgery, infection, age, and alcohol abuse. Alcohol abuse remains the primary culprit in non–war-related hypothermia. Alcohol increases susceptibility to hypothermia by depressing the sensorium and decreasing shivering as well as by causing vasodilation, which further increases heat loss. Age is also a prominent factor in hypothermia. Neonates are especially susceptible because of their high ratio of body surface area to body size. In addition, as age increases, the ability to generate heat from metabolic activity decreases. Inability to mount an appropriate physiologic response to cold is also caused by a decrease in cardiac output, the presence of peripheral vascular disease, and the effects of vasoactive and cardiac medications.

Humans are homeotherms that can independently maintain a core body temperature of 97° to 99°F (36.1°–37.2°C) in the face of ambient variants, which range from 60° to 130°F. The homeostatic core body temperature of 98.6°F (37°C) is maintained by the anterior preoptic region of the hypothalamus. In the face of a mild to moderate decrease in core body temperature to 90° to 94°F (32°–35°C), the hypothalamus initiates a sympathetic and catecholamine response that leads to an increase in cardiac output, basal metabolic rate, oxygen consumption, and intermittent peripheral vasoconstriction. Isometric muscle contractions in the form of shivering generate up to a fivefold increase in peripheral heat production. As core temperature continues to decrease to below 90° to 94°F, a generalized downward metabolic spiral begins. Basal metabolic rate, blood pressure, and cardiac output decrease. Central blood volumes increase as a result of peripheral vasoconstriction, and this, coupled with cold-induced renal dysfunction, leads to a cold diuresis. Hematocrit, creatinine, and blood urea nitrogen levels all increase. Respiratory rate slows, and mental status becomes sluggish. As core temperature reaches 80.6° to 89.6°F (27°–32°C), physiologic abnormalities progress. Shivering stops below 89.6°F. Bradycardia with decreased sinoatrial node response and J (Osborne) waves become evident. Myocardial excitability increases, and atrial fibrillation is common. A continued rise in blood viscosity occurs, which increases viscosity by 2% for each 1°C decrease in temperature. The oxygen dissociation curve shifts to the left. Cerebral oxygen demand decreases 6% for each 1°C fall in temperature. Coagulation abnormalities occur. Platelets are transiently sequestered in the liver and spleen. Impairment of the Na^+-K^+ ATP pump leads to hyponatremia and hyperkalemia. Blood pH falls in response to an increase in lactate production. When severe hypothermia (<80°F [<26.7°C]) develops just before a coma state occurs, peripheral vasoconstriction diminishes and surface rewarming takes place. Patients experience a subjective rewarming phenomenon. After this, further cooling occurs rapidly. Patients may become apneic and exhibit profound bradycardia or asystole. In this setting, ventricular excitability is great. A patient may appear lifeless; however, no patient should be pronounced dead until rewarming to 94°F (35°C) has been completed.

Hypothermia is primarily a diagnosis of suspicion and is confirmed by use of a low-reading thermometer. Prevention is always the best therapy. In the prehospital setting, therapy is directed toward prevention of further heat loss, with removal of wet clothing and wrapping in a dry blanket. Warmed intravenous fluid and warmed humidified oxygen should be administered. High oxygen tension and limited patient movement decrease the likelihood that ventricular fibrillation will occur during transport. Asystolic patients should receive a modified cardiopulmonary resuscitation. Compressions should be longer and slower and have increased relaxation intervals to compensate for the decreased blood flow associated with higher blood viscosity.

Initial resuscitation includes administration of warm humidified oxygen (100% at 42°C). If the patient is apneic, careful intubation should be performed. Pretreatment with 100% oxygen by facemask and intravenous bretylium tosylate, 5–10 mg/kg, decreases the likelihood of ventricular fibrillation. Mechanical ventilation should be instituted and arterial blood gas readings should be corrected for physiologic shifts observed with hypothermia. For each 1°C decrease in temperature from 37°C, pH increases by 0.015, PCO_2 decreases by 5%, and PO_2 decreases by 7%. As such, the alkalotic state noted in hypothermia should be expected and promoted to maintain the intracellular neutrality needed to ensure proper enzymatic and cellular function. Venous access should be obtained, and ECG monitoring instituted as the patient is exposed and then wrapped in blankets. During insertion of central venous catheters, care must be taken to avoid passage of the guide wire or catheter into the ventricle. The use of pulmonary artery catheters is contraindicated. Warmed (42°C) intravenous fluids consisting of normal saline, with or without dextrose, are recommended. Potassium-containing fluids are not recommended. Thiamine and folate should be administered. Patient movement should be kept to a minimum because of cardiac irritability. Laboratory examination of baseline blood values should be performed, and ECGs should be obtained. Resuscitation must be attempted in all hypothermic patients until core temperature increases to 35°C.

Two rewarming techniques can be used—passive and active. Passive rewarming relies on endogenous heat generation and ambient temperature to raise core temperature slowly at a rate of 0.5° to 2°C per hour. Active rewarming implies the use of heat sources to raise core body temperature. External heat sources such as heat shields, warming blankets, and immersion baths can be perilous to a patient. Rapid rewarming of the shell can cause peripheral vasodilation with associated shunting of cold, hyperkalemic, lactate-rich blood to the core. This can precipitate rewarming shock, cardiac arrhythmias, or asystole. Many forms of internal rewarming have been used successfully.

The most basic form of internal rewarming consists of administering heated (42°C), moist oxygen and warm intravenous fluids along with body coverage with a dry blanket. With this method, body temperature should rise 1° to 2°C per hour. Nasogastric and rectal lavage with warmed fluids can increase temperature 5° to 10°C per hour. Bretylium tosylate can be administered prophylactically. In unstable or asystolic patients, more aggressive rewarming may be warranted. Peritoneal lavage with fluids warmed to 45°C raises temperature 15° to 20°C per hour. Unilateral closed pleural lavage accomplishes a similar warming trend with the added advantage of rapid cardiac rewarming. Direct cardiac rewarming by means of median sternotomy and mediastinal irrigation has also proved effective. Extracorporeal bypass using femoral access is an excellent technique for rapid rewarming because it allows for a controlled temperature rise and provides an external pump in the event of cardiac dysfunction. The major disadvantage of this rewarming technique is the need for heparinization. New rewarming techniques include the use of heparinless extracorporeal bypass and a Bio-Medicus pump, continuous arteriovenous rewarming by direct patient pressure, and extracorporeal diathermy.

Cold Urticaria

Cold urticaria is a syndrome in which exposure to cold leads to urticaria and angioedema. In certain subsets, anaphylaxis occurs, causing hypotension, tachycardia, shock, and death. Although limited cold exposure can act as a trigger, most anaphylactic responses are associated with aquatic activity. Diagnosis is confirmed by history and a positive result on the cold stimulation test. Management consists of prevention. Cold tolerance induction and medications such as antihistamines, cyproheptadine, doxepin, ketotifen, epinephrine, corticosteroids, and doxantrazole have all proved effective.

Local Cold Injuries: Frostbite

Frostbite is the most severe of the local cold injuries, and it involves freezing of the affected tissues. Freezing uniformly begins when tissue temperature reaches −2°C; however, the effects of cold exposure can be increased in the presence of wind or moisture. There are two classifications of frostbite injury. The first is clinically based and categorizes injury as superficial (if only the skin and subcutaneous tissue are frozen) or deep (if underlying tissue is frozen). The second classification grades frostbite by degree. First-degree injury consists of hyperemia and edema. Second-degree injury is characterized by hyperemia, edema, and clear blister formation. Third-degree injury displays hyperemia, edema, and hemorrhagic blister formation; fourth-degree injury presents with complete tissue necrosis and gangrene. Risk factors for frostbite are similar to those for hypothermia; however, the effect of wind chill can drastically increase the severity of injury.

As tissue temperature decreases in the face of cold exposure, the body responds with a cyclic pattern of peripheral vasoconstriction followed by vasodilation. This 7- to 10-minute sequence, known as the hunting reflex, helps to minimize heat loss. As core temperature decreases further, this reflex is bypassed because the body preferentially maintains core temperature. At −2°C ice crystals begin to form in the interstitial space, creating an osmotic gradient and a fluid shift from the cell into the interstitium that leads to cellular dehydration. Chondrocytes show direct freeze injury. Vascular integrity is lost. Rapid freezing is characterized by ice crystal formation within the intracellular space, which leads to direct cellular injury and tissue death.

As tissue is rewarmed, reperfusion commences. Ice crystals begin to dissolve, and cellular swelling occurs as a result of intracellular fluid shifts. Endothelial damage spreads into the entire microvascular tree. This leads to a combination of events that increase cellular and tissue death by increasing tissue hypoxia.

Generally, rewarming is contraindicated in a setting in which the potential for refreezing exists because refreezing dramatically increases tissue damage. In the prehospital setting, care should be taken to minimize trauma to the desensitized area.

Hospital care includes rapid rewarming of the frostbitten area by placing the affected part in a warm water bath (42°C) for 30 minutes. A direct heat source should not be used because thermal injury can occur. Narcotics may be needed since rewarming can be extremely painful. Tetanus prophylaxis should be given. After rewarming, the wound should be assessed for possible débridement. Clear blisters can be removed. Hemorrhagic blisters should be left intact. The affected area should be elevated. Use of systemic antibiotics should be limited to patients with documented or suspected infections. Follow-up care consists of active physiotherapy and twice-daily hydrotherapy with judicious wound débridement. Surgical management should be of an expectant nature. Escharotomy is warranted if vascular compromise occurs. Early débridement or amputation may be necessary if the affected tissue is causing uncontrollable sepsis or DIC. Otherwise, surgical intervention consists of débridement and reconstruction 30 to 60 days after injury.

Sequelae of frostbite vary in degree of severity and include hypersensitivity to cold, hyperhidrosis, Raynaud's disease, peripheral neuropathy, possible bone deformity, and atrophy of nails, hair, or muscle.

Immersion Foot and Trench Foot

Immersion foot and trench foot represent a multifactorial process in which conductive heat loss due to moisture combines with poor vascular flow secondary to immobility and constriction to produce cold injury in an extremity exposed to temperatures of 50°F (10°C) or less. Symptoms include numbness, tingling, pain, and itching. Initially, the skin is swollen and red, which gradually gives way to a gray-blue discoloration. After a few days, a hyperemic state sets in. Two to 6 weeks later, these symptoms gradually subside, and the patient is left with a cold-sensitive extremity. Superficial gangrene may be seen. Management is similar to that for a second-degree burn. Limb elevation and careful wound management are essential.

Ophthalmic Cold Injuries

Corneal injury due to freezing associated with high wind chill situations and to exposure to reflected ultraviolet radiation at high altitude can cause keratitis combined with opacification and corneal pitting. Aggressive ophthalmologic intervention with cycloplegia, mydriasis, and antibiotics is essential for a good result. Prevention with appropriate eyewear is the treatment of choice.

THE HYPERTHERMIC SYNDROMES

Fever in the critically ill patient is almost always considered to be a manifestation of infection and a possible harbinger of either sepsis or septic shock. High body temperatures are observed in certain clinical entities such as meningitis, falciparum malaria, cerebrovascular accidents near the hypothalamus, and multiple organ system failure. A body temperature of greater than 106°F (41.1°C) during a period of high ambient temperatures, combined with an early elevation of liver enzyme levels, suggests the possibility of heat stroke. Cooling should be instituted immediately while the diagnosis is being clarified.

Temperature Regulation

Radiation and convection account for 75% of heat losses at room temperature if an individual is undressed. The wearing of clothing significantly decreases such losses. The unique evaporative loss by sweating accounts for only 25% of heat loss at room temperature but becomes the dominant mechanism at high ambient temperatures. High humidity reduces evaporative losses.

When ambient temperatures rise, activation of hypothalamic centers leads to cutaneous vasodilation with shunting of blood away from the liver and splanchnic area in an apparent effort to contain visceral heat production to a limited region. Vasodilation enhances sweat gland activity and permits the loss of up to 1.5 L of sweat per hour in the unacclimated person. Such vasodilation increases cardiac output and stresses the heart. Acclimation occurs after 1 week of prolonged heat exposure and is associated with a substantial increase in sweat volume and a reduction in sweat sodium content. Plasma volume also increases.

Consequences of Exposure in Hot Environments

Three classic heat-related syndromes are heat cramps, heat exhaustion, and heat stroke. Heat exhaustion follows vigorous exercise in young individuals and the failure of an appropriate cardiovascular response in the elderly. Fluid depletion and hemoconcentration are observed. Patients present with a temperature of 100° to 103°F, profuse sweating, postural hypotension, fatigue, and thirst. A relatively normal mental status distinguishes them from individuals with heat stroke. Fluid replacement with normal saline and rest in a cool place are usually sufficient to reverse symptoms.

Acute neurologic abnormalities are the hallmark of heat stroke. Other manifestations include lethargy, fatigue, dizziness, nausea, and vomiting. Body temperatures are greater than 103°F (39.4°C) and may be greater than 107°F (41.6°C). Tissue damage begins with temperatures above this level. At core temperatures of 107°F, uncoupling of oxidative phosphorylation and the failure of enzyme systems occur. Liver damage is extremely common, and early elevation of serum glutamic-oxaloacetic transaminase and serum glutamate pyruvate transaminase is a useful sign of heat stroke. Pulmonary edema, DIC, cardiovascular abnormalities, and acute renal failure are common after initial cooling and stabilization. Fluid management becomes critical. Acute renal failure has been found in up to 35% of patients with heat stroke and can be caused by a combination of direct thermal injury, hypotension, shock from cardiovascular collapse, and rhabdomyolysis. Rhabdomyolysis should be treated with alkalinization and mannitol, furosemide, and fluid therapy. Major electrolyte abnormalities are observed. Hypophosphatemia, hypocalcemia, hypoglycemia, and infections are common.

The high mortality rate observed with delayed treatment can be reduced if the patient is rapidly cooled. Immersion in a tub filled with ice water is the most efficient way to produce rapid cooling, although cold packs or frequent sponging may also be useful. The peripheral vasoconstriction associated with immersion in ice water may have adverse effects in patients with cardiovascular dysfunction and has led to alternative cooling methods. Evaporation of 1 g of water consumes seven times as much heat as does the melting of 1 g of ice and does not produce peripheral vasoconstriction.

Malignant Hyperthermia

Malignant hyperthermia is a genetically inherited disease of muscle metabolism, in which intracellular calcium levels are increased as a result of exposure to certain triggering agents. This results in increased ATP activity, with depletion of ATP; actin-myosin coupling, which causes intense muscle contraction; breakdown of glucose with a sharp increase in oxygen consumption; production of carbon dioxide; and production of heat. Once begun, progression is rapid. Severe acidosis and hyperthermia occur in minutes. Ventricular fibrillation is typically the terminal event. Known triggering agents include the depolarizing muscle relaxant succinylcholine and all of the volatile inhalation anesthetics (ether, halothane, enflurane, and isoflurane). In general, the intravenous anesthetic agents, including the nondepolarizing relaxants such as pancuronium and vecuronium, are not triggers.

Prevention is an important aspect of management. Known triggering agents should be avoided in susceptible patients. Patients with Duchenne-type muscular dystrophy and other rare myopathies also are susceptible.

Diagnosis is by observation. Muscle rigidity, high fever after the administration of triggering agents, hypercarbia despite adequate ventilation, myoglobinemia, myoglobinuria, and marked elevation of creatine kinase values are all typical of malignant hyperthermia. No specific laboratory test for malignant hyperthermia is available.

Treatment includes the use of dantrolene, a hydantoin derivative that inhibits the release of calcium from the sarcoplasmic reticulum. Intravenous administration of dantrolene, 2.5 to 10 mg/kg, immediately aborts the syndrome. Dantrolene may also be given prophylactically at 2.5 mg/kg preoperatively. Nonspecific therapy includes surface cooling and lavage of open body cavities with cold saline.

CHAPTER 11

Central Nervous System

Thomas W. K. Lew, MBBS, MMed(Anes)
Joseph M. Darby, MD

Dedicated neurologic and neurosurgical intensive care units have developed in recognition of the advantages that a specially trained team approach provides in the management of patients with life-threatening brain or spinal cord injury.

The severity of the initial insult determines the degree of primary injury sustained by the central nervous system (CNS) as a result of tissue ischemia and cell death. These primary pathophysiologic processes also trigger mechanical, neurohumoral, and neurophysiologic mechanisms that lead to further or secondary brain injury. These involved mechanisms include raised intracranial pressure, cerebral edema, seizures, hyperemia, vasospasm, and reperfusion injury. Furthermore, systemic perturbations in cardiopulmonary and endocrine functions may occur as a result of deranged neural output from the brain. The brain and spinal cord are unique in their increased susceptibility and vulnerability to systemic insults in comparison with other organ systems. Systemic hypovolemia, hypotension, hypoxia, hypoglycemia and hyperglycemia, even of a relatively brief duration, may have catastrophic consequences.

Neurointensive care thus encompasses, but is not limited to, the prompt and skilled delivery of therapy to reverse or ameliorate the effects of the patient's primary neurologic insult, the utilization of appropriate neurophysiologic monitoring for diagnosis and assessment of therapeutic interventions, and the provision of aggressive and vigilant supportive management to prevent secondary brain injury. The standards of practice developed in neurologic intensive care units are equally applicable to neurologically ill patients in general medical or surgical units when a dedicated neurologic ICU is not available.

General Management

Patients in the neurointensive care unit may be at increased risk of hypoxia, hypercapnia, and pulmonary aspiration due to a deterioration in mental status, loss of ventilatory drive, or impaired protective airway reflexes. Early endotracheal intubation and mechanical ventilation should be considered in patients with respiratory failure, long apneic periods accompanying irregular respirations, and frequent vomiting. Endotracheal intubation should be performed in a controlled fashion to prevent reflex elevation of blood pressure, particularly in patients with elevated intracranial pressure (ICP). This response may be blocked by rapid administration of intravenous (IV) thiopental, 3 to 5 $mg \cdot kg^{-1}$ body weight (BW) and IV lidocaine, 1.5 $mg \cdot kg^{-1}$ BW, followed by the use of a rapid-onset neuromuscular relaxant such as vecuronium or succinylcholine. Someone with the expertise for securing a surgical airway (tracheostomy or cricothyroidotomy) should be available during emergency intubation of the head-injured patient with possible cervical spine or facial injuries. Normocapnia ($PaCO_2$ of 35 to 40 mm Hg) is generally maintained unless hyperventilation with hypocapnia is specifically indicated (see later). Relatively large tidal volumes and slow ventilatory rates favor cerebral venous drainage. Positive end-expiratory pressure can be applied at low levels in patients with good intracranial compliance. Aggressive pulmonary toilet and chest physiotherapy are employed to prevent atelectasis and to reduce the risk of nosocomial pneumonia. However, these maneuvers should not be allowed to induce prolonged or dangerously large increases in ICP.

Reflex sympathetic responses associated with endotracheal suctioning may be effectively blocked by the intermittent administration of intravenous lidocaine (1.5 $mg \cdot kg^{-1}$) a minute or two before the patient is suctioned. The timing of tracheostomy for clearance of secretions and airway protection varies, depending on the prognosis for neurologic recovery. For example, many patients with a stroke recover function within 7 to 10 days, thus avoiding the need for tracheostomy. Deep venous thrombosis and pulmonary embolism prophylaxis using sequential calf compression devices or adjusted-dose heparin are instituted until patients are ambulatory. In the immediate postoperative patient with established deep venous thrombosis for which full anticoagulation is contraindicated, an inferior vena caval filter should be placed. Submassive pulmonary embolism frequently may be overlooked when episodic arterial desaturation is attributed to transient mucus plugging.

Normovolemia and normotension should be maintained unless other specific hemodynamic goals are indicated for the management of conditions such as cerebral vasospasm, in which case a titrated hypervolemic and hypertensive state is induced, or in the prevention of normal perfusion pressure breakthrough bleeding after resection of large arteriovenous malformations, when controlled hypotension is induced (see later). Cautious volume resuscitation and rehydration are initiated in hypovolemic patients with traumatic injuries or in patients who had received diuretics during the acute management of raised ICP. Normalization of electrolytes is important, especially in the latter group of patients who may have hyperosmolality from osmotic diuresis, or hypokalemia and hypomagnesemia from the use of loop diuretics. Hypotonic solutions with excessive free water are avoided to prevent the development of cerebral edema. Hyponatremia may occur secondary to the syndrome of inappropriate antidiuretic hormone (SIADH) secretion or the cerebral salt-losing syndrome. Both syndromes are characterized by hyponatremia, hypotonic serum, inappropriately concentrated urine, and elevated urine sodium excretion, but the cerebral salt-losing syndrome is also associated with intravascular volume depletion and possibly hypotension. SIADH is usually managed with fluid restriction, whereas cerebral salt-losing nephropathy should be treated with volume and salt repletion. Both hypoglycemia and hyperglycemia should be assiduously avoided—the former, because of the brain's dependence on glucose as the sole substrate for metabolism, and the latter, because of its association with a worse outcome in patients with impaired cerebral blood perfusion and resultant cerebral lactic acidosis.

Hyperthermia should be avoided as it imposes increased cerebral metabolic demands on neurologic patients who may already have borderline or impaired cerebral blood supply. Surveillance and early detection of infection, which is the commonest cause of hyperpyrexia, are also important because of immunosuppression in patients with traumatic injuries. Sepsis is a leading cause of late death in the critically ill neurosurgical patient. Meticulous skin care, frequent turning, and the avoidance of pressure on peripheral nerves are needed to prevent decubitus ulcerations, infections, and neuropraxia. Eye shields and methylcellulose artificial tears should be used to prevent corneal desiccation and ulceration. Nutritional support is an integral part of the management of any critically ill patient. Acute brain injury is associated with a hypermetabolic state, and there is evidence supportive of improved outcome in head-injured patients who receive early parenteral nutrition.

Physiology of Raised Intracranial Pressure, Cerebral Perfusion Pressure, and Cerebral Blood Flow

The volume of the intracranial compartment consists of brain (80%), cerebrospinal fluid (10%), and blood (10%). The introduction of a space-occupying lesion results initially in a compensatory reduction in these components. When compensatory mechanisms are exhausted, intracranial pressure (ICP) begins to rise. Displacement of cerebrospinal fluid (CSF) from the intracranial compartment to the spinal subarachnoid space, and a reduction in cerebral blood volume, occur early in response to an intracranial mass. Blockade of CSF flow by tissue shifts (e.g., uncal herniation) leads to a rapid elevation of intracranial pressure (ICP). Intracranial *compliance* is reflected in the magnitude of the change in ICP for a given change in volume and is the slope (dV/dP) of the volume (V) – pressure (P) curve for the intracranial compartment. Once compensatory mechanisms are exhausted and intracranial compliance is low, further small increases in intracranial volume result in large changes in ICP.

ICP is normally less than 10 mm Hg. The *cerebral perfusion pressure* (CPP) is defined as mean arterial pressure (MAP) minus ICP; it normally ranges from 70 to 100 mm Hg and is a major determinant of cerebral blood flow (CBF). CPP levels below 30 to 40 mm Hg result in cerebral ischemia and ultimately neuronal death. Transient and periodic elevations in ICP, known as plateau waves (Lundberg A waves), are due to vasomotor instability and can result in ischemic injury and sudden brain herniation. Once ICP reaches 20 mm Hg, compliance decreases and the brain's ability to tolerate additional increases in volume is reduced. Patients with ICP greater than 40 mm Hg are always associated with clinical neurologic deterioration. Aggressive control of ICP and maintenance of an adequate CPP may thus have a beneficial effect on outcome, especially in patients with head injuries.

Normally, cerebral blood flow is closely coupled to cerebral metabolism. Normal CBF is approximately 50 $ml \cdot 100\ g\ brain\ tissue^{-1} \cdot min^{-1}$. However normal brain function may be maintained with a CBF as low as 18 $ml \cdot 100\ g\ brain\ tissue^{-1} \cdot min^{-1}$, indicative of the amount of reserve blood flow that is normally supplied to the brain. CBF below 18 $ml \cdot 100\ g\ brain\ tissue^{-1} \cdot min^{-1}$ initially results in the cessation of neuronal electrical activity while membrane pump function is maintained. Further reduction in CBF causes membrane pump failure, resulting in ionic gradient breakdown, intracellular edema, and cell death. An increase in CBF is generally accompanied by an increase in cerebral blood volume, raising ICP when brain compliance is low. Physiologic variables that alter CBF include the partial pressures of carbon dioxide ($PaCO_2$) and oxygen (PaO_2), pH, and temperature. There is a linear decrease in CBF when $PaCO_2$ is reduced from 80 to 20 mm Hg. Carbon dioxide crosses the blood-brain barrier rapidly, but the hydrogen ion cannot pass this barrier, resulting in an increase in CSF pH that normalizes over several hours. CBF thus falls initially, then returns to normal over the same time course. PO_2 affects CBF only in its extremes. A PaO_2 of less than 50 mm Hg may stimulate CBF by increasing lactate production. A very high PaO_2 decreases CBF, although the magnitude of this reduction is small. CBF decreases by 6% for every degree Celsius of reduction in temperature, whereas fever increases CBF in a linear fashion up to 42° Celsius. Beyond this temperature, direct toxic injury to the brain occurs. In normal individuals, CBF remains unchanged from a mean arterial pressure (MAP) of 60 to 130 mm Hg (*cerebral autoregulation*) via compensatory changes in vascular tone. This range may be shifted to a higher level in patients with hypertension. Beyond these limits, CBF follows MAP passively, increasing or decreasing significantly in response to blood pressure changes.

Cerebral Monitoring

ICP monitoring, particularly via a ventriculostomy in the lateral ventricle, is of value in patients with moderate-to-severe head trauma, acute hydrocephalus, Reye's syndrome, and encephalitis. The direct measurement of ICP allows for CPP to be determined and the effects of therapeutic maneuvers aimed at maintaining adequate cerebral perfusion and lowering ICP to be evaluated. It may also help the clinician decide on the timing of surgical intervention.

Electroencephalography (EEG) monitoring in the ICU requires constant attention to maintain optimum signals so as to avoid misinterpretation of artifacts. Considerable expertise is required in the interpretation of raw EEG to detect subtle changes. It may be useful in the detection of cerebral ischemia, to monitor for the presence of seizures or electrical status epilepticus and the effects of anticonvulsant therapy on paralyzed patients, and for prognostication after head injury or anoxic-ischemic insult. Processed EEG may be presented as a compressed spectral array or analyzed in terms of spectral edge, content of specific frequencies, or frequency ratios plotted against time.

Evoked potentials are very-low-amplitude electrophysiologic manifestations of the nervous system's response to various types of stimulation. Commonly monitored modalities in the ICU include brain stem auditory evoked potentials (BAEPs) and somatosensory evoked potentials (SSEPs). BAEPs comprise five sequential waves generated from specific brain stem structures along the auditory pathways after a brief auditory stimulus is delivered to one ear. Wave I represents potentials generated by the eighth nerve. Other waves originate from the cochlear nucleus (wave II), the superior olive (III), the lateral lemniscus (IV), and the inferior colliculus (V). The presence of wave I but not II through V implies significant pathology of the brain stem auditory pathways. Unilateral abnormalities suggest localization of lesions to one side. Lesions above the midbrain do not result in BAEP abnormalities unless tissue shifts occur, resulting in the disturbance of lower brain stem function. Brain stem lesions are also rarely found in the context of normal BAEPs. SSEPs are obtained by electrical stimulation of the median, ulnar, peroneal, or tibial nerves. When upper extremity nerves are used, waves are generated from the brachial plexus, upper cervical cord, dorsal column nuclei, ventroposterior thalamus, and sensory cortex. Absence of cortical but presence of dorsal column potentials reflects loss of sensory cortex integrity. BAEPs and SSEPs may be useful in several clinical situations in the neurointensive care unit, including the prognostication of patients with head injury, global cerebral anoxia, or ischemia. Absence of wave II through V on BAEPs or bilateral absence of cortical waves in SSEPs (in the presence of dorsal column potentials) in this group of patients is associated with a poor prognosis since they imply loss of electrical activity in the brain stem or both cerebral hemispheres, respectively. The same findings have been used as confirmatory tests for brain death. Raised ICP causing midbrain compression due to tissue shifts can cause a loss of BAEP wave V, and severe hemispheric ischemia can cause a loss in amplitude or delay in latency of cortical and subcortical SSEPs.

Transcranial Doppler (TCD) ultrasonography is a noninvasive technique for evaluating the intracranial arterial circulation of ICU patients. Insonation of the following vessels using a 2-Mhz ultrasound probe is possible: middle cerebral, anterior cerebral, and posterior cerebral artery via the temporal window; basilar and vertebral vessels via the occipital window; and intracranial internal carotid and ophthalmic arteries via the orbital window. Blood flow velocities detected by TCD may be altered by changes in $PaCO_2$, temperature, hematocrit, and cardiac output. TCD has been used to guide therapy for raised ICP in patients who are poor risks for direct ICP monitoring. Changes in blood flow velocity curves reflect ICP changes. Rising ICP is associated with a decrease in the mean flow velocity, an increase in the pulsatility index (defined as [peak velocity − end-diastolic velocity]/mean velocity) and diastolic flow reversal when ICP approaches MAP. TCDs have also been used as an ancillary tool to support the diagnosis of brain death when blood flow is absent on attempted insonation of multiple intracranial arteries. It has been used to identify occluded intracerebral arteries and to monitor the progress of thrombolytic therapy in the treatment of acute ischemic stroke. Its use in the diagnosis of cerebral vasospasm complicating subarachnoid hemorrhage is described later in this chapter. TCDs have also been used to detect possible changes in middle cerebral artery flow velocities after carotid endarterectomy that may signify hyperemia, reocclusion, or recurrent emboli, necessitating therapeutic intervention.

Treatment of Intracranial Hypertension

In patients with brain injury, the control of ICP is critical to avoid secondary brain damage from tissue shifts and to prevent ischemia. In patients with head injury, raised ICP is associated with poor outcome, and brain death is a common consequence. ICP elevation may simply reflect the extent of underlying brain damage, and no improvement in outcome may be seen after treatment of ICP. However, control of ICP occasionally leads to improvement. Patients with intracerebral hemorrhage and ischemic stroke also have poor outcome when ICP is raised. While the benefits of ICP monitoring and treatment are still unproved, it at least provides a guide for medical therapy and may help the clinician decide on the timing of surgical intervention. The mainstay of conventional medical therapy for raised ICP includes hyperventilation and use of osmotic agents. The underlying principle behind all modalities of therapy is to ensure that the brain remains adequately perfused and oxygenated, *cerebral perfusion pressure being the major determinant of CBF.*

Hyperventilation reduces ICP rapidly by inducing hypocapnia, which leads to cerebral vasoconstriction and a reduction in cerebral blood volume (CBV). Its effect is almost immediate and is maximal after 30 minutes. If the $PaCO_2$ is initially kept at 25 to 30 mm Hg, further hyperventilation is possible for subsequent spikes in ICP. However, once initiated, hyperventilation should be maintained, since a reversion to normoventilation may trigger a rebound elevation in ICP. Paradoxical elevation in ICP may also occur with transmission of increased intrathoracic pressure to the intracranial compartment. Controversy exists regarding the relative risk for cerebral ischemia under circumstances in which regional cerebral blood flow is already compromised. While hyperventilation often improves cerebral oxygen metabolism, especially in patients with post-traumatic cerebral luxury perfusion, it may also adversely affect the outcome of severe head injury, especially when used on an empirical basis. The recent development of monitors of cerebral oxygenation using near-infrared spectroscopy may help identify patients who are at risk for ischemia and allow for a more physiologic titration of this treatment.

Osmotic diureses can also effectively lower ICP in most pathologic conditions. Mannitol, administered in doses of 0.25 to 1 $g \cdot kg^{-1}$ lowers ICP within 15 minutes and maximally at 60 minutes. Mannitol is thought to create a relative osmotic load in the intravascular space and to extract both intracellular and extracellular water from the brain. Growing evidence indicates that mannitol may also induce vasoconstriction by lowering blood viscosity and local oxygen delivery. Normovolemia is maintained to prevent hypotension and a low cardiac output from compromising CBF. An initial increase in serum osmolality up to 300 $mOsm \cdot kg^{-1}$ is usually adequate to reduce ICP. If ICP continues to rise, additional increases in osmolality as high as 320 $mOsm \cdot kg^{-1}$ may provide additional benefit. Volume depletion, hypotension, electrolyte disturbances, and hyperglycemia occur at higher osmolality levels. Mannitol may cause a transient rise in CBF within the first 5 minutes of administration owing to an initial increase in serum osmolality. This effect is not exhibited by *nonosmotic diuretics*, which may also be used to reduce ICP acutely. The combination of furosemide and mannitol may result in a greater and more sustained decrease in ICP than the use of either drug alone.

The *blood pressure* of patients with raised ICP should be controlled to the extent that the cerebral perfusion pressure is maintained within a range of at least 60 to 70 mm Hg. In areas of damaged brain where cerebral autoregulation may be impaired, elevation in blood pressure will increase hydrostatic pressure and contribute to edema formation. Hypotension may reduce ICP but not improve CPP because of the concomitant drop in mean arterial pressure. Mild hypotension can trigger cerebral vasodilatation and plateau waves, resulting in prolonged ICP elevations. Conversely, a hypertensive spike can abort the plateau wave and lower ICP. The use of pressors to raise blood pressure has therefore been advocated, but this is not yet standard therapy for raised ICP.

Drainage of ventricular or *lumbar CSF* can effectively lower ICP, especially when this is secondary to ventricular enlargement. Ventricular drains may be placed at the bedside in the ICU, and drainage may be continuous or intermittent. Complications are intraparenchymal hemorrhage during placement (1%) and CSF infection (2% to 7%).

Brain swelling and intracranial hypertension refractory to all other therapies may respond to *high-dose barbiturates*, especially in global diffuse brain injury with associated cerebral hyperemia and luxury perfusion. Barbiturates act by reducing the cerebral metabolic rate of oxygen ($CMRO_2$), cerebral blood flow, and cerebral blood volume and by preventing further neuronal ischemia. Maintenance of adequate intravascular volume prior to barbiturate loading is essential. Hemodynamic monitoring with central venous or pulmonary artery catheter is recommended. Pentobarbital is usually employed at a loading dose of 3 to 10 $mg \cdot kg^{-1}$ IV, given in aliquots of 50 to 100 mg. The maintenance dose is 1 to 4 $mg \cdot kg^{-1} \cdot hr^{-1}$. Normal arterial pressure is maintained with volume loading and vasopressors. The therapy may be titrated to pentobarbital level (greater than 5 $mg \cdot dL^{-1}$) or EEG evidence of burst suppression (3 to 5 bursts per minute). The slow taper of barbiturates (3 to 5 days) prevents rebound intracranial hypertension. After cessation of therapy, the residual effects of barbiturates may still continue to mask the neurologic evaluation of the patient for an additional 24 to 72 hours.

Systemic steroids are useful in the treatment of vasogenic edema associated with tumors and abscesses. However, they have not been shown to be beneficial after traumatic intracranial hemorrhage or in the treatment of cytotoxic edema, which commonly occurs in ischemic, hypoxic, and traumatic head injuries.

Elevation of the head may also be useful in lowering ICP, but the response may be variable. Occasionally, head elevation results in an elevation of ICP, induced by a shift of brain tissue toward the foramen magnum, thereby impeding the outflow of CSF. Head elevation may also result in a greater decrease in mean arterial pressure at head level than in ICP and will thus produce a net decrease in cerebral perfusion pressure. However, others have demonstrated that in the normovolemic patient, head elevation usually results in a reduction in ICP. Thus, when ICP monitoring is available and CPP can be measured, the degree of head elevation may be individualized.

EVALUATION OF THE COMATOSE PATIENT

Definitions

Consciousness is defined as a state of awareness of the self and environment and requires two intact physiologic components: wakefulness and cognitive function. The vegetative state may be defined as a state of chronic wakefulness without awareness. Patients who exhibit this state for at least 1 month after brain injury are considered to be in a persistent vegetative state. Coma is defined as a state of uninterruptable, sleeplike unresponsiveness. In stupor, only vigorous external noxious stimulation leads to brief periods of arousal. Consciousness depends on the continuous interaction between the mechanisms providing arousal and awareness. Arousal mechanisms arise from the rostral one third of the pontine tegmentum and hypothalamus. Signals are projected via the thalamic relay nuclei (medial, intralaminal, and reticular) diffusely to the cerebral cortex. A self-cycling corticothalamocortical loop further contributes to arousal. The cerebrum provides for cognition and self-excitation. A depressed level of consciousness can result from the dysfunction of brain stem–activating mechanisms or impaired cerebral hemispheres or both. Impaired consciousness and coma may be caused by either structural or nonstructural disorders.

Structural Etiologies for Coma

Structural disorders leading to coma are exemplified by mass lesions located in the supratentorial or infratentorial compartments that cause coma by disrupting brain stem–diencephalic activating mechanisms through tissue shifts or direct compression of deep-lying intracranial structures. The location, size, and acuteness of the lesion determine the degree and rate of loss of arousal. Direct mass effect or a *differential* pressure gradient between compartments (and not the absolute level of intracranial pressure) leads to displacement of intracranial contents, with potentially fatal consequences. Blockage of cerebrospinal fluid outflow may lead to obstructive hydrocephalus, increased intracranial pressure, and herniation of supratentorial contents into the subtentorial compartment. In patients with acute brain lesions, displacement of the *pineal body* seen on computed tomography correlates with the patient's level of consciousness, suggesting that horizontal shifts are also important indicators of level of consciousness.

Two herniation syndromes illustrate the mechanisms by which supratentorial mass lesions produce coma. Downward transtentorial herniation may be predominantly central or unilateral. *Central herniation* accompanies deep or midline supratentorial masses, large hemispheric infarctions, or extra-axial mass lesions. Bilateral, symmetric displacement of the supratentorial structures occurs through the *incisura*, or tentorial notch, into the subtentorial region. Successive pathologic and clinical stages have been described. With deep diencephalic compression, arousal is impaired early, pupils become small (less than 3 mm in diameter) and reactive, and bilateral corticospinal tract dysfunction develops. Periodic (Cheyne-Stokes) breathing, grasp reflexes, roving eye movements, or depressed escape of oculocephalic reflexes often accompanies the process. Decorticate or decerebrate posturing is common. Central herniation will progress to the compression of the midbrain, leading to deep coma and to the pupils becoming midpositioned (3 to 5 mm in diameter) and unreactive to light, signifying both sympathetic and parasympathetic denervation. Spontaneous eye movements cease and become increasingly difficult to elicit by either oculovestibular or oculocephalic maneuvers. Spontaneous decerebrate posturing may occur as midbrain destruction progresses. Once this stage is reached, recovery becomes unlikely. As the wave of downward compression-ischemia advances, it destroys pontine and medullary function, resulting in bizarre breathing patterns and absent reflex eye movements. Eventually, autonomic respiratory and cardiovascular functions cease as medullary centers fail.

Uncal herniation usually accompanies laterally placed hemispheric lesions, producing side-to-side brain displacement as well as transtentorial herniation. Clinical stages are characterized by focal hemispheric dysfunction (e.g., aphasia, hemiparesis, seizure), leading to unilateral (usually ipsilateral) compression, paralysis of the third cranial nerve with pupillary enlargement, and diminished reaction to light. Shortly after the pupil dilates, more severe oculomotor paresis develops, and the eye turns outward and downward. The ipsilateral posterior cerebral artery may become compressed, causing ipsilateral occipital lobe ischemia. Unchecked, the temporal lobe compresses the midbrain, resulting in loss of consciousness and bilateral or contralateral decerebrate posturing. Ipsilateral to the cranial lesion, a hemiparesis may develop if the opposite cerebral peduncle becomes compressed against the contralateral tentorial edge. Brain stem signs then become symmetric, and herniation proceeds in the same pattern as occurs with central herniation, with progressive rostral-caudal brain stem dysfunction.

Posterior fossa lesions can also produce coma by direct destruction or compression of brain stem–activating mechanisms or by upward or downward herniation. Brain stem hemorrhage or infarction is often accompanied by signs of midbrain-pontine damage, such as pinpoint pupils, ocular bobbing, dysconjugate eye movements, nystagmus, and decorticate posturing. Downward compression of the medulla into the foramen magnum results in cardiorespiratory collapse. Thrombosis of the apex of the basilar artery may cause infarction of the midline thalamic nuclei, also producing coma without other obvious brain stem signs.

Other posterior fossa lesions such as cerebellar hemorrhages, infarctions and infection, rapidly expanding cerebellar or fourth ventricular tumors, and subtentorial epidural or subdural hematomas can cause coma by compression of the brain stem or upward herniation.

Nonstructural Disorders

Metabolic or toxic encephalopathy produces coma by diffusely depressing the function of brain stem and cerebral arousal mechanisms (Table 11–1). The onset of coma may be abrupt or gradual, depending on the cause. The commonest distinguishing clinical feature of metabolic encephalopathy is the *preservation of pupillary reflexes;* lack of pupillary reactivity requires a search for an underlying structural lesion.

Exceptions are encephalopathy from overdose of anticholinergic agents or near-fatal anoxia. Table 11–2 lists neurologic manifestations of common drug poisonings.

Vegetative State

Coma is not a permanent state; all patients who survive beyond the stage of acute, systemic complications reawaken and either proceed to recovery (with none or varying degrees of disability) or plateau at a vegetative level. Pathologically, extensive damage to the cortical mantle, thalamus, and cerebellum is seen, usually with limited or no direct brain stem destruction. *Positron-emission tomography* (PET) demonstrates profound depression of glucose utilization of the cerebral cortex. Clinically, vegetative patients are normothermic, exhibit spontaneous eye opening and movement, have stereotypic facial and limb movements, and appear to be awake with a cyclical sleep pattern. They have normal function of the cardiovascular, respiratory, and digestive systems. They are unable to demonstrate speech or comprehension and lack purposeful movement. They show no evidence of cognitive function or learned behavioral responses to external stimulation.

An important differential to the diagnosis of the vegeta-

Text continued on page 581

Table 11–1. METABOLIC OR TOXIC CAUSES OF STUPOR OR COMA

I. Endogenous disorders
   A. Deprivation of substrate
      1. Hypoxia with normal cerebral blood flow
         a) Diminished oxygen tension secondary to pulmonary disease
         b) Diminished oxygen content
            (1) Anemia
            (2) Carbon dioxide poisoning
            (3) Altitude sickness
            (4) Anesthetic accidents
            (5) Cyanide poisoning
      2. Ischemia
         a) Diminished cerebral blood flow to diffuse brain regions
         b) Shock secondary to hemorrhagic hypovolemia, sepsis, cardiac arrest, pulmonary embolism, or diminished peripheral vascular resistance
         c) Increase in cerebrovascular resistance
            (1) Hyperventilation
            (2) Hyperviscosity syndrome
            (3) Vasospasm secondary to subarachnoid hemorrhage
            (4) Vessel occlusion
               i) Disseminated intravascular coagulation
               ii) Vasculitis
               iii) Multiple emboli secondary to subacute bacterial endocarditis, aortic disease, fat
               iv) Cardiopulmonary bypass

II. Abnormalities of osmolality or acid-base status

III. Abnormalities of temperature regulation
   A. Hypothermia
   B. Hyperthermia
      1. Neuroleptic malignant syndrome
      2. Heat stroke

IV. Infections or inflammation of the central nervous system
   A. Encephalitis
   B. Leptomeningitis
   C. Parainfectious encephalomyelitis

V. Seizures and postictal states

VI. Concussion

VII. Exogenous poisons
   A. Alcohol or sedative drugs
   B. Acid poisons
      1. Ethylene glycol
      2. Methyl alcohol
      3. Paraldehyde
   C. Psychotropic drugs
      1. Opiates
      2. Cocaine
      3. Amphetamines
      4. Lithium
      5. Tricyclic antidepressants and anticholinergic agents
      6. Phenothiazines

v) Platelet disorder
vi) Thrombotic thrombocytopenic purpura
(5) Failure of autoregulation
(6) Hypertensive encephalopathy
3. Hypoglycemia
4. Cofactor deficiency
a) Thiamine
b) Vitamin B_{12}
c) Pyridoxine

B. Organ dysfunction with secondary brain dysregulation
1. Liver
a) Hepatic encephalopathy
b) Reye's syndrome
c) Urea cycle disorders
2. Kidney
3. Lung
4. Endocrine
a) Parahypopituitarism
b) Hyperthyroidism or hypothyroidism
c) Hyperparathyroidism or hypoparathyroidism
d) Hyperadrenalism or hypoadrenalism
e) Diabetes
(1) Ketoacidosis
5. Other
a) Porphyria
b) Sepsis
c) Paraneoplastic encephalopathy secondary to cancer

7. Mescaline
8. Monoamine oxidase inhibitors

D. Other
1. Anticonvulsants
2. Salicylates
3. Cimetidine
4. Steroids
5. Cardiac glycosides
6. Ciguatera toxin

VIII. Intensive care unit psychosis

Table 11–2. NEUROLOGIC MANIFESTATIONS OF COMMON DRUG POISONING

Drug	Signs and Symptoms	Diagnostic Test	Treatment
Sedative Hypnotics			
Benzodiazepines Barbiturates Chloral hydrate Meprobamate Ethchlorvynol (Placidyl)	Confusion; lethargy; ataxia; nystagmus; hypothermia; dysarthria; respiratory depression; coma. Pupillary reactions preserved except in instances of deep barbiturate coma. Possible withdrawal seizures	Blood	Supportive care; gastric lavage; flumazenil for benzodiazepine overdose; hemoperfusion for extreme barbiturate intoxication
Glutethimide	As above, except pupils may be fixed at different degrees of dilatation, anticholinergic signs, hyperthermia	Blood	As above
Methaqualone	Agitation; hypertonic; hyper-reflexia; ataxia; hallucinations; convulsions	Blood	As above
Ethanol	Confusion; agitation; delirium; ataxia; nystagmus; dysarthria; coma	Blood, breath	Supportive care; lavage if within 1 hour of ingestion; thiamine; glucose Treat withdrawal with benzodiazepines

Opioids	Lethargy; small reactive pupils; hypothermia; hypotension; urinary retention; shallow, irregular respirations; convulsions	Urine Response to naloxone	Naloxone, 0.4 mg IV or IM; continuous naloxone infusion, if necessary Supportive care with intubation as necessary Lavage if overdose is by ingestion
Stimulants Amphetamine Methylphenidate Cocaine	Hypervigilance; paranoia; violent behavior; tremulousness; dilated pupils; hyperthermia; tachycardia or arrhythmias; focal neurologic signs secondary to CNS stroke or hemorrhage; seizures	Blood, urine	Supportive care; sedation with benzodiazepines Treat hypertensive crisis with sodium nitroprusside or labetalol Watch for rhabdomyolysis
Psychedelics (LSD, mescaline, PCP)	Delirium; delusions; marked agitation; hallucinations; hyperactivity; dilated pupils; hyper-reflexia; nystagmus	Blood Measure PCP levels in gastric juice	Gastric lavage; charcoal Benzodiazepines and haloperidol for sedation

Table continued on following page

Table 11–2. NEUROLOGIC MANIFESTATIONS OF COMMON DRUG POISONING *Continued*

Drug	Signs and Symptoms	Diagnostic Test	Treatment
Antidepressants			
Tricyclic antidepressants	Anticholinergic effects: dry mouth; agitation; restlessness; ataxia; tachycardia or arrhythmias; hyperthermia; hysteria; convulsions; mydriasis	Blood, urine	Cardiac monitoring; gastric lavage; charcoal; mild systemic alkalinization. Physostigmine for refractory arrhythmias Anticonvulsants for seizures
Monoamine oxidase inhibitors	Drowsiness; ataxia; seizures; hypertensive crisis. Hypotension with severe overdose		Symptomatic care; gastric lavage; avoid narcotics
Neuroleptics	Dystonia; drowsiness; coma; convulsions; hypotension; miosis; tremor; hypothermia; neuroleptic malignant syndrome	Urine	Gastric lavage. Treat extrapyramidal signs with diphenhydramine or benztropine mesylate Treat neuroleptic malignant syndrome with dantrolene or bromocriptine
Lithium	Lethargy; tremulousness; weakness; polyuria; polydipsia; ataxia; seizures; coma	Blood	Hemodialysis for delirium, seizures, or coma
Methanol, Ethylene Glycol	Drunkenness; hyperventilation; stupor; convulsions; coma. Blindness with methanol use	Blood	Symptomatic care; gastric lavage; ethanol infusion; hemodialysis For methanol intoxication, 4-methylpyrazole (under investigation)

Antihistamines	Anticholinergic effects: dry mucosa; flushed skin; hyperthermia; dilated pupils; delirium; hallucinations; seizures; coma		Supportive care; gastric lavage; control of seizures with benzodiazepines; physostigmine for life-threatening anticholinergic effects
Organophosphates	Cholinergic crisis; cramps; excessive secretions; diarrhea; bronchoconstriction. Later, tremulousness; fasciculations; weakness; convulsions; hypertension; tachycardia; confusion; anxiety; coma	RBC cholinesterase level	Symptomatic care; decontamination; atropine; pralidoxime
Carbon Monoxide	Confusion; agitation; headache; convulsions; coma; respiratory failure; cardiovascular collapse	History Carboxyhemoglobin level	Remove patient from area; 100% oxygen until carboxyhemoglobin levels fall to <5% Hyperbaric oxygen if central nervous system affected Treat cerebral edema with hyperventilation, diuretics, and cerebrospinal fluid drainage, if necessary

Table continued on following page

Table 11–2. NEUROLOGIC MANIFESTATIONS OF COMMON DRUG POISONING *Continued*

Drug	Signs and Symptoms	Diagnostic Test	Treatment
Salicylate	Tinnitus; hyperpnea; confusion; convulsions; coma; hyperthermia	Blood	Supportive care; gastric lavage; charcoal; systemic alkalinization; hemodialysis for coma or seizures
Cyanide	Agitation; confusion; headache; vertigo; hypertension; hypotension; seizures; paralysis; apnea; coma	Blood	Amyl nitrate; sodium nitrate; sodium thiosulfate; 100% oxygen; hyperbaric oxygen for refractory signs Vitamin B_{12} injection
Anticonvulsants			
Phenytoin Carbamazepine Phenobarbital (see Barbiturates) Valproic acid Primidone Ethosuximide Felbamate Clonazepam (see Benzodiazepines)	Drowsiness; ataxia; nystagmus; tremulousness; coma. Dysrhythmias with carbamazepine or phenytoin overdose	Blood Ammonia level in patients taking valproic acid	Supportive care; gastric lavage; charcoal Watch for withdrawal seizures

(Adapted from Plum F: Disturbances of consciousness and arousal. *In:* Cecil Textbook of Medicine. 19th ed. Wyngaarden JB, Smith LH Jr, Bennett JC [Eds]. Philadelphia, WB Saunders, 1992, pp 2048–2059; Mofenson HC, Caraccio R, Greenshen J: Acute poisonings. *In:* Conn's Current Therapy 1993. Rakel RE [Ed]. Philadelphia, WB Saunders, 1993, pp 1148–1192; Olson KR: Toxicology screens and asymptomatic poisoning. *In:* Current Practice of Emergency Medicine. Callahan ML [Ed]. Philadelphia, BC Decker, 1991, pp 1138–1142, *and* Linden CH: Antidotes in poisoning. *In:* Current Practice of Emergency Medicine. Callahan ML [Ed]. Philadelphia, BC Decker, 1991, pp 1146–1162.)

tive state is the *locked-in state*. In this condition, patients are aware and awake but are unable to communicate because of total muscular paralysis. Pathologically, this may be caused by lesions of the descending motor pathways in the ventral pontine or inframedullary bulbar regions and severe inflammatory acute demyelinating or axonal polyneuropathies. PET demonstrates mild diminishment in central glucose utilization compared with control subjects.

Neurodiagnostic Evaluation

Initial evaluation of the comatose patient is directed toward ensuring cardiopulmonary stability, followed by a focused history, physical examination, and blood studies. Subsequent investigations provide anatomic and physiologic assessment of the central nervous system, locate the lesion, and provide guidance for therapy. Magnetic resonance imaging (MRI) provides earlier visualization of acute stroke, encephalitis, central pontine myelinosis, and traumatic shear injury with greater resolution than computed tomography (CT) scanning. Imaging of the posterior fossa is also not affected by bone artifact inherent in CT scanning. Sagittal MRI views can better document the degree of compartmental herniation and enable intervention before clinical deterioration. Injection of gadolinium helps delineate areas of blood-brain barrier disruption. CT is superior in detecting calvarial fractures and intracranial hematomas (epidural, subdural, intraparenchymal, intraventricular, subarachnoid). It should also be performed prior to *lumbar puncture* for suspected meningitis, encephalitis, and posterior fossa lesions. Injection of iodinated contrast highlights tumors, meningitis, abscesses, and acute or subacute stroke associated with breakdown of the blood-brain barrier. Electroencephalography (EEG) has selective value over brain imaging in differentiating the causes of coma. Focal lesions show focal slow activity or epileptiform discharges whereas toxic or metabolic encephalopathies are usually characterized by symmetric slow or fast wave activity. Focal slowing into the theta (4 to 7 Hz) or delta (1 to 3 Hz) range with paroxysmal triphasic waves is characteristic of hepatic encephalopathy. The EEG is also of great value in the evaluation of nonconvulsive status epilepticus or multiple complex partial seizures. A normal EEG in an unresponsive patient generally excludes organic brain disease and is highly suggestive of psychogenic unresponsiveness. Blood samples are analyzed for glucose level, blood gases, electrolyte level, renal and hepatic function, calcium level, and a complete blood count. Blood and urine are also analyzed for toxic substances.

Management

The emergency therapy for coma involves initial cardiorespiratory stabilization and usually includes early endotracheal intubation and mechanical ventilation. Measures should also be taken to reduce or prevent further elevation of ICP, if this is present, to prevent secondary brain injury. If structural causes of coma are likely, emergency CT scan is indicated and early neurosurgical intervention sought. Patients suspected of having a nonstructural etiology of coma should be given (1) thiamine, 100 mg IM, for Wernicke's encephalopathy, (2) 50% glucose, 50 mL IV, for hypoglycemia, (3) naloxone IV, to antagonize narcotic overdose, and (4) flumazenil IV, to antagonize benzodiazepine overdose, after blood samples have been drawn. Repeat administration of the appropriate antidote may be needed for recurrent lethargy or coma after initial arousal in moderate-to-severe poisoning. Electrocardiography is performed to rule out myocardial infarction or arrhythmias that may have caused cardiac arrest and hypoxic-ischemic brain injury. Subsequent management depends on continued evaluation of the comatose patient. Hypothermia, when present, should be gradually corrected. When infection is suspected, cultures of specimens from blood, CSF, sputum, urine, or other suspected sites are obtained, followed by empirical antimicrobial therapy until sensitivities of organisms cultured are known. Status epilepticus, when present, must be aggressively managed (see later), and specific antidotes for any known drug intoxication, when available, are administered.

Prognosis

Establishment of a highly probable outcome should be made within the first 24 hours. This allows for an early informed discussion with family and loved ones with regard to decisions for discontinuation of intensive therapy in hopeless instances. Overall prognosis of *nontraumatic coma* is poor. Only 16% of 500 patients in one study regained independent life during the first year after presentation. The remainder of this cohort either died without recovery from coma (61%), remained in a persistent vegetative state (12%), or became permanently dependent on others for daily living (11%). The total mortality of this group of patients at 1 year is estimated at 88%. The factors that influence outcome include etiology, severity of brain stem dysfunction on admission, and duration of coma. Patients in coma secondary to cerebrovascular disease or subarachnoid hemorrhage had only a 9% chance of achieving independent function, followed by patients suffering a cardiopulmonary arrest (12%). One third of patients with metabolic dysfunction, particularly hepatic encephalopathy, did well, regaining independent activity.

Exposure to exogenous agents or sedative drug intoxication, in the absence of medical complications, carries an overall good prognosis. The severity of signs of brain stem dysfunction on admission correlates inversely with the chance of good recovery in nontraumatic coma. Absent pupillary responses at any time after onset and absent caloric reflexes 1 day after onset indicate a poor prognosis (less than 2% recovery). No patient with absent pupillary light reflexes, corneal reflexes, caloric or doll's eyes responses, or a lack of a motor response to noxious stimulation at 3 days after onset ever regained independent function. Patients who did recover were those who were able to speak words, opened their eyes to noise, had spontaneous eye movements or nystagmus to caloric testing, had doll's eyes responses, and were able to follow commands at 1 and 3 days. The longer a coma persists, the lower the chance for recovery; patients surviving in coma for a week without confounding variables (e.g., sedation) rarely recover. An EEG pattern of "alpha coma," resembling normal alpha activity but extending over a broader range (8 to 13 Hz) after anoxic-ischemic injury carries an extremely poor prognosis. "Spindle coma," the presence of spindle activity despite unresponsiveness, is associated with a greater likelihood of good outcome.

Traumatic coma carries a better prognosis than nontraumatic coma. Recovery correlates inversely with the Glasgow coma score. Approximately 40% will recover to moderate disability or make a good recovery at 6 months. Poor prognostic indicators include increasing age, associated intracranial hematoma, autonomic dysregulation, nonreactive pupils, and absent eye movements within the first 24 hours. Sustained intracranial hypertension (intracranial pressure greater than 20 mm Hg) occurring after head injury is also associated with increased mortality independent of other factors that are considered predictive of neurologic outcome.

The development of the *vegetative state* also carries an ominous prognosis. Patients whose vegetative state is caused by head trauma or subarachnoid hemorrhage have a more favorable prognosis than those whose vegetative state is caused by asphyxia. One study reported that 14 of 140 trauma patients were vegetative at 1 month but regained independent function; all were younger than 40 years old and none recovered fully. In another study, among 134 men and women whose vegetative state (induced by trauma) persisted 1 month, 54% regained consciousness. Of these, about half managed to care for their daily needs, but only eight became independently employed. The statistics for recovery from nontraumatic coma are even worse, with only 3 of 100 patients studied ever becoming independent in daily living tasks. Forty-six per cent died within the first postonset year, and 68% died within 6 years. The results in both the traumatic and nontraumatic cases provide important information to help physicians and families reach ethical decisions about caring for overwhelmingly brain-damaged patients.

MANAGEMENT OF CEREBROVASCULAR EMERGENCIES

Newer therapies for patients with acute cerebrovascular emergencies requiring emergency intervention may increase the need for management of these patients in the ICU. In addition, intensive care is also needed for the management of both neurologic and non-neurologic complications of stroke. Options for the management of stroke increasingly depend on the physician distinguishing among the pathologies that produce an abrupt onset of brain dysfunction, as occurs when cerebral blood flow is impaired as a result of occlusion or rupture of a cerebral blood vessel. Strokes are generally categorized as being ischemic, hemorrhagic, or due to other more unusual causes (Table 11–3).

Diagnosis and Initial Assessment

The initial assessment involves making the diagnosis of stroke, differentiating between ischemia and hemorrhage and localizing the lesion to the cortex, subcortical region, or brain stem. A diagnosis of stroke should be considered in anyone presenting with (1) abrupt onset of focal cerebral dysfunction, (2) signs of elevated intracranial pressure, or (3) alteration in consciousness. The neurologic examination should be repeated frequently.

The temporal features of presenting signs and symptoms are helpful but not always reliable. The majority of cardioembolic strokes occur abruptly, whereas large artery thrombotic strokes often fluctuate or worsen in a stepwise fashion. Small artery strokes are often preceded by transient ischemic attacks (TIAs) and may be progressive. Subarachnoid hemorrhage (SAH) frequently presents with sudden and extremely severe headache. With intracerebral hemorrhage (ICH), focal symptoms are maximal within minutes. Included in the differential diagnoses of stroke are metabolic and toxic encephalopathies, subdural or epidural hemorrhage, postictal deficit after an unwitnessed seizure, complex migraine, and peripheral neurologic disease.

Initial diagnostic investigations include a complete blood count (CBC), coagulation studies, hepatic function, electro-

Table 11–3. CAUSES OF STROKE

Ischemic
- Large vessel atherothrombosis (35%)
- Small penetrating vessel (lacunae) disease (20%)
- Cardioembolism (25%)
  - atrial fibrillation
  - acute myocardial infarction
  - ventricular aneurysm
  - dilated cardiomyopathy
  - cardiac surgery
  - cardiac catheterization
  - valvular heart disease
  - bacterial endocarditis

Hemorrhagic (15%)
- Subarachnoid hemorrhage (berry aneurysm rupture)
- Intracerebral hemorrhage
  - hypertensive angiopathy
  - amyloid angiopathy (elderly)
  - arteriovenous malformation
  - anticoagulation/thrombolytic therapy
  - drugs (cocaine, amphetamine, phencyclidine)
  - tumors
  - sickle cell disease

Other (5%)
- Fat emboli
- Air emboli
- Carotid or vertebral artery trauma

lyte and metabolic screen, syphilis serology, chest radiograph, and electrocardiogram. A noncontrast computed tomogram (CT) scan of the head is the usual initial diagnostic imaging test used. Intracerebral hematoma, tumor, abscess, subdural hemorrhage, or artery thrombus can usually be detected. Infarctions are evident 6 to 12 hours after onset. Serial CT scans prompted by progression of symptoms may reveal hemorrhagic infarction or mass effect secondary to edema in ischemic strokes or underlying tumor or arteriovenous malformations (AVM) in ICH. Magnetic resonance imaging is superior to CT for an earlier diagnosis of ischemic stroke and localization of lacunar and cerebellar infarcts. It does not however, detect an acute hematoma as readily as the CT scan. Noninvasive studies for atherothrombotic diseases include extracranial carotid artery duplex test, transcranial Doppler, and magnetic resonance angiography. Echocardiography is indicated in patients with a suspected cardiac source of embolization. Transesophageal echocardiography is superior to the transthoracic echocardiography in imaging the left atrium, its atrial appendage, and aorta, as well as detecting septal defects. Lumbar puncture (LP) may be used to establish the diagnosis of SAH when CT is negative or when bacterial meningitis or septic embolism is suspected. Angiography may distinguish between atherothrombotic and cardiac embolic stroke in patients with mild stroke or TIA and detect cervicocephalic dissection, fibromuscular dysplasia, or vasculitis in younger patients presenting with stroke. Angiography is also indicated in the preoperative evaluation for extracranial carotid artery surgery and for resection of AVM or aneurysm clipping.

General Management

Elevated blood pressure following an ischemic stroke usually falls spontaneously within 12 to 72 hours. Mean arterial blood pressure below 140 mm Hg or a systolic blood pressure (SBP) below 200 mm Hg should not be acutely treated since this may result in an inadequate cerebral perfusion pressure (CPP) to injured brain regions where there may already be a loss of autoregulation. However, mortality and rebleeding are increased in patients who have elevated blood pressure untreated following subarachnoid hemorrhage. Antihypertensive agents should be used in this situation, especially if the aneurysm is unclipped, and relief of pain, agitation, hypoxia, and vomiting fail to normalize blood pressure. After ICH, blood pressure control should be carefully balanced between avoiding inadequate CPP and the risk of further bleeding into the hematoma. Parenteral antihypertensives such as labetalol or sodium nitroprusside can be carefully titrated to control blood pressure when necessary. Severe hypertension should be treated in patients with concomitant myocardial, renal, or aortovascular diseases. Dehydration and hypovolemia should be corrected to avoid hyperviscosity and impaired cerebral perfusion. Although studies with hypervolemic or normovolemic hemodilution have not shown clear benefit in acute stroke, volume expansion and venesection should be considered in patients with a hematocrit that is greater than 50%.

Treatment of Ischemic Stroke

The benefit of *antithrombotic therapy* using heparin or warfarin in acute and progressing stroke is uncertain. Heparin has been used after a recent TIA, in the early prevention of recurrent cardioembolism, after acute large vessel thrombosis, in arterial dissection with significant vessel narrowing, after cerebral venous thrombosis, and in small cardioembolic strokes after 48 hours of onset, once hemorrhagic transformation has been excluded by CT scan. Heparin should not be used with large infarctions (greater than two thirds of hemispheric size), because of an increased risk of clinically significant hemorrhage into the infarct. A bolus dose of heparin also is not used when a larger than one third hemispheric infarction is present. The *antiplatelet agents* aspirin and ticlopidine are beneficial in preventing recurrent stroke and stroke after atherothrombotic TIA. The potential benefit of *fibrinolytic therapy* is currently being studied.

Neuroprotective therapy is principally directed at the inhibition of calcium flux into the free cytosol. Free intracellular calcium is known to lead to calcium-activated enzyme cascades that contribute to neuronal death after an ischemic insult. These mechanisms include activated proteases and phospholipases, producing free radicals that destroy cell membranes. Calcium influx into neurones can be triggered by excitatory neurotransmitters (e.g., glutamate) that are released during ischemia; this is presently under intense investigation. The use of glutamate receptor (specifically, N-methyl-D-aspartate, or NMDA) antagonists has been shown experimentally to reduce ischemic neuronal injury. Calcium channel blockers do not appear to be beneficial when administered 12 to 24 hours after the onset of stroke but may be beneficial when given within 6 hours. The efficacy of free radical scavengers such as 21-aminosteroids (lazaroids) is presently under investigation.

Surgical Treatment of Intracerebral Hemorrhage

Currently, the role of surgery for ICH is controversial. Surgery is currently considered for the evacuation of hematomas causing progressive deterioration secondary to mass effect. Superficial lobar hematomas or accessible subcortical intracranial hemorrhages can improve after surgical intervention, but deep-seated, large basal ganglia and brain stem hematomas usually do not benefit. Prognosis is also poor for elderly patients with large hematomas and a decreased level of consciousness. Cerebellar hemorrhage often presents as a surgical emergency, leading to brain stem compression and acute hydrocephalus due to impingement on the fourth ventricle. Surgical evacuation of large cerebellar hemorrhages should be performed before consciousness is greatly decreased. Patients with small cerebellar hemorrhage and no hydrocephalus can be treated by close observation. Intraventricular hemorrhage is not itself an ominous sign but may result in hydrocephalus. Ventriculostomy may be necessary early in patients with acute hydrocephalus and in some patients with intracerebral hematomas whose conditions are deteriorating.

Treatment of Subarachnoid Hemorrhage

The main complications after rupture of an intracranial aneurysm are aneurysmal rebleeding, cerebral vasospasm, and hydrocephalus. Aneurysmal rebleeding occurs most commonly within the first 48 hours, with an associated mortality of 10% to 30%. Prevention of rebleeding by early surgical clipping of the aneurysm results in improved outcome. Patients with mild deficits (Hunt and Hess grades I to III) are usually operated on within the first 24 to 48 hours. Grades IV and V patients can improve significantly with clot evacuation and treatment of hydrocephalus. Presurgical therapy usually involves careful control of blood pressure and administration of mild sedatives, anticonvulsants, and stool softeners. Surgically inaccessible aneurysms can be ablated by balloon occlusion or coil thrombosis.

Cerebral vasospasm is an arteriopathy that results in marked narrowing of the cerebral arteries or arterioles leading to cerebral ischemia. The incidence and extent of delayed-onset cerebral vasospasm following SAH correlate with the amount of bleeding visualized by CT. It is most severe and common after aneurysmal subarachnoid hemorrhage but may also occur after head injury or craniotomies for tumors and unruptured aneurysms. The onset of symptoms of delayed ischemia is usually between 4 and 10 days after SAH. The diagnosis of cerebral vasospasm may be made by cerebral angiogram, clinical signs of neurologic deterioration, or transcranial Doppler (TCD) examination. Vasospasm is demonstrated angiographically in 75% of SAH patients, but the frequency of clinical vasospasm is much lower. TCD diagnosis of vasospasm is suggested by a ratio of flow velocities of 3:1 when comparing the middle cerebral artery to the internal carotid artery. Flow velocities greater than 120 $cm \cdot s^{-1}$ correlate with angiographically visible vasospasm; velocities greater than 200 $cm \cdot s^{-1}$ are usually associated with greater than 50% reduction in arterial diameter. A normal resistance index (defined as [maximum systolic flow velocity − end-diastolic flow velocity]/maximum systolic flow velocity) of less than 0.5 rules out concomitant ICP elevation when TCD is used to monitor the severity of vasospasm.

The general approach to the prevention of vasospasm and delayed ischemic deficits in patients with aneurysmal SAH is to employ strategies that will enhance cerebral perfusion. All patients should receive calcium channel antagonists (nimodipine), which has been shown to reduce the incidence of ischemic deficits. In patients with unclipped aneurysms, euvolemia and normotension are maintained. Following aneurysm clipping, a more aggressive approach, including volume expansion, hemodilution, and mild hypertension is employed. Intracisternal injection of tissue plasminogen activator (TPA) may also enhance clearing of blood from the subarachnoid space and prevent vasospasm. Should these preventive measures fail and signs of vasospasm emerge, induced hypertension using vasopressors and guided hypervolemia are employed in an attempt to reverse or limit ischemic brain injury. Percutaneous transluminal balloon angioplasty can benefit selected patients with persistent arterial narrowing.

Hypervolemia is induced with crystalloid, colloid, or whole blood until central venous pressure (CVP) is 8 to 12 mm Hg or pulmonary wedge pressure (PWP) is 14 to 20 mm Hg. Subcutaneous vasopressin has been used to counteract the diuretic response to induced hypervolemia. Systolic hypertension between 150 and 200 mm Hg may be maintained with vasopressors after aneurysm clipping. Reflex vagal response can be blocked with atropine. Hemodilution to a hematocrit in the range of 33% to 40% may improve cerebral blood flow by decreasing blood viscosity. Its efficacy in the treatment of cerebral vasospasm, however, remains controversial. The exact mechanism of action of nimodipine is unclear, but it may be due to a selective blockade of calcium influx to cerebral vascular smooth muscle cells, resulting in inhibition of contraction or the prevention of calcium-mediated neuronal ischemic cellular death. Various regimens have been utilized (2 $mg \cdot hr^{-1}$ IV for 12 to 14 days, followed by 45 to 60 mg q4h PO for 7 days or alternatively, 60 to 90 mg q4h PO for 21 days). Effects of treatment are difficult to demonstrate on angiographically visible vasospasm, suggesting that nimodipine may act on smaller caliber arteries beyond the resolution of cerebral angiography. Flow velocities using TCD are also seen to be decreased in treated patients.

Hydrocephalus may occur acutely after SAH from intraventricular hemorrhage or bleeding into the basal cisterns. Treatment is immediate *ventriculostomy*. Subacute hydrocephalus in the first few days to a week after SAH is characterized by the gradual onset of stupor. Delayed hydrocephalus may occur 10 days to months after SAH and is characterized by gait apraxia, urinary incontinence, and cognitive dysfunction. *Ventriculoperitoneal shunting* reverses most impairments.

AVMs may be treated by a combination of preoperative endovascular embolization and surgical and radiosurgical techniques. Strict blood pressure control is critical after resection of large AVMs. Intraparenchymal hemorrhage may occur from rupture of tenuously cauterized blood vessels. Normal perfusion pressure breakthrough bleeding can occur in chronically dilated vessels serving areas adjacent to the AVM that were relatively ischemic earlier and are then subjected to increased cerebral blood flow and intravascular pressures. This may result in vascular congestion with severe brain swelling or frank hemorrhage.

Complications of Stroke

Cerebral edema and *transtentorial herniation* are the commonest causes of death within the first week in both hemorrhagic and ischemic strokes. Cerebral edema is often greatest 2 to

5 days after the onset of a stroke. Transtentorial herniation is signalled by a change in the patient's level of consciousness and ipsilateral pupillary dilatation. Early signs of brain stem compression may occur from edema after a large cerebellar infarction. Immediate efforts to lower ICP and surgical resection of an edematous cerebellum may be life-saving. Although the frequency of early focal seizures following stroke is low (2% to 7%), they may be accompanied by neurologic worsening and the later development of epilepsy. Thus, anticonvulsants are indicated.

Non-neurologic complications of stroke include *cardiac arrhythmias* and *myocardial infarction*. Atrial fibrillation occurs in approximately 18% of patients who have a cerebral infarction or hemorrhage. Four per cent of patients have more serious arrhythmias. Acute myocardial infarction occurs concomitantly with stroke onset in up to 3% of patients. *Pneumonia* is the leading cause of death in the weeks after stroke. Aspiration occurs in up to 50% of patients after unilateral stroke. Therapy includes elevation of head, pulmonary toilet, respiratory therapy, and postural drainage. Oral feeding is delayed in patients with impaired oropharyngeal control until aspiration is excluded by examination or barium swallow. Placement of a feeding tube or percutaneous gastrojejunostomy may be required. *Early urinary incontinence* occurs in 60% of patients and may signify increased morbidity and mortality when seen in the first week. *Urinary tract infections* are also frequent. *Hyponatremia* is common after SAH from volume contraction, deranged antidiuretic hormone regulation, and elevation of plasma atrial natriuretic factor.

Secondary Prevention After TIA and Ischemic Stroke

Eleven per cent of patients with atherothrombotic stroke will suffer a recurrent stroke within the first year. One third of patients with untreated TIAs will progress to ischemic strokes, with 20% occurring within a month and 50% within a year. Prevention of recurrent stroke involves directing attention to the risk factors present. Pharmacologic intervention includes *aspirin* (dosages range from 30 to 60 mg qd PO to 325 to 1300 mg qd PO) or *ticlopidine*. Patients with atrial fibrillation should be anticoagulated with warfarin. *Carotid endarterectomy* is indicated following TIA or nondisabling stroke in patients with a high-grade bifurcation stenosis (70% or more).

SEIZURES IN THE CRITICALLY ILL

Seizures complicate the course of about 3% of adult ICU patients admitted for non-neurologic conditions and may be the first indication of a central nervous system complication. Patients with preexisting seizures may also require ICU treatment of other problems. Status epilepticus (SE) occurs in approximately 250,000 patients a year in the United States, with an estimated mortality of 22%, which is frequently attributable to the underlying disease. Certain ICU patients are at higher risk for seizures. Theophylline frequently produces seizures or SE when rapidly loaded or if high concentrations of the drug occur. Occasionally, these complications arise at "therapeutic" levels. Renal failure or an altered blood-brain barrier increases the likelihood of seizures for patients receiving imipenem-cilastin. Transplant recipients, especially those receiving cyclosporine or FK-506, are also at increased risk, as are those who rapidly become hypo-osmolar for any reason. Nonketotic hyperglycemia patients have an unusual predisposition to partial seizures and partial SE.

Overall mortality figures for patients with SE are variable and range from a low of 1% to 2% to as high as 22%. SE lasting longer than 1 hour carried a mortality rate of 32% compared with 2.7% of SE with a duration of less than 1 hour in one study. SE caused by anoxia has resulted in 70% mortality in adults but in less than 10% in children. The commonest causes of SE in adults are stroke, withdrawal from antiepileptic drug therapy, cryptogenic SE, alcohol withdrawal, anoxia, and metabolic disorders. Systemic infection is the commonest cause of SE in childhood, followed by congenital anomalies, anoxia, metabolic problems, anticonvulsant withdrawal, CNS infections, and trauma.

Classification

The most frequently used classification scheme is that of the International League Against Epilepsy. This scheme allows classification based on clinical criteria without inferring cause. Simple partial seizures start focally in the cerebral cortex, without invading other structures. The patient is aware throughout the episode and appears otherwise unchanged. Bilateral limbic dysfunction produces a complex partial seizure; awareness and ability to interact are diminished (but may not be completely abolished). Automatisms (movements that a patient makes without awareness) may occur. Secondary generalization results from invasion of the other hemisphere or subcortical structures. Primary generalized seizures arise from the cerebral cortex and diencephalon at the same time; no focal phenomena are visible, and consciousness is lost at the onset. Absence seizures are frequently confined to childhood; they consist of the abrupt onset of a blank stare that usually lasts 5 to 15 seconds after which the patient abruptly returns to normal. Myoclonic seizures start with brief synchronous jerks, without alteration of consciousness initially, followed by a generalized convulsion. They frequently occur in the genetic epilepsies. In the ICU, they commonly follow anoxia or metabolic disturbances. Tonic-clonic seizures start with tonic extension, evolve to bilaterally synchronous clonus, and conclude with a postictal phase. Application of this classification in the ICU may be hampered by altered consciousness in patients due to drugs, hypotension, sepsis, or intracranial pathology. Metabolic disturbances, postanoxic myoclonus, and psychiatric disturbances may mimic complex partial seizures.

SE is defined by 20 minutes of *continuous* or *recurrent*

seizure activity. Classification of SE is similarly based on observable clinical phenomena (Table 11–4). Secondarily generalized SE implies the presence of a structural lesion. Nonconvulsive SE (NCSE) in the ICU commonly follows partially treated generalized convulsive SE (GCSE). Visible convulsions may stop, but the electrochemical seizure continues. NCSE should be suspected in patients who fail to awaken 15 to 20 minutes after successful termination of SE.

Pathogenesis and Pathophysiology of Status Epilepticus

Seizures follow the opening of ionic channels coupled to excitatory amino acid (EAA) receptors, including the alpha-amino-3-hydroxy-5-methyl-4 isoxazolepropionic acid (AMPA), *N*-methyl-D-aspartate (NMDA), and metabotropic channels. The cellular effects of excessive excitatory amino acid channel activity include (1) toxic levels of cytosolic free calcium, (2) activation of autolytic enzyme systems, (3) production of oxygen-free radicals, (4) phosphorylation of enzyme and receptor systems, (5) generation of nitric oxide, and (6) an increase in intracellular osmolality and neuronal swelling. These events and biochemical evidence of immediate early gene activation and heat shock protein production indicate neuronal injury associated with status epilepticus. Elevated extracellular potassium, the result of sustained depolarizations in SE, potentiates the production of more seizures. Exhaustion of local glucose and oxygen intracellular stores needed to support neuronal ionic pumps leads to lactic acidemia and is a major cause of epileptic brain dam-

Table 11–4. CLINICAL CLASSIFICATION OF STATUS EPILEPTICUS

Generalized Seizures
- GCSE
  - Primary generalized SE
    - Tonic-clonic SE
    - Myoclonic SE
    - Clonic-tonic-clonic SE
  - Secondarily generalized SE
    - Partial seizure with secondary generalization
    - Tonic SE
- NCSE
  - Absence SE ("petit mal" status)
  - Atypical absence SE (e.g., in the Lennox syndrome)
  - Atonic SE
  - NCSE as a sequela of partially treated GCSE

Partial SE
- Simple partial SE
  - Typical
  - Epilepsia partialis continua
- CPSE

Neonatal SE

(Adapted from Lothman EW: The biochemical basis and pathophysiology of status epilepticus. Neurology 1990; 40(Suppl 2):13–23.)

age, of which the hippocampus contains the most vulnerable neurons. Counterregulatory ionic events that may terminate seizure activity are triggered by activation of inhibitory gamma-amino butyric acid (GABA) interneurons and inhibitory thalamic neurons.

Systemic manifestations of GCSE include (1) initially elevated systemic and pulmonary arterial blood pressures, (2) increased circulating epinephrine and cortisol leading to hyperglycemia, (3) intense muscular activity leading to lactic acidemia and hyperthermia, (4) impaired gas exchange from airway obstruction and abnormal diaphragmatic contractions. This combination of respiratory and metabolic acidosis, hypoxemia, and elevated circulating catecholamines frequently results in hyperkalemia and may precipitate epileptic sudden death from cardiac arrest or neurogenic pulmonary edema. Other sequelae of SE include aspiration pneumonitis, rhabdomyolysis leading to renal failure, compression fractures, and other injuries.

Diagnosis and Management of Single Seizures

The partial onset or postictal evidence of language, motor, sensory, or reflex abnormalities indicates *focal* pathology. Cardiovascular disease or a systemic infection should be sought. Drug intoxication occurring in the setting of renal or hepatic failure, and drug withdrawal, are frequent causes of seizures in the ICU. Electrolytes, osmolality, and a drug screen should also be obtained. CT scan of the head is generally indicated to rule out a cerebrovascular, infectious, or neoplastic cause. An EEG is indicated to rule out a focal cause, classify the seizure type, and guide treatment. Emergency EEG may be indicated to rule out nonconvulsive status epilepticus (NCSE).

In general, placement of padded tongue blades or similar items is *not* useful in single seizures and may cause airway obstruction. Medication is also unlikely to influence the course of the seizure before its spontaneous termination. Considerations for initiating anticonvulsant therapy should be based on probable cause of the seizure, likelihood of recurrence, and the efficacy of treatment in preventing recurrence of seizures. *Short-term* anticonvulsant therapy is indicated for convulsions during barbiturate or benzodiazepine withdrawal and in metabolic or drug-induced seizures. Withdrawal convulsions from ethanol are not prevented by the administration of phenytoin. *Long-term* therapy is indicated for patients with seizures and CNS disease, as well as after a first unprovoked seizure to prevent subsequent epilepsy.

Phenytoin is the drug of choice in the ICU because of its ease of administration and lack of sedative effects. A loading dose of 20 mg · $^{-}$kg^{1} is given at a rate of no faster than 50 mg · min^{-1}. Hypotension and atrioventricular block are side effects that can be prevented by slow IV infusion at less than 25 mg · min^{-1}. The commonest adverse effect is hypersensitivity, which is manifested by fever, rash, and eosinophilia. The therapeutic total plasma concentration of phenytoin is in the range of 10 to 20 μg · mL^{-1} (corresponding to a free plasma concentration of 1 to 2 $\mu g \cdot mL^{-1}$). Failure to prevent seizures at concentrations of 25 $\mu g \cdot mL^{-1}$ or more is an indication to add phenobarbital to the regimen. The clearance half-life of phenytoin is 12 to 20 hours (IV) to 24 hours (extended-release capsules), so dosing intervals need not be more frequent than every 12 hours. The free fraction (10%) is metabolized in the liver, and dosages should be decreased in hepatic dysfunction. Renal failure does not affect clearance but will lower total plasma concentration due to a lower bound fraction. Thus, the free phenytoin level should be monitored, as it may be within normal limits even when total phenytoin levels are low. *Phenobarbital* is indicated for persistent seizures after adequate phenytoin administration. A therapeutic serum concentration of 20 to 40 $\mu g \cdot mL^{-1}$ is targeted. Clearance half-life is 96 hours, and the dosing interval should be once a day. Hepatic and renal dysfunction results in reduced metabolism and delayed excretion.

Diagnosis and Management of Status Epilepticus

Status epilepticus is a medical emergency for which concomitant diagnosis and treatment are necessary. Treatment should be started after 5 minutes of continuous seizure activity or after the second or third seizure occurs without recovery between the spells. GCSE may occasionally be confused with decerebrate posturing or tetanic spasm. SE may be entirely masked by pharmacologic paralysis in the ICU. An EEG must be obtained as soon as possible after treatment is started. Continuous EEG monitoring is subsequently recommended in patients with refractory SE or neuromuscular blockade. The management protocol for SE is outlined in Table 11–5.

Prognosis

The effect of a single seizure in medical ICU patients for a non-neurologic reason has been shown to result in a doubling of in-hospital mortality. Mortality rates associated with SE lasting longer than 1 hour increase tenfold compared with SE lasting less than 1 hour. In both instances, the effect on prognosis reflects the underlying cause of the seizures. Survivors of SE often have memory and behavioral disorders out of proportion to the structural damage produced by the cause of their seizures. These data strongly emphasize the need for rapid and effective control of SE.

CONFUSION AND AGITATION

The Acute Confusional State

The acute confusional state (ACS) in the ICU is a common and potentially life-threatening condition that is often misdiagnosed, mistaken for a worsening dementia, or mistakenly called "ICU psychosis." This entity, also known as *"functional" psychosis* in a critical care setting, is rare. It

Table 11–5. SUGGESTED PROTOCOL FOR TREATING STATUS EPILEPTICUS

I. Establish an airway, provide oxygen, and ensure ventilation. If neuromuscular junction blockade is required for intubation, use a short-acting agent (e.g., succinylcholine or vecuronium).

II. Determine blood pressure. If the patient is hypotensive, begin volume replacement or the use of vasoactive agents (or both) as indicated. GCSE patients who present with hypotension usually require admission to a critical care unit. (Hypertension should not be treated until SE is controlled, since terminating SE usually substantially corrects it, and many of the agents used to terminate SE can produce hypotension.)

III. Unless the patient is known to be normo- or hyperglycemic, administer dextrose (1 mg/kg) and thiamine (1 mg/kg).

IV. Terminate SE. The following sequence is recommended (see text for details); be cognizant of the potential of these drugs to eliminate the visible convulsive movements of GCSE when leaving the patient in nonconvulsive SE. Patients who do not begin to respond to external stimuli 15 minutes after the apparent termination of GCSE should be considered at risk for nonconvulsive SE and should undergo emergency electroencephalographic monitoring.

D. Should the patient not be controlled with midazolam, administer pentobarbital, 12 mg/kg at a rate of 0.2–0.4 mg/kg/per minute as tolerated, followed by an infusion of 0.25–2.0 mg/kg per hour as determined by electroencephalographic monitoring (with an initial goal of burst suppression; in some cases, an isoelectric electroencephalogram may be required to eliminate all seizures). Most patients require systemic and pulmonary artery catheterization, with fluid and vasoactive drug therapy as indicated to maintain blood pressure. Other complications of this treatment are discussed in the text.

V. Prevent recurrence of SE. The choice of drugs depends greatly on the cause of SE and/or the patient's medical and social situation. In general, patients not previously receiving anticonvulsants whose SE is easily controlled often respond well to chronic treatment with phenytoin or carbamazepine. In contrast, others (e.g., patients with acute encephalitis) require two or three anticonvulsants at "toxic" levels (e.g., phenobarbital at greater than 100 μg/mL) to be weaned from midazolam or pentobarbital and may still have occasional seizures.

A. Give lorazepam, 0.05–0.2 mg/kg at a rate of 0.04 mg/kg/per minute. This drug should be diluted in an equal volume of the solution being used for intravenous infusion, as it is quite viscous. Most adult patients who respond do so by a total administered dose of 8 mg. The latency of effect is debated, but lack of response after 5 minutes should indicate failure.

B. If SE persists after lorazepam administration, begin phenytoin, 20 mg/kg at a rate of 0.3 mg/kg per minute. If the patient tolerates this infusion rate, it may be increased to a maximum of 50 mg/min. Hypotension and arrhythmias are the major concern. Many investigators believe that an additional 5 mg/kg dose of phenytoin should be administered before the next line of therapy is attempted.

C. If SE persists, administer midazolam, 0.2 mg/kg as a bolus, followed by an infusion of 0.1–2.0 mg/kg per hour to achieve seizure control (as determined by electroencephalographic monitoring). Intubate the patient at this stage if this has not already been accomplished. A patient reaching this stage should be treated in a critical care unit.

VI. Treat complications.

A. Rhabdomyolysis should be treated with vigorous saline diuresis to prevent acute renal failure; urinary alkalization may be a useful adjunct. If definitive treatment of GCSE takes longer than expected because of hypotension or arrhythmias, neuromuscular junction blockade under electroencephalographic monitoring might be considered.

B. Hyperthermia usually remits rapidly after termination of SE. External cooling usually suffices if the core temperature remains elevated. In rare instances, cool peritoneal lavage or extracorporeal blood cooling may be required. High-dose pentobarbital generally produces poikilothermy.

C. The treatment of cerebral edema occurring secondary to SE has not been well studied. When substantial edema is present, one should suspect that SE and cerebral edema are both manifestations of the same underlying condition. Hyperventilation and mannitol may be valuable if edema is life threatening. Edema due to SE is vasogenic in origin, thus steroids may be useful as well.

implies that the environmental features of critical care settings such as sensory deprivation or monotony are capable of causing psychosis. When used as a convenient diagnostic catch-all term for delirium of an unknown cause, it discourages the search for differential diagnoses and their specific treatment. Instead, the ACS may represent the initial or only sign of a serious underlying illness. Acute confusional states may be seen as a complication of a variety of illnesses (Table 11–6) or in the postoperative state (Table 11–7).

Confusion denotes a state characterized by a disturbance of attention. Salient features are disorientation, increased

Table 11–6. DIFFERENTIAL DIAGNOSIS OF BRAIN DYSFUNCTION IN CRITICAL CARE PATIENTS (LUDWIG'S DIFFERENTIAL DIAGNOSIS OF THE CONFUSION-DELIRIUM-DEMENTIA-COMA COMPLEX)

General Cause	Specific Causes
Vascular	Hypertensive encephalopathy; cerebral arteriosclerosis; intracranial hemorrhage or thromboses; circulatory collapse (shock); systemic lupus erythematosus; polyarteritis nodosa; thrombotic thrombocytopenic purpura
Infectious	Encephalitis; meningitis; general paresis
Neoplastic	Space-occupying lesions such as gliomas, meningiomas, abscesses
Degenerative	Senile and presenile dementias such as Alzheimer's or Pick's dementia, Huntington's chorea
Intoxication	Chronic intoxication or withdrawal effect of sedative-hypnotic drugs such as bromides, opiates, tranquilizers, anticholinergics, dissociative anesthetics, anticonvulsants
Congenital	Epilepsy; postictal states; aneurysm
Traumatic	Subdural and epidural hematomas; contusion; laceration; postoperative trauma; heat stroke
Intraventricular	Normal-pressure hydrocephalus
Vitamin deficiency	Deficiencies of thiamine (Wernicke-Korsakoff), niacin (pellagra), vitamin B_{12} (pernicious anemia)
Endocrine-metabolic	Diabetic coma and shock; uremia; myxedema; hyperthyroidism, parathyroid dysfunction; hypoglycemia; hepatic failure; porphyria; severe electrolyte or acid-base disturbances; remote side effect of carcinoma; Cushing's syndrome; Wilson's disease
Metals	Heavy metals (lead, manganese, mercury); carbon monoxide; toxins
Anoxia	Hypoxia and anoxia secondary to pulmonary or cardiac failure, anesthesia, anemia
Depression, other	Depressive pseudodementia; hysteria; catatonia

(From Ludwig AM: Principles of Clinical Psychiatry. New York, Free Press, 1980, p 234.)

Table 11–7. FACTORS ASSOCIATED WITH POSTOPERATIVE CONFUSION

Preoperative Factors: Previous History of:
Transient ischemic attacks
Stroke
Diabetes mellitus
Peripheral vascular disease
Myocardial infarction
Cardiac dysfunction
Depression
Dementia
Old age
Intraoperative Factors
Cardiopulmonary bypass time > 2 hours
Operative time > 7 hours
Low hematocrit
Massive intraoperative bleeding
Perioperative hypotension
Postoperative Factors
Hypotension
Requirements for pressors
Intra-aortic balloon pump
Electrolyte abnormalities
Hypoxemia
Systemic infection

distractibility, inability to register immediate events or recall them later, or maintaining a coherent stream of thought. Symptoms may worsen nocturnally. Irritability and restlessness may also occur. *Delirium* is a confusional state characterized by overactivity of psychomotor and autonomic nervous system functions in which perceptual disturbances are prominent. An example of delirium occurs in patients with alcohol withdrawal, who present with tremulousness, jerky movements, dilated pupils, flushed facies, tachycardia, diaphoresis, hallucinations and delusions.

Clinical, Laboratory, and Imaging Approach

Accurate mental status and neurologic examination must begin before the patient is confused. An accurate history taken from the patient and the family is essential, including questions about prior strokes or mental decline and whether or not the patient balances his or her checkbook, shops alone, or drives a car. Are there any lateralizing findings, such as hemiparesis, that suggest a prior stroke? This information is valuable later, when the physician tries to decipher which physical findings are new. The clinical approach to the evaluation of the postoperatively confused patient is outlined in Table 11–8.

Three neurologic studies are useful in the evaluation of the confused patient: (1) cranial computed tomography or magnetic resonance imaging, (2) lumbar puncture, and (3) electroencephalography. The indication for and information derived from a CT or MRI of the head are discussed in the earlier section on evaluation of the comatose patient and are

Table 11–8. EXAMINATION OF THE CONFUSED PATIENT

History (from Family and Patient)
Baseline mental status (balances checkbook, shops independently, or drives)
Previous medical illnesses (diabetes mellitus, heart disease, or liver disease)
Previous stroke
Previous psychiatric history
Substance abuse (alcohol, sedative-hypnotics)

General Physical Examination
Vital signs (respiratory pattern, e.g., Cheyne-Stokes)
Evidence of acute or chronic systemic illness
Nuchal rigidity
Evidence of head trauma

Neurologic Examination
Mental Status Examination
Level of consciousness (e.g., is hyperalert, alert, lethargic, stuporous, comatose)
Attention (can give months or days in reverse order)
Language (comprehends yes/no questions and conveys meaning without errors)
Memory (remembers details from hospitalization or a short story)
Visuospatial (can draw a clock, shows spatial neglect)
Cranial Nerves
Pupillary reaction and size
Extraocular movements (gaze preference)
Facial symmetry
Motor System
Pronator "drift"
Fine finger movements
Gait (walks on heels and toes)
Spontaneous (e.g., tremor, myoclonus, asterixis)

equally relevant to the patient with confusion and evidence of asymmetries or focal processes on neurologic examination. Lumbar puncture may be life-saving for the diagnosis of bacterial meningitis, which may occur in the absence of a stiff neck. It should be performed in patients with both confusion and unexplained fever, and in patients in whom meningitis is highly suspected, such as those who have undergone neurosurgery. The physician must carefully record the opening pressure before sending the fluid for protein, glucose, cell count and microscopic analyses, and microbial cultures. The EEG is a potentially useful diagnostic test. Not all conditions that cause confusion have the same effect on the EEG, even though slowing of the background rhythm is common in patients with alterations of consciousness. Barbiturate intoxication and effects of other sedatives may induce increased frequency and amplitude on the EEG, whereas delirium tremens and Wernicke-Korsakoff disease cause surprisingly little or no change on the EEG. Bilaterally synchronous, large, sharp "triphasic waves" are characteristic of hepatic encephalopathy but may also appear in patients with renal or pulmonary failure. Sharp waves, or "spikes" (fast waves of high amplitude), may be detected if seizures are present. A normal EEG in a patient whose responses are slow or who is inattentive supports the diagnosis of depression, whereas mild but diffuse slow-wave abnormalities occur with profound dementia.

Other laboratory tests should include determinations of electrolytes, glucose, and calcium levels; white blood cell count; hematocrit; and both urine and serum toxin screening. Additional laboratory tests that may be useful include arterial blood gases, ammonia level, phosphate level, liver and thyroid function tests, coagulation screening, blood and urine cultures, urinalysis, electrocardiography and chest x-ray studies.

Differential Diagnoses

The list of conditions associated with postoperative confusion is extensive. Several conditions are routinely called to mind in the intensive care setting. These are states in which intervention needs to be especially prompt, because prolonged failure to make the diagnosis may result in permanent central nervous system damage: (1) Wernicke's disease, (2) hypoxia, (3) hypoglycemia, (4) hypertensive encephalopathy, (5) intracerebral hemorrhage, (6) meningitis/encephalitis, and (7) poisoning, whether exogenous or iatrogenic. Focal findings on examination are useful for determining the cause of the confusion. Nonfocal findings suggest that the primary source of the ACS lies outside the central nervous system. Infections usually do not cause focal neurologic findings and must be aggressively pursued, even in the absence of fever. Meningeal signs may not be present in the stuporous patient. Neurologic disorders occur in over 50% of transplant recipients, with infection being the most frequent cause. Mental status changes accompanying systemic infection without other organ failure or overt involvement of the brain or meninges is termed *septic encephalopathy.* Clinical or EEG evidence of diffuse cerebral dysfunction and polyneuropathy with difficulty in weaning from mechanical ventilation may also occur in patients with sepsis. Cytokines may be responsible for the direct alteration of brain function via mechanisms that increase procoagulant activity, cause capillary leakage with tissue edema, and alter the blood-brain barrier.

Medications are among the most commonly cited causes of postoperative confusion. Drug toxicity is especially common in the elderly patient with a compensated dementia, impaired renal or hepatic function, or a known increased sensitivity to medications. Drugs commonly associated with postoperative confusion are listed in Table 11–9. Patients with neurologic causes of confusion usually have focal signs, except patients with meningitis, encephalitis, or small, widespread emboli from endocarditis. Two stroke syndromes may present with confusion and few other findings. A *right middle cerebral artery infarction* is associated with confusion, visual field loss, neglect of visual stimuli on the left side of space, slight drift of left arm, and mild left face and hand weakness. *Left or bilateral posterior cerebral artery infarction*

Table 11–9. DRUGS COMMONLY USED POSTOPERATIVELY THAT HAVE BEEN ASSOCIATED WITH CONFUSION

Anticholinergic agents	Methyldopa
Anticonvulsants	Metoclopramide
Antihistamines	Metronidazole
Benzodiazepines	Narcotic agents
Captopril	Nitroprusside sodium
Cephalosporins	Nonsteroidal anti-inflammatory drugs
Cimetidine	Penicillin
Ciprofloxacin	Procainamide
Clonidine	Propranolol
Corticosteroids	Quinidine sulfate
Digitalis	Ranitidine
Imipenem-cilastin	Theophylline
Ketoconazole	Trimethoprim-sulfamethoxazole
Lidocaine	

presents with visual field loss, hemisensory deficit, inability to read but preserved writing, and anomia most severe for colors.

Treatment

Therapy is generally aimed at reversible medical disorders, but symptomatic treatment may also be needed to protect the agitated patient from injury. Polypharmacy should be avoided, and all nonessential drugs, especially those with psychoactive properties, should be withdrawn. Sedative-hypnotic drugs should not be used unless alcohol or benzodiazepine withdrawal is being treated. Agitation is best controlled by nonpharmacologic means, whenever possible. The physician should encourage the presence of a family member, explain all procedures in detail, arrange nursing procedures to maximize uninterrupted sleep, keep the room dimly lit, and replace eyeglasses and hearing aids to avoid loss of sensory cues.

Haloperidol is the drug of choice for rapid control of agitation when nonpharmacologic measures fail, with a few exceptions. It has fewer cardiopulmonary effects compared with the benzodiazepines. The IV route is preferred and is associated with fewer extrapyramidal effects compared with the IM or PO routes, but approval of the hospital's independent review board is needed as the drug is not approved by the Food and Drug Administration for intravenous use. Initial dose varies with the degree of delirium: 0.5 to 2 mg for mild agitation, 2 to 5 mg for moderate agitation, 10 to 20 mg for severe agitation. Onset of action is 10 to 30 minutes. Doses may be repeated after 30 minutes and doubled subsequently every 30 minutes until calm is achieved. After complete lucidity has returned, only small oral doses (e.g., 3 mg) may be needed at night. Extrapyramidal side effects respond to anticholinergic therapy (e.g., diphenhydramine or benztropine). Patients with HIV infection may be more susceptible to extrapyramidal effects and the neuroleptic malignant syndrome. The alternative use of molindone in this group of patients has been advocated. Torsades de pointes may occur with intravenous haloperidol use.

Neuroleptics should not be used for the treatment of anticholinergic delirium, hepatic encephalopathy, or alcohol or benzodiazepine withdrawal. They are also contraindicated in coma. Anticholinergic drugs should be discontinued and supportive care provided for patients with anticholinergic delirium; parenteral physostigmine may be useful in life-threatening cases but can cause side effects, such as cardiac arrhythmias and respiratory depression. In hepatic encephalopathy, a short-acting benzodiazepine that requires little liver degradation (e.g., oxazepam) is recommended. Benzodiazepines are the drugs of choice in the treatment of alcohol or benzodiazepine withdrawal.

Reversal of factors leading to confusion usually results in no permanent residual damage. However, in the elderly, there is a considerable lag time between the resolution of the underlying metabolic derangement or drug effect and the recovery of mental function. Those suffering from anoxic brain damage may not return to a normal mental status or the original level of function.

MANAGEMENT OF SPECIFIC PSYCHIATRIC PROBLEMS

Fear and Anxiety

Fear of death or permanent disability associated with a life-threatening disease or its treatment can cause behavioral changes of verbosity, outbursts of anger, paranoia, or silent withdrawal. Treatment includes medication and reassurance. Routine prescription of benzodiazepines (Table 11–10), the drugs of choice, may be warranted in patients with autonomic lability (e.g., after a myocardial infarction) despite the absence of overt anxiety. Clarification, explanation, and valid assurance have very soothing effects on patients whose fear stems from threatening or erroneous conceptions of their disease. Positive aspects of the treatment plan, particularly those that address the patient's fears, should be mentioned. Equanimity on the part of the caregiver has perhaps the most soothing effect on patients.

Denial and the Threat to Sign Out

Denial allows acutely ill patients to avoid panic by minimizing or precluding the threatening implications of their disease. Threatening to sign out is usually a manifestation of panic. Such patients are often desperate, irrational, and antagonistic to efforts made to detain them. Before talking to patients who threaten to sign out, the family should be mobilized immediately to induce patients to stay. Hysterical patients, even after becoming calm, should be medicated promptly with an antipsychotic (e.g., droperidol). A calm, gentle, and quiet approach to such patients, emphasizing the positive aspects of proposed therapy, is usually most

Table 11–10. BENZODIAZEPINES: DURATION OF ACTION, METABOLIC HALF-LIFE, AND ACTIVE METABOLITES

	Half-Life (Hr)	Onset of Action	Metabolized to
Short-acting			
Oxazepam (Serax)	5–15	Slow	—
Lorazepam (Ativan)	10–20	Intermediate	—
Temazepam (Restoril)	9–12	Slow	—
Alprazolam (Xanax)	12–15	Intermediate	α-Hydroxyalprazolam
Triazolam (Halcion)	2–3	Intermediate	α-Hydroxytriazolam
Estazolam (ProSom)	10–24	Intermediate	4-Hydroxyestazolam
			1-Oxo-estazolam
Midazolam (Versed)	1.5–2.5	Rapid	1-Hydroxymethyl m.
Moderately long			
Diazepam (Valium)	26–53	Rapid	*N*-desmethyldiazepam
Chlordiazepoxide (Librium)	8–28	Intermediate	Desmethylchlordiazepoxide
			Demoxepam
			N-desmethyldiazepam
Halazepam (Paxipam)	14	Intermediate	*N*-desmethyldiazepam (five metabolites)
Clonazepam (Klonopin)	20–80	Slow	
Long			
Clorazepate (Tranxene)	30–200	Rapid	*N*-desmethyldiazepam
Prazepam (Centrax)	30–200	Slow	*N*-desmethyldiazepam
Very long			
Flurazepam (Dalmane)	40–150	Rapid	*N*-desalkylfurazepam
		Rapid	Hydroxyethylflurazepam
		Rapid	Flurazepam aldehyde
Quazepam (Doral)	40–150	Rapid	2-Oxo-*N*-desalkylthorazepam

effective. They should be told that their illness is manageable if they stay in the hospital. As patients calm down, they may respond to questions about the source of their fears. Even if they leave, they should be assured that they are welcome to the appropriate treatment whenever they change their mind and choose to return.

Despondency

Illness-induced acute despondency may be seen in the second or third day of hospitalization when feelings of dread, bitterness, despair, and low self-esteem occur as a result of concerns with work, relationships, career, and personal aspirations. Patients should be allowed to express these concerns and be assured that these are normal emotional reactions to physical illness and will probably disappear as health returns. Discussion of rehabilitation plans while patients are still in the acute phase of recovery is often reassuring. The patient's family and social network is assessed and, when possible, integrated into treatment and support.

Major Depression

Major depression, depression with mania or manic symptoms, and depression with psychotic symptoms require specific treatment in the critical care setting. The diagnostic criteria for depression include sleep disturbances, including insomnia, hypersomnia, and especially early morning awakening; loss of interest in work, hobbies, or social activities; feelings of guilt, self-reproach, or worthlessness; decreased energy and tiredness or exhaustion; impaired concentration, decreased ability to think, slow or mixed-up thinking, and indecisiveness; disturbed appetite with weight gain or loss; psychomotor agitation or retardation; and recurrent thoughts of death or suicide, including the wish to be dead. The presence of at least four of the preceding symptoms for 2 weeks is required to qualify as major depression.

The treatment of major depression begins with the initial use of a psychostimulant (e.g., 2.5 to 20 mg of dextroamphetamine or methylphenidate) for patients who appear to be physiologically recovering from their illnesses but are lethargic, lack motivation, and are disinterested in their caretaking regimen. Addition of a sedative antidepressant may be needed at night for insomnia (e.g., doxepin, 25 mg; nortriptyline, 10 to 25 mg; or trazodone, 50 mg). An adequate sleep dose may need to be titrated. Subsequently, antidepressants are started if there is only partial or ineffective response to psychostimulants. Tricyclic antidepressants (e.g., nortriptyline) may be used, starting at 25 mg PO nightly, increasing weekly by 25 to 75 mg nightly for a therapeutic plasma level of 50 to 150 ng · ml^{-1}. Side effects of tricyclic antidepressants include orthostatic hypotension (especially imipramine, chlorimipramine, amitriptyline, and desipramine), anticholinergic effects (especially amitriptyline and protriptyline), and prolonged cardiac conduction, particularly in the His-Purkinje system. Serotonin-specific reuptake inhibitors are another class of antidepressants that are free of the aforementioned side effects associated with tricyclic antidepressants. They can be given once a day at any time: fluoxetine, 10 mg, paroxetine, 20 mg, or sertraline, 50 mg. These drugs compete for metabolic oxidation by the cytochrome P-450 enzyme system with other drugs (e.g., benzodiazepines), and they may decrease metabolism and increase levels of the latter. Bupropion can be started at a dose of 50 to 75 mg, and given two or three times a day, increased to a total dose of 200 to 400 mg daily.

Anxiety That Inhibits Weaning from the Ventilator

A multimodal approach is needed. A benzodiazepine (e.g., lorazepam) is administered before weaning periods. Haloperidol may be needed for patients in near-panic. Hypnosis or relaxation techniques may also be helpful in distracting patients from the weaning process. Patients will also benefit from the explanation that the weaning process can be expected to cause anxiety.

The Difficult Patient: Refusal to Obey the Rules

Rule violators are often dependent persons who react by hyperindependent behavior when placed in a dependent position. Physicians need to restore a sense of control in these patients whenever possible. Patients should be made to understand that they are respected, that they cannot be forced to do what they do not want to, that their treatment regimen is not intended to be an act of oppression, but that they and *not* the caregivers will be the ones to suffer if they fail to comply with treatment. Compromises may be allowed if not medically contraindicated.

Hostile Patients

The style of expressing anger is molded by a patient's personality. Anger and aggression are usually aroused by threat or damage to self-esteem and are common in patients who have been in the ICU for more than 2 weeks. Anger may be openly expressed as a direct response to disease or indirectly discharged at some tangible targets—e.g., a noisy roommate or the night staff. The physician's response should be to quietly hear out the grievance, gently ask for details, and offer sincere regret for whatever has damaged the self-esteem. Anger should be redirected at the primary culprit, the disease itself.

Subtle hostility and devious aggression are disguised and more difficult to deal with. Physicians are often provoked to annoyance by such patients who are ingratiating, convey demeaning implications, ignore what is being said, and instigate staff conflicts by passive-aggressive behavior. Physicians should first keep their own hostility under control and help such patients admit their hostility by confronting them with evidence of their behavior. They should be gently and firmly reminded that physicians are not to be blamed for the disease and that all treatment is for their benefit, even when a cure cannot be guaranteed.

The assistance of the psychiatrist should be sought for extremely manipulative patients with borderline personality disorders who are habitual help-rejecters and who engage others in conflict-ridden relationships and provoke staff conflicts.

Discharge from the ICU

Transfer from the ICU to a general ward generally implies to the patient reduced coverage and observation. To allay anxiety, patients should be warned well in advance of the discharge date and assured that despite less frequent checks and fewer nurses, intensive care is no longer necessary because of an improvement in their condition.

The ICU environment should be geared toward recovery by addition of windows, clocks, calendars; changing lighting schedules to approximate day and night; noise reduction; addition of music, photos, or ear phones; and the tailoring of visit schedules to meet patients' needs.

BRAIN DEATH CERTIFICATION

Traditional criteria for defining death require the cessation of cardiac and respiratory function. The technologic capacity to sustain cardiopulmonary function after severe brain injury led to the need to address the separation of cardiorespiratory and neurologic survival. Reasons for addressing this separation included justification for making further clinical decisions, such as discontinuation of cardiopulmonary support and the improved survival of recipients after transplantation of organs from donors who were brain dead but had beating hearts.

Uniform Determination of Death Act

This Act is the basis for most statutes in the United States. It concludes: "An individual who has sustained either (1) irreversible cessation of circulatory and respiratory function, or (2) irreversible cessation of all functions of the entire brain, including the brain stem, is dead."

Through practice, public opinion, policy, legal precedence, and statute, the equivalency of a patient's death and the death of all components of the brain has been accepted in most countries of the world. This acceptance is, in part, based on the inability of CNS neurons to replace or regenerate loss due to injury or disease, the lack of an extracorporeal substitute for lost brain function, and the inability to transplant this vital organ. Nonetheless, controversies still revolve around the definition, diagnosis, and certification of brain death. Conflicting viewpoints remain as to whether death should be defined as a physical or philosophical event, the reliability of the testing methods selected to identify confidently when death has occurred, and who may make the clinical diagnosis and certification of death.

Whole Brain Criteria

The equivalency of life to the function of the entire brain forms the basis of these criteria for death. Thus, a person may be declared deceased only when all functions of the entire brain are determined to be irrevocably absent. Implied therein is the permanency of an *irrevocable* state, testing of all parts of the brain, and the assumption that all testing is valid to avoid an unacceptable false determination of death. A large number of criteria have been proposed as valid testing of brain death. All published criteria require that certain agents or conditions known to depress brain function reversibly (Table 11–11) be absent before testing is started. Table 11–12 lists specific criteria and methodologic considerations for testing; these apply not only to whole brain standards but also to brain stem criteria (see later).

Specific evidence of death of the cerebrum is documented by EEG showing absent neuronal function or through the demonstration of a complete lack of cerebral blood flow. Tests dependent on neuronal function are valid only when those confounding factors listed in Table 11–11 are absent. Tests of cerebral blood flow are used when confounding factors (e.g., drugs) may invalidate tests dependent on neuronal function. Additional tests that may be performed in conjunction with the neurologic examination to document absent functions of the entire brain are listed in Table 11–13.

Despite elaborate standards and procedures, considerable evidence shows that in some patients, residual neuronal function continues even though a patient has fulfilled whole brain criteria. Such evidence includes:

1. Maintenance of body temperature (i.e., not all patients become poikilothermic)

Table 11–11. CONFOUNDING AGENTS/CONDITIONS THAT MUST BE ABSENT BEFORE BRAIN DEATH TESTING

Shock/hypotension
Hypothermia <32°C
Drugs known to alter neurologic and/or neuromuscular function or electroencephalographic testing:
- Anesthetics
- Paralytics
- Methaqualone
- Barbiturates
- Diazepam
- High-dose bretylium
- Mecloqualone
- Amitriptyline
- Meprobamate
- Trichloroethylene
- Alcohols

Brain stem encephalitis
Guillain-Barré syndrome
Encephalopathies associated with hepatic failure, uremia, and hyperosmolar coma
Severe hypophosphatemia

Table 11–12. EXAMINATION CRITERIA AND METHODS IN BRAIN DEATH TESTING

1. Absent spontaneous movement, decorticate or decerebrate posturing; lack of seizures, shivering, response to verbal stimuli, response to noxious stimuli administered through a cranial nerve pathway. Spinal reflexes may persist.
2. Absent pupillary reflex to direct and consensual light; pupils need not be equal or dilated. The pupillary reflex may be selectively altered by eye trauma cataracts, high-dose dopamine, glutethimide, scopolamine, atropine, or monoamine oxidase inhibitors.
3. Absent corneal, oculocephalic, cough, and gag reflexes. The corneal reflex may be altered as a result of any type of facial weakness.
4. Absent oculovestibular reflex when tested with 20 to 50 mL of ice water irrigated into an external auditory canal clear of cerumen after elevating the patient's head 30°. Labyrinthine injury or disease, anticholinergics, anticonvulsants, tricyclic antidepressants, and some sedatives may alter responses.
5. Failure of the heart rate to increase by more than 5 beats per minute after 1–2 mg IV of atropine has been used to further assess the vagal nerve and nuclei.
6. Absent respiratory efforts in the presence of hypercapnia (partial pressure of carbon dioxide >50–60 mm Hg) or, in rare circumstances, carefully monitored hypoxemia. Many protocols for apnea testing have been advocated to prevent hypoxemia during testing.

2. Spontaneous depolarizations detected by deeply placed electrodes despite an isoelectric cortical EEG

3. Continuing or inducible pituitary and/or hypothalamic hormone production after four-vessel angiography has shown no flow

4. Resumption of blood flow after relief of obstructing lesions and postmortem examination in patients whose brain

Table 11–13. CONFIRMATORY TESTS IN WHOLE-BRAIN CRITERIA

Evaluate neuronal function:
- Electroencephalogram or cerebral function monitor
- Evoked potentials
- Biochemical tests of cerebrospinal fluid or jugular venous blood

Evaluate intracranial blood flow:
- Contrast angiography, magnetic resonance, or computed tomography imaging
- Radionuclide perfusion studies using technetium cranial radionculide angiography and technetium-HMPAO scintigraphy
- Xenon-enhanced computed tomography
- Digital subtraction angiography/venography
- Ophthalmic artery blood flow
- Transcranial Doppler study

Miscellaneous:
- Intracranial pressure higher than systolic blood pressure
- Sustained cerebral perfusion pressure <5 mm Hg

death was confirmed by the absence of blood flow demonstrated by angiography

Therefore, those who demand the most precise documentation that all cellular function of the entire brain is absent before confirming brain death acknowledge that no set of criteria is sufficiently detailed for that purpose. Most commonly, the potential that residual cellular and tissue function may exist is recognized but not specifically sought.

Cerebral Criteria

Loss of cerebral or "neocortical" function while brain stem function persists has *not* traditionally been accepted as equivalent to death. Proponents of this criterion advocate permanent loss of organized cognition originating from the cerebrum as being equivalent to loss of the essential element of the human quality, or "personhood." Unfortunately, the *permanence* of cerebral dysfunction cannot be predicted in most clinical circumstances, as evidenced by prolonged states of absent cognition followed by awakening among patients in metabolic encephalopathy or persistent vegetative states. Although assessment of cerebral anatomy or neocortical cellular function may diagnose extreme cases of anatomic ischemia or extremely low cerebral oxygen uptake, intermediate levels of injury remain difficult to quantify and accurately predict. There has, however, been legal support for recognizing death in *noncognitive* patients and *anencephalic* infants with absent cortical tissue, since such patients have never experienced cognition and thus could not regain it, nor could they ever acquire any integrated responses.

Brain Stem Criteria

Groups that accept criteria documenting absent brain stem function as equivalent to a patient's death do not require cerebral testing beyond clinical confirmation of noncognition. Interruption of the reticular activating fibers within the brain stem presumes a noncognitive state.

Brain Death in Children

Criteria considered useful in infants and children younger than 5 years of age have been published by the Task Force for the Determination of Brain Death in Children and are outlined in Table 11–14.

Specific Process of Certification

Brain death may be certified by one or more physicians with documented expertise in this area and who may or may not have a primary or consultative relationship with the patient. Concerns with potential conflict of interest for a certifying physician during organ donation may further limit a physician's participation. Specific criteria mandate repeated examination at a specified interval and require a known cause of brain failure to imply irreversibility. All criteria

Table 11–14. GUIDELINES USEFUL FOR BRAIN DEATH EVALUATION IN CHILDREN

Prerequisite to evaluation:
- History of cause of coma eliminates reversible conditions (similar to Table 11–11)

Physical examination criteria:
- Coma (loss of consciousness, vocalization, and volitional activity)
- Apnea using standardized testing
- Absent brain stem function:
  - Midposition or fully dilated pupils unresponsive to light
  - Absent spontaneous eye movements, oculocephalic and oculovestibular reflexes
  - Absent movement of bulbar musculature
  - Absent corneal, gag, cough, sucking, and rooting reflexes
  - Flaccid tone and absent spontaneous or induced movements except for those caused by spinal cord reflexes
  - Findings or examination should be consistent with brain death during entire observation and testing period as below

Age-specific observation period and retesting:
- 7 days of age to 2 months—two examinations and EEGs separated by 48 hours
- 2 months to 1 year of age—two examinations and EEGs separated by at least 24 hours or initial examination plus isoelectric EEG followed by cerebral radionuclide study confirming no cerebral blood flow
- Older than 1 year—two examinations at least 12 hours apart, with EEG and cerebral radionuclide studies optional

(From Guidelines for determination of brain death in children. Arch Neurol 1987; 44:587.)

assume that all reasonable therapeutic interventions have been attempted to treat the underlying brain injury.

NEUROMUSCULAR DISORDERS IN CRITICAL CARE

Recognition of Neuromuscular Respiratory Failure

Patients with neuromuscular respiratory failure typically present with upper airway dysfunction and diminished tidal volume. Upper airway dysfunction is manifested by difficulty in swallowing liquids, including secretions, and a hoarse or nasal voice. Diminished tidal volume occurs most dramatically with diaphragmatic weakness (paradoxical abdominal movement) but also follows injury to the paraspinal intercostal nerves, which maintain chest expansion against negative intrapleural pressure (e.g., in lower cervical spinal cord injuries).

Respiratory manifestations of progressive generalized weakness are initially characterized by the development of diminished tidal volume prior to the development of airway weakness. A compensatory increase in respiratory rate occurs if the patient's ventilatory drive is intact. $PaCO_2$ is thus initially maintained normal or low (35 mm Hg) from subjective dyspnea or hypoxic drive. A subsequent rise in

$PaCO_2$ signifies imminent and abrupt respiratory failure. A reduction in vital capacity (VC) from 65 to 30 $ml \cdot kg^{-1}$ results in a weak cough and difficulty in clearing secretions. At VC of 20 to 25 $ml \cdot kg^{-1}$, impaired sigh, progressive atelectasis, and hypoxemia from ventilation-perfusion mismatch become manifest. With a VC of 15 $ml \cdot kg^{-1}$ and maximum inspiratory pressure (PImax) or negative inspiratory force (NIF) of less than 20 to 25 cm H_2O, respiratory failure is imminent. Indications for endotracheal intubation and mechanical ventilation at this stage include fatigue, hypoxemia despite supplemental oxygen therapy, difficulty in clearing secretions, and a rise in $PaCO_2$. The precise timing of intubation varies with the patient, the underlying condition, and the likelihood of a rapid response to treatment. Under close monitoring, endotracheal intubation may be withheld in spontaneously breathing patients with the use of inspiratory and expiratory positive airway pressure assist devices (e.g., BiPAP). A cautionary note with regard to the measurement of VC or PImax is the possibility of artifactually low values obtained as a result of failure to form a tight seal around the devices' mouthpieces in patients with weakness of the orbicularis oris muscle. This underscores the need for direct patient observation rather than sole reliance on reported measurements.

GUILLAIN-BARRÉ SYNDROME (GBS). This is an acute inflammatory polyneuropathy or polyradiculoneuritis presenting as a motor peripheral neuropathy of acute onset, presumably due to antibodies directed against peripheral nerve components. In 5% of cases, the condition is a primary axonopathy. Antecedent causes include upper respiratory tract, cytomegalovirus, Epstein-Barr virus, human immunodeficiency virus, hepatitis A, B, and C virus, *Campylobacter jejuni*, and *Borrelia burgdorferi* infections.

The initial presentation of GBS is weakness, usually most marked in the legs. No objective signs of sensory dysfunction are usually found despite sensory complaints. Deep tendon reflexes are usually absent a week after presentation. Autonomic dysfunction usually manifests as a hypersympathetic state with unexplained sinus tachycardia, fluctuations in blood pressure, and rarely bradycardia. Autonomic reflexes in response to tracheal suctioning or visceral distention may be dramatic. Analysis of the patient's CSF typically shows elevation in protein by the second week. The presence of pleocytosis may suggest an acute human immunodeficiency virus infection. EMG studies may be normal initially but subsequently show multifocal conduction blocks, slowed conduction velocity, and impaired or absent responses on tests of proximal function.

Mechanical ventilation is usually required for management of ventilatory failure based on the preceding criteria due to a generally slow response to treatment. When a neuromuscular junction blocking agent is used for endotracheal intubation, a nondepolarizing agent (e.g., atracurium or vecuronium) is preferred to avoid transient hyperkalemia. Mechanical ventilation is generally required for less than 4 weeks.

Improvement of VC to greater than 15 $ml \cdot kg^{-1}$ or of NIF to greater than 25 cm H_2O is an indication to wean. Rarely, temporary pacing of the heart may be considered for severe bradycardia arising from autonomic dysfunction. Autonomic stimulation from iatrogenic or nursing procedures should be minimized. When a specific cause (e.g., Lyme disease) is present, appropriate treatment may speed recovery. Otherwise, plasma exchange remains the only specific and accepted treatment of GBS to remove autoantibodies that presumably underlie the peripheral neuropathy. Five treatments are given over 10 days, with albumin being the preferred replacement solution. High-dose intravenous immunoglobulin has been used but is also associated with disease progression and severe relapses. Nursing care is similar to that for other paralyzed ventilated patients. As patients remain lucid, daytime distractions and night-time sleep cycles are important. Sedation may be necessary for severely affected patients. Physical and occupational therapy should be performed frequently. Enteral nutritional support of GBS patients may occasionally be complicated by autonomic dysfunction affecting the gut, necessitating total parenteral nutrition.

MYASTHENIA GRAVIS (MG). This is an autoimmune disease of the neuromuscular junction, causing impaired neuromuscular transmission. Thymus hyperplasia and thymomas occur in the majority of patients. The reported prevalence of MG is 5 per 100,000, but only a small proportion of patients with MG develop respiratory failure. MG patients may present to the ICU in myasthenic or cholinergic crisis, in respiratory failure consequent to aspiration, or with complications from immunosuppression therapy, and for postoperative care after thymectomy.

Indications for *mechanical ventilation*, BiPAP, and weaning in MG are similar to those described for GBS. Anticholinesterase therapy is usually stopped when ventilatory support is expected to be discontinued within a week but is restarted at a lower dose after more than a week of mechanical ventilation. *Plasma exchange* and *corticosteroid therapy* have been useful in managing acute exacerbations. Commencement of corticosteroid therapy is associated with transient worsening of the disease. The value of thymectomy in the long-term management of MG is clear; however, a patient in acute respiratory failure is generally considered a poor operative risk, and the procedure is delayed until a patient's condition has improved. Post-thymectomy pain control and ventilatory function may be improved by epidural opioid administration.

The distinction between *myasthenic* (worsening of disease) and *cholinergic* (overtreatment with anticholinesterase) *crisis* may be made by blinded administration of a short-acting anticholinesterase (e.g., edrophonium, 10 mg) and a placebo, with pre- and post-test measures of strength (VC or NIF) and neuromuscular transmission (by EMG). Means to ventilate and support the airway and interpretation by an experienced neurologist must be available for the test. A positive result (e.g., strength improves) suggests that a higher dose of an anticholinesterase (e.g., pyridostigmine) may be useful. If a patient becomes weaker, the dose should be reduced.

Table 11–15. DRUGS THAT MAY INCREASE WEAKNESS IN MYASTHENIA GRAVIS

Definite	Likely	Rare or Questionable
Neomycin	Gentamicin	Ciprofloxacin
Streptomycin	Amikacin	Atenolol
Kanamycin	Tobramycin	
Lincomycin	Lidocaine	
Quinidine	Phenytoin	
	Propranolol	
	Phenothiazines	
	Lithium	

However, some doubt the ability of oral anticholinesterase agents in usual doses to produce cholinergic crises. A large number of drugs are reported to worsen or unmask MG; the more important ones are listed in Table 11–15. The disease also affects the response to pharmacologic neuromuscular junction blockade; patients are exceptionally sensitive to nondepolarizing agents but resistant to depolarizing agents.

Critical Illness Polyneuropathy and Myopathy

A sensorimotor axonal neuropathy that delays ventilatory weaning in patients who are otherwise recovering from critical illness, most frequently sepsis, has been described. A separate myopathy of critical illness has also been recognized.

CHAPTER 12
Transplantation

John A. Kellum, MD
George V. Mazariegos, MD

HISTORY AND ORGANIZATION OF ORGAN TRANSPLANTATION

In 1954, Murray and associates performed the first successful kidney transplant between two identical twins. Murray and Thomas, who initiated the technique for bone marrow transplantation, were subsequently awarded the Nobel Prize in Medicine in 1990 for their pioneering transplant research. In the 1960s, organ retrieval, surgical technique, and immunosuppression underwent key developments. Advances continued over the next two decades, allowing solid organ transplantation to become a viable form of life-saving therapy for many patients with end-stage organ failure.

Organ Allocation Systems

An important step in the growth of transplantation into a nationally available resource was the development of a national network for equitable organ allocation. The United Network for Organ Sharing (UNOS) has implemented a nationwide organ distribution system.

The fair distribution of available organs is a difficult task. The current system for organ allocation matches organs to recipients in the following manner: kidneys are matched on a point system by ABO compatibility, tissue antigen matching, a negative serum white blood cell cross-match between donor and recipient, age, and waiting time. The point system for cadaveric kidney allocation is listed in Table 12–1. The distribution of livers is based on compatibility of blood type and organ size. Urgency is considered by assigning priority into four categories based on need. The most urgent category is status 1; this includes patients who are hospitalized in critical condition with one of the following criteria: (a) need for mechanical ventilation; (b) renal failure; (c) severe coagulopathy with prothrombin time greater than 25 sec; (d) fulminant hepatic failure; or (e) primary graft nonfunction following organ transplantation. The next most critical category is status 2, which is reserved for patients who require continual hospitalization but do not need to be in an intensive care unit. Status 3 patients are able to be outside the hospital but require continual medical followup, with an anticipated need for a liver transplant within 1 year. Status 4 is reserved for those patients who have been identified as having end-stage liver disease but are not expected to require a transplant within the next 12 months.

Two categories of need are recognized for patients awaiting heart transplantation. Status 1 patients are those in critical condition who are hospitalized and require support-

Table 12–1. UNOS POINT SYSTEM FOR CADAVERIC KIDNEY ALLOCATION

Allocation Factor	Point Values
Time waiting	1 point: waiting longest. Fraction for all others. Additional 0.5 point: each full year of wait time
Quality of HLA match	10 points: 0 ABDR mismatch—mandatory share 7 points: 0 BDR mismatch 3 points: 1 BDR mismatch 2 points: 2 BDR mismatch 1 point: 3 BDR mismatch
PRA level	4 points if more than 79% and negative cross-match
Medical urgency	Physician judgment
Pediatric recipient	3 points: recipient under 11 years of age 2 points: recipient 11 to 17 years of age

ive measures, which may include mechanical support devices or inotropic drug support. Status 2 patients are outside the hospital. Hearts are also matched by ABO compatibility and size. There is no current categorization for those patients awaiting lung transplantation. They are matched solely on ABO and size compatibility with length of waiting time taken into consideration.

Organ distribution is usually carried out in a local, then regional, and finally national manner. Kidneys that are fully matched at the A, B, or Dr locus are shared on a national basis. Organs that are recovered within an organ procurement organization service area are usually offered first to patients waiting for transplant at centers in that region. If organs are not allocated locally or regionally, then they are offered to patients at centers outside that region. Currently, 11 regions are designated throughout the United States.

Current Need in Organ Donation

In January 1995, more than 37,000 patients were waiting for some type of solid organ transplantation. This included more than 26,000 patients waiting for a kidney transplant and more than 3800 patients waiting for a liver transplant. In 1992, 4548 organ donors resulted in 15,213 organ donations. Unfortunately, this is an increase of only 0.4% over 1991. The gap between the number of patients receiving transplants and the number of patients who require this lifesaving therapy continues to increase. Under the current criteria, there are approximately 12,000 potential organ donors in the United States in any given year, but only about 4500 donations actually take place, although several organs may be recovered from each donor. Continued professional and public education is needed to prevent this waste of lifegiving resources.

ORGAN DONOR CATEGORIES AND MANAGEMENT

The retrieval of the viable allograft is a key component of a successful transplantation. The goal of donor management is to provide organs that will function optimally in the recipient. Emphasis on careful donor management may decrease the incidence of primary organ failure in the recipient.

General Considerations

All dying patients may be evaluated as potential donors except those with extracranial malignancy, untreated septicemia, viral hepatitis, active tuberculosis, and positive human immunodeficiency virus serology. Essentially, there are no age criteria because organs from older and younger patients have proved acceptable. Similarly, those donors with chronic diseases such as diabetes or hypertension need not be automatically excluded unless end-organ damage can be documented. Organ donor categories can be divided into heart-beating donors, nonheart-beating donors, and animal donors. Heart-beating donors commonly evaluated today include: (1) living related donors, (2) living unrelated donors, and (3) the conventional brain-dead donor.

Living Related Donors

After the first successful kidney transplant from a living related donor, this type of donor remained a preferred source of organ for kidney transplantation. As cadaveric organ transplantation from heart-beating brain-dead donors improved, the use of brain-dead donors increased. However, 24% of the 10,108 kidney transplants performed in the United States in 1992 were from living donors. The most common living donor is a kidney donor. Evaluation of these living donors is very thorough, and this has resulted in a donor mortality after unilateral nephrectomy of less than 0.1%. Donors of paired organs are fully evaluated for normal function of both organs before procurement. In the case of both liver and kidney donors, this includes laboratory evaluation as well as angiographic evaluation for variant anatomy and evidence of pathology in the organ at question. With living donors, the recipient waiting time for the organ is minimized, and there are minimal procurement and preservation injuries to the transplanted organs, resulting in improved graft function.

Brain-Dead Donors

Head injury continues to be the leading cause of death in more than 75% of brain-dead organ donors. Most of these result from motor vehicle fatalities. Intracranial hemorrhage, brain tumor, and anoxic injury cause brain death in most other donors. (Diagnosis and certification of brain death are discussed in Chapter 11.)

The goal of conventional therapy in the organ donor is to maintain optimal tissue oxygen delivery using invasive hemodynamic monitoring to guide therapy and assure adequate fluid resuscitation. The aggressive correction of impaired oxygen delivery is perhaps the single most important factor in managing the brain-dead potential organ donor. Pulmonary artery catheters may be placed for assessment of right ventricular function and pulmonary artery pressures before lung or heart procurement or if the status of the intravascular volume is unclear.

Hypotension should first be treated by volume expansion with the choice of colloid or crystalloid product depending on the concurrent clinical status and coexisting electrolyte abnormalities. Vasoactive drugs should be used judiciously to avoid vasoconstriction and possible ischemic damage to donor organs. Use of norepinephrine is discouraged because of vasoconstriction of regional vascular beds.

Despite cardiac and pulmonary support, cardiac arrest may occur after brain death. The interval between brain death and cardiac arrest is unpredictable. The failure to reestablish oxygen delivery quickly leads to ischemic damage in the donor organs, and therefore prompt therapy is essential. Atropine is ineffective after the loss of functioning vagal nuclei. Epinephrine, isoproterenol, or transcutaneous pacing may be needed to treat the patient who has sustained cardiac arrest. When cardiac function cannot be established quickly, open cardiac massage, cardiopulmonary bypass, or emergency organ retrieval must be considered. Standard respiratory care is important in management of the potential organ donor. Vigorous pulmonary toilet, maintenance of adequate arterial saturation, and close monitoring of fluid balance to avoid pulmonary congestion are all important in allowing for successful organ retrieval.

Appropriate fluid therapy is essential in the management of these patients. The most common clinical problems encountered in this scenario are hypovolemia and neurogenic diabetes insipidus. Hypovolemia must be treated aggressively and the underlying cause corrected as quickly as possible. Diabetes insipidus may result in significant polyuria leading to hyperosmolality, severe electrolyte abnormalities, and hemodynamic instability. The resulting hypernatremia, in particular, may be detrimental to organ function after reperfusion in the transplant recipient. The patient's free water deficit must be corrected with hypotonic solutions. Dextrose-containing fluids can be used as long as concomitant hyperglycemia is avoided. Electrolyte disturbances such as hypokalemia also need to be corrected. Exogenous vasopressin may be required to replace circulating antidiuretic hormone after brain death. Intravenous desmopressin acetate (DDAVP) is recommended in divided doses of 0.2 to 4 μg daily. A continuous infusion of aqueous pitressin may also be used at a rate of 1 to 3 mU/kg/hr titrated for urine output of 100 to 250 mL/hr.

Hypothermia may confound the diagnosis of brain death and complicate the management of the brain-dead donor. Treatment should be geared toward preventing excessive heat loss, using warming blankets to maintain a temperature at or above 35°C. Warmed intravenous fluids and heated humidified oxygen at 40 to 46°C via the ventilator may be required for donors with a more extreme component of hypothermia.

There is evidence of disseminated intravascular coagulation in a significant proportion of patients with lethal head injuries. Severe coagulopathy with clinical evidence of bleeding should be corrected with appropriate blood component therapy.

Management of the Non–Heart-Beating Donor

The shortage of cadaveric organs has prompted a re-examination of organ procurement from non–heart-beating donors (NHBD). A recent report from Pittsburgh documents experience with liver and kidney allografts from NHBDs. In general, NHBDs can be characterized as uncontrolled or controlled. Uncontrolled NHBDs are patients who have either been pronounced brain dead by standard criteria or are in the process of being pronounced brain dead when they suddenly develop cardiac arrest. Organ retrieval is carried out after the patient has been transported to the operating room. Controlled NHBDs are patients who either do not fulfill brain death criteria or those who have met the criteria of brain death but have families requesting life support withdrawal prior to organ procurement. Recovery of organs from controlled NHBD patients occurs after patients have been transported to the operating room where ventilation is discontinued. Procurement of kidneys from both uncontrolled and controlled NHBDs leads to acceptable graft function, although there is a high incidence of acute tubular necrosis. Livers procured from controlled non–heart-beating donors have had good immediate liver allograft function. However, liver allografts from uncontrolled NHBDs have had a high incidence of primary nonfunction. More studies will be required to determine the appropriate use of NHBDs for liver allograft transplantation.

MULTIPLE ORGAN PROCUREMENT

Individual Organ Assessment: Abdominal and Thoracic Organs

The preoperative assessment of organ function consists of a thorough evaluation of donor history, current physical examination, hospital history including evidence of cardiopulmonary resuscitation and arrest time, and laboratory evaluation of multiple organ function and serologies. In particular, evaluation of the cardiac donor includes a 12-lead electrocardiogram, normal cardiac isoenzymes in the case of chest trauma or if the donor has had cardiac arrest, and transthoracic or transesophageal echocardiography to evaluate for global or segmental myocardial dysfunction. Coronary angiography is helpful in evaluation of donors at risk for heart disease, especially in those with hypercholesterolemia, history of heart disease, diabetes, a history of smoking, and advanced age.

The evaluation of the heart-lung or isolated lung donor

includes careful attention to donor history as well as donor physical dimensions. The physiologic parameters used to assess the donor include the partial pressure of arterial oxygen/fraction of inspired oxygen ratio (PaO_2/FiO_2) at 250 mm Hg or more, as well as peak airway pressure of less than 30 cm H_2O. A bronchoscopy is indicated when there is a question of foreign body aspiration or to obtain sputum for culture to guide antibiotic therapy after transplantation.

Intestinal Donor Considerations

The management of the intestinal donor is similar to that of other organ donors. A bowel preparation regimen is important in the preparation of the intestinal donor. This includes intravenous ampicillin and cefotaxime every 6 hours preoperatively and enteral polyethylene glycol–electrolyte solution (GoLYTELY) administered through the nasogastric tube to flush the intestine. The administration rate is 10 to 30 ml/min for a total of 250 ml in the infant and 2000 ml in the adult. After intestinal flushing, an oral antibiotic mixture of polymyxin E (100 mg), tobramycin (80 mg), and amphotericin B (500 mg) is given through the nasogastric tube every 4 hours until procurement.

Multiple Organ Donor Operation

Coordinated care between anesthetic and surgical teams prior to organ donation is crucial to successful outcome. The anesthesia team, in particular, is given the responsibility of monitoring and maintaining adequate body temperature, muscle relaxation, and optimal ventilation and oxygenation, as well as preserving perfusion of all organs to be procured by maintaining appropriate intravascular volume with the judicious use of vasopressors if needed. Special issues of concern to the anesthesiologist include maintaining adequate diuresis, correction of hypothermia, and treatment of metabolic acidosis.

Metabolic acidosis must be treated by correcting the underlying cause. Sodium bicarbonate use should be limited to those patients who have a significant acidosis with a pH of less than 7.1 in order to prevent myocardial depression or arrhythmia. Hypernatremia is always a concern; therefore, tromethamine (THAM) may be used instead of sodium bicarbonate to correct metabolic acidosis. THAM is titrated for pH control. After cardioplegia and cross-clamping of the aorta are accomplished, mechanical ventilation and monitoring are discontinued.

The major principles of a successful multiorgan donor operation are effective communication between surgical teams, minimal preperfusion dissection, rapid cold perfusion of donor organs by in situ infusion of preservation solutions, and effective post-perfusion dissection and removal of organs. After a complete midline incision from the suprasternal notch to the pubis, a rapid inspection of the thoracic and abdominal organs is conducted. The thoracic team prepares the chest organs for removal by cannulating the aorta for infusion of cardioplegic solution and dissecting the main pulmonary artery if the lungs are to be harvested as well. The abdominal team obtains control of the aorta immediately above or below the diaphragm. The inferior mesenteric vein is encircled and cannulated for infusion of cold portal perfusate. The distal aorta above the bifurcation of the iliac arteries is prepared for cannulation. For liver procurement, a minimal hilar dissection consists of dividing the common bile duct and incising the gallbladder and washing it free of bile to prevent autolysis of the mucosa of the biliary tract. The arterial anatomy of the liver is carefully examined for possible anomalies. This is crucial in preventing errors during the subsequent organ removal.

After both teams have completed their dissections, 300 to 500 U/kg of heparin are given intravenously. The aorta is cannulated after ligating it distal to the inferior mesenteric artery. The thoracic team proceeds to occlude the superior vena cava, and the aorta is simultaneously clamped proximal to the innominate artery and just above or below the diaphragm. Cold perfusion with preservative solutions begins at this time, and the inferior vena cava is vented to prevent venous congestion. The heart is simultaneously perfused with cold cardioplegic solution. The heart and lungs are then removed sequentially, after which the abdominal organs are recovered. The liver, pancreas, intestine, and kidneys can be removed sequentially or en bloc. Iliac artery and vein procurement complete the recovery. Although extreme cooperation and coordination are required, successful multiple organ procurements from a single donor routinely yield viable allografts.

PRINCIPLES OF IMMUNOSUPPRESSION

The basic goal of immunosuppression is to prevent graft rejection with the least possible suppression of the immune system. This may seem a relatively simple task. However, since there are presently no accurate tests to quantify suppression of immunity and since rejection may present in a variety of clinical manifestations, this goal is often difficult to achieve. There are currently four classes of immunosuppressive drugs: corticosteroids, cytokine suppressors, cytotoxic agents, and antilymphocytic antibodies. The backbone of most immunosuppressive regimens is formed by a combination of a corticosteroid and a cytokine suppressor such as cyclosporin A (CyA). In general, more immunosuppression is required early in the post-transplantation period, and this requirement wanes somewhat with time. For reasons that are poorly understood, some patients are able to be completely withdrawn from therapy without rejection.

Any discussion of the control of rejection requires an understanding of basic immunology, especially with respect to cellular immunity. Antigen specificity is the hallmark of the T cell, and it is mediated by the T cell receptor (TCR). During early development, random rearrangements of specific genes create a vast library of TCRs capable of binding to virtually all antigens, both "self" and "nonself." Thymocytes with TCRs directed to self antigens are then destroyed.

Through their interaction with antigen-presenting cells (APCs) such as the macrophage, mature circulating lymphocytes are able to come in contact with foreign proteins that have been "processed." This processing by the APCs includes the production of major histocompatibility complex (MHC) molecules that display the foreign antigens. Once the lymphocyte with the right TCR comes in contact with the antigen, the MHC stimulates the lymphocyte to produce clones of itself. This antigen-directed proliferation of T cell clones is absolutely required for an effective immune response. Thereafter, a multiplicity of substances that modulate the immune response are also brought to bear. Chief among these substances are the cytokines. Cytokines attract and activate other leukocytes (including B cells), upregulate cellular adhesion molecules, and activate distant organ responses, such as the hepatic acute-phase response, bone marrow phagocyte synthesis, and stress hormone release by the endocrine system. Once the antigen is consumed or removed, the process downregulates. A number of sensitized memory T cells remain and contribute to the stronger secondary response seen with rechallenge. In humans, two distinct subsets of helper T cells appear to exist, Th1 and Th2. Th1 cells drive cellular immunity, whereas Th2 cells stimulate the humoral response.

The main focus of immunosuppression in the early post-transplantation period is on acute cellular rejection (ACR). Humoral rejection may play a role in some patients but is less common and less understood. Chronic rejection appears to be a different process entirely, and its manifestations vary depending on the organ involved. All the immunosuppressive agents currently in use, as well as several experimental agents, are shown in Table 12–2. In practice, these agents are used as part of the treatment of acute rejection and then are reduced or changed to other agents as maintenance therapy. Alternative regimens have been devised like "sequential therapy," which uses one therapy (such as OKT3) early on when the risk of toxicity from standard agents (such as CyA) is highest, and then uses these agents later.

CRITICAL CARE OF KIDNEY TRANSPLANT RECIPIENTS

Nearly 10,000 kidney transplantations are performed annually in the United States. Graft survival rates at 1 year are currently 75% to 90% for cadaveric and significantly higher for living related donor organs. In addition to the benefits to the patient in quality of life, the procedure is cost effective. Most patients receiving a kidney transplant do not require ICU admission. Those with specific medical conditions or complications arising from the surgery or immunosuppression may require ICU management.

Preoperative Evaluation

Preoperative evaluation of patients for kidney transplantation is usually done on an outpatient basis. Strict attention

Table 12–2. IMMUNOSUPPRESSIVE AGENTS

Agent	Indications	Dosage Range	Mechanism of Action	Toxicity
Corticosteroids				
Prednisone (and others)	Acute rejection Maintenance	250–1000 mg bolus 20–200 mg/d (or less)	Broad-spectrum anti-inflammatory, blocks IL-1 and IL-2 production, reduces lymphocyte traffic and circulating Ig levels, inhibits leukocyte adhesion	Infection, hyperglycemia, poor wound healing, GI ulceration, adrenal insufficiency, bone demineralization, etc.
Cytokine Suppressors				
Cyclosporin A (CyA)	Acute rejection Maintenance	3–6 mg/kg/d IV 3–20 mg/kg/d PO (adjusted by levels)	Inhibition of synthesis of several cytokines including IL-2, IL-3, IL-4, and interferon-γ; inhibition of GM-CSF	Acute reversible and chronic irreversible nephrotoxicity, hypertension, hirsutism, minor neurotoxicity (common), major neurotoxicity (rarely), hepatic cholestasis
Tacrolimus (FK-506)	Acute rejection Maintenance Chronic rejection	0.05–0.15 mg/k/d IV 0.15 mg/kg/d PO (adjusted by levels)	Inhibition of calcineurin phosphatase, decreases IL-2 (blocks transcription of m-RNA)	Acute reversible nephrotoxicity, hypertension (less than CyA), neurotoxicity (similar to CyA), QT prolongation (rare), hyperkalemia
Rapamycin (RPM)	Undetermined	Undetermined	Inhibits DTH and both B and T cell responses to alloantigen, inhibits RNA translation of cytokine genes	Unknown

Table continued on following page

Table 12–2. IMMUNOSUPPRESSIVE AGENTS *Continued*

Agent	Indications	Dosage Range	Mechanism of Action	Toxicity
Cytotoxic Agents				
Azathioprine (AZA)	Maintenance	0.5–5 mg/kg/d PO 1-2 mg/kg/d IV	Antimetabolite, inhibits purine metabolism (required for DNA and RNA synthesis), inhibits generation of antigen-specific T cell clones?	Myelosuppression (pancytopenia), nausea/vomiting, and hair loss; reversible hepatitis and rare hepatic veno-occlusive disease; pancreatitis; hypersensitivity
Cyclophosphamide (CPM)	Maintenance Acute (humoral?) rejection	3–5 mg/kg/d PO	Alkylating agent; nonspecifically damages cellular macromolecules, particularly in DNA; greatest effect on B cells	Nausea/vomiting and hair loss, hemorrhagic cystitis, SIADH, cardiac toxicity (15%)
Antilymphocyte Antibodies				
Antithymocyte globulin (ATG)	Acute rejection	10–15 mg/kg/d IV	Equine polyclonal antibody to lymphocytes	Febrile reactions, leukopenia, thrombocytopenia, skin rash, anaphylaxis (<1%)
OKT3	Acute rejection, "sequential therapy"	5 mg/d IV	Murine antibody to CD3 (a T cell protein in close proximity to the TCR), effect is to dramatically reduce circulating levels of effective T cells	Fever/chills, tachycardia, hypo- or hypertension, GI distress with the first few doses (steroid pretreatment helpful), viral infection, lymphoproliferative disorders

Other Agents				
Mycophenolic acid (RS-61443)	Undetermined	Undetermined	Inhibits inosine monophosphate dehydrogenase (which is involved in GMP synthesis), interferes with expression of leukocyte adhesion molecules?	GI toxicity, mucositis, leukopenia
Mizoribine	Maintenance	50–300 mg/d PO	Adenosine analog, inhibits inosine monophosphate dehydrogenase	Unknown
Brequinar	Undetermined	Undetermined	Inhibits dihydrorotate dehydrogenase, which is involved in pyrimidine synthesis	Thrombocytopenia, desquamative dermatitis
15-Deoxyspergualin	Undetermined	80–220 $mg/m^2/d$ IV 3–5 mg/kg/d IV	Unknown	Facial dysesthesias, GI upset, marrow suppression, hypotension

Abbreviations: DTH, delayed-type hypersensitivity reaction; GM-CSF, granulocyte-macrophage colony-stimulating factor; GMP, guanosine monophosphate; SIADH, syndrome of inappropriate antidiuretic hormone; TCR, T cell receptor.

is paid to comorbid medical conditions, and, because of the high incidence of coronary artery disease in this population, stress or adenosine thallium tests are frequently done. This is especially true of diabetic patients. Cardiac catheterization is also performed if necessary. Active infection or malignancy is an absolute contraindication for transplantation. Also, psychosocial evaluation is enormously important.

Serologic studies for hepatitis A, B, and C, cytomegalovirus (CMV), and HIV are routinely checked. HLA typing and panel-reactive antibody (PRA) testing are also performed. The results of this entire work-up are then presented to the evaluation committee, which decides whether the patient should be listed for a transplantation. There is no absolute age limit: recipients have ranged from 8 to 78 years of age. As with other types of transplants, organs are allocated according to a computerized point system that considers antigen matching, PRA levels, and time on the list.

Perioperative Management

When a kidney becomes available, the patient is immediately admitted to the hospital and evaluated. Preoperative dialysis is done for volume overload or hyperkalemia. Preoperative monitoring is usually noninvasive, though central venous lines are used in most cases. Diabetic patients and those with other underlying organ dysfunction may require more invasive monitoring techniques. Unless there is a specific indication for nephrectomy, the native kidneys are not removed. The graft is placed in the iliac fossa. The renal vessels are anastomosed, usually end-to-side with the iliac vessels. Intravenous furosemide (1 mg/kg) and mannitol (1 g/kg) are given, and the ureter is implanted into the recipient's bladder. Antibiotic prophylaxis with a first-generation cephalosporine, both systemic and topical, is routine.

In the immediate postoperative period, urine output is extremely variable, and fluid replacement is regulated accordingly. If urine output is greater than 300 mL/hour, 80% of this volume is replaced with either normal saline or D5/NS. If urine output is less than 300 mL/hour, all the volume is replaced with either solution. General postoperative care is otherwise similar to that of nontransplantation patients. Skin staples are generally left in longer, however (3 weeks), to take account of slower wound healing because of steroid medication.

Immunosuppression usually consists of cyclosporine (CyA), azathioprine (AZA), and prednisone in various combinations. Tacrolimus (FK-506), OKT3, and antithymocyte globulin (ATG) are also used for rejection (or as primary immunosuppression in some centers). Anti-infection prophylaxis with nystatin, acyclovir, and trimethoprim-sulfamethoxazole is also routine.

Indications for ICU Admission

Most patients do not require admission to the ICU. Those who do can be divided into early and late admissions.

Early admissions (within the first 3 months) are typically secondary to problems arising from cardiopulmonary dysfunction, renal failure, rejection, or technical complications. Late admissions are usually for infection or gastrointestinal or neurologic complications.

Patients with left ventricular ejection fraction of less than 30% or significant coronary artery disease usually require perioperative hemodynamic monitoring with pulmonary artery and arterial catheters. The femoral vessels on the same side as the allograft are avoided for such purposes. These patients are at higher risk for volume overload, and this may lead to pulmonary dysfunction. In general, patients without underlying lung disease do not require mechanical ventilation postoperatively.

Severe hypertension can also complicate the perioperative management. This is usually a result of fluid overload or withdrawal from antihypertensive medications or from CyA. Most patients can be managed without intravenous treatment. If nitroprusside is used, thiocyanate levels must be followed. Beta-blocker therapy is also used but can cause hyperkalemia.

Allograft dysfunction is a frequent indication for admission to the ICU. Oliguria in the early postoperative period may occur secondary to ischemia (during procurement and transportation), hypovolemia, vascular thrombosis, or hyperacute rejection. Also, obstruction of the ureter from a hematoma or even the Foley catheter may be the cause. Allograft function usually improves over the first 7 to 21 days if the cause is acute tubular necrosis. Patients with hemodynamic instability or severe hypoxemia may not tolerate standard hemodialysis. Continuous venovenous hemofiltration (with or without dialysis) is much better tolerated in such patients.

Rejection is a common cause of allograft dysfunction, occurring in 50% or more of patients. Rejection is categorized into hyperacute, accelerated, acute, or chronic. Hyperacute rejection is mediated by preformed antibodies and should never occur with the availability of pretransplant cross-matching techniques. When it does occur, the graft fails in minutes and immediate removal is required. Accelerated rejection occurs in the first few days after transplantation and usually leads to irreversible graft thrombosis and destruction. Acute rejection is much more common; it occurs from 1 week to several months after transplantation. It can manifest as a rise in creatinine with or without change in urine volume. Biopsy is required for definitive diagnosis. Treatment consists of high-dose steroids and/or OKT3 (or ATG). Chronic rejection occurs late after transplantation. It is poorly understood and difficult to treat.

Technical complications are unusual but need to be recognized early. Bleeding may occur from inadequate hemostasis or from platelet dysfunction secondary to uremia. The latter is effectively treated with DDAVP (0.3 μg/kg) and/or intravenous estrogens (0.6 mg/kg each day for 5 days). Hemodialysis and cryoprecipitate may also be required. Vascular complications include thrombosis, stenosis, and disruption.

Ureteral complications include stenosis or anastomotic leak. This can be secondary to technical error or ischemia. These complications usually require operative repair. Another complication is a lymphocele secondary to lymphatic disruption. This may manifest as unilateral leg edema and fluid collection around the allograft. Lymphocele is usually drained via a surgically created peritoneal window.

Late complications requiring admission to the ICU are most often related to immunosuppression and its complications. Infection is the most significant and will be discussed separately. Other complications include gastrointestinal and neurologic problems. Gastrointestinal complications include every organ of the digestive system. Esophagitis from *Candida* infection (discussed later) and reflux can be exacerbated by steroids. Similarly, peptic ulcer disease occurs more frequently in these patients. Routine prophylaxis with H_2-blockers or sucralfate appears to reduce this risk. Gastroparesis may occur in the diabetic patient, prompting the use of metoclopramide. Erythromycin may also be used for this indication. For the intestines, large bowel complications are more common than small bowel complications. Pseudo-obstruction of the large bowel (Ogilvie's syndrome) may be seen, particularly in patients with a failing allograft. This complication tends to occur earlier and can lead to perforation with sepsis or even death. Early decompression via colonoscopy is the treatment of choice, though surgery is often required.

Liver and gallbladder disease is also significant in this population. Immunosuppression may exacerbate new or preexisting disease such as viral hepatitis. CyA may cause cholestasis, and gallstone formation is not uncommon. It is important to note that if biliary drainage is required, an open T-tube will significantly decrease CyA levels since CyA is excreted by the liver into the bile. Pancreatitis, either secondary to gallstones, drugs, or hypercalcemia, can be a serious problem. Withdrawal of the offending agent and supportive care are usually effective. Somatostatin may be useful in the treatment of severe pancreatitis.

Neurologic complications are usually related to drug toxicity or infections. Metabolic encephalopathy, hypertensive encephalopathy, cerebral vascular events, and new-onset seizures have all been reported. Caution is needed when phenobarbital or phenytoin is used for seizure, as these drugs induce cytochrome P-450 and can markedly reduce circulating cyclosporine levels if the dose is not adjusted accordingly.

Infectious Complications

Infection remains the most common complication and the leading cause of death in kidney transplantation. Infectious complications are similar among patients receiving various types of transplantation and are covered in more detail in Chapter 8. Infections that are more important to specific types of transplants will be discussed in the section covering that type of transplant.

The first few months following transplantation is the period of highest risk. About one third of renal transplant recipients will acquire infection in the first 4 years. In life-threatening infection, it is important to remember that the transplanted kidney is expendable; immunosuppression is routinely stopped in this setting. Roughly half of all infections occurring in the renal transplant patient are viral. Four main types of viruses are recognized: the herpes viruses (Epstein-Barr, CMV, zoster, and simplex), adenovirus, papovavirus, and hepatitis virus. CMV is the most common. To prevent CMV infection, patients receive acyclovir prophylaxis (dose-adjusted for renal function) for the first 6 months. Also, CMV-seronegative recipients receiving seropositive grafts are given anti-CMV hyperimmune globulin. When prophylaxis fails, gancyclovir is used for treatment. The clinical spectrum of CMV infection ranges from asymptomatic to serious systemic disease, although mortality is now rare with gancyclovir. CMV can occur as a primary infection or as reactivation. The presence of CMV early antigen in the bronchoalveolar lavage (BAL) fluid or in the gastric biopsy specimen with compatible clinical features is an indication for gancyclovir treatment. If CMV infection is severe (especially with pneumonitis), immunosuppression should be stopped.

Herpes simplex infections usually present as mucocutaneous lesions and respond well to intravenous acyclovir. Herpes zoster infections (shingles) also respond to acyclovir. Epstein-Barr virus is often associated with post-transplant lymphoproliferative disorder (PTLD), which can result in serious systemic complications, multiple organ failure, or death. Immunosuppressive therapy is withdrawn, and high-dose acyclovir or gancyclovir is administered. Established PTLD also requires cytotoxic chemotherapy.

Bacteria account for about one third of all infections in renal transplantation patients. Urinary tract infections are common, and prompt, effective treatment is required to prevent ascending infections; bladder catheterization should be avoided, if possible. Mycobacterial infections are unusual but can be life-threatening. Patients with a positive skin test (PPD) should receive isoniazid for 1 year after transplantation. Patients presenting with pulmonary infections should be placed in respiratory isolation until three negative sputum samples are obtained. Treatment of active tuberculosis includes three- or four-drug therapy and cessation of immunosuppression. *Legionella* pneumonia may also occur in this population. Ciprofloxacin or ofloxacin are both effective, as well as erythromycin. Infections with *Pneumocystis carinii*, a protozoa, can be virtually avoided with prophylactic use of trimethoprim-sulfamethoxazole (80/400 mg per day) or inhaled pentamidine (300 mg once a month).

Fungal infections are also a source of morbidity and mortality in the transplant patient. *Candida* is the most common fungal pathogen. Other organisms such as *Mucor, Aspergillus,* or *Cryptococcus* may also produce serious disease. Systemic amphotericin B remains the mainstay of therapy.

CRITICAL CARE OF LIVER TRANSPLANT RECIPIENTS

Orthotopic liver transplantation (OLTx) has become a recognized therapeutic option for patients with end-stage liver disease (ESLD). Although OLTx is expensive, it may well be more cost effective than conventional medical care for terminally ill liver failure patients. Significant progress has been made since the first OLTx in humans was performed by Starzl in 1963. With the introduction of CyA in 1981, the procedure became medically feasible. Currently, sophisticated surgery, anesthesia, and critical care management have afforded 1-year survival rates of nearly 90%.

Candidate Selection

In addition to good general medical status, the risk of recurrence of the primary disease should be low in patients considered for OLTx. Although patients who are at highest risk for surgery are also likely to have the most to gain by a successful outcome, such patients have a higher mortality and require significantly greater resources—particularly intensive care and rehabilitation. In general, centers with more experience are called on to care for patients with higher risk.

Organ availability also plays a pivotal role. When organs are scarce, or not distributed according to need, patients who are at high risk may die before a transplantation can be performed. Patients who are already in the ICU and those with prior right upper quadrant abdominal surgery (particularly biliary reconstruction) tend to have worse outcomes. Patients with cirrhosis and underlying hepatocellular carcinomas may still be candidates for OLTx provided the disease is very limited. The high recurrence rate of chronic viral hepatitis has led some centers to exclude these patients. At present, patients with evidence of active viral replication are currently considered poor candidates for OLTx.

Surgical Procedure

The recipient operation has become a highly refined surgical procedure. It may be divided into three phases: hepatectomy phase, anhepatic phase, and reperfusion phase. Each phase involves special consideration by the anesthesiologist and surgeon. The vascular anastomoses can be varied according to the size and condition of the donor vessels. The donor and recipient caval veins are usually anastomosed end-to-end above and below the liver. The biliary anastomosis is fashioned after the vascular anastomoses are completed and the graft reperfused. Two options currently used are a duct-to-duct anastomosis with T tube drainage or creation of a midjejunal Roux-en-Y limb with a choledochojejunostomy. The former, though faster, has a higher stenosis rate. In approximately 10% of patients, reperfusion is accompanied by cardiovascular collapse (reperfusion syndrome), usually of short duration. The exact mechanism for this syndrome is undefined, although hypocalcemia may play a role in some cases. Monitoring of the coagulation activity is greatly aided by the use of the thromboelastograph. It provides a rapid, quantitative assessment of the coagulation status, indicating the presence or absence of fibrinolysis, and assesses the effects of intervention with protamine or epsilon-aminocaproic acid.

Postoperative Liver Function

The function of the transplanted liver is the dominant factor in the recovery of the patient. In the ICU, early graft function is usually assessed by measurement of total levels of bilirubin, transaminases, canalicular enzymes, and clotting factors. However, no single variable can be identified that adequately predicts graft function in an individual patient. Therefore, the overall status of the patient, including the function of other organs, is a useful guide to assess graft function. Typically, an elevated bilirubin in the first few days reflects preoperative values and the consequence of procurement ischemia. In the absence of severe harvest injury, bilirubin levels typically fall to normal during the first week. Transaminases (alanine and aspartate aminotransferases) often show an injury pattern, with elevations during the first 3 days that slowly return to normal. Canalicular enzymes (gamma-glutamyl transpeptidase and alkaline phosphatase) usually rise to four or five times normal and return to normal over the next few weeks. Unless the graft is severely damaged, synthetic function will normalize after the third day. Occasionally graft dysfunction may be evidenced only by the patient's failure to thrive. In particular, multiple organ system failure may develop or fail to resolve. Retransplantation may be the only option.

When evidence suggests graft dysfunction, a thorough diagnostic work-up must be undertaken even when patterns suggest a certain diagnosis. Technical problems should always be ruled out before other mechanisms are incriminated. The diagnostic work-up should include a Doppler ultrasound examination to determine vessel patency, and concern about the adequacy of flow should prompt an angiogram. Arterial and venous complications present differently. Early occlusion of the hepatic artery may be approached surgically with a nearly 50% graft salvage rate. It presents with a precipitous deterioration in the patient's hemodynamic status, abrupt development of respiratory failure (ARDS, adult respiratory distress syndrome), severe coagulopathy, and marked transaminase elevations. Enteric bacteremia is another common manifestation. Late hepatic artery thrombosis is often less dramatic in its presentation, with some patients actually asymptomatic. Others show destruction of the biliary duct system with multiple intrahepatic strictures, bilomas, and intrahepatic abscesses. Recurrent bacteremia, in the absence of another source, may be the only indication suggestive of hepatic artery thrombosis.

The presentation of portal venous thrombosis may be more subtle. In the early postoperative period, the most frequent manifestation is persistent ascites. Mesenteric congestion and bleeding as a consequence of portal hypertension may also occur. Later, a thrombosed portal vein should be considered if the patient presents with variceal hemorrhage. Stenosis at the lower anastomosis of the inferior vena cava is manifest solely by lower extremity edema and renal dysfunction. Stenosis at the upper anastomosis may present as a syndrome similar to Budd-Chiari syndrome, with marked passive congestion of the liver, ascites, lower extremity edema, and renal failure. The approach to this problem is usually surgical, but balloon dilatation has been accomplished in some cases. Competency of the biliary tract should be confirmed by cholangiography when elevated canalicular enzymes or persistent jaundice is present. Disruption of the biliary anastomosis is rare but typically occurs near the end of the first week and may indicate thrombosis of the hepatic artery. It may be heralded by developing sepsis syndrome and a disproportionate rise in the bilirubin.

Graft rejection may occur at any point following OLTx. Hyperacute rejection is quite rare, if it occurs at all with OLTx. More commonly, acute cellular rejection (ACR) develops. This is often evident after the first week but has occurred within the first few days and after several years. In a graft with stable function, acute rejection is typically associated with a new rise in bilirubin and elevation of the transaminase and canalicular enzyme levels. Other clinical findings include fever, hematologic abnormalities (thrombocytopenia, hemolysis, eosinophilia), diarrhea, and increased ascites. Occasionally, full-blown sepsis results. Like ACR, chronic rejection is also a misnomer as it may occur at any point. Its pathology is that of arteriopathy and vanishing bile ducts. Its presentation is insidious, and signs of terminal liver disease may develop slowly. Liver biopsy and clinical context are used to make the diagnosis of both types of rejection. Immunosuppression for OLTx is accomplished with FK-506 (or CyA) and corticosteroids. Cross-match negative recipients usually can be managed with slightly less immunosuppression. ACR is usually treated with high-dose steroids and increased FK-506 (or CyA), but AZA and OKT3 may also be used for resistant ACR. Systemic illness, especially infection, may also compromise liver function.

ICU Management

ICU management frequently begins preoperatively. Patients with end-stage liver disease (ESLD) severe enough to make them eligible for OLTx often deteriorate precipitously and require admission to the ICU. Common precipitants include infection (particularly pneumonia and spontaneous bacterial peritonitis) and gastrointestinal bleeding (from esophageal and gastric varices, portal hypertensive gastropathy, gastric and duodenal ulceration, and so on). Such events may prove fatal for patients with ESLD. Because the failing liver has such a profound effect on other organ systems, concurrent organ failure is common in this population. Although certain conditions outlined earlier contraindicate OLTx, success has been achieved with patients requiring dialytic support for renal failure, requiring mechanical ventilation, or suffering from severe encephalopathy (grade IV), profound coagulopathies, and multisystem organ failure (MSOF). Usually, with good graft function, these complications will resolve.

The postoperative management of the OLTx recipient is largely governed by the preoperative condition, the adequacy of the donor organ, and the details of the intraoperative course. The characteristic hemodynamic changes of ESLD resolve slowly after liver transplantation. A vasodilated, hyperdynamic state is typical and rarely normalizes completely within the immediate postoperative period. Patients who are unable to mount a hyperdynamic response have much higher mortality. Marked elevation in right-sided cardiac pressures compromises allograft function. Careful management of intravascular volume, combined with judicious use of inotropes, is therefore required. Hepatic congestion results in hyperbilirubinemia and elevated portal pressures (perhaps resulting in bacterial translocation and endotoxemia with further graft dysfunction). Similarly, a depressed cardiac output causes decreased hepatic arterial and portal flow and allograft ischemia. Marked arterial vasodilation, which requires treatment with vasopressors, particularly when it occurs in the face of improving graft function, should prompt an evaluation for a focus of inflammation (infection, pancreatitis, and graft rejection). A low (or even normal) cardiac output, occurring early in the postoperative course, raises the concern for myocardial ischemia or cardiac tamponade. Hypertension commonly reflects inadequate analgesia or sedation, impaired gas exchange, or hypoglycemia. It may also occur as a result of CyA or less commonly FK-506.

Pulmonary complications of ESLD are common and include atelectasis, pleural effusions, reduced functional reserve capacity, and limited vital capacity related to ascites. Fortunately, long-term pulmonary sequelae are rare, and most patients have improved pulmonary function tests when studied more than 1 year after OLTx. However, the prompt evaluation of pulmonary infiltrates in these patients is mandatory. In addition to infection, pulmonary edema and ARDS are commonly seen. ARDS may result from infection (especially abdominal), pancreatitis, or graft failure from any cause. When liver failure, per se, is identified as the cause, ARDS will resolve after transplantation. ARDS may also develop during treatment of rejection with OKT3. Bronchoscopic techniques such as BAL and protected brush (PB) are often used to establish the diagnosis. Despite the severe derangements of coagulation present in such patients, these procedures can usually be performed safely. Quantitative cultures from BAL specimens are sensitive but less specific for the diagnosis of pneumonia. Although there is some increased risk of bleeding with the use of PB, this technique is more specific.

Patients with liver disease may also develop two specific pulmonary complications: the hepatopulmonary syndrome (HPS) and pulmonary hypertension (PHTN). HPS is characterized by hypoxemia, cyanosis, and clubbing in a patient with ESLD. The precise mechanism responsible for these findings is unclear. Intrapulmonary shunting has been found in patients with HPS. However, most patients improve with oxygen and, instead of having pure shunt physiology, appear to exhibit a diffusion defect caused by the presence of dilated intrapulmonary capillaries. Patients with HPS also have impaired hypoxic pulmonary vasoconstriction. The diagnosis can be established most easily by contrast echocardiography. Such patients may be successfully transplanted with resolution of HPS, though more than a year may be required for complete resolution.

PHTN occurs more commonly in patients with cirrhosis than in noncirrhotics. No precipitant has been identified. The picture may become clouded when the process evolves to right ventricular failure with secondary hepatic congestion. Whereas patients with mild PHTN (mean PA pressures of less than 35 mm Hg) undergo OLTx without significant complications, the picture is bleak for those with moderate to severe PHTN. Right ventricular overload and failure develop abruptly, particularly upon reperfusion of the graft. This rapidly compromises the graft, resulting in massive liver and bowel congestion. Low cardiac output results in graft ischemia. These patients succumb quickly in the face of acute multiple organ failure. Such patients are not currently considered candidates for liver transplantation.

Mechanical ventilatory support for patients following OLTx is generally routine with the exception of two issues. First, in the setting of hypoxemia when airway pressure is efficiently reflected in central venous pressure, as in the patients with intrapulmonary shunt, increasing the FiO_2 may be safer than raising the airway pressure. This is because airway pressure is reflected in the hepatic venous and portal venous pressures. The second issue is that of extubation. An increased risk is associated with aspiration pneumonia in this population. Therefore, the patient should have a clear mental state and improving liver function values prior to extubation. The median duration of intubation after transplantation is between 2 and 3 days.

Renal dysfunction in patients with liver disease is frequently unrecognized. Liver dysfunction and malnutrition make elevations in BUN and creatinine unimpressive despite significant derangements in glomerular filtration. In the post-transplant period, medication such as CyA and FK-506, vasopressors, aminoglycosides, and amphotericin may complicate this picture further. In addition, liver allograft dysfunction may lead to a functional impairment of the kidneys analogous to the hepatorenal syndrome. Dialytic support is required in approximately 10% of patients but is usually temporary.

Patients with minimal pretransplant hepatic encephalopathy who have an uncomplicated operation and receive a good graft usually have rapid normalization of neurologic function after the effects of general anesthesia have resolved. Changes in mental status in such patients require aggressive evaluation. Most commonly, side effects of immunosuppressives such as CyA and FK-506 may be identified and resolve with adjustment of medication. The differential diagnosis also includes other medications (analgesics, sedatives, OKT3, and haloperidol), electrolyte abnormalities (hyponatremia and hypomagnesemia), and hypoglycemia. Focal deficits make embolic or hemorrhagic complications a concern. Intracranial infection is rare in the early postoperative period but must be ruled out in the patient who presents at a later date with headache and confusion.

Infections in this population are similar to those of other transplant groups. Fungal infections may be more common in the OLTx population, and fungal colonization is common. Patients with prolonged, difficult surgical procedures who are heavily transfused seem to be at higher risk for fungal infection, as are patients who undergo retransplantation. The routine use of low-dose amphotericin (10 to 20 mg/day) postoperatively for 14 days may be beneficial.

Hyperglycemia is common in the early postoperative period and reflects the combination of stress and administration of corticosteroids and FK-506 (or CyA). Patients are routinely managed with continuous infusions of insulin, with the dose adjusted according to a sliding scale. Hypoglycemia may be precipitated by liver allograft failure as gluconeogenesis is impaired. The sudden development of marked hyperglycemia or symptomatic hypoglycemia that is not iatrogenic should prompt an evaluation for infection. However, secondary adrenal insufficiency may occur in these patients when steroids are abruptly discontinued or they are subjected to supraphysiologic stress. Also, the adrenals may be affected by direct injury during OLTx, or from infection (CMV) or hemorrhage. Thyroid dysfunction, particularly hypothyroidism, is common in patients with primary biliary cirrhosis and in autoimmune hepatitis.

Fulminant Hepatic Failure

Fulminant hepatic failure (FHF) is defined as liver failure with encephalopathy in a patient without previously known liver disease, developing within an 8-week period. FHF is increasingly being managed with OLTx. With this surgical option, the survival has improved from 20% to 75%. Such patients are often critically ill at the time of transplantation. They require intensive monitoring (described later) before, during, and after OLTx. Although some patients may improve with supportive care, most will not. Progressive encephalopathy with sustained intracranial hypertension resulting in inadequate cerebral perfusion precludes successful OLTx, as brain death will result. Such patients are also prone to develop pancreatitis, which, when severe, makes OLTx an unacceptably high risk. Cardiovascular instability, arrhythmias, and respiratory insufficiency are common complications of FHF and make the operative risk significantly higher. Patients who require high-dose vasopressor support and those with severe ARDS are also at unacceptable operative risk.

Patients with FHF require special neurologic consideration because of the risk of elevated intracranial pressure (ICP) and cerebral edema. When such patients develop grade III or IV coma, they should be monitored with an epidural ICP monitor. Measurement of cerebral blood flow via inhalation xenon CT and cerebral oxygen consumption via jugular bulb catheter can be used to guide management. Continuous EEG monitoring may also be needed if pentobarbital is required for the control of elevated ICP. Patients are considered viable candidates for OLTx as long as EEG activity is preserved and adequate cerebral perfusion pressure can be maintained with sustained cerebral blood flow. Intraoperative monitoring includes the preceding measures, combined with the transcranial Doppler. Although the initial period of graft reperfusion is the most hazardous, cerebral hyperemia and intracranial hypertension may persist for several days postoperatively.

CRITICAL CARE OF CARDIAC TRANSPLANT RECIPIENTS

Cardiovascular disease is responsible for over 800,000 deaths in the United States each year. Over the last decade, significant advances have been made in the field of cardiac transplantation. Currently, survival at 1 year exceeds 80%. These successes have prompted the development of numerous centers that now offer this procedure. Over 150 such centers are in existence in the United States today, compared with only 5 in 1981. With this growth has come an appreciation of the importance of perioperative support specific to these unique patients.

Patient Selection

Ischemic heart disease is the most common etiology of heart disease in recipients of cardiac transplantation. With the advent of new immunosuppressive drugs (CyA, FK-506), improved surgical technique, and perioperative support, many patients previously classified as noncandidates can be successfully transplanted. Age, for instance, is no longer an absolute barrier to transplantation; in selected cases, recipients may be older than age 65 years. However, high pulmonary vascular resistance (PVR) remains a contraindication. Obviously, patients with severe dysfunction of other vital organs are also poor candidates for cardiac transplantation.

Postoperative Care

During the initial postoperative phase, cardiovascular monitoring and support are extremely important. Interpretation of the electrocardiogram requires an understanding of the postoperative anatomy (see Figure 178–2 in the *Textbook of Critical Care*). The remnant of the native atria may produce a second (nonconducted) P wave. Anatomic considerations are also important for therapy because the denervated heart will not respond to vagal stimuli, as such medications (e.g., atropine) or maneuvers that alter vagal tone will not affect the transplanted heart. Initially the intrinsic rate of the denervated heart may be quite slow. Ventricular contractility is also impaired as a result of hypothermia, preservation injury, and possible ischemia. For these reasons, initial cardiac output is very low, and thorough invasive monitoring is required. This typically includes a right ventricle ejection fraction Swan-Ganz catheter, arterial catheter, and pulse oximeter. Transesophageal echocardiography is also frequently employed to evaluate ventricular size and regional wall motion.

Support for the newly transplanted heart first consists of both inotropic and chronotropic stimulation. Combined β_1 and β_2 agonists such as dobutamine and isoproterenol are the usual agents chosen. The goals of therapy are to increase the heart rate to more than 90 beats/min and the cardiac index to more than 2.5 $L \cdot min^{-1} \cdot m^{-2}$. Dobutamine appears to be superior in this setting because it causes less peripheral vasodilatation. Patients are typically started on doses of 5 to 10 $\mu g \cdot kg^{-1} \cdot min^{-1}$. Other agents such as epinephrine, dopamine, amrinone, and levarterenol are used infrequently. None of this, however, should obscure the fact that the transplanted heart is exquisitely preload-dependent. This underscores the importance of close monitoring of the intravascular volume. In addition, despite the inherent risks of transfusion, current practice is to maintain hemoglobin concentrations above 10 g/dL to maintain optimal oxygen delivery. All such therapy must, of course, be individualized. Occasionally, aggressive support with intra-aortic balloon counterpulsation or ventricular assist devices may be deemed appropriate. However, enthusiasm for these maneuvers has waned in recent years in light of the risk of infection and limited success rates.

One major complication requiring the use of specialized supportive care is that of recalcitrant pulmonary hypertension. The newly transplanted heart may suffer acute RV failure when exposed to these high pressures. The use of prostaglandin E_1 has been beneficial for some patients with pulmonary hypertension secondary to mitral valve disease. Occasionally an "oversized" donor heart is used when elevated pulmonary vascular resistance (PVR) is known preoperatively, and this has reduced the risk of early postoperative RV failure. However, a transpulmonary gradient in excess of 15 mm Hg generally suggests a poor prognosis. Heterotopic heart transplantation (connecting the new heart in parallel) has also been used in this setting but carries with it its own unique complications, such as compression of the right lower lung and thrombus formation in the native heart.

Certain surgical complications should be mentioned. Atrial septal defects may occur if the atria are placed under too much tension. A patent foramen ovale may also open postoperatively and, therefore, is looked for intraoperatively. Other complications such as pulmonary artery torsion, delayed cardiac tamponade, and RV perforation secondary to endomyocardial biopsy are relatively rare. The risks of RV perforation and coronary artery fistula formation are highest, however, with the first biopsy, and therefore this is usually done in the operating room.

Antiarrhythmic therapy can also be challenging in this population. Because the transplanted heart is denervated, the most frequent rhythm exhibited in the early postoperative period is sinus bradycardia or low-grade AV block. Also, denervation means that drugs such as atropine and digoxin, which affect vagal tone, will have no effect on the heart rate. Consequently, bradycardia must be treated with β-agonists and atrial arrhythmias with direct-acting agents (Table 12–3).

Pulmonary support is tailored to the clinical situation, with attention to details such as hypothermia, which markedly reduces metabolic rate. As the patient is rewarmed, minute ventilation must be increased to avoid respiratory acidosis. Shivering is usually treated with judicious administration of sedation and neuromuscular blockers as it is associated with a marked increase in oxygen consumption. Most patients will meet routine criteria for extubation within 12 to 18 hours of surgery. Unilateral diaphragm paresis, particularly on the left, is associated with hypothermic injury to the phrenic nerve. The problem usually resolves within 7 to 10 days and does not typically exclude extubation unless bilateral. However, occasional cases of prolonged, severe dysfunction have occurred. Pulmonary dysfunction may also occur secondary to parenchymal disease. This problem almost always prompts aggressive measures to exclude infection (including fiberoptic bronchoscopy with bronchoalveolar lavage and/or transbronchial biopsy) because the risks of infection in the immunosuppressed host are significant.

Pulmonary infections are most often caused by gram-negative bacilli, and broad-spectrum antipseudomonal coverage is generally started while cultures are pending. Despite their relative rarity, close attention to opportunistic infections, including *Pneumocystis*, *Aspergillus*, and CMV, is always appropriate. Pulmonary edema may also masquerade as infection and may herald rejection. Sepsis syndrome from any source may produce ARDS and may be difficult to distinguish from primary pulmonary infection. Atelectasis is common (especially of the left lower lobe), and the resultant hypoxemia may be exaggerated by use of vasodilators that blunt the normal hypoxic vasoconstriction. Positive end-expiratory pressure (PEEP) and chest physiotherapy are usually effective in treating atelectasis, although rarely therapeutic bronchoscopy is also required.

Common metabolic considerations include hypomagnesemia and hypo- and hyperkalemia. These derangements may produce cardiac arrhythmias, exacerbate myocardial dysfunction, and produce coronary artery spasm and CNS or renal dysfunction. Hypophosphatemia may also occur and further impair cardiac performance as well as having effects on platelet, CNS, and pulmonary function. Respiratory alkalosis is common early in the postoperative period, followed by a metabolic alkalosis.

Although extensive hemorrhage requiring reoperation is rare, some bleeding is common in the postoperative period, and this requires prompt evaluation and treatment. Coagulation factors should be replaced, and consideration should be given to use of protamine, DDAVP, increased PEEP, and surgical re-exploration. Caution is needed when protamine is used, though severe adverse reactions (hypotension, pulmonary edema, bronchospasm) are rare. Titration of protamine to an activated clotting time of 100 to 120 seconds is

Table 12–3. ANTIARRHYTHMICS

Agent	Use	Comments
Atropine	None	To increase heart rate in the denervated heart, β-agonists (e.g., dobutamine, isoproterenol) are used instead
Digoxin	Chronic atrial arrhythmias	Not useful in the control of acute atrial arrhythmias
Lidocaine	Ventricular arrhythmias	Toxicity may occur more commonly in the transplant population due to decreased clearance
Phenytoin	Ventricular arrhythmias	Decreased clearance, increases metabolism of CyA and FK-506
Quinidine	VT, SVT	Acceleration in heart rate typical of this drug is not seen in the denervated heart
Procainamide	VT, SVT	Toxicity common especially with renal insufficiency, negative inotropism more apparent in the transplanted heart
Bretylium	VT	Unpredictable and rarely used in transplant population
Verapamil	SVT	Effective but severe negative inotropic effects limit use
Diltiazem	SVT	May be better tolerated than verapamil, especially as a continuous infusion
Esmolol	SVT	β-Blocker therapy is best avoided; however, when indicated, this agent's short half-life allows for effective titration

Abbreviations: SVT, supraventricular tachycardia; VT, ventricular tachycardia.

recommended. Persistent bleeding at rates more than 200 mL/hour or drainage hematocrit greater than one half the circulating blood hematocrit is generally accepted as an indication for re-exploration.

Immunosuppression is first achieved by use of AZA and steroids. CyA is usually started 12 hours after the operation. Some centers prefer to use ATG or OKT3, usually beginning on day 3. FK-506 is also under evaluation for use as primary immunosuppression in cardiac transplantation, and early results are encouraging.

Infection complications are similar to those seen in other patients with immunosuppression, with certain exceptions. Mediastinitis occurs in approximately 3% of cases (and is much higher when ventricular assist devices are used). This problem frequently occurs late and can be almost asymptomatic. *Staphylococcus* or gram-negative bacteria are the usual pathogens, although *Mycoplasma hominis* has also been implicated. Abdominal complications, including bowel perforation, are common in this population and may present with subtle clinical findings. Toxoplasmosis may be transmitted when a seronegative patient receives a seropositive organ. Prophylaxis with either clindamycin or a combination of sulfadiazine and pyrimethamine is indicated in such cases.

CRITICAL CARE OF LUNG TRANSPLANT RECIPIENTS

Over the past 30 years, significant advances have been made in preservation, surgical technique, and immunosuppression so that lung transplantation is now being performed more frequently.

Preoperative Evaluation

Potential candidates for lung transplantation are generally younger than age 60 years (50 years for heart-lung) and are in good general medical condition. Patients with cardiac dysfunction are poor candidates for lung transplantation unless this is limited to the right side of the heart. A left ventricular ejection fraction of less than 35% suggests the need for heart-lung transplantation. Cardiac catheterization is undertaken for those at risk for coronary artery disease. Potential candidates are also thoroughly evaluated for renal and hepatic disease and undergo serologic screening as for other types of transplantation.

Pulmonary parenchymal disease (especially cystic fibrosis), emphysema, and idiopathic pulmonary fibrosis are the most common indications for lung transplantation. The timing of transplantation depends on the physical condition of the patient and the natural history of the disease. Transplantation should be postponed as long as possible but not so long that the patient develops severe functional limitation or multisystem dysfunction. Previous thoracotomy is generally considered a contraindication to heart-lung transplantation because of the presence of adhesions and risk of life-threatening bleeding.

Operative Issues

Preservation is more difficult and less understood for the lung than for most other organs. Hypothermic preservation allows for 4 to 6 hours of ischemia time and is the current standard of practice. Preservative solutions used still vary by institution; common ones include modified Euro-Collins and University of Wisconsin solutions. A variety of anti-inflammatory agents have also been tried, including prostaglandins, corticosteroids, and free radical scavengers.

The choice of which transplant to do (heart-lung, double lung, single lung) for each patient must be individualized. The indications for heart-lung transplantation include incorrectable congenital heart and lung disease or reversible pulmonary disease with significant left ventricular dysfunction. Double lung transplantation is indicated for cystic fibrosis, primary pulmonary hypertension, and certain patients with bullous emphysema. Single lung transplantation is by far more common, especially given the scarcity of organs.

The use of cardiopulmonary bypass is decreasing as surgical techniques that do not require it are refined. Currently, bypass is reserved for patients who are unable to tolerate single lung ventilation. Heart-lung transplantation is performed through a standard median sternotomy whereas single lung transplants are done via a lateral thoracotomy. Double lung operations are done using a bilateral thoracotomy or "clamshell" incision, which includes transverse division of the sternum. Tracheal anastomoses are fraught with difficulties related to ischemia (since tracheobronchial arteries are not anastomosed) and are reserved for heart-lung transplants. Therefore, lung transplantation (even double lung) is currently performed with bronchial anastomoses. Generally, the airways are joined by telescoping the mainstem bronchus of the donor airway into that of the recipient to reinforce the juncture.

Postoperative Management

Patients who were hypercapnic preoperatively initially may remain so after transplantation. The $PaCO_2$ gradually normalizes over several weeks. The majority of patients can be extubated within 48 hours. However, respiratory failure can occur as a result of several factors. *Preservation and reperfusion injuries* are apparent as infiltrates and hypoxemia in the immediate postoperative period. The transplanted lung is particularly susceptible to *pulmonary edema* because of disruption of the pulmonary lymphatics and altered capillary permeability in the early postoperative period. For this reason, fluid administration is minimized and diuretics are begun as early as possible. Pulmonary venous obstruction must also be considered in such situations. In single lung recipients, *ventilation-perfusion mismatch* can result in significant impairments in gas exchange. Patients with pulmonary hypertension are at particular risk, and the presence of infiltrates on the allograft side further worsens this problem. Single lung recipients with emphysema are also at risk of developing *hyperinflation* of the native lung due to gross differences in the respiratory mechanics for each side. Severe hyperinflation may compress the allograft side and affect hemodynamics. Management by differential lung ventilation using a double-lumen tube is often required. *Pneumonia* is also a common problem secondary to immunosuppression, impaired ciliary function, and altered lymphocyte traffic from disrupted lymphatics. Episodes of acute *rejection* during the first 30 days are also common. Transbronchial biopsy is required to establish the diagnosis and distinguish rejection from infection. Finally *phrenic nerve injury* may complicate postoperative pulmonary function.

Infection is a significant problem in this population. The use of antimicrobial prophylaxis has significantly reduced the number of infections seen. Infections in the lung transplant population are similar to those in other transplantation groups except that the frequency (and significance) of pulmonary infections is greater. This may occur for several reasons, including bacterial colonization in the donor. In single lung recipients, infection may also result from colonization in the native lung (especially in patients with cystic fibrosis). Resistant pseudomonal organisms, such as *Pseudomonas cepacia*, are difficult to manage.

Other postoperative complications include hemorrhage, which is reduced significantly by avoiding cardiopulmonary bypass and thus heparinization; renal dysfunction secondary to CyA and worsened by the need to minimize fluids; and gastrointestinal complications such as bleeding and pancreatitis.

Immunosuppression for the lung transplant recipient consists of corticosteroids, azathioprine, and CyA (or FK-506). Some centers also use OKT3 or ATG as part of the primary regimen. Also, some centers prefer to limit steroids, as they feel that they impair healing of the airway anastomoses.

Late Complications

Infection remains a significant risk long after transplantation. After the first month, nonbacterial infections become more common. CMV is a particular threat to the lung transplant patient and may manifest as a systemic disease. Fungal infections can also be a serious problem, especially *Aspergillus*.

Chronic rejection can occur insidiously, with dyspnea and cough. The chest radiograph may be clear despite a decline in pulmonary function. The pathology of chronic rejection is apparent on biopsy as bronchiolitis obliterans. This condition is a major source of late morbidity and mortality, with an incidence of 20% to 40%. The pathogenesis of chronic rejection is incompletely understood. Infection, particularly with CMV, appears to play a role.

Other late complications include stricture of the airway anastomosis and PTLD. Strictures are treated with either stenting of the airway or laser treatments to remove the granulation tissue or both.

PANCREAS AND ISLET CELL TRANSPLANTATION

Both pancreatic solid organ transplantation (PTX) and islet cell transplantation (ITX) are becoming more common. More than 600 procedures were performed in 1990. The current 3-year graft survival rate is 57%, with a patient survival of 80%. PTX comprises the great majority of these procedures, as ITX is still in its infancy. PTX is most commonly performed in combination with kidney transplantation for patients with diabetes mellitus and end-stage renal failure. Other multivisceral combinations (such as liver-pancreas) are occasionally done.

For PTX, the graft is usually placed in the peritoneal space to allow for absorption of secretions. Most commonly, the graft drains into the bladder via a cuff of donor duodenum. The donor superior mesenteric artery and celiac axis are connected to the iliac artery, and the donor portal vein is anastomosed to the iliac veins. ITX, by contrast, is performed by separating the islet cells and injecting them directly into the portal vein for hepatic implantation. Other sites have been tried but currently this is the location of choice and is associated with minimal complications. When successful, PTX normalizes glucose and hemoglobin A_{1c} levels. PTX also appears to improve counterregulation of glucose through improved glucagon control. ITX has been less successful at achieving glucose control.

Rejection is difficult to detect in PTX recipients. For a variety of reasons, including accessibility, risk of bleeding, and risk of ductal leakage, biopsy is not a practical technique in PTX. Similarly, endocrine function is a poor guide, as this becomes impaired only late in the course of rejection. Commonly, therefore, urinary amylase is measured, taking advantage of the drainage of the graft into the bladder. Interpretation of this test, however, is by no means straightforward. Urinary amylase will also vary with urine output and nutritional status. Thus, the diagnosis of rejection after PTX and ITX can usually be supported only by the concurrent diagnosis of rejection in organs that can be biopsied. Although this is the only practical method in use today, a 10% to 20% incidence of isolated rejection of the pancreas has been reported. Clearly, therefore, there is a need for more definitive methods for diagnosis of rejection in PTX and ITX.

ICU Management

The principles of management for PTX and ITX patients include routine ICU care, especially nutrition, strict glucose control, and monitoring for rejection and infection. Avoidance of hyperglycemia in the early period following ITX seems to be important for graft survival. This can be quite challenging since CyA, FK-506, and steroids all cause hyperglycemia. Overtreatment can also be problematic, especially in combined liver and pancreas transplants, since hypoglycemia is a significant risk. It is not clear that PTX recipients require such close scrutiny of blood sugar levels.

The usual immunosuppressive regimen for PTX (or ITX) is a combination of CyA (or FK-506), prednisone, and AZA. Much however, depends on what other organs are transplanted. The management of nutrition in these patients is controversial. In Pittsburgh, all patients receive parenteral nutrition beginning early in the postoperative period. They are switched to enteral nutrition as soon as possible.

INTESTINAL AND MULTIPLE ORGAN TRANSPLANTATION

Loss of intestinal function with its associated pathophysiology has led to trials evaluating the role of intestinal and multiple organ transplantation in these patients. In 33 patients at the University of Pittsburgh who underwent composite and isolated intestinal transplantation, the leading indication in adult patients was short gut syndrome secondary to surgical loss after Crohn's disease, trauma, or mesenteric thrombotic disorders. Pediatric patients most commonly presented with a history of necrotizing enterocolitis, gastroschisis, volvulus, and pseudo-obstruction. Decisions regarding the transplant allograft composition are made based on the integrity and anatomy of the remaining gut as well as the function of the other abdominal organs. Patients with hepatic abnormalities documented by biochemical dysfunction, fibrosis or cirrhosis on biopsy, and the presence of portal hypertension are considered for concomitant liver transplantation, in addition to small bowel or multivisceral transplantation. The patients with protein S, protein C, or antithrombin III deficiency are considered for combined liver and small intestine allograft because of the propensity for venous thrombosis and mesenteric venous hypertension following a successful transplantation.

Recipient Operation

Multiple variants of the intestinal and multiorgan transplantation have been described depending on anatomic and technical factors. Immunosuppression is achieved with FK-506 and methylprednisolone. Postoperative care is similar to that administered to other critically ill transplant recipients. However, three areas of note are infection control, nutritional support, and the assessment of graft status.

Recipients of isolated or composite small bowel grafts receive prophylactic, broad-spectrum intravenous antibiotics. They also are treated with selective bowel decontamination using amphotericin B, gentamicin, and polymyxin E. Quantitative surveillance stool cultures performed every 3 days are used to guide antibiotic therapy if the patient demonstrates signs of systemic sepsis or presumed translocation. Translocation can be a particular problem during episodes of acute rejection when the mucosal barrier protective function of the allograft has been lost due to immunologic mechanisms. These patients are at high risk for the usual bacterial, viral, or fungal infections that can occur in an immunocompromised patient.

Total parenteral nutrition is tapered as enteral feedings are begun. Tube feedings are usually instituted with isotonic dipeptide formulas that contain medium chain triglycerides and glutamine. Surveillance of intestinal graft rejection and function focuses on clinical evaluation and examination of the allograft using endoscopic means. An allograft ileostomy is usually part of the transplant procedure and allows for routine enteroscopy. Enteroscopy can be supplemented by histologic evaluation of biopsy specimens to guide therapy. Other important assessments of small bowel function include absorption studies of D-xylose and quantitative fat studies in the ileostomy output.

Graft Rejection

Intestinal allograft rejection usually is heralded by clinical symptoms that may include fever, abdominal pain and distention, nausea, and increases in stomal output. Gastrointestinal bleeding may occur in cases of uncontrollable rejection in which ulcerations with sloughing of mucosa occur. Translocation of bacteria or fungi during rejection may present as clinical sepsis and bacteremia or fungemia. The endoscopic appearance is that of hyperemia or dusky mucosa that is hypoperistaltic. The mucosa may also become friable, and diffuse ulcerations may appear. Mononuclear cell infiltrates and cryptitis with apoptosis and regeneration are required to establish a diagnosis of acute rejection. Treatment is carried out with bolus steroid therapy of methylprednisolone with steroid tapers used in cases of moderate to severe rejection. Adequate FK-506 levels are assured by either the oral or intravenous route. OKT3 is used to treat steroid-resistant rejection. Chronic rejection is usually marked by villous blunting and ulcerations with obliterative thickening of intestinal arterioles on histologic examination. The bowel takes on a tubular pattern with strictures and loss of a normal mucosal pattern.

Technical Complications

The extensive dissection required in most patients who require transplant for short gut syndrome may lead to postoperative bleeding. Postoperative management is centered on controlling coagulopathy by directed replacement of appropriate clotting factors.

Biliary leak or obstruction may occur in patients with manipulation of the bile duct. The key to diagnosis is a high index of suspicion and prompt evaluation with radiographic techniques using cholangiography if needed. Surgical correction has been the mainstay of therapy for these complications.

Major arterial or venous complications are usually acute, dramatic clinical problems, manifested by clinical deterioration, sepsis, and mental status changes. Vascular patency is rapidly confirmed by Doppler ultrasonic examination, followed by angiography if needed. Although attempts at revascularization may be carried out, major vascular thrombosis is usually associated with graft loss.

Anastomotic dehiscence is more common in pediatric patients than in adults. It is usually accompanied by sepsis. Confirmation is obtained with radiologic contrast imaging, and surgical revision, evacuation, abdominal lavage, and reexplorations are often required to eliminate any persistent focus of sepsis.

Infectious Complications

Intestinal recipients are subject to similar bacterial, fungal, and virus infections as in other solid organ transplantation. CMV infection poses a significant problem in adult intestinal graft recipients, usually involving the allograft intestine. Key strategies have been to avoid the use of CMV-positive grafts in CMV-negative recipients and to reduce immunosuppression while treating with ganciclovir and CMV immunoglobulin.

BONE MARROW TRANSPLANTATION

This section will highlight the management of patients following bone marrow transplantation (BMT), focusing on diagnosis and management of complications after this treatment modality. Allogeneic BMT refers to an infusion of normal stem cells from a human leukocyte antigen (HLA)-identical sibling or a partially or fully HLA-identical related or matched unrelated donor. The stem cells are given after ablative chemo- or radiotherapy to the host. Syngeneic BMT refers to donor cells harvested from a twin donor. Autologous BMT refers to the use of the recipient's own bone marrow or blood-derived stem cells.

The indications for bone marrow transplantation are still increasing and now include acute leukemia, lymphoma, chronic myelogenous leukemia, and aplastic anemia, with increasing experience in BMT for myelodysplastic syndrome, germ cell tumors, metastatic breast cancer, and ongoing trials in other solid tumors, such as high-dose chemotherapy with BMT or peripheral stem cell rescue in patients with ovarian cancer or neuroblastoma.

Various techniques such as tumor cell purging, T cell depletion, and elutriation are used to provide the maximal benefits of graft lymphocytes with optimal engraftment and antileukemic effect while preventing serious consequences of BMT such as graft-versus-host disease (GVHD).

Graft-Versus-Host Disease

BMT is characterized by several unique complications, one of the most serious being GVHD, which is rarely significant in solid organ recipients. Clinically significant GVHD occurs in 25% to 75% of patients receiving HLA-identical sibling BMT and in virtually all recipients of incompatible or unrelated donor BMT. The risk factors for development of GVHD are HLA disparity, female donor to male recipient, and older age.

Acute GVHD generally occurs within the first 100 days

after allogeneic transplantation and may affect the skin, gastrointestinal tract, and the liver. The first manifestation is an erythematous maculopapular rash that involves the face, neck, palms, and soles and is associated with pain or tingling of the extremities. The rash varies from a localized eruption to a diffuse process with bullae and desquamation. Acute GVHD is usually accompanied by fever or flulike symptoms. A skin biopsy confirms the diagnosis and demonstrates epidermal necrosis and dyskeratosis as well as perivascular mononuclear cell infiltration of the dermis and lower epidermis. Most of these mononuclear cells appear to be T lymphocytes, although natural killer cells have also been observed. The intestinal component of GVHD may present as a secretory, bloody diarrhea with cramping abdominal pain, nausea, and vomiting. Upper and lower endoscopic biopsies usually demonstrate the presence of GVHD.

Liver involvement often occurs simultaneously or follows the onset of rash by several days with elevated bilirubin and alkaline phosphatase levels, and subsequent elevation of transaminases. Clinical staging of acute GVHD takes into account the skin, liver, and intestinal involvement, as listed in Table 12–4. Grades III and IV are associated with significant mortality.

Many trials of GVHD prophylaxis have been carried out. However, the treatment for GVHD is less than satisfactory. Corticosteroids and intravenous cyclosporine are the usual first-line treatments. However, they carry an overall response rate of less than 50% for grades III and IV GVHD. Second-line therapies include FK-506, OKT3, and antithymocyte globulin (ATG).

Octreotide acetate (Sandostatin), the synthetic somatostatin analog, has been beneficial as an adjunctive therapy for acute GVHD of the intestine. Total parenteral nutrition and institution of enteral diet when tolerated are important for the nutritional support of these patients.

Chronic GVHD is a later complication of allogeneic BMT and occurs in 60% of patients who survive more than 100 days after transplantation. This syndrome is characterized by lacrimal and salivary gland dysfunction, with dry eyes and mouth, as well as skin fibrosis that can damage adnexal structures with hyper- or hypopigmentation of the skin. Table 12–5 lists the characteristics of chronic GVHD. Mus-

Table 12–4. CLINICAL STAGING OF ACUTE GRAFT-VERSUS-HOST DISEASE

Grade	Skin	Liver	Gut
I	<25% body surface area	Bilirubin 2–3 mg/dL	Diarrhea 0.5–1 L/day
II	25%–50% BSA	Bilirubin 3–6 mg/dL	Diarrhea 1–1.5 L/day
III	Generalized	Bilirubin 6–15 mg/dL	Diarrhea >1.5 L/day
IV	Desquamation	Bilirubin >15 mg/dL	Ileus

Table 12–5. CHRONIC GRAFT-VERSUS-HOST DISEASE

Limited

Localized skin involvement
Hepatic dysfunction

Extensive

Generalized skin involvement
Local skin and/or hepatic dysfunction with
- Liver histology of cirrhosis or chronic aggressive hepatitis
- Eye involvement
- Oral mucosa or salivary gland involvement
- Other target organ involvement

cles, joints, and the gastrointestinal system may all be affected. Pulmonary involvement with bronchiolitis obliterans is the most severe manifestation of chronic GVHD. Treatment consists of steroids and CyA or FK-506.

Other Noninfectious Complications

Other noninfectious complications of bone marrow transplantation arise primarily from the toxicity of the chemotherapy and irradiation that is used in the BMT induction regimens. Neurologic complications are a frequent problem after BMT, affecting as many as 70% of both adults and children, and usually present as acute CNS toxicity due to the initial cytoreductive protocol. Chemotherapy, including mechlorethamine and carmustine, are particularly toxic. Busulfan can cause seizures, and two thirds of patients show epileptiform activity on electroencephalography.

Oral and GI mucositis are frequent and severe complications of cytotoxic chemotherapy. Pain in the oral pharynx can be disabling, requiring narcotic analgesia. These complications are usually self-limited and resolve when adequate neutrophil and platelet levels return. Treatment is directed toward pain control and topical antibiotic treatment to suppress bacterial, fungal, and viral colonization.

Although most pulmonary complications are infectious in etiology, significant pulmonary toxicity can be attributed to chemotherapy or radiation directly. Interstitial pneumonia may complicate the use of total body irradiation or be secondary to drugs such as cyclophosphamide, carmustine, or busulfan. Treatment for this complication is supportive in nature and includes ventilatory support, but the outcome is generally fatal. Diffuse alveolar hemorrhage produces a syndrome of dyspnea, hypoxia, and diffuse consolidations on chest radiograph and usually has a very early onset in the post-BMT course. Hemorrhage on BAL is a diagnostic finding. BAL is also important to rule out a coexisting infectious component. This complication is generally fatal, but reversal has been documented with high-dose corticosteroids.

The major cardiac complications are related to the cytotoxic therapy used in these patients. Cyclophosphamide may cause myocardial edema, fibrosis, and hypertrophy, as well as fibrinous pericarditis. Ifosfamide may also result in congestive heart failure, usually in the first 2 weeks after bone marrow transplant. A significant component of congestive heart failure may reverse with time, but the presence of myocardial fibrosis usually leads to a baseline deficit that can be exacerbated by fluid overload or other compromised pulmonary function. Strict attention to fluid management and consideration of more invasive hemodynamic monitoring, such as by pulmonary arterial catheterization, are appropriate.

Hepatic veno-occlusive disease results in severe liver injury that is characterized by fibrous obliteration of the lumina of intrahepatic central venules that leads to centrilobular hepatocyte degeneration and sinusoidal fibrosis. The clinical syndrome of hepatic veno-occlusive disease is that of weight gain, followed by abdominal pain, hepatomegaly, ascites, and progression to liver failure. Hepatic veno-occlusive disease usually develops within the first 2 weeks after BMT. Risk factors for development of veno-occlusive disease include hepatitis, older patient age, use of AZA, and hematologic malignancy other than acute lymphocytic leukemia. Therapy is supportive; however, reports of thrombolytic therapy with recombinant human tissue plasminogen activator have been published that show reversal of established severe veno-occlusive disease.

Renal complications from drug toxicity are common following BMT. Hemorrhagic cystitis is a frequent complication of cyclophosphamide that affects not only the bladder but the renal pelvis and the ureters as well. The use of mesna (sodium-2-mercaptoethane sulfonate) during cyclophosphamide administration decreases the incidence of this complication.

Hemolytic-uremic syndrome is characterized by intravascular hemolysis, thrombocytopenia, and renal failure, seen in association with CyA and FK-506. Treatment is recommended with vincristine and plasma exchange, but the outcome in severe cases is usually fatal. A more common difficulty encountered is thrombocytopenia that requires platelet matching to allow for adequate support. Human leukocyte antigen–matched platelets are usually required to treat thrombocytopenia that is clinically significant.

The clinician caring for the bone marrow transplant patient must have a high index of suspicion for hypothyroidism as well as adrenal insufficiency that may occur in these patients. Attention to proper metabolic support using a combination of parenteral and enteral nutrition is important to maintain positive nitrogen balance. Glutamine supplementation may be important to attenuate the fluid retention that is normally seen with the standard parenteral formulations.

Infectious Complications

Infections remain the most frequent cause of morbidity and mortality after BMT. They relate to specific time periods after BMT, as listed in Table 12–6. The early period after BMT comprises the first 30 days and is marked by severe

Table 12–6. PEAK INCIDENCE OF INFECTIONS AFTER BONE MARROW TRANSPLANTATION

Early (<30 Days)	Middle (30–100 Days)	Late (>100 Days)
Staphylococcus	*Aspergillus*	*Pneumococcus*
Streptococcus	*Pneumocystis carinii*	*Haemophilus influenzae*
Gram-negative enterics	*Toxoplasma gondii*	Varicella-zoster
Candida albicans	Cytomegalovirus	
Herpes simplex	Adenovirus	
	JC virus	

neutropenia, lymphopenia, mucositis, and gastroenteritis, owing to chemotherapy and radiation therapy toxicities. The immunosuppression used to prevent acute GVHD also increases the infectious risk in allogeneic BMT. The common pathogens are gram-positive organisms, as well as *Candida* and herpes simplex virus (HSV). Neutropenic patients may be especially prone to infections due to gram-negative bacteria. Neutropenic patients following BMT are covered immediately with broad-spectrum antibiotic coverage at the first sign of fever. Regimens used to treat these patients prophylactically include a semisynthetic penicillin or antipseudomonal cephalosporine combined with an aminoglycoside. Empiric therapy may also be carried out with imipenem-cilastatin or double beta-lactam protocols that have been shown to be as effective while avoiding the renal toxicity of aminoglycoside therapy.

Prophylaxis against gram-negative infection is usually carried out with ciprofloxacin, which is given until the first neutropenic fever attack, at which time broad-spectrum coverage is initiated, or until neutropenia resolves if a patient remains afebrile.

The middle period (30 to 100 days) after BMT is characterized by infections due to CMV, *Pneumocystis carinii*, or *Aspergillus* species. The herpes viruses are the most frequent causes of viral infection in BMT recipients, and the most common cause of infectious death after allogeneic BMT is CMV infection. CMV infection is documented by culture as well as biopsy of affected organs. The use of antigenemia assays has been helpful in making an early diagnosis of CMV. CMV pneumonia is the most serious manifestation of this disease. The treatment consists of intravenous ganciclovir, 5 mg/kg every 12 hours, adjusted for renal function, as well as intravenous immunoglobulin. Another herpes virus infection often seen is caused by HSV. With the institution of acyclovir prophylaxis, HSV infection is usually encountered only after prophylaxis has ended. The BK virus and JC virus are occasional causes of cystitis after bone marrow transplant during the middle period of infectious risk. BK viruria is more common and is associated with hemorrhagic cystitis. Adenovirus may be associated with interstitial pneumonia and follows the same time course as CMV. Respiratory syncytial virus may cause upper respiratory tract infections. There is preliminary experience with ribavirin to treat this infection. Protozoan infections with *Pneumocystis carinii* usually occur in the middle period after BMT. The diagnosis is made by BAL or lung biopsy. Treatment with trimethoprim-sulfamethoxazole is usually effective. Toxoplasmosis is an occasional cause of morbidity after BMT. It requires a high index of suspicion to diagnose the patient who presents with central nervous system symptoms such as hemiplegia, meningitis, or confusion accompanied by fever. Nearly every case occurs in those who are seropositive for *Toxoplasma gondii* before BMT. Reactivation of recent infection appears to be the principal cause of disease. Diagnosis is confirmed by parasitemia or brain biopsy.

In the late period of infectious complications (more than 100 days), pulmonary pneumococcal infections may occur because of functional asplenia. Prophylaxis with trimethoprim-sulfamethoxazole several days a week prevents this complication. Varicella-zoster infection with shingles generally occurs during the late period after BMT in one third of BMT recipients who are seropositive for varicella-zoster. Acyclovir is effective therapy and should be given intravenously in complicated cases.

GENERAL SURGICAL COMPLICATIONS IN TRANSPLANT PATIENTS

General surgical complications frequently occur in transplant recipients and are significant causes of morbidity and mortality. Common problems are more frequent in immunosuppressed patients. Problems unique to the transplant recipient can be subtle. This section will review the common general surgical complications that occur by system as well as post-transplant lymphoproliferative disorders.

Esophagus

Esophagitis is common in transplant recipients and produces symptoms of dysphagia and epigastric discomfort. It rarely requires surgical intervention, and management is similar to that of nontransplant patients, consisting of antacids, histamine receptor antagonists, or proton pump antagonists. Esophageal ulcerations may be due to a viral or fungal cause. Viral ulcerations in the esophagus occur typically as discrete lesions with raised edges, whereas *Candida* esophagitis is diagnosed when endoscopy shows typical lesions consisting of white plaques with overlying friable erythematous mucosa. Treatment of both of these consists of specific antiviral or antifungal therapy as well as lowering of immunosuppression medication as tolerated.

Stomach and Duodenum

Peptic ulcer disease is common in transplant recipients. Histamine receptor antagonists are used as prophylaxis. Gastroduodenal ulcerations may be due to either infectious or peptic causes. Peptic ulcer disease has a high incidence in renal transplant recipients, although the pathogenesis of this is unclear and may be multifactorial. CMV as well as herpes virus may also cause gastric and duodenal ulceration.

Patients who present with epigastric pain or discomfort or with upper GI bleeding require an evaluation that includes prompt esophagogastroduodenoscopy. Biopsy specimens are obtained from ulcers and appropriate antiviral or antifungal therapy is added if an infectious cause is identified. A biopsy also allows the detection of lymphoproliferative disorder or other neoplasms involving the stomach. Bleeding or perforation requires aggressive evaluation and consideration of surgical treatment as in other nontransplantation patients.

Biliary Tract

A high incidence of cholelithiasis among organ transplant recipients has been noted. In most instances, symptomatic cholelithiasis in transplantation candidates should be treated by cholecystectomy if the patient's condition permits. Most nonthoracic organ transplant candidates such as potential kidney recipients can tolerate cholecystectomy without difficulty; laparoscopic techniques combined with endoscopic methods have hastened recovery and improved the postoperative course. Cholecystectomy in patients with cirrhosis should be avoided. All medical means should be used to prevent complications of bleeding and liver failure that are often encountered, if a cholecystectomy is undertaken in the cirrhotic patient. Cholecystectomy in thoracic organ transplant candidates likewise carries high morbidity and may best be performed after transplantation when the patient's cardiac and pulmonary functions are improved.

The treatment of asymptomatic cholelithiasis in transplant recipients is controversial. In general, it is recommended that all patients be screened for cholelithiasis and that elective cholecystectomy be performed in kidney transplant candidates when possible. Pretransplant cholecystectomy if the patient's condition permits is preferable, because the complications of infection in the face of ongoing immunosuppressive therapy, as well as potential danger to the transplanted organ, are avoided.

Pancreas

Acute pancreatitis is a serious complication following solid organ transplantation. The etiologies of acute pancreatitis after organ transplantation include all common causes of acute pancreatitis such as gallstones, alcohol, and specific drugs. Immunosuppressive therapy, specifically corticosteroids and AZA, has been implicated in the development of acute pancreatitis. Hypertriglyceridemia and hyperlipidemia are also associated with the development of acute pancreatitis. Acute pancreatitis in the early postoperative period after heart or lung transplantation may result from cardiopulmonary bypass.

Early diagnosis and treatment of acute pancreatitis are essential in transplant recipients. Appropriate imaging studies of the pancreas consist of dynamic computed tomography (CT) performed by rapid bolus infusion of intravenous contrast. Dynamic CT scanning permits differentiation of acute interstitial pancreatitis from necrotizing pancreatitis in which areas of pancreatic necrosis fail to enhance. Acute pancreatitis is treated by immediate withdrawal of oral intake and administration of intravenous hydration. Careful attention to metabolic and organ support is essential because of the fluid shifts and metabolic derangements that occur. If possible, it is important to discontinue drugs that may be related to the development of pancreatitis, such as corticosteroids, AZA, and possibly sulfa. Aggressive management of necrotizing pancreatitis is important. This includes a high index of suspicion for infection and operation when infection is confirmed or if the patient's clinical condition continues to deteriorate despite appropriate nonoperative therapy. Pancreatic debridement with abdominal lavage and re-exploration or open abdominal wound care has been successful in treating these patients. Management of complications of acute pancreatitis such as pancreatic pseudocysts should be carried out as with nontransplant recipients.

Small Intestine, Colon, and Rectum

A very diverse range of surgical complications involving the small and large intestine may arise in transplant recipients. Three specific problems are lower GI bleeding, colon perforation, and lymphoproliferative disorder. Lower GI bleeding in transplant patients is uncommon but carries a high mortality. Most episodes of lower GI bleeding are caused by opportunistic infection by fungi or CMV. These are managed by withdrawal of immunosuppression, appropriate antiviral or fungal therapy, and early operative intervention for significant continued bleeding.

Clostridium difficile colitis may also occur in transplant recipients and presents as GI bleeding or sepsis. Fecal studies for *Clostridium difficile* toxin and colonoscopy are diagnostic. CT scans characteristically demonstrate diffuse colonic wall thickening. Initial treatment consists of enteral vancomycin and parenteral metronidazole. Total abdominal colectomy with an ileostomy should be considered if a patient develops hemodynamic instability or signs of clinical sepsis with failure to respond promptly to medical therapy.

Colonic perforation is most commonly caused by diverticular disease. Prompt resuscitation, intravenous antibiotics, and laparotomy are needed to manage diverticular disease and its complications, particularly perforation, successfully. Diverticulitis without evidence of perforation or abscess can be treated successfully by antibiotics, with surgery considered for patients who undergo recurrent episodes of diverticulitis or experience a complication of acute diverticulitis.

Post-Transplant Lymphoproliferative Disorders

Post-transplant lymphoproliferative disorder (PTLD) may arise throughout the body, including the transplanted organ, and is commonly of B cell origin. When it occurs in the small and large intestine, it may result in obstruction, perforation, or bleeding and require surgical intervention. The risk factor for PTLD is chronic immunosuppression; infection by Epstein-Barr virus is an important cofactor in the development of these tumors. Three patterns of clinical presentation have been described for PTLD: (1) fulminant progressive polyclonal disease; (2) single or metastatic clonal tumors that progress despite withdrawal of immune therapy; or (3) single or multiple clonal or nonclonal tumors that respond to immune modulation. The mainstay of therapy is reduction of immunosuppressive therapy, with acyclovir, ganciclovir, and interferon-alpha used as adjunctive therapy. Chemotherapeutic regimens have been used in monoclonal PTLD, which has a clinical course that resembles lymphoma.

Surgical intervention is indicated for perforation, bleeding, or obstruction and involves limited resection of the affected bowel area.

FUTURE OF TRANSPLANTATION

Immunologic advances, innovations in support systems and artificial organ technology, and xenotransplantation hold promise to further the growth of organ transplantation in the near future.

Immunologic Advances—Chimerism

The basis for graft acceptance has been difficult to understand. Recent investigations based on prior observations support the theory that the mutual engagement of migratory immunocytes from the graft to the recipient results in microchimerism, and that this is the key event in graft acceptance. Technologic advances have allowed the detection of small numbers of donor cells outside the grafted organ within the recipient tissues. This migration of donor organ–derived cells after transplantation has been shown to occur in experimental models as well as human organ transplant models, using techniques of immunostaining or polymerase chain reaction (PCR).

Long-term survivors of liver transplantation were studied systematically by obtaining biopsy specimens of the patient's transplanted organ, skin, lymph nodes, and other tissues. Using immunostaining and PCR, it was possible to determine the origin of cells within the tissue as being from the organ donor, the recipient's own body, or both. In a group of 22 surviving liver transplant recipients, all demonstrated systemic tissue microchimerism. It is hypothesized that the immunologic tolerance of a graft is in part mediated by the dendritic cell component of that organ. Allografts with a large dendritic cell component may be expected to be immunologically more privileged because they are able to establish this microchimeric state more easily. A number of other factors, however, determine the ultimate effect of the migratory donor cells on allograft survival. It is thought that sufficient immunosuppression is required in the early phases after transplantation to prevent these cells from becoming immunogenic and accelerating a rejection process. If the balance is turned in the other direction and the recipient is made immunoincompetent either by cytoablation or other means, GVHD may occur.

These findings have led to trials of augmentation of the donor leukocyte load with a perioperative infusion of nondepleted organ donor bone marrow in solid organ recipients of liver and kidney allografts. The early results have demonstrated good organ function and easily detectable blood chimerism without significant GVHD. It is hoped that this therapy may result in improved graft acceptance with the potential for withdrawal of immunosuppressive therapy.

Extracorporeal Liver Assist Devices

Research into extracorporeal liver assist devices has been prompted by the prevalence of both acute and chronic liver insufficiency. The shortage of organ donors has limited therapy for many of these patients, who succumb before a suitable organ is found. Several proposed systems have been developed to attempt to provide support to the failing liver. One system developed by Demetriou and coworkers consists of plasma separation and perfusion through a charcoal filter and hollow fiber cartridge, using porcine hepatocytes attached to microcarrier beads that are placed into the extracapillary space of a porous hollow fiber module. Plasma is passed through the intracapillary space, and the hepatocytes are separated from the plasma by the cartridge membrane. In a case report of a patient treated with total hepatectomy and extracorporeal liver support by this mechanism for fulminant hepatic failure, there appeared to be reversal of neurologic dysfunction and normalization of intracranial pressure, as well as decreased serum ammonia levels. The patient went on to successful transplantation.

Other investigators have developed a rat hepatocyte system that isolates these hepatocytes in a collagen gel matrix that is placed in the lumen of hollow fiber cartridges. A third system is based on the use of a clone of a human hepatoblastoma cell line that expresses near-normal levels of several central metabolic pathways and has the morphology characteristic of human hepatocytes. This cell line can be grown in hollow fiber cartridges. A limited investigation has been carried out in humans with fulminant hepatic failure and advanced encephalopathy. The initial results warrant continued investigation.

Xenotransplantation

Discordant donors for cross-species transplantation are characterized by the presence of preformed antibody in the recipient, usually at high titers, that may cause hyperacute rejection of the donor organ. Concordant combinations of cross-species transplantation are characterized by a low concentration of preformed antibodies. Primate-to-human transplantation is considered concordant, whereas transplants from a pig into a human are discordant. Liver xenografts may be envisioned as temporary support until the failing native liver recovers from injury, as a bridge to transplantation until an appropriate human liver is found, or as permanent orthotopic replacement of the diseased liver. The immunosuppressive therapies that have been considered experimentally and clinically deal with minimizing the effect of preformed cytotoxic antibodies and minimizing the inflammatory cascade that occurs in these patients. In patients with highly cytotoxic antibodies, depletion of these antibodies can be effected theoretically by immunoabsorption or by plasmapheresis. After reducing the preformed antibody load, low titers of cytotoxic xenoantibody levels would be maintained by pharmacologic means.

The second consideration is to minimize the inflammatory

cascade that is amplified by the complement system. Agents that interfere with the cascade and subsequent inflammatory mediators must be developed.

The third area of concern in xenotransplantation immunotherapy is to obtain sustained suppression of cell-mediated rejection in order to minimize the long-term damage to the xenograft that may occur via lymphocyte-derived cytokines. Other key areas that will determine the success of xenotransplantation are compatibility of proteins between donor and recipient species, as well as risk of potential zoonoses associated with animal donors.

Conclusions

There has been tremendous growth in the field of transplantation in the 40 years that have followed the first successful human transplant. Advances in multiple disciplines have enabled the evolution of transplantation into an accepted therapeutic option. The critical care of transplant recipients is extremely challenging, and the scarcity of donor organs has encouraged the development of new strategies for meeting this need. Advances in immunotherapy and artificial organ support systems, as well as xenotransplantation, are likely to characterize the next decade of transplantation.

CHAPTER 13
Patient Care, Organization, and Ethics

Joann I. Lamb, MSN, RN-C, FCCM

PART A
Issues in Patient Care

ASPECTS OF CRITICAL CARE NURSING: LOOKING BACK TO FACE THE CHALLENGE OF THE FUTURE

In its infancy, critical care practice was an unknown science attracting practitioners who were intrigued by the uncharted waters of intensive care. In the earliest intensive care units (ICUs), the sickest patients were grouped together for close visual observation, rudimentary ventilatory support, and consolidation of nursing care. Now, technologic advances in pharmacology, space age diagnostic and therapeutic interventions, widespread transplantation of multiple organs, and interfaced computer applications at the bedside have replaced mere patient proximity with a highly technical environment. Because of the often chaotic nature of this environment and the mandates of managing intricate technology, humanistic care is often a problem. Rather than moving into the next century with undefined goals, it is time to look back and use what we know about selected aspects of critical care nursing practice to face the challenge of the future.

In 1969, Meltzer and colleagues suggested that "the goals of the ICU team are, first, the preservation of life; second, the restoration of the patient to his maximal functional capacity; and, third, a decrease in overall morbidity" (see *Textbook of Critical Care,* 3rd ed, Chapter 189). Despite a span of nearly 30 years, these goals are still applicable. The complex aspects of critical care practice have increased markedly in the past decade, however, and some of these conspire to make outcomes less predictable:

- Legislative and judicial decisions about patient care
- Resource allocation in an era of cost containment
- Growing numbers of Americans without health insurance or access to care
- Deferred preventive healthcare by people without insurance
- High cost of healthcare, cost of living, and higher salaries in urban areas
- Diagnosis-related grouping (DRG) compression forcing many rural and smaller community hospitals to close

- More acute patient mix increasing demand for more nursing hours
- Patients that are older and younger than ever before, requiring increasingly complex care of multisystem problems
- Expectation of ICUs by the institution, the public, and caregivers
- Downsizing professional and nonprofessional nursing care staff to meet higher salary demands
- Inadequacies of ancillary patient services, increasing the number of non-nursing tasks required by professional nurses, which often leads to professional dissatisfaction

Critical care practice hones exceptional clinical and managerial skills, and experienced critical care nurses are a welcome addition to other fields. For recruitment and retention purposes, hospitals offer tuition benefits for further education. Critical care nurses who acquire advanced education may develop a desire for change, such as opening an independent practice or accepting a promotion that takes them away from direct patient care. When an experienced critical care nurse leaves a unit, the loss is not just another nurse, but an expert who the field can ill afford to lose.

Although the emphasis on patient-centered care in the current milieu implies flexibility, institutions and departments of nursing are relatively inflexible. Dissatisfaction with the critical care environment has been voiced by patients and families, administration, and the medical community. A nursing manager who anticipates, communicates, collaborates, and plans for change becomes a facilitator who ensures that critical care nursing practice is constantly evolving while remaining grounded in scientific theory based on relevant research. How a critical care nurse leader maintains this multiple focus and still achieves outcomes mandated by public policy, institutional needs, and regulatory agencies is a riddle. The answer lies in the commitment of the leader to use a combination of theory, skill, and expectations based on the single-minded philosophy that quality nursing care is the only product provided by the unit.

If nursing practice, as it is applied to critically ill patients, is to evolve in the future, it must be supported by personnel, resources, and an expanded body of knowledge based on research. As practice evolves, critical care nursing standards can lead the way toward a better understanding of how patient outcomes are affected when the standards are implemented appropriately. Ways to ensure clinical competency and performance and to measure productivity are unresolved. Nursing academe and service continue on a dichotomous course. The resolution of this problem will contribute to the survival of nursing as a strong profession within the healthcare field in the next century. The interface of critical care documentation to the hospital information system is developing rapidly (see *Textbook of Critical Care,* 3rd ed, Chapters 196 and 197), but research into the best way of storing and evaluating the abundance of information gleaned from continuous monitoring of many parameters is still in its infancy. Nursing research focused on the outcomes of the care provided is necessary to ensure that practice is based on scientific inquiry and that this practice justifies the cost of care provided. Patient outcomes related to independent nursing practice, including ambulation, feeding, hygiene, and rest and sleep patterns of critically ill patients, are not fully understood and require investigation. As cost containment compresses the healthcare delivery system even more in the future, finances will necessitate that varied levels of technical and professional personnel work together in the critical care unit. Growth and change with cooperative practice will provide holistic care for patients and families in an exciting, safe, but challenging workplace for caregivers.

IMPACT OF HEALTHCARE AND TECHNOLOGY TRENDS ON CRITICAL CARE PRACTICE

Worldwide societal and economic changes are occurring at an accelerating rate. The globe continues to shrink as communication technology advances. The way international business is conducted and the way scientific advances are implemented in one country are quickly adapted elsewhere. Diseases, too, spread rapidly. Medical and nursing innovations in healthcare and the accompanying technology will continue to have both regional and global implications.

Critical care in the United States can be divided into six subject areas:

1. Trends related to the financial climate
2. Changes in healthcare services
3. Technologic advances
4. Changes in healthcare management
5. An emerging concept of an "ethical environment"
6. A mushrooming legal environment

Triage, resource allocation, and rationing occur in various forms. Overall healthcare trends include downsizing of American hospitals, increased patient acuity, increased complexity of home care, increased use of ambulatory services, and delivery to more underprivileged people. Reimbursement policies have changed the way healthcare is delivered, because reimbursement for ambulatory procedures has increased but that for hospital procedures has decreased. Noninvasive technologic devices are on the increase, thereby decreasing costs and risks related to invasive procedures. Major directions in biotechnology today affect critical care nursing and include genetic manipulation of crops and farm animals, identification and manipulation of inherited characteristics, and genetic engineering to conquer diseases for which there are no known cures.

A decade of cost containment has done little to slow spiraling heathcare costs and problems related to widespread lack of insurance, and an aging population and immigration waves of low-income minorities make restructuring of the American healthcare system inevitable. Critical care services have already expanded to home care of patients with ventilators, vasoactive drugs, central nutrition lines, and other high-technology procedures like dialysis. Left ventricular assist devices, until recently seen only in cardiac ICUs, are now battery operated and used at home. Problems that affect financial trends in our current healthcare system include lack of universal access to care, cost shifting (disguised as cost containment), increasing use of technology with limited assessment of new technology, and lack of motivation in Congress to change the system. Recent societal changes have occurred in attitudes toward access to care, infallibility of physicians, death and dying, extent of extraordinary invasive care, informed consent, and the handicapped. Our society has returned to the concept of reduced access to professional or in-hospital care, with patients wanting and having personal responsibility to provide for their own care. The Patient Self-Determination Act of 1991 requires that patients receive information on advance directives; this should result in patients' wishes being followed when they are unable to make decisions. Surrogates will be more readily identified, thus shortening delays in decision-altering care and withdrawal of care.

Technologic advances have leaped beyond society's ability to cope with the financial, legal, and ethical dilemmas that have been induced. Although new therapies can be awesome and can provide help for many patients, they also require tremendous investments in highly skilled personnel and costly adjunct equipment to support them. A growing trend in critical care, for example, is expansion of the field of organ transplantation. It has become the standard of care for some end-stage kidney, heart, lung, and liver diseases. As the benefits of transplantation have become increasingly apparent and the medical barriers have fallen, the demand for transplantation has grown rapidly, far exceeding the supply of organs. As transplantation options expand, the need for critical care nurses in the field of transplantation increases. Although 15,000 people die each year in the United States under circumstances that would allow them to become organ donors, fewer than 4000 organ donations have occurred annually in recent years.

Once one subset of the population has access to a technology, society finds it intolerable to see people dying in need of it. Within hospitals, there is also a similar compulsion to use high-technology interventions. Administrators blame a pervasive American infatuation with technology and continue to purchase new items as they become available. Profits from the use of new technologies are very high, and many large hospitals rush to be the first to have the latest in the technologic arsenal. Inadequate assessment of the device or technique often results. A model for technology assessment in critical care should include technologic capability, range of possible uses, therapeutic impact, diagnostic and therapeutic accuracy, and patient outcome.

New technologies do not decrease costs at all. For, example, a computed tomographic scanner or magnetic resonance imager may be much more accurate than conventional radiography at detecting blood clots in the brain, but physicians more often than not use two, or even all three, of these tests. Another need related to the introduction of new technology is the planning and regulation of standards for training those who use it. It is time-consuming and expensive, for example, to train surgeons, critical care nurses, and adjunct personnel in the execution, postoperative care, and outcome assessment of a newly introduced surgical technique such as laparoscopic cholecystectomy. However, the patient has heard of its advantages, the surgeon wants to do something new and different, and the hospital has bought the equipment—so the procedure begins. Although lip service is given to regional sharing of expensive technologic equipment, the current environment of competition among hospitals soon puts that possibility to rest. Provision of new devices and services precludes or prevents planning for and purchasing everyday equipment.

The future will demand answers to many healthcare technology questions:

- How much do Americans want?
- How much are we willing to pay for?
- Will it come at the expense of the elderly, the disabled, and others who need less glamorous care?
- Can we accept cost containment in healthcare?
- Can we establish an *equitable* process of rationing?
- Will we allow it to drive our healthcare system?
- Will fair assessment be possible?
- Will healthcare institutions use mechanisms of technology assessment?

Clinical practice is the essence of patient care. To manage it, factors that create a patient-centered environment must be present. By implementing management strategies, resource use can be maximized and patient care can be enhanced.

Building Bedside Collaborative Practice

Physicians have traditionally directed all aspects of care through a vertical hierarchy in which communication and planning are unidirectional. In this arrangement, allied health professionals had a restricted scope of activities and depended on the physician's direction for providing various aspects of care. Changing practice environments, however, have led to a greater reliance on the knowledge, expertise, and services provided by other practitioners, especially professional nurses. In fact, patients are often admitted to the hospital because they require nursing care.

Both nurses and physicians have come to realize that communication and a collegial relationship are essential for effective practice. In the late 1960s and early 1970s, the social dimension of the nurse–physician relationship was explored in numerous studies. In response to the developing interest in collaboration, the American Medical Association and the American Nurses Association formed the National Joint Practice Commission (NJPC) in 1972 to identify factors that promote close working relationships. Following the NJPC's lead, the Society of Critical Care Medicine and the American

Association of Critical Care Nurses established a task force in 1982 to identify factors necessary to foster collaboration in the intensive care environment. This task force, the Interorganization Liaison Group, meets at intervals and has prepared several position papers that have been adopted by each parent organization. Endorsement of a multidisciplinary approach to critical care also came from a consensus conference held at the National Institutes of Health in 1983. In addition, the Joint Commission on Accreditation of Hospital Organization recognized the value of integrated practice by mandating a multidisciplinary approach to the management of critical care units.

Objective assessment of improved patient outcome through collaboration has been infrequently reported. A few studies, however, have shown significant differences in patient outcomes that were not predicted on the basis of the severity of illness of the patient alone; rather, they were influenced by administrative structure. Those units with the highest degree of staff involvement and physician–nurse interaction demonstrated the most favorable mortality ratios, suggesting that the *process* of care influenced patient outcome. In one study, the results revealed a strikingly favorable difference from the anticipated mortality for the demonstration unit, supporting the belief that organizational characteristics can significantly affect outcome (see *Textbook of Critical Care,* 3rd ed, Chapter 191). When patient and nursing opinions about these units were gauged by various measurement tools, a high degree of satisfaction was demonstrated in both groups. This finding translated into lower-than-expected turnover in nursing staff and a decreased use of nurse-controlled consumable supplies. Additionally, patients and families appear more likely to be satisfied and to trust caregivers in an atmosphere of cooperative enterprise. Achieving these goals remains an active area of investigation for nursing and administrative researchers. Despite empirical and objective support for collaborative practice, implementation of collaborative models on a larger scale has been slow. Enduring patterns of physician dominance and nurse deference, together with a heightened sense of competition between professional groups, have retarded progress in this area.

In the critical care environment, the nursing profession has responded to these challenges principally through educational initiatives and team building, thereby leading to a greater sense of autonomy and clarity of purpose. The character of nursing practice is evolving through the use of nurse practitioners, primary care nurses, and clinical nurse specialists. Physicians—unlike their nursing counterparts, who are enjoying a professional ascendancy—have witnessed the erosion of their historical prerogatives on many fronts. The consumer is demanding a greater say in healthcare decisions. The legal profession and the healthcare insurance industry are increasingly reviewing patient management and outcomes. Cumbersome government regulations and changing reimbursement patterns are also affecting the manner in which physicians deliver care. Additional sources of conflict come from administrators who regulate these areas, both within and outside the hospital setting. Thus, the previously preeminent rule of the doctor is diminished. In this modern environment, some physicians are threatened by collaborative practice.

Within the past few years, physicians have become increasingly forced to adapt to multidisciplinary efforts. Currently, many work in groups, and they frequently interact not only with other physicians but also with other healthcare providers. This trend appears to be gaining momentum. Physicians may therefore be more likely to accept a collaborative, mutually respectful relationship with the professional critical care nurse now than they were a few years ago. Increasing contact leading to collaboration often evolves whether consciously pursued or not. Communication is much more likely to be optimal, however, when it reflects a deliberate effort to identify and clarify goals and mutually overlapping roles. In the process of developing such a relationship, the team members in each unit should discuss issues, shared values, and potential areas of conflict. They should develop a mission statement to define the practice model, create standards of care, outline admission and discharge criteria, and develop protocols for caring for patients with difficult problems such as severe or recurring pain or terminal illness. Other steps endorsed by the NJPC include integration of the patient record, encouragement of nurses' decision making, and creation of joint care review panels. A strong, ongoing commitment from administration and the nursing and medical departments is essential for the continued development of such a practice model. Joint practice committees charged with the continuous monitoring of nurse–physician relationships and the evolution of strategies that support joint practice should also be created. These committees should have a balanced rotating membership to decrease the opportunity for any one group to dominate the team's agenda.

Minimizing the inevitable effects of individual conflicts and personal biases is particularly difficult in the ICU, where the self-assurance of nurses and physicians attracted to the specialty is typically quite high. These professionals are accustomed to independent decision making and have a high sense of accountability. Sensitivity to each other's perspectives can be fostered by role-playing activities incorporated into unit retreats, orientation of new nurses and physicians, grand rounds presentations, and basic critical care education. The effectiveness of these policies and techniques have been demonstrated in numerous settings and can be expected to be a common feature of future hospital environments as providers explore ways to control costs, provide comprehensive care, promote professionalism, and ensure patient and family satisfaction.

Preventing Complications in the Intensive Care Unit

Foreseeing and preventing all complications in an ICU is, of course, impossible. Minimizing complications, however, demands that ICU personnel adopt an aggressive approach in managing what are sometimes considered the mundane aspects of patient care, such as skin care or line maintenance. Successful complication prevention requires a multidisciplinary commitment to the development and monitoring of standards of care with a preventive focus. Standards of care should reflect current research findings and should be appropriate for the population of the unit. These standards should incorporate nationally or internationally set standards when available or applicable, for example, international standards for safety in the ICU or the Society of Critical Care Medicine's *Standards of Care for Patients With Acute Respiratory Failure on Mechanical Ventilatory Support* (see *Textbook of Critical Care,* 3rd ed, Chapter 192). In addition to being theoretically sound, these standards must also be continually evaluated through a unit-based program (e.g., continuous quality improvement).

Preventing complications in the ICU must be initiated as early as possible in the patient's stay or before admission (e.g., in patients undergoing elective surgery) when feasible. Standardized admission order forms are useful to ensure that certain procedures are routinely carried out, especially in settings in which a significant learning curve exists, such as in teaching hospitals.

The variety and number of potential complications in critically ill patients are tremendous. Some occur commonly, are pertinent to most critically ill patients, and are predictable and therefore usually preventable. These complications can include the following:

Skin and mucosal breakdown

- Pressure ulcers over bony prominences or around body openings secondary to immobility, decreased oxygen delivery or consumption, poor nutrition, extremely young or old age, obesity, cachexia, edema, diabetes mellitus, immunocompetence, infection, decreased level of consciousness, impaired sensation, hyperthermia or hypothermia, preexisting illness, incontinence, use of vasopressors, and invasive procedures (e.g., intravenous lines)
- Endotracheal tubes at point of entry (lip or nares) or at the site of the intratracheal balloon exacerbated by secretions and fastening ties or tape
- Tracheostomy tubes at point of entry (neck) or at the site of the intratracheal balloon exacerbated by secretions and securing ties
- Feeding tubes and oral, nasal, or gastrostomy sites made worse by leaking or improper taping or tying in place
- Rectal tubes causing mucosal breakdown near the internal retention balloon
- Wound or fistula drainage that leaks onto intact adjacent skin

Musculoskeletal injury

- Contractures and footdrop

Pulmonary complications

- Atelectasis
- Nosocomial pneumonia
- Unplanned extubation

Nosocomial infections due to patient-to-patient cross contamination or staff-to-patient exposure
- Lung
- Surgical wounds
- Urinary bladder or kidneys
- Intravenous or intra-arterial sepsis

ICU psychosis

Other patients develop less common complications secondary to their illness or treatment, including cardiac arrhythmias, pneumothorax, fluid overload, bleeding, stress ulcers, and pulmonary embolism. These complications are covered in the chapters in this book that address the primary illness that may have lead up to the particular complication in question.

Preventing complications in the ICU requires the concerted efforts of a highly skilled multidisciplinary group. Unit-based standards of care and a preventive approach are important for ensuring that early assessment and intervention are carried out for all patients. Ongoing evaluation of these standards through quality-improvement monitoring is needed to ensure that the desired patient outcomes are achieved.

STRESS MANAGEMENT FOR STAFF, PATIENTS, AND PATIENTS' FAMILIES AND BARRIERS TO CARE

A person–environment transaction is stressful if the person feels that his or her well-being is threatened or that coping resources are strained or surpassed. People perceive an event as stressful only if they determine it to have an impact on them. Whether or not a single event becomes a stressor depends on the nature of the stressor itself (harm, threat, or challenge), on whether the event is perceived as stressful, and on the availability of situational supports and effective coping mechanisms.

Maslow's hierarchy of needs can be used as a framework to assess the status of patients, families, and staff in the critical care environment. Physiologic needs require no definition, but employees who are tired, hungry, or thirsty cannot function optimally. This is equally true for family, visitors, and physicians. An environment that is safe and secure is needed before staff can focus on providing quality critical care to patients. When the ICU is not physically safe or when staff believe they are not safe, these factors emerge. Frequent needlesticks, low back injuries, or staff complaints about low wages are red flags that suggest that safety and security needs of the staff are not being fully addressed. Additionally, to perform at their best, staff in a critical care unit must feel as if they are part of a team and belong to the unit. When staff believe that the work they do is valued, they are proud and self-motivated.

Coping strategies are thoughts and acts that the person uses to handle the demands of stressful person–environment transactions; they are considered to be the mediators between the stressful event and its outcome. Most persons tend to use both problem- and emotion-focused strategies during stressful life events. Problem-focused coping involves the confrontive (interpersonal) and cognitive (intrapersonal) forms. Emotion-focused strategies include distancing, escape–avoidance, self-control, positive appraisal, and acceptance of responsibility. When people seek social support (emotional, informational, or tangible aid from another person), they are using a combination of problem- and emotion-focused strategies. People faced with physical health threats seek social support as their primary coping behavior, followed in frequency by wishful thinking, avoidance, and self-blame.

Constant sensitivity to families, who may be overwhelmed by the physical care needs of the critically ill patient, can help to sustain the humanistic and compassionate side of critical care providers' work. Physicians can explain to families the medical plan of care, the patient's response to that plan, and the risks and benefits of treatment modalities for continued care. Nurses orchestrate the timing of critical care, nurturing patients and assisting them in mobilizing their own strengths toward recovery. Nurses can aid families by explaining the hospital's layout, the unit's appearance, and the patient's appearance, as well as by providing information, comfort, and support throughout the patient's critical care experience. Other healthcare professionals, including social workers, psychiatrists, and psychologists, can make important contributions to the care of families. Social workers can guide the family through the maze of clinical and administrative rules and policies. If the family has a religious affiliation, a chaplain or layworker from that denomination can be a valuable source of support and can also be a safe conduit between the family and the physicians and nurses. When death occurs in the ICU, the family needs support from both their own social support network and the direct care providers and psychologic-social-spiritual team of providers interacting with the family.

The recent attention to advance directives, or living wills, and durable powers of attorney may alleviate some of the ethical decision making expected of families of critically ill patients. Living wills go into effect when the patient has no reasonable hope of recovery and is unable to participate in decisions for care. The durable power of attorney provides for a surrogate decision maker in the event of the holder's requiring critical care. The surrogate can provide as much guidance as the person (patient) has allotted him or her before the critical illness or injury (sometimes determined even by chance remarks made by the person prior to becoming a patient).

Neonates

Many potential environmental, physiologic, and procedural neonatal stressors have been identified in the neonatal ICU (see references in *Textbook of Critical Care,* 3rd ed, Chapters 193 and 194), including bright lights, high levels of noise, and sensory deprivation. Routine nursing procedures, such as heel sticks and ventilator weaning, have been shown to cause physiologic stress in the neonate. Stress-reducing techniques include intermittent, gentle tactile contact by the caregiver, non-nutritive sucking, and oscillating waterbeds. While all families experience some disruption of role relationships during critical illness, parents of neonates in ICUs said the most stressful aspect of that environment was the alteration in their parental role. Mothers interviewed 6 months after their babies were discharged from a neonatal unit agreed that their memories were more painful if the infant had been seriously ill, if they had had problems dealing with neonatal ICU staff, or if they experienced less attachment with their infants. In contrast, mothers who retained pleasant memories reported having found a purpose for the hospitalization.

Children

A critically ill child perceives hospitalization as a stressful event, involving both physiologic and psychologic stressors. Behavioral indictors of psychologic stress in hospitalized children vary from appearing passive and withdrawn (showing fear, bewilderment) to kicking, screaming, and biting (showing anxiety, distress). Postoperatively, school-age children use inactive behavior and attempts to control as means of coping. Nurses can support the coping mechanisms of critically ill children by using stress immunization and relaxation techniques. The presence of supportive parents is essential. Absence of the nuclear family from the ICU has been shown to be detrimental to the child's adaptive coping. Parents are able to provide emotional, tangible (physical care), and informational support. Care providers support families by recognizing the tremendous changes the family is experiencing, both for themselves and for the patient. Parents may experience fear, surprise, or revulsion at the sights, sounds, and smells surrounding the child. Nursing interventions should be centered around supporting parents as they resolve three major issues: coping with loss, overcoming barriers to bonding, and obtaining adequate information about the child's course and future needs. Parents reported need for information and for assurance of good care similar to those reported by families of critically ill adults. In addition, parents' being recognized in their child's recovery and helping with the child's physical care were seen as important. Care providers and administration should critically assess the family waiting area for adequacy of size, comfort, food availability, privacy, and toileting facilities. Parents resent restricted visiting; they prefer having open visiting privileges and being allowed to be involved with care of their child (mutual participation model).

Adults

Common indices of injury severity used as predictors of survival in trauma patients have not been useful for estimating their long-term psychosocial adjustment and functional disability. Patients' stress is related to the family environment and to the employment and financial consequences suffered as a result of the injury. Of all demographic and socioeconomic variables that have been evaluated, educational level was the only variable found to be positively related to better long-term functioning. Patients recovering from coronary artery bypass grafting were found to use fewer coping strategies 6 weeks after the bypass than they did 1 week after the bypass. The coping behaviors used most frequently included seeking social support, being problem focused, blaming self for unhealthy behaviors, and engaging in wishful thinking and avoidance.

Interest in the effect that critical illness has on the family began when it was realized that many family needs were not being met in critical care units. Of necessity, nurses' energies are directed toward the patient, leaving little time to help families cope with the threatening event. The impact that the ICU admission has on the family and the patient includes the following:

- Lack of communication
- Protection of children from harmful information
- Perceived overwhelming threat
- Disruption of normalcy at home
- Change in family relationships
- Role conflict and overload

In interviews, nurses appeared to understand little of the impact that critical illness has on family members (see *Textbook of Critical Care,* 3rd ed, Chapter 193). Critical care nurses' responsibilities should include assessment of the family's needs, identification of families at risk for ineffective coping, and identification of strategies to support the psychologic needs of the family. A dysfunctional family may demonstrate high levels of independence, low levels of individual self-esteem, ineffective coping styles, and extremely rigid family relationships. Better patient outcomes occur in families with more cohesion and expressiveness and less conflict. Other family characteristics found to be helpful are independence, intellectual–cultural orientation, active–recreational orientation, and organization. Even well-functioning families may require help with the long-term adjustment to the stress caused by a severe injury. Early referral to counseling services may assist them in functioning more adaptively during the crisis and postcrisis periods.

Staff

The most severe stressors reported by nurses, regardless of work area, were in patient care. Too many interruptions, lack of respect or consideration from physicians, and need for rapid decision making due to physicians not arriving soon enough in a crisis contributed to stress levels. Interruptions and slow laboratory results contributed more to overall stress than did the more severe major work events (work overload and dealing with dying patients). Social support and coping were found to have a direct effect on the work situation. Those who received more social support in the work setting experienced higher job satisfaction and significance and reported fewer health complaints. Factors that have been shown to improve self-actualization include the institution of decentralized decision making, primary nursing, clinical ladder advancement, encouragement of collaborative practice by managers, and provision of incentives for school attendance. The increased emphasis on patient autonomy (e.g., the Patient Self-Determination Act of 1991) comes in the midst of this clash between experienced, opinionated care providers and inexperienced but intimately concerned families. Patients may want freedom from suffering, comfort, and palliation. Families on the other hand may want the patient's survival and continued life support. Care providers want to prevent failure at all costs while espousing commitment to the patient's quality of life and sensible use of available resources.

PART B
Organization and Management of Critical Care*

USE AND ALLOCATION OF CRITICAL CARE RESOURCES

The specialty of critical care medicine is coming of age at a time when all health care in the United States is undergoing dramatic change. The confluence of multiple forces—aging population, a battered economy, technologic advances, and a general awareness that the per capita cost of healthcare in America far exceeds that of other nations—has acutely forced a reassessment of healthcare delivery. Indeed, the military-industrial complex of the 1950s and 1960s has now been replaced by the medical-industrial complex as arguably the single predominant industry in this country. Whereas the restructuring of this industry has been ongoing for some years now, resulting in a free-market melange of private practice, health maintenance organizations (HMOs), preferred provider organizations, and managed care associations, the demand for change will only accelerate in the immediate future. By its nature an expensive, technology-driven specialty, critical care will be at the center of the vortex of evolution.

The demand for reform of healthcare is driven by two powerful forces. The first, and perhaps most potent, is the

*Note to readers: The following two sections of this chapter frequently cite scientific studies and medical publications. For a comprehensive list of references the reader should consult the parallel chapters contained in *Textbook of Critical Care,* 3rd ed.

rapidly escalating cost of healthcare delivery, clashing with an economy in flux. The second is an aging but educated population that has come to know few limits and whose expectations of the miracles of modern science border on the unrealistic. Healthcare costs in the United States are increasing at a rate several times that of inflation. This has caused the public and legislators to take serious notice and many echo the sentiments of a former Governor of Colorado, Richard Lamm, who said: "Medical care is a fiscal black hole into which a nation can pour endless wealth. We should not transfer more national assets to health care."

Serious federal attempts to reform healthcare and control costs began in the early 1970s. One of the major efforts was the passage of the Health Planning and Resource Development Act by Congress in 1974. This gave states and local agencies the authority to review hospital capital expenditures through "certificates of need." The goal was ostensibly to reduce costs by eliminating duplication of services and by generally making institutions think twice before they undertook major capital purchases or engaged in new construction. It has been estimated that this process has slowed the rate of increase of expenditures by 2% to 3% at best and has significantly increased bureaucracy. Despite all efforts, including the introduction of the Medicare Prospective Payment System in 1983, healthcare expenditures continued to rise at a rate estimated at three to five times that of inflation. Despite these extraordinary expenditures, the United States ranked 9th in hospitalizations per capita of 11 Western industrialized nations examined, 9th in life expectancy at birth for women (11th out of 11 for men), and 11th of 11 for both infant mortality and the incidence of low infant birthweight. Indeed, Sweden's infant mortality rate was 58% that of the United States.

Since critical care accounts for over 20% of acute care hospital charges and for about 1% of the nation's gross domestic product, it is inevitable that it will come under the most careful scrutiny of any segment of the medical industry. As the intensity of the healthcare crisis has increased, discussion of rationing healthcare services has become widespread and now permeates the literature. Although the rationing of healthcare services remains a politically dangerous concept, de facto rationing by practitioners and policy makers is generally conceded to be common. National public policy seminars have addressed the issue, and Oregon is engaging in what has been described as "social experimentation" with the rationing of Medicaid expenditures. In 1993, Oregon obtained a federal waiver that allowed it to proceed with the reallocation of Medicaid funds to do the following:

- Extend Medicaid eligibility for all persons with incomes below the national poverty level
- Define a basic minimal healthcare package based on a rank-ordered listing of 709 paired medical conditions and treatments
- Provide a liability shield for medical providers that protects them from both criminal and civil prosecution as well

as from professional disciplinary action when they do not provide those services that the legislature has chosen not to fund

The Oregon Health Plan has great implications for how critical care is provided, regardless of its ultimate success or failure. It has already significantly raised public consciousness of the problems that arise from an increasing demand for a supply of resources that is no longer unlimited. The term *rationing* has now become part of the public policy lexicon and has become the subject of much media attention. It is now common to discuss openly and rationally sensitive issues that were commonly avoided just a few years ago.

Critical care is an expensive resource that must be managed effectively if the compromising of the quality of care delivered is to be avoided. Although there is general agreement about this, there is little agreement and less information about what constitutes quality care and, even more so, cost-effective care. Consequently, rationing not only exists but is growing. Medical ethicists have taken up the issue of rationing and the allocation of resources; the proliferation of papers on the subject attests to this. It is the attending physician, nurse, and patient, however, who are caught between the hammer of reality and the anvil of policy, and this is even more true for the nurse and physician directors of critical care units. Their primary responsibility in managing the units is to ensure the appropriateness and quality of care and, ultimately, the allocation of care and valued scarce resources.

Appropriateness of Care

Appropriate care can be defined as care whose benefits exceed its cost or negative consequences. The definition and measurement of benefit and cost remain elusive yet important goals. Numerous studies and commentaries in the area of medical ethics have been made that include the withdrawal and withholding of care and the difficulty of defining "futile" care. How mortality prediction models such as the Acute Physiology and Chronic Health Evaluation (APACHE) and the Mortality Probability Model (MPM) tools figure into the decision-making process remains to be seen, but they have already contributed significantly to the debate. The applicability of statistical tools that may be 95% or 99% reliable to real-world decisions raises thorny moral, ethical, and social issues (see further discussion on versions of APACHE and MPM later in this chapter).

Utilization of Critical Care Units

It is more than likely that some populations of patients admitted to critical care units could be cared for in less costly environments. Many patients admitted to ICUs never receive any intervention and are admitted strictly for monitoring purposes, receive significantly fewer interventions if they have low APACHE scores, and are admitted because they are thought to be at risk for postoperative complications. The organization and design of critical care units should include provisions for these low-intervention patients, possibly in the form of intermediate or step-down monitoring units. The key to improved utilization is a better understanding of the prognosis by physicians, patients, and their families to reduce the amount of futile care. Surveys have shown, however, that most patients who want to communicate with their physician about life support have not done so.

Measuring and assessing the quality of care delivered are essential components of the utilization of critical care units. The MPM II provides information about the likelihood of survival at the time of admission to the ICU based on 15 objective variables. APACHE III assesses severity of illness and the probability of survival and length of ICU stay based on 17 physiologic variables, age, and 7 comorbid conditions occurring during the first day of ICU stay. The Pediatric Severity of Illness Measure (PRISM) has been used to compare and assess pediatric ICUs (see *Textbook of Critical Care,* 3rd ed, Chapter 198). Although these tools have been extensively tested, they are not widely used in practice, and there is no consensus as to how they should be used. The organizational practices in some of the ICUs that have been studied were related to a patient-centered culture, strong medical and nursing leadership, effective communication and coordination, and open, collaborative approaches to solving problems and managing conflict. Some of these units had strong, shared visions; empowered nursing staffs; ongoing educational programs; a strong sense of collegiality among nurses, physicians, and administrative staff; supportive visible leadership; and a generally defined concept of collaborative practice. However, efficacy was not necessarily related to efficiency, nor were efficacy and efficiency necessarily related to organizational characteristics.

The legitimate demand for ICU care occasionally exceeds the supply. The responsibility to triage—that is, to ensure adequate care and the appropriate allocation of scarce resources—falls directly on the shoulders of the unit directors. This is an important point to stress in an environment in which the allocation of ICU resources is often performed in an ad hoc manner and not necessarily with consideration of the best interests of the patient or the population as a whole. One study observed that during times of overcrowding, surgical attending physicians rarely used other open in-house ICU beds when surgical ICU beds were unavailable. Political power, medical provincialism, and income maximization overrode medical suitability in the provision of critical care services. The great difficulty for ICU directors is that triage and rationing place them in a position in which a serious potential for conflict of interest exists, especially if the director is personally caring for patients in the critical care unit.

Managing Units

As the problems of ensuring appropriate care, quality care, and the allocation of resources are examined, it is apparent not only that these issues have economic, medical, legal, and ethical implications but also that they are closely interrelated. None of these issues can be considered in isolation. Rather, they are systematic problem areas that are closely interconnected and interdependent. To deal with these issues in a timely manner, the ICU must be viewed as a single system, an organization with multiple constituents, and stakeholders embedded within the larger framework of the hospital and its stakeholders, which in turn constitute the regional and national healthcare economies. Every critical care unit has a particular culture that resists change, as do the practices of medicine and nursing themselves. Patient-focused care, or even acceptance of the idea of employing a full-time intensivist or director of critical care, requires a significant change in thinking—that is, a change in the organizational culture of not only the ICU but also of the medical staff, the nurses, the ancillary staff, and the hospital administrators. The forces of change, driven by the healthcare economic crisis, mandate that critical care units can no longer be managed in the laissez faire mode of the past. The future requires that a comprehensive, multidisciplinary, systematic approach be taken to the management of all health care, but especially to those areas that demand the most resources. Critical care specialists must provide the leadership to ensure the optimal use and allocation of these vital resources.

COMPUTERS IN THE INTENSIVE CARE UNIT

As a result of their medical problems, patients in ICUs are monitored with elaborate bedside consoles and are subjected to a wide variety of laboratory tests. Therapy is complex, timing of treatment is critical, and careful documentation of the care given is essential. A large volume of data must be stored, processed, and used for clinical decision making. The tremendous growth in the volume of medical information, the demand for cost-effective care, and the need to document and justify clinical decisions have placed a large burden on the medical care team. Patients, payers, the public, and healthcare policy makers are increasingly demanding accountability, insisting that complete and accurate records be kept by physicians, nurses, and therapists who care for the critically ill.

Since the late 1960s, rapid development in business computer technology has occurred, with remarkable reductions in computer cost (from $500,000 to less than $5,000) and size (from room-sized units to laptop models), as well as an almost 1,000-fold improvement in computing speed and a reduction in power consumption. With the increasing capability and decreasing cost of computing, the possibility of using computers to help solve the problem of data collection, storage, and decision-making support needs of the ICU is attractive.

Computerized Record Keeping

The medical record remains the principal instrument for ensuring the continuity of patient care. In complicated cases, the conventional handwritten record is less helpful than a structured flow chart. In one study, detailed records were kept of the data used by physicians to make treatment decisions during teaching rounds in a shock-trauma ICU. It was a surprise to find that laboratory values (42%) were the most frequently used data (clinical laboratory: 33%; blood gas values: 9%), since physiologic bedside monitors have become synonymous with the modern ICU. Drug and fluid balance data were next (22%), followed by clinicians' observations (21%). The bedside physiologic monitor accounted for only 13% of the data used in making therapeutic decisions during teaching rounds. These findings also provide evidence that data from several sources, not just from the traditional physiologic bedside monitoring devices, must be communicated and integrated into a unified medical record to permit effective decision making and treatment in the ICU.

Integrated Intensive Care Unit Computer Records

Computer charting in the ICU must support multiple types of data collection to be effective. For computer charting systems to be successful, they must be able to collect a wide variety of data from bedside monitors as well as from nurses and physicians at the bedside. Many computer systems disregard these requirements and unwittingly force double-charting. Communication of information to other departments within a hospital is mandatory. Convenient and timely access to clinical and administrative information from a physician's home or office by means of a modem and a personal computer link is essential. A computerized record allows this type of communication. Because the computerized ICU record is stored in the system, it is also readily available for concurrent or retrospective research purposes. Although excellent progress has been made in the field of computerization in the ICU, many challenges have yet to be overcome:

- Development of better data entry techniques, including mouse and floating cursor, light pens, touch-sensitive monitor screens, and charting by exception
- Standardization of data transfer among computers, such as for laboratory results
- Creation of a medical information bus, a device to connect bedside monitors together to aggregate data
- Better quality control methods for alerting, reminding, and directing staff

The mark of a good physician is the ability to make sound clinical judgments. Medical decision making has traditionally been considered an artful and intuitive process rather than a scientific process. In recent years, however, computerized medical decision making has gained greater acceptance.

Until 1993, the development of computerized patient data management systems took place primarily in universities and medical schools and their affiliated hospitals. As a result of the interest and excitement of having computer-assisted care in the ICU, several commercial vendors became interested in the marketing of such systems. A number of commercially available computerized ICU systems that have decision-support capabilities are now becoming available.

A Healthcare Scenario of the Future

While driving a new car, John Smith, a hypothetical patient, was involved in a severe head-on collision with a tree. The incident occurred at a remote location on a state turnpike. The transit times for police and rescue crews were optimally short because John's car was equipped with a crash alarming system. The system transmitted the exact location of the crash based on global positioning coordinates.

John was the sole occupant of the car and was found unconscious at the scene. Fortunately, he carried his healthcare record on a "smart card," which is like a credit card. Using the rescue vehicle's card reader, an emergency medical technician was able to obtain critical information about John's history of arrhythmias and his current treatment regimen. All the observations and interventions at the accident site were entered into a pen-based computer:

- An electronic pen replaces the keyboard and the pointing device.
- The user interface includes a menu of choices whenever possible.
- Selections are made by pointing to the menu choices with the pen.
- The computer recognizes handwritten letters and numbers.
- Diagrams can be drawn on the screen and stored as part of the record.

The locations of John's injuries were entered on anatomic diagrams that were brought up on the screen. The cardiac and blood pressure monitors provided direct input to the computer. All data were simultaneously sent to the receiving trauma center by radio transmission.

The police used a similar computer to report the crash information. Electronic images of the scene and of the interior and exterior of the vehicle were obtained. Relevant views were transmitted to the trauma center, providing graphic documentation of the positioning of the occupant before extrication from the vehicle as well as data on the magnitude of the crash forces. At the trauma center, all data from John's medical history, including recent radiographic images and the police and rescue crew information, were available. Monitored data and interventions, such as fluid infusions, were electronically entered into the computer system.

In this future system, nurses chart observations and interventions such as medication infusions using radio-linked, pen-based computers. A coding system allows descriptions of diagnoses and procedures to be chosen from menus. These detailed descriptions form a problem list, which summarizes the care process. The vocabulary in the menus is easy to understand but also detailed. Translations are made by the computer system to other standardized nomenclatures, such as the internal Classification of Diseases, the Abbreviated Injury Score, and the Current Procedural Terminology. The standardized nomenclature is also used for performing searches of computerized literature. Other features of the system include the following:

- Unstructured comments are dictated.
- The system reviews all dictation for content. (It informs the clinician who is dictating whenever codifiable diagnoses of procedures contained in the dictation are not included in the data base.)
- All radiographs, scans, and ultrasound examinations are maintained in the system.
- High-resolution electronic "viewstations" throughout the trauma center allow multiple images to be reviewed simultaneously.
- The data "superhighway" permits consultation on diagnostic images with geographically distant experts.
- Orders are entered into the computer system. Complex software can evaluate orders for completeness, appropriateness, and cost-effectiveness.
- Dosage of an ordered drug can be checked.
- Patients can be included in research protocols much more easily. The system can review each patient's description to determine eligibility for various protocols.

Ultrasound evaluation had quickly confirmed a hemoperitoneum, and the accident victim, John, was taken to the operating room a short time after his arrival at the trauma center. There:

- Anesthesiology workstations have hands-free voice-entry for data.
- Electronically recorded operating room data are entered directly.
- Inventory management system is updated each time supplies are used.
- Replacement materials are automatically ordered as needed.
- Nurse, surgeon, and anesthetist records all identify the same times, diagnoses, procedures, and participating personnel.
- The surgeon uses ceiling-mounted and laparoscopic cameras to document the operative procedure.
- The dictated (and electronically transcribed) operative report is supplemented by a description of the diagnosis and procedures that is based on the standardized nomenclature system.

In the ICU of the future, all of this patient's previously obtained data will be available. In this case, it was useful to have a complete record of fluid and medication interventions used during resuscitation and in the operating room. All information was computerized, and nursing tasks, monitoring data, and laboratory results were readily available. Patient care both in the ICU and on the patient care floors will be improved for several reasons:

- Clinicians can review the literature on similar problems stored in electronic libraries.
- Case histories on similar cases can be reviewed.
- Quality assurance and utilization review are byproducts of the system.
- Professional and hospital bills emanate from the clinical data base.
- Discrepancies can be eliminated, reducing medicolegal risks.
- Multimedia inservice education can be provided.
- Self-evaluation can be performed.
- Electronic reference materials like the *Physicians Desk Reference* can be reviewed.

Technology in Transition

In the past, it would have been impossible to develop large-scale information systems with the complexity and scope described in this scenario. Impediments to building useful computer-based patient records (CPRs) are quickly disappearing as reliability, speed, multiuser functions, huge data bases, vast supplies of software, and availability of remote workstations become reality. It is not clear what costs hospitals will incur to computerize medical record keeping, but estimates run $20,000 to $30,000 per ICU bed. It is unknown whether hospitals will be willing to take on the expense of installation and maintenance of such units, not to mention the costs of training personnel to use it. Hospitals spend a significant portion of their operating costs on current paper and radiographic record keeping, but whether these costs can be offset by the costs of a computerized system is unknown. Although advantages of computerization include instantaneous data availability, readily available copies, retrieval of data for reporting demands, reduction of medicolegal risks, and obviation of indecipherable handwriting, future approaches are not clear.

Data Server Technology

In the new generation of computer technology, data are maintained on optimized "servers," in which everything is stored in digitized form, such as on commonly available compact disks. In a similar fashion, radiographs, color pictures of histologic preparations, and even motion-based images such as ultrasound examinations and angiograms can be stored. A server capable of supporting hundreds of users simultaneously while managing vast quantities of stored data can be bought for a few thousand dollars. Servers can provide uninterrupted availability of data.

The Network Link

The second part of the client-server technology is the network that links the hundreds of workstations and the data servers needed in even medium-sized hospitals. Current technology supports data transmission rates of up to 10 megabytes per second (roughly equal to 1 million single letters or numbers). The technology of the future will likely use the "asynchronous transmission mode," which will handle hundreds of millions of bytes of data per second. (To achieve truly paperless and filmless CPRs, advanced communication technologies like the asynchronous transmission mode will be necessary.) For example, many clinicians will need to simultaneously view their patients' radiographs at workstations throughout a hospital. Each image will be equivalent, minimally, to a 1 million–byte record. For all the images to appear instantaneously, the network capacity must be very high. Traditional approaches use only wires or fiberoptic cables for transmission, whereas wireless communication typically employs radiofrequency technologies. Advantages include movable and untethered terminals, high-speed communication, and the unlimited number of clients that can be serviced.

American medicine may be about to embark on a journey into a new way of operating. In the future, the management of resources may be as critical as the care of patients. However, optimization of the system of care will occur only if educational and management strategies that take advantage of the potential are developed.

SEVERITY OF ILLNESS INDICES AND OUTCOME PREDICTION: DEVELOPMENT AND EVALUATION

A desirable outcome is often perceived differently by physicians, patients, and society. Modern clinical trials are designed to assess the impact of medical intervention on one or more traditional endpoints, typically survival or a quantifiable measure of disease activity, such as cardiac ejection fraction. These endpoints, however, are not what concerns patients the most. Whereas physicians focus on chances for disease-free and overall survival, patients may be more concerned with the potential of returning to baseline function, of being chronically disabled, or of being a burden to their family. For many, some of these alternative outcomes are worse than death.

Defining acceptable outcomes for individuals is particularly relevant for critical care because modern life-sustaining therapy often succeeds in postponing death but may be ineffective at restoring health. As the science of outcome prediction matures, qualitative outcomes, rather than mortality alone, will be increasingly measured. Efforts are ongoing and will provide data so that physicians can offer informed treatment options. Until better data are available, physicians learning to incorporate predictive models into their practice must bear in mind the limitations of using mortality as an endpoint.

Improving Accuracy of Medical Decisions

Medical decisions are made in a fashion that is analogous to the way individuals make everyday decisions and are based on a hypothetical-deductive model, heuristics, or rule-based behavior. Probability estimates generated by predictive instruments help guard against errors introduced by standard clinical decision making by providing objective estimates based on a representative patient sample. Most ICU patients require multiple diagnostic and therapeutic interventions, and construction of a basic decision tree using probability estimates derived from a predictive model provides a way to present outcomes for different treatment options scientifically rather than empirically. Most physicians are not yet ready to incorporate formal decision models or predictive instruments into everyday practice, and they remain skeptical of the accuracy of these instruments. These instruments have generally performed as well as or better than clinicians in discriminating outcome (i.e., predicting who will live or die). Clinicians are adept at selecting patients at high risk for mortality (frequently stated as >90% chance for death) but provide less accurate predictions for patients with moderate illness.

Statistics, Patient Autonomy, and Futility in Medicine

Although probability estimates are generated using scientific principles, statistical considerations can introduce considerable uncertainty about their accuracy. A study of prognosis in 500 patients with nontraumatic coma used neurologic findings to predict outcome with excellent accuracy. However, opponents of using these data point out that even this relatively large study had a 5% false-positive rate in predicting chronic vegetative state, a condition that occurs in 1% of cases. This disparity implies that 7 patients of the next 90 identified to have no recovery or severe disability instead could have moderate disability or good recovery.

Even if a prognostic system were able to generate statistical accuracy, many physicians would still be unable or reluctant to act on this information. Our society emphasizes the autonomy of each patient, and some patients want every intervention, no matter what the chances. Thus, for physicians who value life above all other considerations, even if outcome data were 100% accurate, life support would not be withdrawn or limited for the 99 patients destined to die if the 100th patient is destined to survive. As already discussed, however, cost considerations are mandating a change in the paradigm, and although patient autonomy will always be respected, patients are unlikely to be able to insist on an intervention that is unlikely to benefit them. Recent efforts to define futility in medicine are important indicators of the desire to provide guidelines to practitioners as to when they might consider continued treatment of a given case "futile." One proposed definition of futility is treatment that has not benefited or has failed in the most recent 100 patients to whom it has been offered. Defining a treatment as futile does not preclude the possibility that it could benefit a given patient, but it does provide a rationale for withholding the treatment. Although attempts to develop a numeric definition of futility oversimplifies a complex concept, objective estimates of outcome will be important in providing information that can be used for these difficult medical decisions. It will always be important to remember, however, that probability estimates are best used to support clinical decisions, not to make them.

Outcome Prediction Models

Outcome prediction models can be broadly classified as disease specific or general. Prognostic indices for specific diseases include the Ranson criteria for acute pancreatitis, the Child-Turcotte classification for cirrhosis, the Burn Index, the Injury Severity Score System, the Glasgow Coma Scale for assessing neurologic function, and the Hunt-Hess scale for subarachnoid hemorrhage. Prognostic indices developed for specific diseases have a conceptual advantage over general systems because they focus on predictors that are specific or peculiar to that entity. A general prediction model (e.g., APACHE III), however, is intended to estimate prognosis for a broad variety of diseases. Since general prognostic systems have the widest applicability, readers are encouraged to familiarize themselves with these systems and their uses.

Mortality Prediction Model

The MPM was designed to estimate the probability of hospital mortality at ICU admission, 24 and 48 hours after admission, and at other intervals during ICU stay. The methods used to develop the MPM differ substantially from those used for APACHE II. Instead of using an expert panel to select and weight predictors according to perceived severity and impact on survival, the MPM is based on objective statistical modeling. Information was obtained on a large number of variables, followed by identification of a smaller subset of the strongest outcome predictors derived from statistical reduction techniques. The MPM has been used to estimate probability of hospital mortality for ICU patient groups and for identifying charts for ICU quality assessment review. The MPM is not recommended for assessing prognosis for an individual patient. Refinement is continuing, with the aim of improving the MPM's accuracy and usefulness.

Acute Physiology and Chronic Health Evaluation

The original APACHE system was introduced in 1981 and consisted of two parts: (1) a scale that reflected the degree of physiologic derangement and (2) a chronic health evaluation that reflected the patient's status before the acute illness. This scale was developed by an expert panel of physicians who selected and weighted 34 laboratory and clinical measurements based on their perceived impact on mortality. APACHE provided a reliable and valid method for severity measurement and risk stratification but was complex and required multihospital validation. APACHE II was introduced in 1985 and incorporated major changes in the original APACHE system. The number of physiologic variables was reduced from 34 to 12, and a higher score was assigned to acute renal failure and coma to better reflect their prognostic impact. Scoring for operative status, such as emergency surgery, was added, and chronic health evaluation was changed to reflect the impact of aging; immune deficiency; and chronic cardiac, pulmonary, renal, or liver disease. Finally, an equation was developed to estimate prognosis based on information collected during the first 24 hours in the ICU.

APACHE III was introduced in 1991 to expand and improve the prognostic estimates provided by APACHE II. APACHE III re-evaluated the selection and weighting of physiologic variables using objective statistical modeling; expanded the size and representative nature of the reference data base; examined how outcome is related to patient selection for, and timing of, ICU admission; and clearly distinguished the use of predictive estimates for patient groups from mortality estimates for individuals.

The APACHE III system consists of two parts: an APACHE III score and a series of predictive equations linked to diagnosis and the APACHE III data base. The APACHE III score consists of points for physiologic abnormalities, age, and chronic health status.

Scoring is based on the degree of abnormality in 17 physiologic variables, which reflect values for vital signs, laboratory tests, and neurologic status. In addition, points are added based on age and seven comorbid conditions shown to have a significant impact on short-term mortality. The sum of points for APACHE III's components yields a numeric score that theoretically ranges from 0 to 299; physiologic scoring contributes most (0–252) of the score, compared with age (0–24) and chronic health evaluation (0–23).

The APACHE III score can be used to measure severity of disease and to stratify patients by risk within a single diagnostic category or independently defined patient group. This is because an increasing score is associated with an higher risk of hospital death.

Future Applications of Prognostic Systems

It is expected that, in the future, the use of prognostic systems for clinical research, quality improvement, and utilization review will become more common and more sophisticated. These systems will be used to assist in decision making about ICU admission and discharge, but their exact role in individual patient care decisions is uncertain. ICU clinicians could obtain and use probabilities at the patient's bedside in much the same way the results of laboratory tests are currently used. Unlike the results of a blood test, however, a risk probability is derived indirectly from patient characteristics and a reference data base.

Conclusions

Important social and financial considerations are changing American medicine. Physicians are, and should remain, uncomfortable with making treatment decisions based solely on financial factors, but the influence of these factors can no longer be avoided. In 1992, an estimated $809 billion was spent in the United States on health care, representing 13% of the gross national product. Current practices will continue to escalate these expenditures, hence the mandate for change.

For financial, ethical, and medical reasons, intensive care is likely to be heavily scrutinized as part of any new health care delivery proposal. Policy analysts point at studies that suggest that 8% of ICU patients, the "high-cost admissions," consumed as many resources as the remaining 92%. Of the 8% designated as high-cost patients, 70% died in the hospital. Results of such studies, combined with a general societal concern about the amount of healthcare costs spent during the last year of life, add to the perception that we are wasting substantial resources.

Cost control should never dictate withholding or withdrawal of care, and physicians must strive to maintain their role as a patient advocate. Physicians also need to recognize, however, that financial considerations are not necessarily at odds with their primary scientific and ethical obligations. Predicting who will and who will not benefit from ICU care is an important new step in refining use of the very expensive therapy.

PART C
Ethical Decision Making in Critically Ill Patients

LEGAL ISSUES INVOLVED IN THE DELIVERY OF CRITICAL CARE MEDICINE

With the advent of advanced and complex medical technology, and with the ever-increasing concern over patients' rights to make informed medical decisions, it is not surprising to see a concomitant increase in litigation about medical care decisions. These are not, however, the traditional medical malpractice cases that most American courts are familiar with. Rather, these cases involve complex ethical, legal, and medical issues concerning a patient's right to die and right to demand or reject appropriate medical care. Moreover, it is unfortunate that the American legal and legislative systems have so much involvement in the making of what many would argue are medical decisions best left to the patient and to his or her attending physician.

Indeed, judicial cases in this area have become so numerous that the federal government recently enacted a new law, the Patient Self-Determination Act of 1991, in an attempt to reduce the number of patient and medical provider controversies being resolved in the courts. The Patient Self-Determination Act requires all hospitals, skilled nursing facilities, home health agencies, hospice programs, and HMOs that receive Medicaid or Medicare funding to give written information to all incoming patients on a patient's right to create a living will or a medical power of attorney under applicable state laws. The act does not require that a medical facility actually assist the patient in making these advance directives, but it does require that each medical facility have a written policy informing its patients of the assistance they can receive in adopting or rejecting these advance directives.

Because these advanced directives are created by state law, the federal Patient Self-Determination Act has a secondary purpose of encouraging the state legislatures to reassess their own living will statutes—if they have them—and, it is hoped, to revise prior state legislation in light of the newer empirical, ethical, and legal trends in medical decision making.

Although most states have living will statutes, some do not, and even among the states with living will laws the individual state statutes differ significantly. Moreover, despite the greater availability of state laws allowing more people to create living wills, few people choose to do so. In addition, because those who have living wills seldom carry them on their person or make reference to them, hospital emergency departments and ICUs treating trauma patients usually do not have written documents to rely on.

Accordingly, despite these important state and federal laws, which were created largely to avoid litigation, many medicolegal conflicts must still be resolved by the courts. And although these judicial controversies deal with medical, legal, and ethical issues, they can all be classified within general conceptual categories that assist the reader in understanding how the courts are attempting to resolve these troubling controversies.

Medical Decisions Made by a Competent Adult Patient

A competent adult patient generally has the legal right in most states to refuse medical treatment and to be free of medical intervention, even at the risk of his or her death, and this legal right of a patient's self-determination normally outweighs the state's interest in preserving life or in safeguarding the integrity of the medical profession. Moreover, an incompetent patient can express this intent through a prior living will document or through the surrogate decision making of a relative.

Medical treatment involving minors, however, is a very different matter, and numerous judicial cases have held that when medical treatment involves little risk to the child, but a failure to provide treatment would substantially endanger the child's life or health, the state can step in, acting under its *parens patriae* power, and order such medical treatment over the objection of the child's parents.

Once an appropriate decision maker has been designated, another category of judicial opinions deals with what legal standards are involved in the making of the decision itself.

The elements normally include the risks and benefits of treatment, the alternatives to treatment, and the consequences of foregoing such treatment.

Medical Decisions Made on Behalf of an Incompetent Adult Patient

Making medical decisions for an incompetent patient is a different matter entirely. Five tests for competency have been proposed in the literature or have been inferred from judicial commentary:

- *Evidencing of a choice:* the unconscious patient or the mute psychiatric patient
- *"Reasonable" outcome of choice:* the patient's capacity to reach the "right" or "responsible" decision
- *Choice based on the patient's "rational" reasons*
- *Ability to understand the information:* even if the patient weighs the information differently from the caregiver
- *Actual understanding:* the physician's responsibility to educate the patient and to ascertain whether he or she has understood the risks and benefits of medical treatment or nontreatment.

Once a determination is made that the patient does not have the capacity to make medical decisions, the courts must apply additional legal tests to determine who will make such medical decisions in lieu of, and on behalf of, the incompetent patient.

Surrogate Medical Decision Making

If the patient is deemed incompetent but once had the capacity for decision making, the surrogate assigned to make the medical decision on the patient's behalf is required to make his or her decision based on what the patient would have wanted. This legal standard for surrogate decision making is call the *substituted judgment test.* This means that treatment can be withheld or withdrawn from an incompetent patient when the particular patient would clearly have refused the treatment under the circumstances involved.

Under a *limited objective test,* life-sustaining treatment can be withheld or withdrawn from a patient when trustworthy evidence exists that the patient would have refused the treatment and the decision maker is satisfied that the burdens of the patient's continued life with the treatment clearly outweigh the benefits of life to him or her. Under a *pure objective test,* net burdens of the patient's life with the treatment should clearly and markedly outweigh the benefits the patient derives from life. Further, the recurring, unavoidable, and severe pain of the patient's life with the treatment should be such that the effect of administering life-sustaining treatment would be inhumane. It has been held in at least one case that decision making based on assessments of the personal worth or social utility of another's life or on the value of that life to others could not be authorized.

Thus, a surrogate decision maker attempts to establish as

accurately as possible what decision the patient would make if he or she were competent to do so. He or she tries to determine the following:

- Expressed preferences of the patient
- Religious convictions of the patient
- The impact on the family
- The probability of adverse side effects

Traditionally, physicians and the courts look to the patient's family as appropriate surrogate decision makers because the family usually is the most concerned about the good of the patient; is the most knowledgeable about the patient's goals, preferences, and values; and deserves recognition as an important social unit. The state should be reluctant to intrude. Consulting with family members also neutralizes the possibility of subsequent medical malpractice claims, and this element also accounts for its current popularity.

Problems still arise, however, when family members disagree about what constitutes appropriate medical treatment for an incompetent patient, when they may not be acting in the best interests of the patient, or when the patient has never had the capacity to make medical decisions. For these patients, many courts are increasingly using a *best interests test.* In the same manner that many Americans evidence a general denial of death, however, many courts have a difficult time conceding the reality of an impending death. The debatable logic is that any prolongation of life is a better "interest" than is death and any act that can be performed to prolong life, despite the medical futility of such an act and despite the suffering of the patient, is defined as being in the best interests of the patient.

Limitations on a Patient's Medical Choices

A patient must decide whether he or she wants a particular medical treatment before a physician can treat the patient. A patient's right to decide whether he or she wants medical treatment is meaningless, however, unless the patient has information about the risks and benefits of the proposed medical treatment. This is the concept of informed consent, and it constitutes the legal basis for the medical, legal, and ethical principle of patient autonomy. Complete patient autonomy is not always possible, because a patient cannot possess all of the medical knowledge held by his or her physician.

Various courts throughout the United States have affirmed a group of state interests that could supersede a patient's right to choose or refuse medical treatments:

- Preserving life
- Preventing suicide
- Protecting innocent third persons, such as children
- Preserving the integrity of the medical profession
- Encouraging the charitable and humane care of afflicted persons

Courts have always taken a strong interest in the protection of children. Therefore, when parents refuse to consent for medical treatment deemed necessary to save the life of a child, courts often overrule the patients' desires, whether they be based on religious convictions or other reasons. When parents cannot agree on a treatment decision for a terminally ill child, for example, the hospital can request a hearing and appointment of an independent guardian.

Taking into account all of these countervailing interests (including patient autonomy versus appropriate medical treatment), current medical and ethical thought, buttressed by numerous influential judicial decisions, strongly suggests that physicians now have the moral and legal responsibility to respect the wishes of competent patients and the wishes of surrogate decision makers for incompetent patients in regards to the termination of life-sustaining medical treatment or futile medical care.

The troubling corollary to patient autonomy and right-to-die cases is the scenario of a patient's right to demand medical care, even though the attending physician believes that such medical treatment would be futile. Here again, limits to patient autonomy exist, and patients have never had a generally recognized legal right to demand unlimited medical care. As America moves toward a national health system that surely will place more limitations on the type and the amount of medical care that Americans will receive, however, more legal controversies in this area are likely. When people do not get what they want, they increasingly resort to the courts. Health care rationing, or the process of making rational choices for medical care under new budgetary and personnel restrictions, will thus undoubtedly constitute the next horizon of judicial involvement in this medicolegal brave new world.

Positive Versus Negative Rights and the Integrity of the Medical Profession

It is a fallacy to believe that because patients have a moral right to refuse life-sustaining treatment they have an unqualified right to demand it. The negative right to refuse treatment is found in the constitutional rights of privacy and liberty or in the common law right against battery. Positive rights to have treatment may exist, but, if they do, they must be understood and justified separately from the right to refuse treatment.

The doctrine of informed consent specifies that patients have a right to an informed choice or a refusal of treatments offered to them within the standard of medical care; it does not say that they have a right to ask for any and all treatments at a physician's disposal. Society has entrusted physicians with the responsibility for making clinical judgments, and the patient's ability to exercise positive rights to treatment is limited by those judgments. In fact, judgments form the basis of the medical profession, and medicine has goals that the physician must promote—above all, to benefit patients and do them no harm. The act of offering a futile intervention sends a mixed message that may actually undermine patient autonomy. After all, why would a physician offer a treatment if it were not going to be helpful?

MEDICAL FUTILITY

Futility must always be discussed in relation to an identified goal. Potential goals include postponing the moment of death, extending life for a specific period, and achieving an acceptable quality of life. It may also be defined by the *probability* of a given intervention's achieving a goal. Below a certain probability, an intervention would be considered futile. The further away from physiologic futility the decision makers get, the more value judgments are introduced about the worthiness of the goals that can be achieved, or the probability that distinguishes an unacceptably low chance from a chance worth taking. The physician has a responsibility to restrict the alternatives made available to patients, employing value judgments that will benefit the patient as a whole. The goal of medicine is to achieve a benefit above a certain minimal *qualitative* or *quantitative* threshold.

Several other concerns have been raised about a physician's using futility as a rationale for unilaterally limiting treatment, since determinations of futility are so value laden. Until standards are set for the profession as a whole, definitions of futility will likely vary from physician to physician. Some argue that condoning unilateral decision making by physicians would set back shared decision making between patient, family, and physician, returning us to an earlier era of unbridled paternalism that our society has found unsatisfactory. Concern exists that rationing and futility are becoming confused. This issue is important because futility and rationing have different meanings, moral implications, and methods for resolution.

Motives for Demanding Futile Treatment

Rather than learning to understand the reasons that patients and their families demand futile interventions, physicians can use medical futility as an easy explanation for nontreatment. Understanding what motivates people to ask for or demand futile therapy offers physicians an opportunity to provide optimal care for dying patients and their families and to promote shared decision making.

The reasons that patients and families demand futile care include the following:

Failure to set timely treatment goals, which can include

- Restoring the patient to a previous satisfactory quality of life.
- Achieving a reduced but still satisfactory quality of life.
- Helping patients and families realize that a goal is not achievable.
- Discussing death and dying, which is often difficult and time-consuming.

- Planning to keep the patient comfortable while allowing death to occur.

Ignorance

- Patients or families simply do not understand the facts.

Confusion

- Patients have been given inconsistent and contradictory information.
- Attending physicians on the case do not agree on a treatment plan.
- Multiple consultants may give information on isolated body systems only.
- Monthly rotation of house officers or shift changes of nurses breaks continuity of care.

Mistrust

- Some patients are habitually mistrusting.
- Previous medical predictions have not come to pass.
- Socioeconomic or racial diversity affects perceptions and attitudes.

By understanding the motives that lead to requests for futile treatment, physicians can take steps to prevent a confrontation near the end of a patient's life. By creating treatment goals with staff, patients, and family members giving full disclosure about prognoses and by providing consistent care, the level of mistrust can be minimized.

As more institutions and professional societies develop medical futility policies, our society perhaps will recognize the difference between the negative right to refuse treatment and the positive right to demand it, letting physicians make more professional judgments about how to determine when end-of-life interventions offer little or no benefit.

FOREGOING LIFE-SUSTAINING THERAPY IN INTENSIVE CARE

In *The Art,* Hippocrates stated that the role of medicine was "to do away with the sufferings of the sick, to lessen the violence of their diseases, and to refuse to treat those who are overmastered by their diseases, realizing that in such cases, medicine is powerless." Thus, the physician must try to cure those who may be cured, decrease morbidity of diseases where possible, and when unable to do so, ensure a patient's comfort. Finally, when a disease has "won" and a patient will die, the physician is obligated to recognize this and to ease the dying process. This characterization remains peculiarly pertinent to intensive care more than two millennia after Hippocrates.

Although the attempt to forestall death has been present in physicians' actions throughout time, it was not until the recent past that they could significantly affect the prevention of death without influencing the likelihood of recovery. That is, with the advent of techniques that support failed organs for a potentially indefinite time, machines can now breathe, pump blood, excrete wastes, and provide nutrition for patients. Thus, a new category of patient was created as a result of medical advancement—the "nearly dead," those who are alive only because they are receiving life support in the ICU.

When ICUs were first created, they were filled not with the elderly but rather with young patients who were more likely to benefit from the interventions they provided. As the benefits became more apparent, older and sicker patients were also treated in these ICUs. The new dilemma of how to deal with incurable life-supported ICU patients was recognized. Physicians have no obligation to treat diseases from which there is no hope of recovery. If they agree, physicians and patients are now widely accorded the ability and right to withdraw futile therapy in the face of terminal illness.

Distinction Between Withholding and Withdrawing Support

Withholding support is defined as never providing the patient with a particular therapy; *withdrawing* support refers to discontinuing therapy that has already been instituted. The phrase *foregoing therapy* refers to both withdrawing and withholding therapy. Both of these approaches result in the unimpeded progression of the disease; the two focuses of foregoing therapy are considered ethically equivalent. However, many families feel uncomfortable terminating support because of the temporal relation between the removal of support and the patient's death, if it occurs soon thereafter.

Interventions *intended* to hasten death directly are considered *active euthanasia,* which is illegal in the United States. An example of active euthanasia is the delivery of a lethal intravenous dose of potassium chloride, which causes cardiac arrest.

Assisted suicide refers to the practice of helping a person to take his or her own life but not of directly performing the action that causes death. An example would be placement of an intravenous catheter into a patient, supplying the lethal medication, and instructing the patient in how to use it to commit suicide.

Withdrawing Mechanical Ventilatory Assistance

Removing respiratory support requires special attention because of its emotive nature and the significant distress that it can cause for the patient, his or her family, and the professional staff. The major goal of the removal of ventilatory assistance is the withdrawal of unwanted therapy while maintaining a patient's comfort. Patients who have their ventilatory assistance withdrawn are likely to suffer respiratory distress unless their physicians anticipate this occurrence and act to prevent and treat it. Sedation in the form of narcotics administration (to suppress feelings of dyspnea) and the use of anxiolytics (to suppress anxiety) are almost always necessary. In dosing these medications, it is important to remember the therapeutic goals. It is crucial that comfort be maintained, even if providing the needed medication also hastens death. This has been referred to as the *double effect*. For example, a hypotensive patient who has respiratory discomfort should still receive narcotics, even though his or her blood pressure may decrease further as a result and death may occur sooner. The physician's *primary* intent—to relieve suffering—is crucial to the legitimate giving of medication that may also hasten death.

Most physicians choose to give morphine or diazepam, or both, to relieve anxiety and to prevent dyspnea before they initiate therapy withdrawal. As withdrawal of mechanical ventilation progresses, more sedation is usually required. Physicians and nursing staff watch carefully for signs of distress and alleviate them immediately. It is important to recognize that respiratory drive is a potent force in the cause of this distress. Many ICU patients have developed some tolerance to opioids and sedatives. Therefore, very large doses of these medications may be required. Some patients may need hundreds of milligrams of morphine if adequate control is to be achieved. Experienced physicians are able to titrate the sedation to prevent rather than to relieve discomfort, and this is a laudable practice. As long as the patient remains comfortable, weaning from ventilatory support can proceed, but the rate of progression depends on patient tolerance. The decision of whether to extubate the patient must be considered by the medical team, the patient, and the family. If the tube is removed, care must be taken to prevent acute airway obstruction, which can cause the patient significant distress. Use of an oral or nasal airway is usually sufficient for this purpose.

Most commonly, the physician remains at the bedside to titrate the medications. Careful documentation of dosage and of the rationale for the medication is warranted. Some nurses who are experienced in the withdrawal of support are able to enact terminal weaning orders as long as an experienced physician is readily available to oversee and assist this activity.

The physician must actively choose not to try to prevent death (when appropriate) and in fact must help facilitate it if the autonomy or dignity of the individual is threatened. Osler demonstrated this when caring for his patients and at the time of his own death, when he turned from the use of medications for his chronic bronchitis to the use of opium, which made him comfortable. He recognized the importance of dying as a process, which must be physiologically and, if necessary, medically supported to eliminate pain—whether it be spiritual, physical, or mental.

It is important to include the nursing staff in family discussions and the decision-making process. Without such a discussion, the ordered (intended) therapy may not be the same as the delivered therapy. The nursing staff may give less or more medication than required based on their own interpretation, which may be different from the physician's intent.

Patient preferences for ICU care clearly support the desire to live, if that outcome is reasonably likely. No physician was ever found liable for terminating treatment at the request of a competent adult. This is because all interventions require consent, which reflects the voluntary nature of the patient's participation. This effectively precludes the physician from liability. Still, physicians may fear litigation. It is the responsibility of hospitals to design policies about the management of such problems. On the other hand, by *not* complying with a request to terminate treatment, the physician does become vulnerable to a new type of legal action. The right-to-die suit. In fact, doctors of a patient in such a situation have been found liable for pain and suffering caused by unwanted care.

When weaning a patient from his or her ventilator, intermittent mandatory ventilation is often used. Pressure support, inspired oxygen concentration, and end-expiratory pressure can all be reduced gradually or rapidly.

Withdrawing Nonventilatory Life Support

In addition to mechanical ventilation, other forms of life-sustaining support can be foregone. Therapy with antibiotics, blood products, and antiarrythmic agents is usually discontinued abruptly. There seldom is great controversy or difficulty in foregoing most of these forms of therapy. Removal of other therapies, however, may be more emotive because of some special symbolism or significance. Discontinuation of hydration and nutrition have been particularly difficult to rationalize for some, but most physicians and opinions of the courts and the public equate all therapy. The difference between such therapies as mechanical ventilation and nutrition is the immediacy of the effects of their deprivation on a patient.

For therapies that can cause distress when removed, the physician must anticipate this possibility and treat or, preferably, prevent the distress. For example, hunger may be caused by the discontinuation of feedings. Another example is the anxiety potentially experienced by patients who understand that treatment is being discontinued. However, these problems can be treated or prevented through the use of narcotics, sedatives, or anxiolytics, which are able to suppress those sensations. One should always administer anxiolytics and narcotics to patients who *possibly* may experience such sensations, even if the distress is unlikely to occur.

Euthanasia

The rationale for foregoing therapy has been framed in terms of enhancing patient autonomy and avoiding futile (nonbeneficial) therapy, while allowing death to occur with dignity and the greatest possible comfort at the end of the patient's life. Euthanasia arguments are virtually the same but differ in extent.

Euthanasia has received greatest acceptance when it is considered for patients who have terminal illness and who are unresponsive to therapeutic interventions. These patients commonly suffer from pain or unremitting psychologic anguish. Some people now believe that physicians and surrogates must be ready and willing not to intervene in the dying process and indeed to hasten it when they see the autonomy and dignity of patients are threatened. Hastening death remains an illegal action in the United States, however. Unfortunately, current legality depends on intentions and semantics. Other people think that the difference between euthanasia and letting the patient die by withdrawing or withholding treatment is merely a moral quibble.

Groups such as the Hemlock Society, which has more than 38,000 members, have formed to support social acceptance and foster legislation permitting euthanasia. They have been active in promoting the same goals for foregoing support as well. Euthanasia has received considerable media attention. Jack Kevorkian, a retired pathologist, has become renowned for aiding several people to commit suicide. His actions have caught the attention of lay people, legislators, and ethicists. The interest kindled may prove to set the stage for further debate and change.

Hospital Policy Formation

In the United States, legislation requiring hospitals to adopt policies about advance directives has given further impetus to the development of policies concerning withdrawal of support. (Refer to *Textbook of Critical Care,* 3rd ed, Chapter 202, for more information as well as an example of such a medical center policy.)

Situations in which families and physicians cannot reach an agreement about further provision of care are arising with increasing frequency. When patients or families want care to be provided and the physician believes that the therapy is not indicated, a stalemate of sorts may ensue. A policy may explicitly state that patients and surrogates cannot compel a physician to provide therapy that is against his or her judgment. Therefore, some institutions have policies or committees that serve as a mechanism to withdraw care without the family consent or over family refusal. They usually require third-party review by another physician and by an ethicist, as well as some sort of formal presentation of the problem for discussion. The formalization of the process and the assurance that it seems to provide physicians appear to have resulted in lifting a burden from families unable to reach these decisions on their own.

Foregoing therapy in the ICU is common in the United States and an accepted practice in most countries. The physician must be aware of the rationale for foregoing support and must be able to effectively prevent pain and distress as the end of life approaches. Physicians must be just as prepared to approach the making of such decisions as they are in approaching other medical dilemmas. Many resources available to caregivers can facilitate the decision-making process. Effective ICU care includes creating appropriate policies and using a team approach to deal with decisions of an ethical nature. A team can variously include nurses, physicians, social workers, clergy, patient representatives, and even the patients themselves.

OUTCOME PREDICTION FOR SPECIFIC CONDITIONS

Subtle differences in disease presentation can have a profound impact on a patient's outcome. For example, treatment recommendations can vary greatly for two patients with fulminant hepatic failure and similar serum biochemical abnormalities treated at the same institution. Because of the importance on outcome of age, cause of liver failure, and differences in prothrombin time, one patient may be treated conservatively and the other transferred to a liver transplant facility. Current data for predicting outcome for some conditions deserve special emphasis. These conditions include nontraumatic coma, inhospital cardiac arrest, metastatic and hematologic malignancy, acquired immunodeficiency syndrome (AIDS), cirrhosis, and multiple organ dysfunction syndrome.

Coma

Mental status changes are frequent in critical illness and have important prognostic implications. Coma is particularly important because of its prevalence, negative impact on survival, and the possibility for severe chronic disability.

Despite conflicting opinions, rational prognostication for coma patients is possible. Relevant considerations include the following:

- Poor quality of life (e.g., persistent vegetative state)
- Length of time from date of injury or insult
- Self-fulfilling prophecy (do not withdraw care before it is time)

The most useful prognostic estimates for *nontraumatic* coma were developed from multi-institutional studies that included 500 patients whose comas lasted at least 6 hours after admission, whose serial neurologic examinations outcomes were analyzed, and whose treatment decisions were made by their own physicians. Neurologic outcomes were defined and patients were classified according to the best condition achieved, regardless of other outcome (even death). Causes of coma included subarachnoid hemorrhage, hypoxia-ischemia, other cerebrovascular disease, hepatic encephalopathy, infection, mass lesions, and metastatic disturbances.

The study's general findings included a lack of importance for age as a predictive variable, a tendency for almost all surviving coma patients to awaken after 2 to 4 weeks, and improvement on serial examinations. Although physicians may not be willing to prognosticate as early as 6 hours after admission, the guidelines presented for 1, 3, and 7 days are similarly accurate and allow time to ensure the absence of reversible factors and to permit discussions with the family to take place. The study verified the accuracy of brain stem reflexes, best motor responses, and predictive value of formal vestibulo-ocular reflex testing. However, clinical features, such as seizure and myoclonus, and other tests, like electroencephalography and somatosensory evoked potentials, have contributed little to overall prognostication.

Patient demographics were similar, but a detailed analysis of the first 310 patients entered into the study revealed that three times as many laboratory tests (e.g., scans) were performed on patients in the United States as those in the United Kingdom. Overall outcomes were similar, although a higher percentage of the total deaths occurred within the first 72 hours in the United Kingdom than in the United States. (Mortality rates at 1 month were not different.)

Cardiopulmonary Resuscitation in Hospitalized Individuals

Cardiopulmonary resuscitation (CPR) has achieved the unique position of a treatment that *will* be administered unless there are specific orders to the contrary. These orders, known as *do-not-resuscitate* (DNR) orders, have become a subject of intense debate concerning patient autonomy versus a physician's right to withhold ineffective therapy. In reality, CPR is a medical treatment with specific benefits and indications that was never intended to be used on all patients dying in a hospital.

Overall, 40% to 50% of patients undergoing CPR have vital signs restored, but only 5% to 15% live to be discharged from the hospital. Most deaths occur within the first week after CPR. Cardiovascular patients with ischemic heart disease or arrhythmias have the best outcome; success rates are higher for patients in coronary care units and lowest for those in ICUs and general medical or surgical wards. In large part, underlying disease, response times, and the number of witnessed versus unwitnessed arrests account for these differences. Patients with poor prognostic reserve because of age, chronic disease, and multiple organ dysfunction have a dismal prognosis, with a 0% to 5% survival rate at discharge.

Other studies verify the uniformly dismal prognosis after CPR for patients with chronic disease, particularly those with malignancy, cerebral vascular accidents, chronic renal or hepatic failure, chronic obstructive pulmonary disease, and AIDS. In addition, patients with asystole, continued arrest after 15 minutes of CPR, or a history of more than one cardiac arrest do not survive to be discharged.

Although studies reveal earlier and increased use of DNR orders in ICUs since the mid-1980s, prolonged, futile efforts are a continuing problem. It is hoped that the public discussion and implementation of federally mandated notification about advance directives will improve opportunities for communication. Although better communication allows physicians to make decisions based on knowledge of a patient's preferences and values, accurate information about the likelihood of success of CPR is also essential to decision making.

Acquired Immunodeficiency Syndrome

Early experience with respiratory failure in AIDS patients due to *Pneumocystis carinii* pneumonia (PCP) demonstrated an 84% to 100% hospital mortality rate, with many of the survivors dying within 6 months. Subsequent articles and editorials discussed the futility of mechanical ventilation and ICU admission for these patients but also emphasized that non-AIDS patients with a similar prognosis (e.g., metastatic cancer) were routinely offered ICU care. They also emphasized that it would be unethical to triage individuals with AIDS differently than patients with other disorders and warned about promoting a self-fulfilling prophecy for AIDS patients by providing less aggressive care, thereby ensuring a continued high mortality rate. In the late 1980s, these concerns proved prophetic as hospital survival rates for patients with PCP and respiratory failure increased to 38% to 55%. Improved survival was not due to differences in patient selection, and speculation about the reasons for improved prognosis included the impact of zidovudine (AZT), better nutrition, improved antibiotic treatment of PCP, and the use of steroids for patients with respiratory failure. The improved outcome experience with AIDS patients demonstrates the pitfalls of using historical data to predict current outcome for a new disease that is the focus of dynamic research and new treatments.

With improved prophylaxis for PCP, an expanding patient population at risk, and the emergence of other infections, such as multiple drug-resistant tuberculosis, the increase in ICU admissions for human immunodeficiency virus–infected individuals will continue. Given the huge number of patients at risk and the substantial financial impact of providing them with critical care, accurate prognostication is essential.

Critical care is often withheld more frequently from those with AIDS than from those with other terminal diseases. One reason for this is because an AIDS patient is more likely to request therapeutic limits, through either a living will or a surrogate. Although AIDS is a horrible contagion, it has taught us many important lessons. Many patients have seen loved ones die of the disease and are knowledgeable about and willing to discuss the effectiveness of medical intervention. This has resulted in an open, informed environment in which physicians, patients, and their representatives discuss therapeutic options and the advisability of life support measures. Agreement about what represents futile therapy is common, and many terminally ill patients die without receiving artificial ventilation, CPR, or intensive care. Advance directives and power of attorney for healthcare decisions are frequently granted to others should the need arise.

Multiple Organ Dysfunction Syndrome

A typical scenario is a septic or trauma patient admitted to the ICU who has severe physiologic abnormalities. Despite initial control of the inciting event and optimal support, the patient develops, over days or weeks, sequential dysfunction of multiple organ systems (MODS), which frequently terminates in death. Although the syndrome has been recognized since the early 1970s, its cause remains uncertain. In many ICUs, MODS is the most frequent cause of death; patients have protracted ICU stays, consume inordinate amounts of resources, and generate enormous costs. Studies of prognosis in MODS have demonstrated that the death rate rises as the number of organ failures increases. The mortality rate increases from 5% to 30% for single-organ failure, from 40% to 60% for double-organ failure, from 60% to 80% for triple-organ failure, and from 95% to 100% for those with failure of four or more organs.

One study, reported in 1990, demonstrated the potential value of prognostic data in MODS. Daily estimates of risk for hospital mortality for patients with organ system failure were provided to ICU physicians. The type, frequency, and reason for limiting or stopping therapy were then compared with the same for a control period when probability estimates were not available. Compared with the control period, a small but significant increase in decisions to stop active treatment and provide comfort care was limited to patients with three or more organ system failures. Although the number of patients affected was small, this study demonstrated how probability estimates can be used to supplement clinical decision making in MODS.

Acute and Chronic Liver Disease

Cirrhosis

The scoring system developed by Child and Turcotte (the CTC or Child's criteria) and a subsequent modification by Pugh and coworkers are the most familiar and useful measures of severity and prognosis in liver disease. The CTC uses the extent of abnormality for five variables—serum bilirubin, albumin, ascites, neurologic dysfunction, and nutritional status—to classify patients into groups that reflect increasing severity of disease (see *Textbook of Critical Care*, 3rd ed, Chapter 203). Child's criteria have also been used to risk-stratify cirrhotic patients undergoing other types of elective or emergency surgery, but use of the criteria as a prognostic tool has significant limitations.

Of the few studies that have specifically examined the prognosis of cirrhotic patients admitted for critical care, the most useful have focused on the efficacy of mechanical ventilation. In one study of 100 intubated and ventilated patients with cirrhosis and severe complications, the overall mortality rate was 89%, but three variables—severe cirrhosis, septic shock, and hepatic coma due to superimposed acute hepatitis—were associated with a 100% mortality rate.

These studies provide effective guidance in selecting cirrhotic patients for ICU care and for subsequent management decisions. Patients admitted with a problem isolated to a single organ system, such as upper gastrointestinal bleeding, deserve a trial of therapy because hospital and 2-month mortality rates for patients with severe upper gastrointestinal bleeding range from 26% to 68%. Patients who present with or subsequently develop MODS or who require artificial ventilation have a poor prognosis, and decisions to limit or withdraw therapy are often appropriate.

Fulminant Hepatic Failure

Fulminant hepatic failure is due to acute massive liver necrosis and is characterized by progressive neurologic deterioration within 8 weeks of onset. The average mortality rate for this syndrome is about 80%, despite the fact that it often afflicts previously healthy young individuals. Identification of variables that predict outcome early in the syndrome is important because hepatic transplantation has resulted in improved survival for some patients. Onset of grade 4 hepatic encephalopathy and a prothrombin time greater than 100 seconds are independently associated with a mortality rate exceeding 95%. Other important prognostic factors include age, bilirubin level, and the cause of the fulminant hepatic failure (the outcomes of patients with acetaminophen overdosage and hepatitis A are better than those of patients with other causes).

Metastatic and Hematologic Malignancies

The overall mortality rates from ICU care for patients with malignancy range from 22% to 55%, but overall mortality figures are not relevant, because many of these ICU admissions are postoperative, are for local or limited disease, or are for a specific, acute, reversible problem such as hypercalcemia. In all the studies cited (see *Textbook of Critical Care,* 3rd ed, Chapter 203), the mortality rate was markedly increased for patients with metastatic disease and multiorgan dysfunction, particularly those with respiratory disease who required mechanical ventilation.

Until further information is available, how is the physician to interpret and use existing outcome data for patients with malignancies? Many patients develop reversible problems that can be treated with a high likelihood of success. These patients should be treated aggressively in the ICU. But what about the patient with metastatic cancer or hematologic malignancy in relapse who develops multiorgan dysfunction or respiratory failure? At many institutions, this type of patient causes considerable friction and disagreement between critical care specialists and oncologists. This is understandable because the same patient is perceived differently. Oncologists often see an individual with whom they have a longstanding relationship that developed under difficult circumstances. Treatment options were discussed, promises made, and expectations developed. The intensivist has no prior relationship with the patient but is aware that the need for life support, particularly mechanical ventilation, dramatically alters prognosis regardless of prior expectations. The intensivist perceives a chronic incurable illness with a low probability for survival and a high probability of prolonged dying. The potential for conflict is obvious.

Additional studies need to focus on identifying variables that accurately predict prognosis for cancer patients admitted to ICUs, but until more information is available, a solution to this dilemma requires cooperation and mutual education. The intensivist must rely on the oncologist to provide an accurate prognostic estimate for the malignancy, concentrating on expected survival after ICU discharge. The oncologist must depend on the intensivist for an accurate prognostic estimate for the acute process and likelihood of ICU discharge. Only with accurate input from both parties can a reasonable and beneficial decision be reached.

CRITICAL CARE PRACTICE IN THE ERA OF CONSUMERISM

The vocabulary of healthcare has become firmly centered around access, quality, and cost. *Access* clearly embraces supply and demand, whereas *quality* and *cost* are universally understood consumer concerns. We live and practice in the era of medical consumerism.

Critical care has evolved rapidly into one of the ultimate consumer products: it is both high risk and high volume; it is extraordinarily expensive; every American is a potential and likely consumer; and it often involves literally life and death.

The problem is not as simple as providing expensive care to a large number of patients while maintaining quality. The paradox of contemporary critical care is that, although meaningful prolongation of life is not always possible, the postponement of death frequently is. Thus, end-of-life issues have moved increasingly to the forefront for both consumers and providers alike.

Resources

In 1992, a Task Force of the Society of Critical Care Medicine (SCCM) conducted an extensive survey of all American Hospital Associated hospitals with at least one ICU. Their description was based on 40% of such hospitals (4233), representing 32,850 ICU beds and 25,871 patients from 2,876 units in 1,706 institutions. These data relate a great deal of information about the quantity and quality of the critical care resources available to American consumers. The study shows a wide disparity in the characteristics that most would agree describe an adequate ICU. Less than half of ICUs meet relatively permissive criteria. The unexpected occurrence of critical illness or injury finds individuals unprepared and unable to "shop" for the unit most appropriate to his or her needs. After admission, insufficient opportunity often exists for the patient and his or her family to have a partnership role with physicians and nurses to exert their own autonomy.

Access, cost, and quality are inextricably woven together in an ICU. Inappropriate admissions imply poor quality. Unnecessary costs are experienced, and beds are denied to patients who might benefit from the specialized care available. Critical care professionals must work together to ensure the general availability of high-quality care.

The Consumer

Eighty per cent of all Americans experience the need for critical care at some time in their lives, either as a patient or as a family member. The experience is usually unanticipated and unplanned. Because the issues are frequently matters of life and death, and because the decisions usually involve loved ones, opinions and values are often vehemently expressed. The courts become involved because of the intensity and ambiguity of the issues, but, as with individuals, legal precedent is not consistent. One person's desire for critical care and life support may be quite different from that of another under remarkably similar circumstances.

One study concluded that about 70% of people would decide against life-sustaining treatments if they were incompetent and had a poor prognosis. These data have meaning as information about consumer preferences but have no potential to guide policy, since they imply that 30% of people would want critical care even under what others consider the worst of circumstances.

Another study indicated that the percentage of consumers who would want life support is 90% if they could be restored to health; 30% if they could not care for themselves; 16% if their condition were hopeless; and 6% if they would remain in a persistent vegetative state.

The data from the SCCM Task Force indicate that, nationally, bed occupancy in ICUs averages 87%. The number of chronic patients averages 2.2 in the smallest of hospitals and increases to 21 in hospitals with more that 500 beds. Unavailability of a lower acuity bed is the largest single reason for inability to transfer ICU patients appropriately, but between 8.6% and 20.3% of units, depending on type, cite other reasons, including patient, family, or physician unwillingness, and medicolegal concerns.

Frankl and coworkers concluded that patients base their preferences for life support on perceived outcomes. A singular or small number of anecdotal experiences, which may not have been firsthand, often represent the consumer's only frame of reference. It is clear, however, that if the consumer exercises his or her individual rights in the fashion and proportions indicated by published surveys, consumer perceptions is one of the most powerful forces shaping the issues of access, cost, and quality in critical care.

In 1992, the Foundation for Critical Care gathered preliminary data from elderly consumers regarding their knowledge base, experiences, and preferences with respect to critical care issues. The results reveal the nature of American consumers who may desire treatment that they either know little about or believe to be infrequently successful. For example, 77% indicated that they knew what CPR means, whereas only 26% knew what DNR means. Thirty-five per cent believed that CPR is usually successful, and 84% wanted CPR for themselves in at least some circumstances. Similar apparent contradictions exist about attitudes toward respirator use and critical care in general.

Patient Self-Determination Act of 1991

As discussed previously in this chapter, the Patient Self-Determination Act of 1991 encourages and empowers people to formulate advance directives. The decisions involved are nonetheless profound and likely to be difficult. Writing an advance directive should represent the culmination of a process that begins with the gathering of objective information, the formulation of reasonable expectations for certain scenarios, and the blending of those expectations with personal values.

Specific concerns have been raised about the implementation of this statute, focusing on how and by whom a person is informed of his or her rights. The most serious concern related to advance directives is that they will not be honored in detail or that they will be ignored. Studies have shown that advance directives may be ineffective as much as 25% of the time, and that some providers may give higher priority to other considerations than to patient autonomy.

Conclusions and Recommendations

The issues of access, cost, and quality are in sharp focus in critical care. For them to be optimized, critical care physicians should be encouraged to do the following:

1. Support the SCCM paradigm of the well-trained critical care physician and encourage full-time, coordinated, collaborative unit management by credentialed medical and nursing directors.
2. Participate in healthcare reform to ensure that critical care is properly considered in basic benefits packages and that accountable health partnerships foster appropriate critical care management.
3. Support efforts to regionalize critical care for major trauma and the most intensive and expensive technologies (such as extracorporeal membrane oxygenation) while working to upgrade both the standard and the consistency of critical care in community hospitals.
4. Support the Foundation for Critical Care in its efforts to educate consumers about critical care and to help them plan effectively for an ICU experience.
5. Support the optimal implementation of the Patient Self-Determination Act in their own institutions by taking part in consumer and professional education, developing hospital policies, and participating in the hospital's ethics committee.
6. Develop a unit environment that fosters humane caring for both patients and families, facilitates communication among all caregivers and consumers, and is founded on realism and patient advocacy.

Relman has defined good, cost-effective medical care as "the care provided by a competent and compassionate physician who has no incentive to do more or less that is judged appropriate in each case." Critical care physicians can realistically approach this paradigm in the delivery of critical care. In the era of medical consumerism, it is required that they embrace their roles in political process, hospital policy, unit management, ethics committees, public and professional education, patient advocacy, and family support with the same passion that has achieved such substantial success at the bedside of the critically ill and injured.

ETHICS OF RESOURCE ALLOCATION IN THE INTENSIVE CARE UNIT

Although ethicists, attorneys, and others worry about the legal and ethical bases for rationing care, intensivists practice rationing of ICU resources on a daily basis. The demand for well-staffed and well-equipped ICU beds frequently exceeds the local supply, and physicians must provide ICU care for some, knowing that in the process they may deny care to others. Using only their professional knowledge and a sense of equity, intensivists regularly decide whether to admit one more patient to a crowded ICU, transfer a patient to a less well-staffed unit in favor of one who shows greater promise of benefiting from ICU treatment, or transfer a patient who now shows little promise of benefit from ICU treatment. Because these patients are seriously ill, the reason for rationing is almost always based on the scarcity of resources rather than on the insurance status of the patients.

Hospitals are placing greater responsibility on clinicians in the following ways:

- Reorganization: Allocation decisions are delegated to front-line health professionals.
- Creation of programs to provide cost information to physicians.
- Changing physician behavior through utilization management programs.

Physicians assigned to these new roles are frequently unprepared for the ethical consequences of such resource allocation decisions. They are traditionally trained to be advocates for individual patients, and their frame of reference emphasizes patient and professional autonomy. Frequently, their insistence on individual patient needs comes into conflict with the financial needs of the institution.

Allocation, Rationing, and the Business of Healthcare

Healthcare services have never been considered a basic American right. Instead, healthcare is considered to be a commodity that is, just like any other commodity, allocated and rationed through the marketplace. Services are available to those who can afford healthcare; those who cannot afford it frequently go without. The long-delayed move to healthcare reform has been fueled in large part by the belief held by many Americans that it is unfair and unjust to link access to healthcare to socioeconomic status.

Important distinctions between allocation and rationing can be made. *Allocation* decisions determine to what extent a society devotes its resources to a particular service. *Rationing* is usually a "micro" level issue because decisions are made about who receives resources for a particular purpose. Obviously, allocation decisions affect rationing decisions. The more resources allocated for a given clinical problem, the more profitable it is to provide such services. Hospitals attempt to increase their market share of well-reimbursed services by vigorously promoting their programs in transplantation or cardiac surgery, but not in poorly reimbursed services like treatments for multiple injury.

A major emotional distinction exists between statistical and identifiable lives when rationing is under consideration. Governments and insurers make decisions whether to pay for a specific procedure on the basis of population statistics and the number of lives that might be spared or lost as a result of these decisions. In contrast, when a child who requires organ transplantation dies while his or her family is trying to raise funds for the procedure, the child becomes a very identifiable individual. Healthcare reform will almost certainly create more litigation in the healthcare industry than has been seen under the present system, in which most legal action is related to the allegation of medical malpractice.

Impact of the Legal System on Allocation and Rationing

Physicians and hospitals are gravely concerned about the rising frequency and severity of medical malpractice claims. Physicians are held to a standard of care for all patients. How well the courts will consider and incorporate the realities of rationing and allocation into their decisions is not clear yet. Physicians rightly fear that the limitation of ICU beds at any given moment will not be fully understood by the courts when a physician is forced to deny a patient access to one of these beds.

Physicians are required only to provide the standard of care that is appropriate under the circumstances, and sometimes understaffing, fly-by status, or the need to triage patients for limited ICU beds requires physicians to refuse to admit patients to their unit. The development of criteria for admission is important but controversial. Most physicians agree that the likelihood of potential benefit should guide such decision making, but issues of patient desire, gender, income, age, preexisting illness, and social worth frequently make it almost impossible for them to develop universally acceptable criteria.

Theories of Justice

Although physicians make clinical decisions based on the ethical concepts of patient autonomy, nonmaleficence, beneficence, and confidentiality, management decisions regarding allocation and rationing are heavily premised on theories of distributive justice. This principle states that benefits and burdens should be distributed equitably, that resources should be allocated fairly, and that one should act in such a manner that no one person or group has a disproportionate share of benefits or burdens. Physicians frequently wonder whether it is morally right to prioritize patient admissions based on a criterion such as potential benefit.

Many formulations of rationing draw heavily on the concept of justice put forth by John Rawls in his many writings and in his comprehensive work *A Theory of Justice*. Rawls begins by discussing "justice as fairness" and suggests that "society is well-ordered when it is not only designed to advance the good of its members but when it is also regulated by a public conception of justice." He points out that most people agree with the need for a general code of justice but frequently disagree over what principles should determine the assignment of "basic rights and duties" and "the proper distribution of the benefits and burdens of social cooperation." Because part of the disagreement over the distribution of societal goods is based on each individual's position in society, Rawls suggests that such decisions be made behind a "veil of ignorance," when one does not know whether he or she will be rich or poor, healthy or ill.

Rawls goes on to suggest that these principles of justice be embodied in a social contract between the body politic and the social institution or country. He summarizes his views in two principles of justice:

- Each person is to have an equal right to the most extensive basic liberty compatible with a similar liberty for others.
- Social and economic inequalities are to be arranged so that they are both reasonably expected to be to everyone's advantage and attached to positions and offices open to all.

He insists that "social and economic inequalities, for example inequalities of wealth and authority, are just only if they result in compensating benefits for everyone, and in particular for the least advantaged members of society." Rawls' interpretation of justice as fairness is based on Kant's notion of autonomy and Kant's "idea that moral principles are the objects of rational choice." It is little wonder, therefore, that Kantian ethical theories have achieved predominance in the field of bioethics.

Applied Justice in Healthcare Policy

Norman Daniels, in his provocatively titled book *Just Health Care*, suggests that Rawls' approach to justice as fairness can be applied to healthcare by claiming that such care, like education, is necessary to ensure equality of opportunity. He points out that each individual's genetic makeup provides him or her with a "normal opportunity range." It is considered "morally acceptable that there are winners and losers, even in races where the prize is a share of important social goods, provided the race is *fair* to all participants." Disease and disability reduce the range of available opportunities, and measures that reverse or moderate these disadvantages can be morally justified because they help provide a more "level playing field." However, society cannot provide every healthcare service that an individual might like; thus, agreement on what are *essential* healthcare services is necessary.

President's Commission for the Study of Ethical Problems

As the United States and other countries embark on the road of major healthcare reform, a full national debate on access to such care and related issues is needed. A 1932 report of the national Committee on the Costs of Medical Care pointed out that "many persons do not receive services which are adequate either in quantity or quality, and the costs of services are inequitably distributed." In 1974, the President's Commission for the Study of Ethical Problems in Medicare and Biomedical and Behavioral Research was created. It found that "we discern in our country's traditional commitment to fairness an ethical obligation on the part of society to ensure that all Americans have access to an adequate level of health care without the imposition of excessive burdens." It appears to suggest that the withholding of potentially beneficial care for certain individuals is ethical because it exceeds the definition of what is adequate. The fact that some people are believed to be poor because of their own actions and that others become ill because of smoking, drinking, reckless driving, inappropriate sexual activity, or other risky behavior makes it attractive to create a class of "undeserving poor" or "undeserving ill" who might be excluded from governmentally funded healthcare services. It is doubtful, however, whether American society is ready to withhold care from those who have squandered their ability to obtain health insurance because it seems "inhumane, and indeed indecent, to let someone suffer or die for lack of easily available care."

State governments, perhaps, have made more significant progress toward consensus on bioethical issues, particularly those dealing with allocation of medical resources, than has the federal government. A year after the President's Commission completed its report, the state of New York developed its own Task Force on Law and Life. This task force has released several comprehensive reports. Although other states have followed New York's lead in developing interdisciplinary commissions, Oregon is perhaps best known for its attempt to actually implement rationing of care to its poorest citizens. The Oregon plan ran into considerable opposition on both political and moral grounds. It uses an arbitrary ranking system to redistribute healthcare resources among the poor. Current Medicaid recipients receive less care, the uninsured poor receive more care, and the insured continue to receive their same level of benefits. In 1993, a federal court maintained that Medicaid had to fund all children in need of transplants, thus adding unanticipated millions into state Medicaid budgets. It is anticipated that litigation for patients' rights of access to federal programs will only increase during healthcare reform.

Theories of Justice and the Practice of Critical Care Medicine

Theories of justice are most useful in making mesoethical and macroethical decisions but have limitations when clinician managers are faced with the decision of whether to admit an individual with a myocardial infarction and unstable blood pressure or a gunshot victim to the last monitored bed in the ICU. These physicians are making distributive decisions, and such decisions are almost always based on the chances of clinical benefit to the patient. If survival rates appear to be similar, physicians usually start considering the patient's preexisting health status and age and the likelihood of full restoration of health.

Justice and Cost

The concept of "health," to use the jargon of the economist, is clearly elastic. Since the presence of symptoms leads to physician intervention, it is essential to distinguish between the "ill" and the "worried well." The total cost to the nation of all healthcare depends as much on how much care is given to those without serious illness as to the 20% of Americans who are ill. It could, for example, cost the nation far more to treat headaches with aspirin than to perform heart, kidney, lung, and bone marrow transplantation on relatively few patients. Thus, total cost is elastic to the perception of medical need and the cost of medical intervention, but the usual market expectation of demand driving down cost almost never occurs. Little has been written, in a market-organized economy, to emphasize how much the competition to perform expensive and presumably useful techniques has raised the cost of healthcare.

Toward an Ethic for Resource Allocation

It is important for institutional interdisciplinary committees to create written policies about major rationing and allocation choices. Such policies should specify not only who makes such decisions but also the criteria on which these decisions are based. These policies should become part of the medical standard of care, thereby decreasing liability for physicians and hospitals that follow such policies. The role of hospital ethics committees should be extended from the traditional emphasis on individual patient care decisions to one that analyzes the way that institutions respond to the complex moral issues that they regularly encounter. The stakes in allocation ethics are high, and, to the most practical extent possible, such policies should be published and debated within the population served by the hospital. Objective information is critical to resource allocation and to decision making on the part of both health professionals and their patients. Only when accurate assessments of the outcomes of treatment on the duration and quality of subsequent life are available will it be possible to allow society to adopt the morally appealing principles of providing potentially beneficial care to all who require it.

The relations among access to care, cost of such care, and appropriate levels of care for any given population should be freely debated by the public. Cost issues cannot be ignored, of course, and common sense always dictates a less expensive approach if the same outcome can be achieved. Relating the cost of treatment to the reductions in the cost of illness is a measure of cost-effectiveness, relating cost to resultant outcomes is a measure of cost benefit, and relating cost to the utility of a treatment is measured in terms of increases in quality-adjusted life years. Reducing cost and increasing the precision of medical decision making will permit society to adopt the morally appealing principle of providing potentially beneficial care to all who require it. In addition to clinical ethical dilemmas, institutional ethics committees need to address the ethical dilemmas that they face as part of their business planning. Finally, academic institutions training hospital administrators and clinicians must include training in allocation ethics in their curricula. The substantial benefits anticipated in the brave new world of healthcare reform will be realized only if structural change is accompanied by broad interdisciplinary training of the individuals who are expected to perform roles that extend far beyond the traditional health professional–patient relationship.

CHAPTER 14

Pediatrics

Christiane C. Corriveau, MD

An unknown number of children are cared for in nonpediatric emergency rooms and intensive care units. This chapter is designed to identify several conditions that require urgent care. Ideally, the pediatric patient is best served in a setting dedicated to meeting the medical, developmental, and social needs of children and their families. Transport to a setting with pediatric critical care capabilities, if possible, should occur upon stabilization of the child.

The readers are referred to the chapters in the *Textbook of Critical Care* for detailed pathophysiology and therapeutics of pediatric critical illness.

RESUSCITATION

A. Cardiopulmonary Resuscitation (CPR)
   1. Most frequently performed on very young (<1 yr) patients. Definitive therapy cannot occur until resuscitation and stabilization are complete.
   2. Respiratory arrest is most common, circulatory arrest is rare in children; with prompt establishment of airway, circulatory insufficiency improves.

B. The Neonate
   1. Apgar score is used to assess physiology at birth (1 and 5 minutes) (Tables 14–1, 14–2, and 14–3).
   2. Initial evaluation follows recommendations by the American Heart Association (Fig. 14–1).

Table 14–1. THE APGAR SCORING SYSTEM*

	Apgar Score		
Variable	*0*	*1*	*2*
Heart rate	Absent	Less than 100 bpm	More than 100 bpm
Respiratory effort	Absent	Slow, irregular	Good, crying
Color	Blue, pale	Body pink, extremities blue (acrocyanosis)	Completely pink
Reflex irritability (response to insertion of a nasal catheter)	Absent	Grimace	Cough, sneeze
Muscle tone	Limp	Some flexion of extremities	Active motion

*Each variable is evaluated individually and scored from 0 to 2 at both 1 and 5 minutes of age. The score of each time period is the sum of the scores of the individual variables. A score of 10 is perfect.

Table 14–2. APGAR SCORE (AT 1 MINUTE)

	<2	3–4	5–7	>8
Dx:	Severely asphyxiated	Moderately depressed, cyanotic, poor respiratory effort	Mild asphyxia	Normal
Rx:	Immediate resuscitation Tracheal intubation Ventilate 30–60 breaths/min 100% oxygen	Bag-mask ventilation 100% blow-by oxygen	Blow-by oxygen Tactile stimulation Suction	Dry, warm Tactile stimulation

Note: Resuscitation efforts should begin immediately if indicated by inadequate heart rate or respirations.

3. Wean FiO_2 to maintain PaO_2 at 50–70 mm Hg and oxygen saturation at 87% to 95%.
4. Normal lungs should not require >25 cm H_2O of pressure to expand. Sufficient pressure should be applied during inspiration to move the chest wall. Excessive airway pressure is the major cause of pulmonary gas leaks; use of an in-line manometer is helpful.
5. Thick "pea soup" meconium requires tracheal suctioning through an endotracheal tube. Thin, watery meconium does not require removal at delivery.
6. Vascular access—Umbilical arteries and umbilical vein provide readily available access.
7. Volume resuscitation—60% of asphyxiated preterm infants are hypovolemic at birth. At-risk infants include those with abruptio placentae, accidental placental transection, and umbilical cord occlusion.
   a. Crystalloid (lactated Ringer's), 10 mL/kg
   b. Colloid
      (1) Albumin 5%, 5–10 mL/kg
      (2) Albumin 25%, 2–4 mL/kg
      (3) O negative low titer crossmatched against mother's blood type—10 mL/kg
      (4) Placental artery blood (sterile) is an immediate source of the newborn's own blood.

Table 14–3. INTUBATION EQUIPMENT

Weight *(kg)*	Laryngoscope Blade *(Size)*	ID *(mm)*	Suction
<1.5	0	2.5	5 Fr
1.5–2.5	0	3.0	6 Fr
2.5–3.5	0	3.5	6–8 Fr
4.0	1	4.0	8 Fr

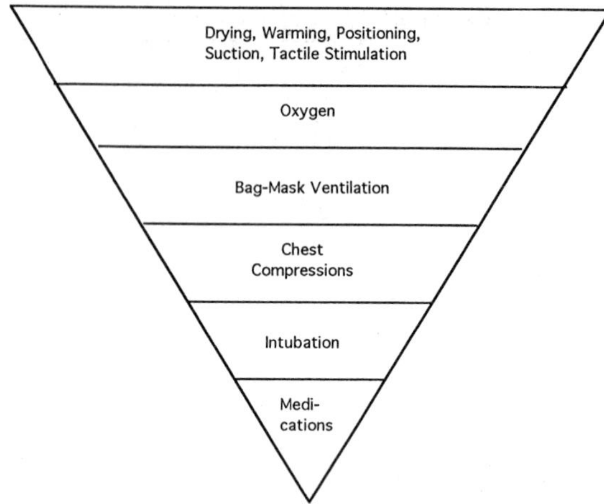

Figure 14–1. Inverted pyramid reflecting the approximate relative frequencies of neonatal resuscitative efforts. Note that a majority of infants respond to simple measures. (Reproduced with permission from Textbook of Pediatric Advanced Life Support, 1988, 1990. Copyright American Heart Association.)

Note: The volume required to raise the blood pressure to normal may require replacement of up to 50% of neonates' blood volume. Avoid overexpansion of the intravascular volume and hypertension, which increase the risk of intracranial hemorrhage.

8. Electrolyte/metabolic disturbances—Hypocalcemia, hypomagnesemia, and hypoglycemia are common causes of hypotension.
9. Cardiac resuscitation—Initiate cardiac massage if heart rate (HR) <100 beats per minute and fails to increase with 100% oxygen delivery by bag and mask.
   a. Technique
      (1) Position two fingers placed over sternum, one fingerbreadth below the intermammary line. Alternate method is hands encircling the chest and thumbs used to compress the chest at midsternum.
      (2) Depth, 0.5–1 inch
      (3) Rate at least 100 times per minute
   b. Drugs used (Table 14–4)

C. Pediatric. Arrest in children >1 year of age is usually the result of trauma or is seen in critically ill children in the intensive care unit.
   1. Basic CPR (1–8 years of age)
      a. Airway
      b. Breathing with 2 initial breaths then 15 breaths/minute
      c. Circulation

Table 14–4. DRUGS USED DURING NEONATAL RESUSCITATION

Drug	Indication	Dose	Route	Response	Complications
Atropine	Bradycardia	0.03 mg/kg; minimum dose, 0.15 mg	IV	Increased heart rate	Marked tachycardia, diminished cardiac output
Calcium gluconate	Low cardiac output, documented hypocalcemia	100 mg/kg over 5–10 min (ECG monitoring)	IV	Improved cardiac output	Bradycardia, dysrhythmias
Sodium bicarbonate	Metabolic acidosis despite adequate ventilation, pH <7.1	1–2 mEq/kg slowly	IV	Improvement in critical pH; monitor ABGs; improved cardiac output at pH >7.2	Hypertonic solution requires dilution; intracranial hemorrhage
Glucose	Blood sugar <40 mg/dL	$D_{10}W$, 4 mL/kg	IV		Hyperglycemia increases risk for intracranial bleed

(1) Check carotid pulse.
(2) Position palm of hand along lower one third of sternum.
(3) Depth 1–1.5 inches
(4) Rate 100 times per minute

2. Vascular access
   a. Children <5 years:
      (1) Attempt peripheral access for 90 seconds, then proceed to intraosseous (IO) line.
      (2) IO line established along medial portion of tibia at the level of tibial tubercle.
      (3) Central access (femoral, internal, or external jugular or subclavian veins) attempted promptly if IO fails.
   b. Children >5 years: Proceed to central access or venous cutdown if peripheral intravenous attempts fail. IO lines not readily placed in this age group.
3. Volume resuscitation. Goal is to titrate an amount to restore adequate blood pressure by constant assessment of pulses, breath sounds, liver size, and skin color.
   a. Crystalloid: Lactated Ringer's or normal saline, 10–20 mL/kg
   b. Colloid: O Rh negative, whole blood or packed red blood cells
   c. Albumin 5%, 10 mL/kg or fresh-frozen plasma, 10 mL/kg
4. Electrolytes/metabolic disturbances: Dextrose administration for documented hypoglycemia <60 mg/dL, $D_{25}W$ at 4 mL/kg bolus
5. Drugs (see Table 14–5)

CARDIOVASCULAR SYSTEM

A. Acute Hypertension. Malignant hypertension is rare in children. Hypertensive encephalopathy is most common manifestation of uncontrolled hypertension in children.
   1. Presentation. Signs and symptoms related to the rate of increase in blood pressure.
      a. Infants may present with poor feeding, irritability, and vomiting.
      b. Older children present with headaches, anxiety, and dizziness.
      c. Chronically hypertensive children may have no acute changes; asymptomatic.
      d. Hypertensive encephalopathy
         (1) Early signs include headaches, nausea, diplopia, blurred vision.
         (2) Late signs include mental confusion, varying levels of consciousness, and focal neurologic abnormalities or seizures.
         Note: Retinal hemorrhages and papilledema (Keith-Wagener retinal changes) are less frequent in pediatric patients.
   2. Etiology (see Table 14–6).

Table 14–5. DRUGS USED DURING PEDIATRIC RESUSCITATION

Drug	Indication	Dose	Route	Effect
Epinephrine	Asystole, sinus or junctional bradycardia	Initial *dose 0.02 mg/kg (0.2 mL/kg of 1:10,000 solution; double the dose on subsequent administration)	IV, IO, ET	$Alpha_1$, $beta_1$, and $beta_2$ stimulation–vasoconstriction–positive inotropy–chronotropy
Atropine	Sinus or junctional bradycardia Slow idioventricular rhythms	0.01 mg/kg; minimum dose 0.15 mg to a maximum dose of 1 mg	IV, IO, ET, IM	
Sodium bicarbonate	Cardiac arrest with: Hyperkalemia Metabolic acidosis Refractory shock	1–2 mEq/kg; subsequent doses 0.5 mEq/kg every 10 min	IV, IO	Excessive CO_2 accumulation, depressed spontaneous cardiac activity
Calcium chloride	Documented: Hypocalcemia Hyperkalemia Hypermagnesemia Calcium channel blocker overdose	10 mg/kg calcium chloride; or 100 mg/kg calcium gluconate	IV, IO	

*Recommendations JAMA 1992; 268:2251.
Abbreviations: ET, endotracheal; IM, intramuscular; IO, intraosseous; IV, intravenous.

Table 14–6. CAUSES OF SEVERE HYPERTENSION IN CHILDREN

Renal Acute glomerulonephritis (poststreptococcal, Henoch-Schönlein, and so on) Hemolytic-uremic syndrome Chronic glomerulonephritis (all types) Acute and chronic pyelonephritis Congenital malformations (dysplasia, hypoplexia, cystic diseases) Tumors (Wilms', leukemic infiltrates, and so on) Postrenal transplantation with rejection Oliguric renal failure Trauma Obstructive uropathy After genitourinary surgery Blood transfusions in children with azotemia	**Endocrine** Pheochromocytoma Neuroblastoma Adrenogenital disease Cushing's syndrome Hyperaldosteronism Hyperthyroidism Hyperparathyroidism
Cardiovascular Coarctation of the aorta Renal artery abnormalities (stenosis, thrombosis, and so on) Takayasu's disease	**Iatrogenic** Intravascular volume overload Sympathomimetic administration (epinephrine, ephedrine, and so on) Corticosteroid administration **Miscellaneous** Immobilization (fractures, burns, Guillain-Barré syndrome) Hypercalcemia (hypervitaminosis D, metastatic disease, sarcoidosis, some immobilized patients) Cocaine use Hypernatremia Stevens-Johnson syndrome Increased intracranial pressure (any cause) Dysautonomia Postresuscitation

3. Management. Goal is the immediate control of blood pressure.
   a. Acute hypertensive encephalopathy requires aggressive management.
   b. Chronic hypertension requires gradual 20% to 30% reduction in blood pressure over days; do not want to sacrifice cerebral perfusion.
4. Pharmacologic agents: See Table 14–7. Urgency requires the use of parenteral or sublingual agents.
5. Outcome. Signs and symptoms of hypertensive encephalopathy or renal failure resolve with the decrease in blood pressure. Residual neurologic abnormalities such as seizures, blindness, cranial nerve palsies, and hemiplegia may persist.

B. Congestive Heart Failure (CHF). Unlike adult causes of CHF, coronary vascular occlusion generally is not the cause of CHF in infants and children.
   1. Presentation. Common etiologies of CHF are summarized in Table 14–8.
      a. All ages present with cardiac enlargement, tachycardia, and tachypnea.
      b. Neonates/infants may have hepatomegaly and poor feeding.

Table 14–7. PHARMACOLOGIC CHARACTERISTICS OF ANTIHYPERTENSIVE DRUGS AVAILABLE FOR PARENTERAL AND SUBLINGUAL ADMINISTRATION TO PEDIATRIC PATIENTS

	Administration			Effect			Removal by Dialysis*				
Drug	*Route*	*Preparation*	*Dosage*	*Onset*	*Peak*	*Duration*	*H*	*P*	Adverse Effect	Relative Contraindication	Comments
Sodium nitroprusside**	IV infusion	50 mg of lyophilized powder in D_5W	0.5 $\mu g \cdot kg^{-1} \cdot min^{-1}$ titrated to a max of 10 $\mu g \cdot kg^{-1} \cdot min^{-1}$	Within 30 sec		Length of infusion	+	+	Nausea/vomiting Vasodilation sx† Neurologic sx‡ Apprehension, restlessness	Hepatic insufficiency	Solution good for 24 hr Photosensitive (wrap in foil) Monitor blood thiocyanate if used longer than 72 hr (D/C for thiocyanate >10 mg/dL)
Labetalol HCl**	IV bolus injection	20-mL vial containing 100 mg (5 mg/mL)	Bolus: 0.5 mg/kg over 2 min. For nonresponse, double dose and repeat every 10 min to a max dose of 5 mg/kg	1–5 min	5 min	Variable	–	–	Postural hypotension Neurologic sx‡ Nausea/vomiting	Bronchial asthma, CHF	Keep supine for 3 hr after administering drug Ambulate gradually Use cautiously in pheochromocytoma and diabetes Synergistic with halothane (hypertension)

Table continued on following page

Table 14–7. PHARMACOLOGIC CHARACTERISTICS OF ANTIHYPERTENSIVE DRUGS AVAILABLE FOR PARENTERAL AND SUBLINGUAL ADMINISTRATION TO PEDIATRIC PATIENTS *Continued*

	Administration			Effect			Removal by Dialysis*				
Drug	*Route*	*Preparation*	*Dosage*	*Onset*	*Peak*	*Duration*	*H*	*P*	Adverse Effect	Relative Contraindication	Comments
Diazoxide**	IV bolus injection	20-mL ampule containing 300 mg (15 mg/mL)	1–3 mg/kg repeated every 5–15 min until BP controlled (minibolus)	1–5 min	1–5 min	Variable, usually less than 12 hr	+	+	Arrhythmias Hyperglycemia Sodium and water retention Vasodilation sx† Neurologic sx‡	Thiazide sensitivity Severe tachycardia Diabetes Coarctation	Ineffective in pheochromocytoma Give diuretics to decrease sodium retention Hypoproteinemia potentiates effects Prolonged use (weeks) often reinstates sensitivity to oral medication

Hydralazine	30-min IV infusion or IM	1-mL ampule containing 20 mg	0.15–0.2 mg/kg every 6 hr	10–20 min	10 min–1.5 hr	3–6 hr	–	–	Headache Nausea/vomiting Tachycardia palpitation headache Vasodilation sx†	Hypersensitivity to hydralazine ("hyper-dynamic syndrome") Concomitant use of β-blocking drugs and cimetidine	Undergoes color changes in most infusion fluids, which does not indicate loss of potency Dose can be withdrawn from capsule with 1-mL syringe and squirted sublingually
Enalaprilat**	IV over 5 min	2-mL vials (1.25 mg/mL)	0.04–0.8 mg/kg every 4–6 hr	15 min	1–4 hr	Variable	+	–	Hypotension when ECFV is contracted Hyperkalemia Oliguria	Renal failure Dehydration	Treat hypotension with volume expansion
Phen-tolamine	IV bolus injection	5 mg of lyophilized powder reconstituted with diluent	0.05–0.1 mg/kg	Within 30 sec	2 min	15–30 min			Tachycardia Arrhythmias Marked hypotension		Specific for pheochromocytoma

*Removal of drug by dialysis relates to the need to supplement a dose after dialysis. It does not apply to the use of dialysis to treat drug overdose.
**Manufacturer's warning: Safety in children not established.
†Vasodilation symptoms include sweating, flushing, feelings of warmth, orthostatic hypotension, tachycardia, palpitations, nausea, and vomiting.
‡Neurologic symptoms include headache, blurred vision, dizziness, and lightheadedness.
Abbreviations: sx = symptoms; max = maximum; BP = blood pressure; D_5W = 5% dextrose in water; H = hemodialysis; P = peritoneal dialysis; CHF = congestive heart failure; + = removed by dialysis; − = not removed with dialysis; IV = intravenous; D/C = discontinue; HCl = hydrochloride; IM = intramuscular; ECFV = extracellular fluid volume.

Table 14–8. CAUSES OF CONGESTIVE HEART FAILURE IN INFANTS AND CHILDREN

Congenital cardiac malformations
Congenital arteriovenous malformations
Anomalies of aortic arch
Endocardial fibroelastosis
Anomalous origin of left coronary artery
Cardiomyopathy
Myocarditis
Anemia
Congenital heart block
Tachyarrhythmias
Rheumatic fever
Kawasaki's syndrome
Endocarditis
Cardiac surgery

Note: Sepsis may be accompanied by cardiogenic shock with low cardiac output, hypotension, and impaired contractility.

c. Older children present with history of exercise intolerance and excessive fatigue.

2. Congenital heart disease (CHD). Frank cardiogenic shock presenting with metabolic acidosis, hypotension, poor perfusion, thready pulses, and diaphoresis is a common presentation of CHD. Ductal dependent lesions such as coarctation, hypoplastic left-sided heart syndrome, interruption of the aortic arch, and critical aortic stenosis present in the newborn period.
3. Treatment. See Table 14–9.

Table 14–9. STRATEGIES TO TREAT CONGESTIVE HEART FAILURE

Goal	Agents
1. Augment contractility	Digoxin Catecholamines Dopamine Dobutamine Epinephrine Amrinone
2. Reduce myocardial work	Mechanical ventilation, oxygen, PEEP Sedation Pain relief/anxiolytics Neuromuscular blockade Fever control Pharmacologic afterload reduction β-Blockers Aortic balloon counterpulsation ECMO, ECLS, LVAD, RVAD
3. Volume expansion*	Colloid/crystalloid

**Note:* Most patients will be dehydrated due to decreased PO intake. Volume resuscitation is well tolerated in children with CHF.

Abbreviations: ECMO, extracorporeal membrane oxygenation; ECLS, extracorporeal life support; LVAD, left ventricular assist device; RVAD, right ventricular assist device.

4. Outcome. CHF is an unstable situation. Prompt stabilization is required with age-specific treatment.

RESPIRATORY SYSTEM

A. Proximal Airway. Airway pathology is a common problem for physicians taking care of pediatric patients.

1. Anatomy. Several anatomic differences exist among infants, children, and adolescents.
   a. Nose: Infants <6 months of age may be obligate nose breathers.
   b. Tongue: Tongue is relatively large in relation to the mandible in children <2 years of age.
   Note: The tongue is a common cause of upper airway obstruction in children <2 years old.
   c. Larynx: Infant's laryngeal inlet is at the level of cervical interspace C3–4 (adults, C4–5).
   d. Epiglottis: Infant: Stiff U or V shaped, angulated 45° from anterior pharyngeal wall. Adolescent: Resumes flattened, flexible adult configuration.
   e. Airway diameter: Infants and children <8–10 years, the narrowest portion is usually at the laryngeal outlet, the interior ring portion of the cricoid cartilage. Total lung resistance is 6–20 times greater in children <2 years vs. adults, largely owing to the proximal airway diameter.
2. Presentation. Stridor and wheezing are the hallmarks of respiratory obstruction.
   a. Stridor indicates abnormality above the thoracic inlet.
      (1) Inspiratory stridor—obstruction above larynx.
      (2) Inspiratory and expiratory stridor indicates obstruction below the larynx.
   b. Wheezing indicates intrathoracic pathology.
   c. For common causes of obstruction, see Table 14–10.
3. Management. If signs of acute upper airway obstruction such as stridor, retractions, and tachypnea are present, secure an airway with endotracheal intubation prior to development of life-threatening edema.
4. Etiologies
   a. Infection
      (1) Acute epiglottitis (AE). Life-threatening, sudden onset, ill-appearing child with high fever, drooling. Maintain the patient with the parents, always attended by medical professional skilled in airway management. Direct visualization of airway in operating room only.
      Pathogens: *Haemophilus influenzae,* group A beta-hemolytic streptococci
      (2) Laryngotracheobronchitis (LTB). Usually a mild illness, rarely requires critical care. Symptomatic treatment with humidified air. Dexamethasone, 0.6 mg/kg/day, may be beneficial.
      Pathogens: Parainfluenza virus, adenovirus, respiratory syncytial virus, influenza virus, and measles.

Table 14–10. COMMON CAUSES OF UPPER AIRWAY OBSTRUCTION IN PEDIATRIC PATIENTS

Congenital Obstruction	Acquired Obstruction
Choanal atresia	Infection
Craniofacial dysmorphologic features (with micrognathia and glossoptosis)	Supraglottitis
Pierre Robin syndrome	Laryngotracheobronchitis
Treacher Collins syndrome	Retropharyngeal abscess
Macroglossia	Bacterial tracheitis
Bechwith's syndrome	Trauma
Congenital hypothyroidism	Foreign bodies
Down's syndrome	Iatrogenic
Laryngotracheomalacia	Postextubation
Subglottic stenosis	Postinstrumentation
Vocal cord paralysis	Postoperative
Laryngotracheoesophageal webs	External trauma
Vascular rings and slings	Thermal and chemical burns
Tracheal anomalies	Neoplasia
Tumors and cysts	Laryngeal papillomatosis
Metabolic hypocalcemia	Miscellaneous tumors and nodes
Neurogenic: Reflex laryngospasm	CNS dysfunction
	Head trauma
	Drug overdose
	Increased intracranial pressure

(3) Bacterial tracheitis. Symptoms and presenting features overlap between AE and LTB (Table 14–11). Gradual onset of respiratory complaints progressing to high fever and respiratory distress.
Pathogens: *Staphylococcus aureus, H. influenzae,* or alpha-hemolytic streptococci

b. Trauma. Second most common cause of upper respiratory tract obstruction in children.
(1) Foreign bodies:
Toddlers most affected.
Wheezing due to obstruction distal to larynx.
Removal requires trained personnel.
(2) Mechanical trauma:
Edema resulting from airway instrumentation.
(3) Ingestion: Laryngeal and tracheal edema secondary to ingestion of alkalis, acids, and corrosive chemical substances in addition to inhalation of hot air, steam, smoke, or chemicals. Endoscopic examination of airway and esophagus may be indicated. Admit for observation and monitoring.

B. Distal Airway. Diseases of the lower airway, distal to the carina, account for much of the morbidity and mortality associated with pulmonary disease. Bronchiolitis and asthma rank among leading causes of acute reversible respiratory failure in infancy and childhood.
1. Bronchiolitis
a. Acute lower airway disease, occurring in infants and toddlers.

Table 14–11. COMPARISON OF LARYNGOTRACHEOBRONCHITIS (LTB), ACUTE EPIGLOTTITIS (AE), AND BACTERIAL TRACHEITIS (BT)

	LTB	AE	BT
History			
Age	2 months–3 years	3–7 years (usually)	All ages
Onset	Gradual	Rapid	Gradual
Respiratory disease	None to moderate	Marked	Moderate to marked
Symptoms			
Dysphagia	0	2+	+1−
Dyspnea	+1−	2–3+	2+ −
Sore throat	+1−	4+	+1−
Signs			
Sound	Bark, stridor	Muffled, guttural	Bark, stridor
Secretions	Normal for age	Drooling	Normal for age
Position	Lying, sitting, standing	Sitting, leaning	Sitting
Temperature	37–38°C	38°C+	38°C+
Facies	Normal	Anxious, distressed, toxic	Anxious

b. High-risk infants:
Congenital heart disease
Bronchopulmonary dysplasia
Prematurity
Immune deficiency

c. Etiologies:
Viral most common
Respiratory syncytial virus (RSV) 50% to 75%
Parainfluenza, adenovirus, rhinovirus, and mumps virus

d. Presentation
(1) Cough, low-grade fever, rhinorrhea, wheezing, and tachypnea
(2) Nonobstructive apnea is common; up to 20% of hospitalized patients present with apnea.
(3) Hypoxemia due to $\dot{V}/\dot{Q}$ mismatch

e. Management
(1) Humidified oxygen
(2) Trial of nebulized sympathomimetic drugs (albuterol, terbutaline)
(3) NPO for respiratory rate >60
(4) Ribavirin administration controversial; may benefit high-risk patients (see 1b).
(5) Intubation for acute respiratory decompensation or apnea is common, 7% to 38% of all admitted patients will be intubated.

f. Outcome. Mortality is approximately 2% for hospitalized children (higher in at-risk patients). Long term: Increased incidence of lower respiratory tract infections, hyperactive airways, and asthma.

2. Asthma. Lower airway disease characterized by reversible airway obstruction, airway inflammation, and hyperresponsiveness. Status asthmaticus denotes a severe attack that is unresponsive to routine medication, including continuous aerosolized beta-agonists in conjunction with intravenous corticosteroids.
43% increase in incidence in age group <20 yrs; mortality is increasing, largest increase in children ages 5 to 14 years.
Sudden death due to asthma appears to be increasing; risk factors include history of intubation, withdrawal from or decrease in steroids, and depression.

a. Presentation. Marked dyspnea, intractable bilateral wheezing, the use of sternocleidomastoid, supraclavicular, and scalene muscles, thoracic hyperinflation, and pulsus paradoxus. Altered or depressed levels of consciousness, decreased or absent breath sounds, and cyanosis denote acute respiratory failure.

b. Work-up. Includes complete history and physical, chest roentgenogram, CBC, serum electrolytes, and theophylline level (if indicated).

c. Therapy goals
(1) Increase airway conductance by relaxing smooth muscle, decrease amount and viscosity of secretions, and reduce mucosal edema.

(2) Support vital functions until bronchospasm resolves.
Note: Correction of hypoxemia with oxygen constitutes the single most important factor in preventing cardiac arrest and major central nervous system damage. Hypoxic encephalopathy continues to be a major complication and cause of death in children with a severe asthmatic episode.

(3) For management strategies, see Tables 14–12 and 14–13.

(4) Mechanical ventilation. Use only in severe, life-threatening cases. Duration usually minimum of 12–24 hours. Continue aggressive management with continuous aerosolized and intravenous $beta_2$ agonists. Primary goal is reversal of hypoxemia and insurance of adequate oxygen delivery to heart and brain. Reduction of $PaCO_2$ is a secondary goal.

(5) Complications
Seizures, premature ventricular contractions, theophylline levels >20 mg/L
Myocardial ischemia secondary to continuous $beta_2$ agonists in presence of hypoxemia
Hypokalemia secondary to $beta_2$ agonists, steroids
Extrapleural air—up to 20% incidence of pneumothorax or pneumomediastinum in mechanically ventilated children

Table 14–12. MANAGEMENT OF SEVERE ACUTE ASTHMATIC EPISODES: FUNDAMENTAL THERAPY

Oxygen (with humidity)
Maintain PaO_2 between 90 and 120 mm Hg (SpO_2 95%–99%), fraction of inspired oxygen usually 0.30–0.50
Intravenous Fluids
Up to twice maintenance rates until urine flow ≥ 2 $mL \cdot kg^{-1} \cdot hr^{-1}$; then maintenance rates
Bronchodilators
Primary
Albuterol aerosolized 0.15–0.25 mg/kg per dose every 1–2 hr (0.03–0.05 mL/kg per dose in 2 mL saline)
Secondary
Aminophylline (IV), 3–6 mg/kg initially, 0.5–1.5 mg/kg^{-1} continuous infusion; target serum level 15 μg/L
Corticosteroids
Methylprednisolone (sodium succinate) IV, 1–2 $mg \cdot kg^{-1} \cdot 6\ hr^{-1}$ for 24 hr; then 1–2 $mg \cdot kg^{-1} \cdot d^{-1}$ for 3–5 days total
Buffers
Intravenous sodium bicarbonate ($NaHCO_3$), 1–2 mEq/kg initially, followed by doses adjusted according to base deficit and administered as necessary to maintain arterial pH >7.30*
Antibiotics
If bacterial infection suspected (fever, pulmonary infiltrates)

*Dose $NaHCO_3$ (mEq) = base deficit × 0.3 (body weight in kilograms).

Table 14–13. MANAGEMENT OF SEVERE ACUTE ASTHMATIC EPISODES: RESPIRATORY FAILURE MANAGEMENT

Continuous albuterol aerosol inhalation (0.5 mg · kg^{-1} · hr^{-1}) and/or
Continuous intravenous beta-adrenergic infusions
Terbutaline (10 μg · kg^{-1} bolus, followed by infusion 4–8 μ · kg^{-1} · min^{-1})
Isoproterenol (0.1 μg · kg^{-1} · min^{-1} to a maximum of 6.0 μg · kg^{-1} · min^{-1})
Nebulized anticholinergic agent (ipratropium bromide, glycopyrrolate, atropine)
Mechanical ventilation for respiratory failure

Adrenocortical insufficiency if stress steroids are not given to patients on chronic steroids.

C. Parenchymal Disease. Disorders of structure and function of the respiratory system are frequent causes of admission of children to the pediatric intensive care unit. Respiratory failure accounts for 31% of all admissions.
   1. Presentation
      a. Respiratory rate and pattern of breathing are key to recognizing respiratory failure. Respiratory rates vary greatest during infancy (Table 14–14).
      b. Respiratory distress presents with use of accessory muscles of respiration, flaring of alae nasi, and paradoxical respiratory movements. The use of accessory respiratory muscles and audible grunting (to maintain functional reserve capacity) are among the most reliable clinical signs of respiratory distress.
      c. Altered mental status such as restlessness, irritability, and mood changes may signify hypoxia.
      d. Serial evaluation of physical examination and arterial blood gases helps determine the need for mechanical ventilation.
      e. Intubation criteria are similar to those of adults:
         $PaCO_2$ >50–60 mm Hg or a rise greater than 5 mm Hg/hr
         PaO_2 <60 mm Hg or FiO_2 >60% (Fig. 14–2)

Table 14–14. NORMAL RESPIRATORY RATES

Age	Breaths per Minute
Newborn (after 7 days)	30
6 months	28
1 year	24
3 years	22
5 years	20
8 years	18
12 years	16
15 years	14

Table 14–15. BACTERIAL CAUSES OF RESPIRATORY SYSTEM DISORDERS

Neonate *Up to 6 weeks*	Child *1 month to 6 years*	Adolescent *Older than 8 years*
Group B streptococci Gram-negative enteric bacilli Chlamydiae	*Streptococcus pnemoniae* *Haemophilus influenzae* type B	*Mycoplasma pneumoniae* *S. pneumoniae*

Note: Because of the associated risks of bacteremia, blood cultures should be obtained from any child suspected of bacterial pneumonia.

2. Etiologies
   a. Respiratory viruses
      (1) Majority of cases, 80% to 85% of pediatric infections
      (2) Common agents include respiratory syncytial virus, parainfluenza type 3, and influenza viruses.
      (3) Symptoms include high fever, dry hacking cough, myalgia, and headache.
      Note: Adenovirus types 7, 14, and 21 are associated with severe necrotizing pneumonia, mortality rate of 10% to 17%, usually seen in infants <18 months.
   b. Bacterial (Table 14–15) causes
      (1) Pathogens vary with the age and immune status of the patient.
      (2) Staphylococcal pneumonia (*S. aureus*). Rapidly progressive illness, acute medical emergency. Pneumothorax, pyopneumothorax, and bronchopulmonary fistula are not uncommon. Empyema is a universal finding. Mortality is high, most deaths occur in children <1 year. Radiographic abnormalities may persist for weeks; prognosis for full pulmonary recovery is excellent.
      (3) Pneumococcal pneumonia (*Streptococcus pneumoniae*). Organism most frequently responsible for bacterial pneumonia. Presents with cough, fever, and chills. Chest radiograph shows patchy bronchopneumonia. 25% to 33% of patients develop bacteremia; extrapleural complications include empyema, pericarditis, and meningitis.

ACUTE RENAL FAILURE

Acute renal failure (ARF) is the sudden impairment of homeostatic renal function characterized by the retention of

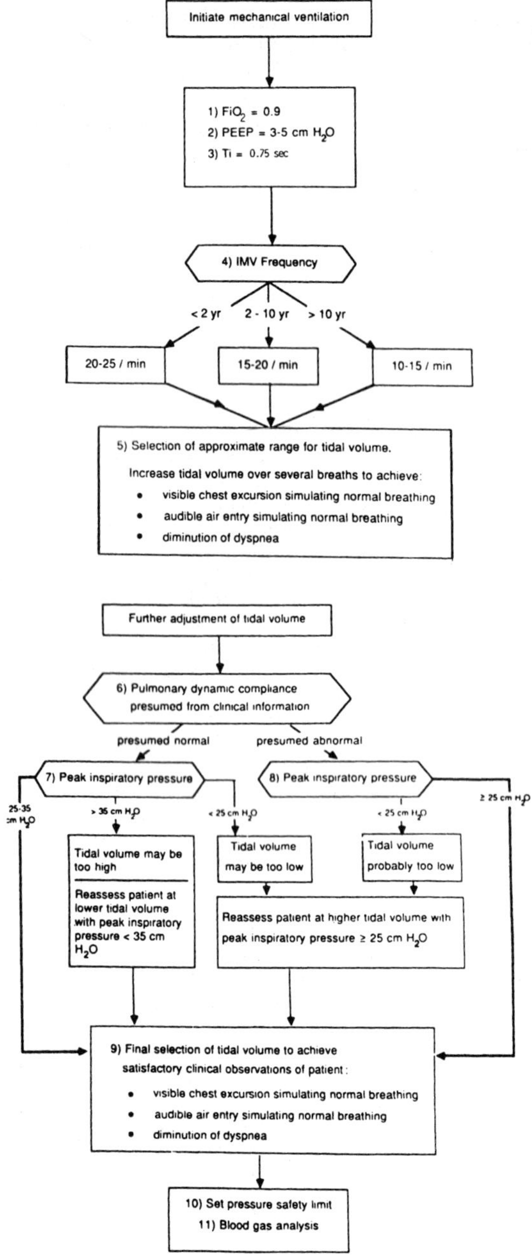

Figure 14–2. Algorithm for the initiation of mechanical ventilation in the pediatric patient. (From Kanter RK: Evaluation and stabilization of the critically ill child. Clin Chest Med 1987; 8:576–577.)

nitrogenous wastes. Common causes in pediatrics in industrialized nations include hemolytic-uremic syndrome, surgery, drug toxicity, and trauma.

A. Etiologies
   1. Cardiovascular. Decreased cardiac output due to sepsis, dehydration, congestive heart disease, or dysrhythmias.
   2. Immunologic. Most common causes in children result from postinfectious glomerulonephritis.
   3. Toxic. The kidney is uniquely sensitive to a number of chemicals and biologic agents (Table 14–16). Prompt recognition of these compounds and their withdrawal can lead to return of normal renal function.
   4. Renovascular
      a. Bilateral renal vein occlusion; common in newborns/infants (dehydration, congestive heart disease, birth asphyxia)
      b. Bilateral renal artery thrombosis; rare complication of umbilical artery catheterization
   5. Microvascular
      a. Medullary necrosis secondary to sickle cell disease or acute pyelonephritis
      b. Microvascular thrombosis secondary to disseminated intravascular coagulation (DIC), hemolytic-uremic syndrome
B. Presentation
   1. History and physical examination are important in guiding diagnostic work-up.
   2. Diagnostic algorithm (Fig. 14–3)
   3. Laboratory tests
      a. BUN is affected by factors other than nitrogen excretion by the kidney. It is an **unreliable** single indicator of renal function.
      b. Serum creatinine is a function of muscle mass, which is affected by age, gender, and body build.

Estimation of Glomerular Filtration Rate Using Creatinine Clearance

$$C_{cr} = \frac{f \times \text{height in cm}}{Cr}$$

$$C_{cr} = \text{mL/min } 1.73\ \text{m}^2$$

$$Cr = \text{serum Cr mg/dL}$$

$$f = 0.55$$

   4. Laboratory tests may help differentiate functional versus parenchymal acute renal failure (Table 14–17).
C. Management. Goal is to correct underlying disorder (shock, dehydration, and so on) when possible.
   1. Sodium and water imbalance. Correct initial deficits estimated from calculated or measured insensible losses. Goal is zero balance.
      a. Oliguric patients should receive Na-free replacement, insensible losses only.

Table 14–16. DRUGS AND TOXINS MOST COMMONLY ASSOCIATED WITH ACUTE RENAL FAILURE IN CHILDHOOD

	Associated Manifestations	Therapy
Immune Reaction or Hypersensitivity		
Penicillins Sulfonamides Cephalosporins	Fever, rash, serum sickness, eosinophilia, eosinophiluria, exfoliative dermatitis (sulfonamides)	Supportive corticosteroids, dialysis
Direct Toxicity		
Heavy metals (mercurials, lead, bismuth, gold, iron, copper)	CNS, GI, circulatory collapse (iron), hemolytic anemia (copper)	Emesis, albumin, charcoal chelation, supportive dialysis
Glycols	CNS, cardiac failure, pulmonary edema	Immediate hemodialysis, gastric lavage
Organic solvents (carbon tetrachloride, turpentine)	CNS, hepatic, GI	Gastric lavage, catharsis, supportive
Aminoglycosides	Ototoxicity, exacerbated by poor hydration	Hydration
Amphotericin B	Hypokalemia, non-oliguric renal failure Toxicity dose-related; exacerbated by poor hydration	Hydration
Mushrooms (especially *Amanita phalloides*)	GI, shock, severe liver dysfunction	Dialysis, hemoperfusion (within 24 to 36 hours), supportive
Salicylates	Tinnitus, hyperpnea, acidosis, GI, hemorrhage, CNS depression	Alkalinization of urine, hydration, gastric lavage, dialysis
Methoxyflurane, enflurane	Acute renal failure frequently non-oliguric; toxicity may be accentuated by aminoglycosides, tetracycline, and obesity	Supportive, possibly early dialysis to remove fluoride
Supportive or hyperuricemic agents (pancreatic enzymes, furosemide, salicylates, radiographic contrast media, antineoplastic agents)		Supportive, diuresis, alkalinization, hemodialysis

Abbreviations: CNS, central nervous system; GI, gastrointestinal.

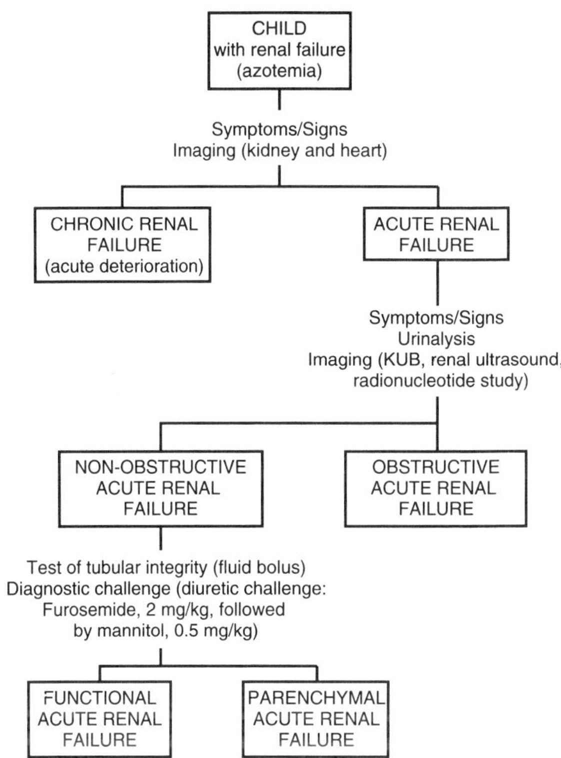

Figure 14–3. A systematic approach to the child with renal failure.

b. Non-oliguric patients should have measured losses replaced.

Sodium Replacement

$([Na^+] \text{ desired} - [Na^+] \text{ present}) \times \text{Weight (kg)} \times 0.6 = [Na^+] \text{ needed in mEq}$

2. Hyperkalemia (Table 14–18)
   a. Potentially fatal complication of ARF
   b. Treatment depends on level of $[K^+]$ mEq/L (Table 14–18).
   c. Begin treatment for levels >6.5 mEq/L or if ECG changes.
3. Acidosis
   a. Mild metabolic acidosis (serum bicarbonate >15 mEq/L): No treatment necessary.
   b. Moderate metabolic acidosis (serum bicarbonate levels 10–15 mEq/L): Replacement therapy indicated.
   c. Severe metabolic acidosis (serum bicarbonate <10 mEq/L): Dialysis.

Table 14–17. LABORATORY TESTS TO DISCRIMINATE FUNCTIONAL FROM PARENCHYMAL ACUTE RENAL FAILURE

Test	Calculation	Expected Results		Discrimination
		Functional ARF	*Parenchymal ARF*	
Tests of Tubular Sodium Absorption				
Urine sodium concentration	Direct measurement	<20 mEq/L	>40 mEq/L	Poor
Fractional excretion of sodium (Fe_{Na})	$U/S_{Na} \div U/S_{cr} \times 100$	<1	>1*	Good
Tests of Tubular Water Reabsorption				
Urine specific gravity	Direct measurement	>1.020	<1.010	Poor
Urine osmolality	Direct measurement	>500 mOsm/kg	<350 mOsm/kg	Poor
Urine-serum osmolality ratio	Direct measurement	>2	<1.1	Fair
Free water clearance (CH_2O)	Urine vol − C osm [C osm = (U osm × U volume) ÷ S osm]	Negative values	Positive values	Good
Urine-serum creatinine	Direct measurement	>40	<20	Fair
Urine-serum urea ratio	Direct measurement	>20	<10	Fair
Renal excretory index	U/S urea × (24-hr urine vol ÷ 100)	>200	<84	

*Some investigators use 3 on the cutoff value.
Abbreviations: U = urine; S = serum; Na = sodium; cr = creatinine; vol = volume; osm = osmolality; C = clearance.

Table 14–18. TREATMENT OF HYPERKALEMIA

Agent	Action	Dose	Onset/Duration	Remarks
Calcium gluconate (10%)	Stabilization of membrane potential	0.5 mg elemental Ca^{+2}/kg IV over 2–4 min	Rapid (min) / transient (hr)	Monitor electrocardiograph for bradycardia during administration May be repeated once; further repetition not recommended
Glucose (50%)	Promotes cellular uptake of K^+	1 mL/kg IV by slow push	1–2 hr/transient (hr)	Do not use in diabetics
Glucose (50%) and insulin	Promotes cellular uptake of K^+	1 mL/kg of glucose with 0.1 U regular insulin/kg IV by slow push or rapid drip	Rapid (30 min)/transient (hr)	*Never* give insulin alone
Sodium bicarbonate (7.5%)	Promotes cellular uptake of K^+	2.5 mEq/kg (~3 mL/kg) by slow push or rapid drip	Rapid (30 min)/transient (hr)	May be repeated with caution, although often ineffective
Albuterol	Promotes cellular uptake of K^+	0.1 mg/kg by aerosol	Rapid (30–45 min)/transient	May repeat every 30–60 min. Can synergize with glucose/insulin
Sodium polystyrene sulfonate (Kayexalate, Breon Labs, NY)	Cation exchange resin	1 g/kg PO (with 3–4 mL of 70% sorbitol/g of resin) or PR (with 10 mL of 70% sorbitol/g of resin)	Hours/days	Unpalatable Enemas should be retained at least 30 min Oral administration more effective/effect delayed Rectal administration less effective/effect rapid Also chelates Ca^{+2} and Mg^{+2}

Abbreviations: K^+, potassium; Ca^{+2}, calcium; IV, intravenous; PO, perioral; PR, perirectal; Mg^{+2}, magnesium.

Bicarbonate Replacement

$$([\text{NaHCO}_3] \text{ desired} - [\text{NaHCO}_3] \text{ measured}) \times \text{weight (kg)} \times 0.5 = [\text{NaHCO}_3] \text{ mEq needed}$$

4. Hypocalcemia/hyperphosphatemia. Treat by reducing serum phosphorus level with aluminum hydroxide or calcium carbonate.
   Note: Do not administer supplemental calcium **before** controlling serum phosphorus level.
5. Anemia. Usually not severe enough to require blood cell transfusion; monitor for congestive heart failure and hypertension if transfusion is necessary.
6. Hypertension (HTN). Most frequently seen with glomerulonephritis or excessive IV fluid or sodium administration. See Cardiovascular System for management of acute HTN.
7. Dialysis. Indications include:
   a. Congestive heart failure
   b. Symptomatic uremia (bleeding, altered mental status)
   c. Life-threatening electrolyte disturbances (hyperkalemia, profound metabolic acidosis)
   d. Uncontrolled hypertension (if volume sensitive). Modalities include hemofiltration, hemodialysis, and peritoneal dialysis for infants and children.
8. Oliguria
   a. Hydration; if oliguria continues, proceed with diagnostic work-up (see Fig. 14–3) and clinical challenge.
   b. Furosemide, 2 mg/kg IV or PO, followed by mannitol, 0.5 g/kg over 5 minutes. Urine output should increase in functional (prerenal) renal failure.

D. Outcome
1. Infection is the leading cause of death, up to 2/3 of all mortalities.
2. Gastrointestinal hemorrhage occurs in up to 20% of adults with acute renal failure (ARF), unknown percentage of children with similar presentation.
3. Postsurgical ARF has a mortality rate of 25% to 75%. Risk factors include young age, poor nutritional state, and prolonged low cardiac output.
4. Oliguric forms of ARF have higher morbidity and mortality compared with nonoliguric form of ARF.

CENTRAL NERVOUS SYSTEM

A. Status Epilepticus (SE), defined as seizure activity lasting longer than 30 minutes.
1. Presentation
   a. Diverse etiologies (Table 14–19)
   b. 5% of all children with febrile seizures will progress to SE.
   c. 25% of all cases of SE are related to infection.
2. Management

Table 14–19. CAUSES OF STATUS EPILEPTICUS IN CHILDREN

No History of Seizures and Normal Neurologic Development
Fever with no central nervous system infection (febrile seizure)
Central nervous system infection
Toxic/metabolic
Head trauma (accidental and nonaccidental)
Familial epileptic syndrome
Idiopathic

No Seizure History and Abnormal Neurologic Development
V-P shunt obstruction
Ex-premature infant with a history of intracranial bleeding
Previous central nervous system infection
Previous traumatic brain injury
Chromosomal abnormality/syndrome
Congenital brain maldevelopment or infection
Cerebral palsy

History of Seizures and Normal Neurologic Development
Nontherapeutic blood levels of anticonvulsant
Superimposed acute illness

History of Seizures and Abnormal Neurologic Development
Nontherapeutic blood levels of anticonvulsant
Superimposed acute illness
Intractable epilepsy
Progressive degenerating neurologic condition
Idiopathic

a. ABCs of resuscitation (see earlier section on Resuscitation).
b. Drug therapies are similar to those of adults (Tables 14–20 and 14–21).

3. Outcome
   a. Mortality rate for childhood SE is 3% to 7%
   b. Patients with febrile SE have a 10% to 21% chance of developing unprovoked seizures; 30% go on to develop epilepsy.

B. Neurosurgical Emergencies. Most are a result of increased intracranial pressure (ICP). Resuscitation of the patient (ABCs) remains the first line of therapy. If increased ICP is suspected, endotracheal intubation, hyperventilation, and 30-degree head of bed elevation should be initiated while diagnostic evaluation is begun.
   1. Trauma
      a. Traumatic lesions requiring surgery are rare; 20%

Table 14–20. DRUG MANAGEMENT OF STATUS EPILEPTICUS

Intravenous	Dose
Lorazepam	0.1 mg/kg
Diazepam	0.3 mg/kg
Phenytoin	20 mg/kg
Phenobarbital	15 mg/kg

Table 14–21. EFFECTIVE DRUGS FOR CHILDHOOD STATUS EPILEPTICUS WHEN AN INTRAVENOUS LINE CANNOT BE PLACED

Drug	Dose
Diazepam (IV solution)	0.5 mg/kg PR
Lorazepam	0.5 mg/kg PR
Paraldehyde	0.3 mL/kg PR (mixed 1:1 with oil)
Valproate	20 mg/kg PR (mixed 1:1 with water)
Carbamazepine	5 mg/kg NG

Note: If IV access is not available, PO/PR drugs are equally effective.
Abbreviations: NG, nasogastric; PR, per rectum.

to 30% of children with Glasgow Coma Score of 8 or less have a surgically treatable lesion.

b. Acute loss of consciousness is a neurologic emergency (diffuse axonal injury), not necessarily a neurosurgical emergency.
c. Potential surgical lesions include:
   (1) Compound depressed skull fractures; open wounds of brain that require urgent debridement.
   (2) Epidural hematoma
   (3) Subdural hematomas are the most common injury in children hospitalized for trauma. Note: The combination of subdural hematoma and retinal hemorrhage is pathognomonic of intentional trauma (child abuse).
d. Intracerebral hematomas and contusions are associated with severe head injury and diffuse axonal injury. These patients are at increased risk for elevated ICP but usually do not require surgical intervention.

2. Vascular lesions
   a. Vein of Galen aneurysm—not a true aneurysm. Presents as congestive heart failure in infancy (see CHF Section in Cardiovascular System).
   b. Arteriovenous malformations
      (1) Four times as likely to be the cause of intracranial hemorrhage in children vs. aneurysms.
      (2) Patients present with the sudden onset of severe headache (HA) or loss of consciousness.
      (3) Mortality as high as 24% with initial bleed. Rarely rebleeds, urgent surgery not indicated.
   c. Aneurysm
      (1) Congenital or mycotic malformations
      (2) Patients present with a history of stiff neck, photophobia, and unendurable HA.
      (3) Diagnosis made by history and lumbar puncture.
      (4) Rebleeds common in first 24–48 hours.
      Note: Trauma victims at risk for traumatic aneurysm of internal carotid artery; presentation

includes acute hemorrhage from nose, mouth, or ear.

3. Hydrocephalus
   a. Congenital or acquired
   b. Presentation includes signs of increased ICP, episodic HA, vomiting, visual disturbances. Physical examination may be normal at the time of evaluation due to intact cerebral autoregulatory mechanisms.
   c. CT scan or MRI is diagnostic.
   d. Therapies will depend on the etiology.
4. Infection
   a. Brain abscess requires drainage for diagnostic and therapeutic purposes.
   b. Ventriculoperitoneal shunt infections do not require removal of shunt. Usually they can be managed with a diagnostic tap and appropriate antibiotics. Infection with *Staphylococcus* requires removal of the shunt.

BLEEDING DISORDERS (Fig. 14–4)

A. Postnatal development of the homeostatic system occurs during the first 3–4 years of life. Failure to account for those differences (specific age-related normal coagulation values) may lead to a misdiagnosis and mismanagement of the child with excessive bleeding.

B. Disorders of Primary Hemostasis
   1. Disorders of platelet production
      a. Wiskott-Aldrich syndrome
      b. Thrombocytopenia with absent radii (TAR) syndrome
      c. Fanconi's aplastic anemia
   2. Disorders of platelet function—von Willebrand's disease (vWD)
      a. vW factor (vWF) is a large, multimeric molecule that circulates in a noncovalent complex with Factor VIII.
      b. Decreased levels of vWF can result in low levels of Factor VIII and a prolonged activated partial thromboplastin time (aPTT).
      c. Evaluation of a patient with suspected vWD is outlined in Table 14–22. Type I comprises 80% of all patients, most subtle presentation.
      d. Presentation. vWD is a group of disorders in which quantitative or qualitative abnormalities in vWF cause impaired adhesion of platelets.
         Patients may present with easy bruisability, recurrent epistaxis, or other mucous membrane bleeds. Type III presents with hemarthrosis similar to hemophilia (Table 14–23).
      e. Treatment. Goal is to restore serum vWF levels promptly.
         (1) Cryoprecipitate is an exogenous source of vWF. Dosage: 1 bag/5 kg of body weight to a maximum of 8 bags in 8–12 hours.

Text continued on page 738

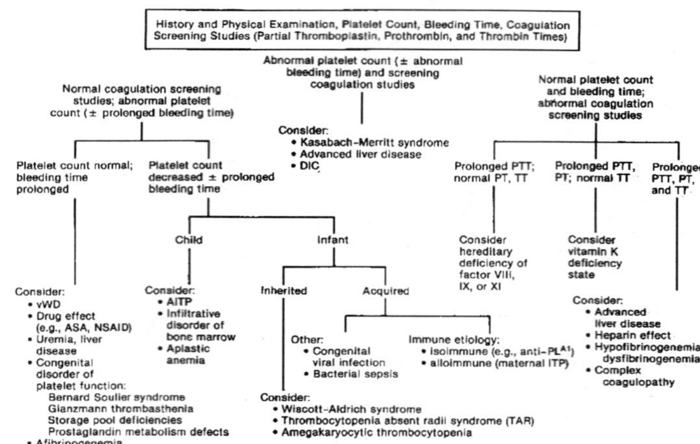

Figure 14–4. Algorithmic approach to the infant or child with a suspected bleeding disorder. (From Bray GL: Inherited and acquired disorders of hemostasis. *In*: Textbook of Pediatric Critical Care. Holbrook PR [Ed]. Philadelphia, WB Saunders, 1993, p 799.)

Table 14–22. RESULTS OF LABORATORY STUDIES IN PATIENTS WITH VON WILLEBRAND'S DISEASE

	von Willebrand's Disease			
Laboratory Test	*Type I*	*Type IIa*	*Type IIb*	*Type III*
Bleeding time	Normal or prolonged	Usually prolonged	Usually prolonged	Always prolonged
Factor VIII:C	Normal or mildly decreased	Normal or mildly decreased	Usually normal	Always markedly decreased*
vWF antigen (Laurell assay)	Normal or mildly decreased	Normal or mildly decreased	Usually normal	Usually absent
Ristocetin-induced platelet aggregation	Usually normal	Usually decreased	Increased†	Markedly decreased to absent
Ristocetin cofactor activity	Normal or mildly to moderately decreased‡	Moderately or markedly decreased	Usually mildly to moderately decreased	Markedly decreased to absent
vWF multimeric analysis in SDS agarose gels	All MW multimers present and decreased proportionately	Absence of high and intermediate MW multimers; normal or increased low MW multimers	Absence of high and intermediate MW multimers; normal or increased low MW multimers	Lack of *all* MW multimers (high, intermediate, and low)

*Levels of Factor VIII:C in most patients with type III vWD are comparable with those exhibited by patients with moderate-to-severe Factor VIII deficiency.
†A diagnostic feature of type IIb vWD is the ability of low concentrations of ristocetin (0.2–0.3 mg/mL) to cause aggregation in platelet-rich plasma.
‡Patients with type I vWD usually have proportionate decreases in plasma levels of VIII:C, vWF antigen, and ristocetin cofactor activity.
Abbreviations: MW, molecular weight; SDS, sodium dodecyl sulfate; vWD, von Willebrand's disease; vWF, von Willebrand factor.
From Bray GL: Inherited and acquired disorders of hemostasis. *In:* Textbook of Pediatric Critical Care. Holbrook PR [Ed]. Philadelphia, WB Saunders, 1993, pp 783–801.

Table 14–23. TREATMENT OF SPECIFIC HEMORRHAGES IN HEMOPHILIA

Type of Bleed	Hemophilia A	Hemophilia B
Hemarthrosis*	20 U/kg FVIII concentrate†; 15 U/kg if treated early. Repeat dose the following day if bleed is severe	30 U/kg FIX concentrate‡; 20 U/kg if treated early
Muscle or significant subcutaneous hematoma	20 U/kg FVIII concentrate; may need treatment every other day until bleed is well controlled	30 U/kg FIX concentrate; may need treatment every 2 or 3 days until bleeding is well controlled‡
Mouth, deciduous tooth, or tooth extraction	20 U/kg FVIII concentrate; antifibrinolytic therapy; remove loose deciduous tooth	30 U/kg concentrate; antifibrinolytic therapy§; remove loose deciduous tooth
Epistaxis	Pressure for 15–20 min; pack with petroleum jelly gauze; antifibrinolytic therapy; 20 U/kg FVIII concentrate if aforementioned therapy fails	Pressure for 15–20 min; pack with petroleum jelly gauze; antifibrinolytic therapy; 30 U/kg FIX concentrate if aforementioned therapy fails (4 hours after antifibrinolytic dose)
Major surgery, life-threatening hemorrhage (e.g., CNS, GI, airway)	50 U/kg FVIII concentrate, then 25 U/kg q 12 hr or continuous infusion to maintain FVIII >50 U/dL for 5–7 d, then >30 U/dL for 5–7 d	80 U/kg FIX concentrate, then 20–40 U/kg every 12–24 hr to maintain FIX >40 U/dL for 5–7 days, then >30 U/dL for 5–7 days‡

Iliopsoas hemorrhage	50 U/kg FVIII concentrate, then 25 U/kg every 12 hr until patient is asymptomatic, then 50 U/kg every other day for a total of 10–14 d‖	80 U/kg FIX concentrate, then 20–40 U/kg every 12–24 hr to maintain FIX >40 U/dL until patient is asymptomatic, then 30 U/kg every other day for a total of 10–14 days‡‖
Hematuria	Bed rest; 1½ × maintenance fluids; if bleeding is not controlled in 1 or 2 days, 20 U/kg FVIII concentrate; if bleeding is not controlled, prednisone if patient is HIV-negative	Bed rest; 1½ × maintenance fluids; if bleeding is not controlled in 1 or 2 days, 30 U/kg FIX concentrate; if bleeding is not controlled, prednisone if patient is HIV-negative

*For hip hemarthrosis, orthopedic evaluation for possible aspiration is advisable.

†For mild or moderate hemophilia, DDAVP, 0.3 μg/kg, should be used instead of FVIII concentrate if patient is known to respond with a hemostatic level of FVIII; if repeated doses are given, monitor FVIII levels for tachyphylaxis.

‡If repeated doses of FIX concentrate are given, add heparin, 100 U per 500 U of FIX; monitor antithrombin III and DIC parameters; when highly purified FIX concentrates are available, they are preferred.

ξDo not give antifibrinolytic therapy until 4–6 hours after a dose of FIX concentrate.

‖Repeat radiologic assessment before discontinuation of therapy.

Abbreviations: CNS, central nervous system; DDAVP, desmopressin acetate; F, Factor; GI, gastrointestinal; HIV, human immunodeficiency virus.

From Gill JC, Montgomery RR: Principles of therapy for hemostasis factor deficiencies. *In:* Hematology of Infancy and Childhood, 4th ed. Nathan DG, Oski FA [Eds]. Philadelphia, WB Saunders, 1993, p 1799.

(2) DDAVP (desmopressin): stimulates endogenous stores of vWF.
Dosage: 0.3 μg/kg over 15–30 minutes IV or SC.
Rapid increase in vWF antigen, Factor VIII, and ristocetin cofactor activity.
(3) Factor VIII concentrates that contain large amounts of vWF represent a third therapeutic option.

3. Acquired thrombocytopenia. Several etiologies contribute to qualitative or quantitative platelet defects in pediatric patients.
   a. Neonatal thrombocytopenia
      (1) Immune mediated
      (2) Infectious—TORCH,* human immunodeficiency virus–1 (HIV-1), bacterial
      (3) Consumptive—birth asphyxia, congestive heart disease, respiratory distress
   b. Immune thrombocytopenic purpura (ITP)
      (1) No gender predilection in pediatrics
      (2) 80% of patients present with platelet count $<40 \times 10^9/L$.
      (3) Coagulation profile normal
      (4) Bone marrow aspiration normal
      (5) Presentation includes epistaxis (25%–30%), GI bleeding (5%), and CNS bleeding (0.5%–1%).
      (6) Physical examination remarkable for purpura and petechiae.
      (7) Natural history of disease includes up to 80% remission within months of initial presentation.
      (8) Ongoing debate whether or not to treat ITP in children. Indications include:
      Acute bleeding
      Intravenous gamma globulin (1 g/kg/d) × 1–3 d; response in platelet count in about 1 week.
      Prednisone (2 mg/kg/d) × 1–3 weeks if platelets $<20–30 \times 10^9/L$.
      Platelet transfusion indicated only for life-threatening hemorrhage or CNS bleed.
   c. HIV-related thrombocytopenia. Common manifestation of HIV-1 infection. Management and presentation similar to ITP as outlined earlier.

4. Hemophilias (Table 14–23):
Present with bleeding into joints and muscles after minimal or no trauma. Bleeding is a result of delayed thrombin generation, which results in deficient clot formation.
   a. Hemophilia A
      (1) Factor VIII deficiency
      (2) 80% to 85% of all cases of hemophilia; occurring in 1 in 5000 male births
      (3) One third of new cases have no family history of bleeding.
   b. Hemophilia B

---

*toxoplasmosis, rubella, cytomegalovirus, and herpes simplex

(1) Factor X deficiency
(2) 10% to 15% of all cases of hemophilia; occurring in 1 in 25,000 males

c. Life-threatening bleeding emergencies
(1) CNS: Incidence 3% to 13% with a fatality of 20% to 50%. Head trauma is a common cause. Chronic neurologic deficits include seizures, and cognitive losses occur in up to 50% of survivors. Diagnosis made by CT scan.
(2) Retropharyngeal: May lead to asphyxia secondary to extrinsic compression of upper airway (especially infants and small children). Older children may complain of sore throat, dysphagia, and hoarse speech.
(3) Retroperitoneal: Occur most commonly after blunt trauma. Patients may present in shock due to large blood loss. Present with flank pain and tenderness over back and abdomen. Diagnosis made by CT scan or ultrasound.
(4) Limb-threatening compartment syndromes: Secondary to expanding hematoma in soft tissue and muscle.
(5) Therapies aimed to restore factor level to 80% to 100% of normal, followed by maintenance of factor level at 50% to 100% of normal for days to weeks after the event. Obtain serum factor levels prior to therapy and after specific interventions.

C. Acquired Coagulopathies
1. Vitamin K deficiency
   a. Newborn
   b. Cystic fibrosis
   c. Celiac disease
   d. Ingestion of warfarin-containing compounds
   e. Treatment includes:
   Vitamin K (SC or IV), 1–5 mg
   Life-threatening hemorrhage: fresh-frozen plasma (FFP), 10 mL/kg to rapidly replace vitamin K–dependent factors
2. Liver disease. Treatment includes FFP and cryoprecipitate for hypofibrinogenemia.

PEDIATRIC TRAUMA

Trauma causes more deaths among children ages 1–14 years than all other illnesses combined. Eighty per cent of those with fatal injuries die before hospitalization. Trauma accounts for 10% of all pediatric hospitalizations and 15% of all pediatric intensive care unit (PICU) admissions.

A. Mechanisms
1. Blunt injury exceeds penetrating injury 7:1.
2. 7% blunt injury due to assault; 3% to physical abuse.
3. Major causes of pediatric trauma, see Table 14–24.

B. Anatomic and Physiologic Considerations (Table 14–25)
1. Head

Table 14–24. CAUSES OF INJURY IN MAJOR PEDIATRIC TRAUMA

	By Circumstance	
	Frequency (%)	*Mortality (%)*
Accident	89	3
Assault	7	5
Child abuse	3	12
Self-injury	1	26
Other	1	8
	By Type	
	Frequency (%)	*Mortality (%)*
Blunt	86	3
Penetrating	12	5
Crush	1	6
Other	1	18
	By Mechanisms	
	Frequency (%)	*Mortality (%)*
Fall	27	4
Motor vehicle occupant	18	5
Motor vehicle pedestrian	15	5
Bicycle	9	2
Sport	5	<1
Gunshot wound	5	10
Stabbing	5	1
Struck	4	2
Beating	3	7
Motorcycle	1	4
Animal bite	1	<1
All-terrain vehicle/ recreational vehicle	1	2
Other	5	7

From DiScala C, Brooke MM, Barlow B, et al: National Pediatric Trauma Registry BiAnnual Report. Boston, Tufts University Rehabilitation and Childhood Trauma Research and Training Center, 1993.

a. Great importance of central neuraxis in pathophysiology of injury
b. Child's head is proportionately larger than adult's; receives larger impact of injury.
c. Cervical spine more flexible, less spinal vertebral injury; **more** spinal cord injury
d. Traumatic brain injury (TBI)
   (1) Cerebral swelling
   (2) Diffuse axonal injury (white matter)
   (3) Major intracranial hemorrhages are uncommon.
   Note: Subdurals in infants may represent traumatic intentional injury.

2. Chest
   a. Forces transmitted to underlying structures due to plasticity of ribs (cartilage)
   b. High incidence of pulmonary and cardiac contusion
   c. Increased risk of hemodynamic compromise from

Table 14–25. FREQUENCY AND MORTALITY OF INJURIES IN MAJOR PEDIATRIC TRAUMA

	By Body Region	
	Frequency (%)	*Mortality (%)*
Multiple	43	5
Extremities	20	0
Head and neck	18	5
External	12	0
Abdomen	3	1
Face	2	0
Thorax	1	3
	By Anatomic Diagnosis	
	Frequency (%)	*Mortality (%)*
Head injury	29	*
Fracture	23	*
Open wound	16	*
Superficial wound	11	*
Contusion	8	*
Thoracic/abdominal injury	8	*
Spine injury	2	*
Other	5	*

*Cannot be accurately determined, because there are 77,480 diagnoses among the 32,574 patients enrolled in the National Pediatric Trauma Registry-2 as of October 1993.

From DiScala C, Brooke MM, Barlow B, et al: National Pediatric Trauma Registry BiAnnual Report. Boston, Tufts University Rehabilitation and Childhood Trauma Research and Training Center, 1993.

tension pneumothorax secondary to mobile mediastinal structures

3. Abdomen
   a. Multiple organ involvement due to limited protection by small, pliable ribs
   b. Increased incidence of pancreatitis
   c. Lower incidence of surgical lesions
4. Bones
   a. Femur and tibia are most frequent long bone injuries in pedestrian motor vehicle accident trauma.
   b. Periosteum more elastic, higher incidence of incomplete fractures (greenstick).
   c. Isolated femur fractures rarely associated with significant blood loss.
5. Airway. Most important differences between adults and children (see Respiratory Section A).
   a. Airway narrower, more susceptible to obstruction by mucus, blood, particulate matter, and tongue if altered level of consciousness.
   b. Goals are to prevent secondary injury resulting from hypoxia.
6. Hypovolemia
   a. Children can compensate for up to 25% to 30% loss of circulatory blood volume.

b. **Hypotension** is a **late** sign of shock in children.
c. Watch for other signs such as tachypnea, tachycardia, and metabolic acidosis secondary to poor tissue perfusion.

C. Management. The approach to resuscitation of child trauma victims is similar to that for adults: Initial attention to airway, breathing, and circulation, including control of bleeding and treatment of shock.

1. Primary survey/resuscitation
   a. Delivery of high-concentration oxygen via either nonrebreathing mask or assisted ventilation
   b. Stabilize cervical spine in neutral position.
   c. Intubation and hyperventilation if Glasgow Coma Score is less than 8. Oropharyngeal route is preferred. Needle or surgical cricothyrotomy is rarely required.
   d. Life-threatening chest injuries—tension pneumothorax
   e. Control of external hemorrhage
   f. Volume resuscitation guided by hemodynamic response:
      (1) Crystalloid: Up to 40 mL/kg
      (2) Colloid: 10 mL/kg of packed RBCs if severe shock present or frank hemorrhage; repeat as needed to maintain Hcts 30%.
      (3) Antishock trousers not useful in initial resuscitation
   g. Orogastric tube to relieve gastric dilatation
2. Secondary survey. Once the primary survey is complete and resuscitation is under way:
   a. Complete exposure of the child; avoid hypothermia.
   b. Head-to-toe physical examination
   c. Laboratory tests to include serial hematocrits, serum transaminase and amylase (liver and spleen injury), urine analysis, and arterial blood gases
   d. Radiographic examination
      (1) Lateral radiograph of the spine **not** necessary prior to intubation because it cannot rule out spinal cord injury or odontoid fracture.
      (2) Skull radiographs are a poor marker of brain injury and are not necessary in the initial evaluation.
      (3) CT scan of head for Glasgow Coma Score <13, history of unconsciousness >5 minutes, or signs of increased intracranial pressure.
      (4) CT scan of the cervical spine if vertebral injury is suspected.
      (5) Double-contrast CT scan of the abdomen when the mechanism of injury suggests intra-abdominal bleeding or shock is present.
   e. Diagnostic peritoneal lavage is rarely helpful. True determinant for laparotomy is the ongoing transfusion requirement or persistent hemodynamic instability. Its use is reserved for patients undergoing general anesthesia for operative treatment of intracranial or musculoskeletal injuries.

D. Outcome. Overall morbidity and mortality of major pediatric trauma are closely linked to the functional outcome of brain injury. Optimal resuscitation of the brain is the primary goal of all phases of initial pediatric trauma management. Most children with major blunt trauma can be managed by nonoperative means in conjunction with pediatric surgical consultation.
   1. Head
      a. Closed linear skull fractures managed expectantly.
      b. Open fractures and depressed fractures that invade the cranial vault require intravenous antibiotics and operative treatment.
      c. Basilar skull fractures with CSF leaks should not routinely be treated with antibiotics.
      d. Impact seizures require no specific treatment unless they recur.
   2. Spinal cord
      a. Cervical region most affected
      b. 50% of injured die prior to reaching the hospital.
      c. Survivors remain disabled despite high-dose methylprednisolone.
         (1) 30 mg/kg IV over 15 minutes; followed by 5.4 mg/kg/hr continuous IV
      d. High incidence of spinal cord injury without radiographic abnormality (SCIWORA)
   3. Chest
      a. Most injuries can be managed expectantly or by tube thoracostomy.
      b. High incidence of pulmonary contusions; no specific therapies indicated
      c. Higher incidence of traumatic asphyxia in children due to extreme severity of blunt forces applied to the chest
   4. Abdomen (Table 14–26)
      a. Acute management of intra-abdominal and genitourinary injuries in children, chiefly nonoperative
      b. Pancreatic pseudocyst occurs with greater frequency in children. Symptoms include a tender epigastric mass 3–5 days after upper abdominal trauma. Treatment includes 6–8 weeks of complete bowel rest and total parenteral nutrition.
   5. Skeleton
      a. Operative treatment is required for open fractures, displaced supracondylar fractures, and major or displaced physeal fractures.
      b. Compartment syndromes occur and require fasciotomy if tissue pulp pressure exceeds 40 cm H_2O.
      c. Fat embolism and rhabdomyolysis as sequelae to severe crush injury rarely occur; supportive treatment of both conditions is indicated.
   6. Penetrating injuries. Encountered in increasing numbers. Children should be referred to a trauma center with pediatric capabilities if possible.

E. Interhospital Transport. If primary transport to a trauma center with pediatric capabilities is not possible, secondary transport from the receiving hospital to a pediatric trauma center may be necessary. Interhospital transport

Table 14–26. INDICATIONS FOR EARLY OPERATION IN PEDIATRIC ABDOMINAL TRAUMA

Blunt
Hemodynamic instability despite adequate volume resuscitation
Transfusion requirement >50% of estimated blood volume
Physical signs of peritonitis
Endoscopic evidence of rectal tear
Radiologic evidence of intraperitoneal or retroperitoneal gas
Radiologic evidence of gastrointestinal perforation
Radiologic evidence of intraperitoneal bladder rupture
Radiologic evidence of pancreatic transection
Bile, bacteria, stool, or >500 WBCs / mm^3 on peritoneal lavage
Penetrating
All gunshot wounds
All stab wounds associated with evisceration; blood in stomach, urine, or rectum; physical signs of shock or peritonitis; radiologic evidence of intraperitoneal or retroperitoneal gas
All suspected thoracoabdominal injuries (unless precluded by laparoscopy or thoracoscopy)
Bile, bacteria, stool, or >500 WBCs/mm^3 on peritoneal lavage

Abbreviation: WBCs, white blood cells.

teams should be staffed by physicians and nurses trained in pediatric critical care and transport as required by patient's condition.

NEAR-DROWNING

A. Drowning is a submersion injury causing death within 24 hours of the incident. Near-drowning is a submersion injury after which the patient survives for at least 24 hours.
   1. Near-drowning ranks as the fourth most common cause of injury-related death in all age groups, the third in toddlers, and the second in unintentional injury among adolescents.
   2. Most pediatric victims are <5 years of age. Drowning generally occurs during unsupervised swimming in pools, lakes, or rivers.
   3. Risk factors include epilepsy, drug ingestion, alcohol, and child abuse.

B. Pathophysiology
   1. Pulmonary. Aspiration of fresh or sea water decreases pulmonary compliance, leading to hypoxia, atelectasis, and pulmonary edema.
   2. Cardiovascular
      a. Bradycardia either due to hypoxia-induced dysfunction or from physiologic diving reflex in cold water
      b. Intense vasoconstriction may be present secondary to hypothermia or as a response to high levels of circulatory catecholamines.
      c. Asystole may occur.
   3. Central nervous system

a. The primary injury is due to hypoxia and ischemia that occur from immersion until adequate resuscitation. Extent of injury depends on the duration of submersion and the rapidity of resuscitation.
b. Irreversible brain damage begins after 4 minutes of anoxia.
c. Normothermic brain is unlikely to recover after 8–10 minutes of anoxia.
d. The prognosis for patients who arrive at emergency departments awake or with blunted level of consciousness is excellent. 40% to 50% of children who arrive in emergency rooms comatose survive normally.

4. Electrolyte abnormalities. Unlikely that surviving patients will have aspirated a sufficient volume of water to cause fluid and electrolyte disturbances.

C. Management. Goal of therapy is to restore ventilation, perfusion, arterial blood gas tensions, and acid-base status to normal as soon as possible.

1. Initiate CPR, insure adequate ventilation.
2. Pulmonary support
   a. Mechanical ventilation with positive end-expiratory pressure (PEEP) to overcome intrapulmonary shunt
   b. Spontaneously breathing patients may benefit from continuous positive airway pressure (CPAP).
   c. Treat bronchospasm with aerosol bronchodilator agents as necessary.
   d. Treat pulmonary edema with PEEP.
   e. Routine use of antibiotics and steroids not indicated
   f. Adult respiratory distress syndrome (ARDS) is most likely a complication of contaminated water aspiration.
3. Cardiovascular support
   a. Intravascular monitoring to include intra-arterial and central venous catheterization
   b. Adequate volume resuscitation
   c. Pulmonary artery catheter as needed (recommended if high PEEP is necessary)
   d. Inotropic support
4. Neurologic support
   a. Rule out neck and spine trauma.
   b. Therapy is directed at **prevention** of secondary CNS injury.
      (1) Ensure adequate volume and cardiovascular support.
      (2) Control oxygenation.
      (3) Fever control to decrease cerebral metabolic rate
      (4) Seizure control as necessary

      Note: Strict control of ICP has not altered outcome. Aggressive ICP monitoring and pentobarbital coma no longer recommended. Moderate hyperventilation ($PaCO_2$ 25–32 mm Hg), head elevation, and maintenance of cerebral perfusion pressure are the goals of cerebral resuscitation.

D. Outcome. No true single predictors of a meaningful neurologic recovery are available. Ominous symptoms include ongoing CPR upon arrival at hospital, Glasgow Coma Score of 3 or less, and abnormal evoked potentials.

POISONING

A. Overview. Poisoning remains a serious public health concern. Children represent 4% of all reported fatalities due to ingestions. 85% to 90% of pediatric poisoning occurs in children younger than 5 years of age.

B. Treatment
   1. ABCs and adequate seizure control necessary before specific decontamination and antidotal therapy are instituted.
   2. Surface decontamination of eyes and skin of external poisonings
   3. Gastrointestinal tract decontamination (Table 14–27)
      a. Emesis with syrup of ipecac
      b. Activated charcoal
      c. Cathartics
   4. Enhanced elimination of poisons from blood and tissue
      a. Forced diuresis with/without alteration of pH

Table 14–27. GASTROINTESTINAL DECONTAMINATION

Therapy		Contraindications
Emesis—Syrup of Ipecac		
Dosage: (repeat × 1)		*Caustic agents*
Infant <1 yr	10 mL	Petroleum distillates
Young children	15 mL	Stupor/coma
Adolescents	30 mL	CNS depressant drugs, e.g., tricyclic antidepressant
Lavage		
Need large-bore orogastric tube to accommodate pill fragments		*Corrosive caustic agents*
		+/− Petroleum distillates
Lavage with saline or ½ N saline until clear		Stupor/coma unless airway protected
Activated Charcoal—Give After Emesis		
Dosage:		Corrosive agents interfere with endoscopy
Children	1 g/kg	
Adults	50–100 g	Acetaminophen ingestion: Reduces the absorption of *N*-acetylcysteine
Cathartics		
$MgSO_4$, 250 mg/kg dose, mixed with activated charcoal × 1 dose		Do not use in renal failure
		Corrosive agents
Sorbitol magnesium citrate		

b. Dialysis
c. Hemoperfusion
5. Antidotal therapy—see Table 14–28. Only a small proportion of poisoned patients can be helped by antidotal therapy.

C. Poisons. The following section discusses frequently encountered pediatric ingestions. The reader is referred to Chapter 130 in the *Textbook of Critical Care* for an extensive review of poisoning and its management.

1. Iron. The leading cause of pediatric accidental ingestions, accounts for 65% of all unintentional pharmaceutical ingestion fatalities in children <6 years.
   a. Physiology. Ferrous iron (Fe^{2+}) is absorbed from the GI tract mucosa, is oxidized to ferric ion (Fe^{3+}), and binds to ferritin. Severity of ingestion is directly related to the amount of elemental iron ingested.
   b. Clinical presentation—see Table 14–29.
   c. Evaluation
      (1) Laboratory tests include serum iron and total iron-binding capacity 2–4 hours after ingestion, serum Fe cleared from serum in 6 hours.
      (2) Ancillary tests include arterial blood gas, electrolytes, BUN, coagulation, CBC, glucose, and liver function tests (aspartate aminotransferase, alanine aminotransferase).
      (3) X-ray film of the abdomen for pill fragments
   d. Prediction of toxicity
      (1) Based on the history of the amount of elemental iron, symptoms, and peak iron level 3–6 hours after ingestion
      (2) Serum iron levels are normally 50–100 μg/dL; levels >300 μg/dL are considered toxic.
      (3) Deferoxamine challenge test. May help determine the need for chelation therapy when serum iron levels are not readily available in symptomatic patients.
      Administer 40 mg/kg IM or 15 mg/kg IV for 1 hour. Vin rose–colored urine indicates presence of free iron in excess of iron-binding capacity. Continue chelation therapy until urine is clear.
   e. Therapy
      (1) Gastrointestinal decontamination (see Table 14–27). Lavage if pills appear in stomach on x-ray film.
      (2) Chelation therapy with deferoxamine if challenge is positive (see preceding section), or if serum iron level >350 μg/dL or serum iron level > total iron-binding capacity.
2. Acetaminophen. This drug is present in many over-the-counter analgesics and antipyretic compounds. A dose of >140 mg/kg is considered toxic.
   a. Clinical presentation
      (1) First 12–24 hours, patients are either asymptomatic or develop nausea, anorexia, and vomiting.

Table 14–28. ANTIDOTES TO COMMON TOXINS

Poison	Antidote	Indications	Dosage
Acetaminophen	*N*-Acetylcysteine	Serum acetaminophen levels in hepatotoxic probable range (Rumack-Matthew nomogram)	140 mg/kg PO followed by 17 mg/kg × 17 doses
Anticholinergics	Physostigmine salicylate	Severe anticholinergic poisoning (seizures, hallucinations, hypertension, arrhythmias)	Child: 0.5 mg/kg IV q 10 min Adult: 1 mg IV q 10 min until desired effect
Benzodiazepines	Flumazenil	Suspected benzodiazepine overdose without proconvulsant coingestants	0.01 mg/kg to a maximum of 0.125 mg, may repeat 0.01 mg/kg
Carbon monoxide	Oxygen	Carbon monoxide levels >5–10%	100% FiO_2; consider hyperbaric oxygen
Cyanide	Cyanide antidote kit: 1. amyl nitrite inhalant 2. sodium nitrate 3. sodium thiosulfate	Suspected cyanide or hydrogen sulfide intoxication	Child: <25 kg sodium nitrate and sodium thiosulfate; doses depend on hemoglobin concentration Adult: amyl nitrite inhalation pending IV; sodium nitrate, 300 mg, then sodium thiosulfate, 12.5 g

Ethylene glycol Methanol	Ethanol	Ethylene glycol or methanol ingestion level >20 mg/dL or osmolar gap and metabolic acidosis	Loading dose: 7.6–10 mL/kg 10% ethanol in D_5W, and maintenance infusion 1.4 mL/kg/hr to a level of 10 mg
Iron	Deferoxamine	Symptomatic patients Serum Fe levels >300 μg/dL or serum Fe > TIBC Positive desferrioxamine	20–40 mg/kg IV given over 4-hr period; maximum 15 mg · kg^{-1} · hr^{-1} followed by 20 mg/kg of 4–8 hr until urine color is normal or level <300 μg/dL
Methemoglobinemia	Methylene blue	Symptomatic patients Methemoglobin level >30–40%	1–2 mg/kg IV
Opiates	Naloxone hydrochloride	Respiratory depression	0.01 mg/kg IV; repeat at 10 × dose if no response in probable narcotic overdose
Organophosphates	Atropine	Cholinergic crisis	0.05 mg/kg IV; repeat q 10–30 min to achieve atropinization followed by pralidoxime
	Pralidoxime (2-PAM)		25–50 mg/kg IV; repeat in 8–12 hr prn

Abbreviations: TIBC, total iron-binding capacity.

Table 14–29. CLINICAL PRESENTATION OF IRON POISONING

Stage	Time from Ingestion	Symptoms
I	30 min–2 hr	Nausea, vomiting with hematemesis, abdominal pain, lethargy
II	6–12 hr	Quiescent phase; patient may be asymptomatic
III	12–48 hr	Life-threatening metabolic acidosis, increased lethargy, coma, vasomotor collapse, GI bleeding
IV	2–4 days	Liver failure
V	Late onset, 4–6 weeks	Gastrointestinal scarring with potential obstruction

(2) Next 12–24 hours, resolution of earlier gastrointestinal symptoms

(3) After 72 hours, liver injury may develop, with marked elevation of serum transaminases and prolonged prothrombin time and partial thromboplastin time. Fulminant liver failure may occur.

b. Laboratory tests

(1) Prediction of toxicity based on acetaminophen levels. Likely with ingestion >140 mg/kg

(2) Rumack-Matthew nomogram (Fig. 14–5) de-

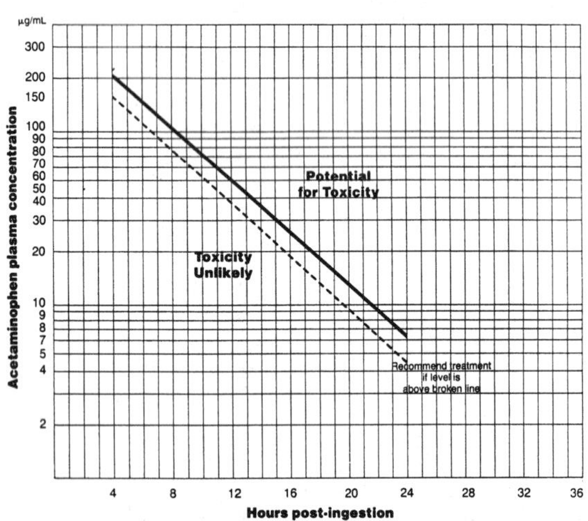

Figure 14–5. Nomogram: Plasma or serum acetaminophen concentration as it relates to the time after acetaminophen ingestion. (Adapted from Rumack BH, Matthew H: Acetaminophen poisoning and toxicity. Pediatrics 1975; 55:871–876. Adapted by permission of Pediatrics.)

fines the risk of hepatic damage from the time of ingestion. Applicable only in **acute** intoxication

c. Management
   (1) Gastrointestinal decontamination (see Table 14–27).
   (2) Do not administer activated charcoal; it reduces the absorption of *N*-acetylcysteine.
   (3) Administer antidote up to 24 hours after ingestion if ingestion is in the possible or probable hepatotoxic range; may consider administration if presentation occurs after 24 hours.
   (4) Treat with antidote if levels are not readily available.
   (5) *N*-Acetylcysteine dosing (PO): 140 mg/kg, followed by 70 mg/kg every 4 hours × 17 doses.

3. Cyclic antidepressants. Responsible for the largest absolute number of fatalities of all exposures in 1992. Approximately 70% of individuals who have taken fatal overdoses are pronounced dead before medical assistance can be provided.
   a. Clinical presentation. Manifestations of cyclic antidepressant overdose are based on the four toxic mechanisms:
      (1) Direct muscarinic receptor blockade (anticholinergic)
      (2) Neurotransmitter blockade (adrenergic excess)
      (3) Alpha-adrenergic receptor blockade
      (4) Type I antiarrhythmic action ("quinidine-like")
   b. Management
      (1) Gastrointestinal decontamination (see Table 14–27), including multidose activated charcoal (interrupts the enterohepatic circulation of tricyclic antidepressants) and lavage (early stages). Ipecac has no role in treatment.
      (2) Alkalinization (serum) with sodium bicarbonate and hyperventilation. Data support the preferred use of sodium bicarbonate to achieve effective serum alkalinization. Initiate therapy at the first sign of electrocardiogram abnormality.
      (3) Arrhythmias (Table 14–30). Prophylactic administration of phenytoin does not prevent cardiotoxicity.
      (4) Seizures (Table 14–30)
   c. Outcome. All patients should be monitored for 24 hours after resolution of all signs and symptoms. Late complications are usually the result of aspiration, prolonged seizures, and anoxia.

4. Salicylates. Incidence of overdose has decreased over the past 2 decades; however, acute and chronic salicylism remains a major problem. Aspirin and acetylsalicylic acid are available alone or in combination in many over-the-counter preparations. Other forms include methylsalicylate (oil of wintergreen) and salicylic acid (keratolytic).
   a. Clinical presentation. Fever is the hallmark of pedi-

Table 14–30. CLINICAL MANIFESTATIONS AND TREATMENT OF TRICYCLIC ANTIDEPRESSANT TOXICITY

System	Signs or Symptoms	Treatment
CNS	Seizures	Benzodiazepines, phenytoin, and phenobarbital. Refractory seizures may require paralysis and pentobarbital coma
	Depressed CNS, myoclonus, pyramidal tract signs	Supportive care
Cardiovascular	Tachycardia	Fluid administration
	Hypotension	Vasoactive drugs with direct alpha-adrenergic activity (Neo-Synephrine, norepinephrine)
	Arrhythmias	Alkalinization (pH 7.45–7.55) with $NaHCO_3$ or hyperventilation
	Ventricular tachycardia	
	Ventricular fibrillation	Lidocaine or phenytoin
	Supraventricular tachycardia	Propranolol for supraventricular tachycardia
	Premature ventricular beats	Do not use quinidine or procainamide
	Heart block	Pacing, beta-agonist (epinephrine)
Peripheral anticholinergic effects	Pupillary size unreliable, dry skin and mucous membranes, urinary retention, and hyperthermia	Supportive physostigmine *contraindicated* because of its cardiotoxic effects

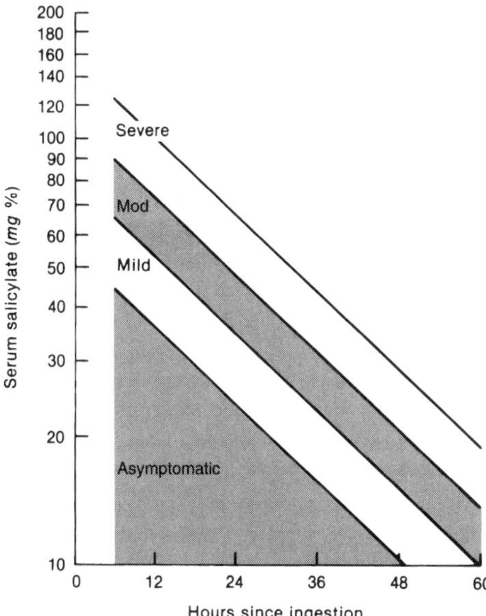

Figure 14–6. Nomogram relating salicylate concentration and expected severity of intoxication at varying intervals following the ingestion of a single dose of salicylate. (From Done AK: Salicylate intoxication. Pediatrics 1960; 26:800. Reproduced by permission of Pediatrics.)

atric salicylism. Levels of salicylates predict toxicity. Measure levels at 6 hours after acute ingestion. Done nomogram clinically useful guide to assess and predict severity of salicylism (Fig. 14–6).
Note: Watch units, mg/dL.
(1) Mild intoxication: Mild confusion, tinnitus, and decreased auditory acuity
(2) Moderate intoxication: Increased central nervous system symptoms. Agitation or lethargy, vertigo, convulsions, hyperventilation, and metabolic acidosis
(3) Severe intoxication: Noncardiogenic pulmonary edema is rare in pediatrics; refractory seizures and death common.

b. Metabolic disturbances
(1) Respiratory alkalosis secondary to direct stimulation of medulla to increase rate and depth of respirations
(2) Increase in intracellular metabolism leads to formation of lactate, pyruvate, and organic acids, creating an anion gap metabolic acidosis.
(3) Overall combined respiratory and metabolic acidosis

c. Fluids/electrolytes

(1) Dehydration
(2) Hypokalemia
(3) Hypocalcemia
(4) Hyper- or hypoglycemia

d. Management
   (1) Gastric decontamination (see Table 14–27), multidose activated charcoal.
   (2) Urinary alkalinization, pH 7.5–8.0, until serum salicylate levels decrease.
   (3) Correct dehydration, rehydrate with sodium bicarbonate in fluids.
   (4) Consider hemodialysis in patients with serum level of 100–200 mg/dL or with refractory metabolic acidosis, altered mental status, seizures, or noncardiogenic pulmonary edema.
   (5) Vitamin K for hemorrhagic complications

Index

Note: Page numbers in *italics* refer to illustrations; page numbers followed by t refer to tables.